Interventional Cardiology and Cardiac Catheterisation

Interventional Cardiology and Cardiac Catheterisation

The Essential Guide

Second Edition

Edited by

John Edward Boland BSc Hons, MSc (Pathology)

Department of Cardiology, St Vincent's Hospital
School of Medical and Applied Science, Central Queensland University
Sydney, Australia

David W. M. Muller, MBBS, MD, FRACP, FACC

Cardiac Catheterisation Laboratories, St Vincent's Hospital
Sydney, Australia

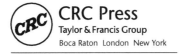

CRC Press
Taylor & Francis Group
Boca Raton London New York

CRC Press is an imprint of the
Taylor & Francis Group, an **informa** business

CRC Press
Taylor & Francis Group
6000 Broken Sound Parkway NW, Suite 300
Boca Raton, FL 33487-2742

First issued in paperback 2020

© 2019 by Taylor & Francis Group, LLC
CRC Press is an imprint of Taylor & Francis Group, an Informa business

No claim to original U.S. Government works

ISBN-13: 978-1-138-48151-0 (hbk)
ISBN-13: 978-0-367-72931-8 (pbk)

Library of Congress Cataloging-in-Publication Data

Names: Boland, John, MSc., editor. | Muller, David W. M., editor.
Title: Interventional cardiology and cardiac catheterisation : the essential guide / [edited by] John Boland, David W.M. Muller.
Other titles: Cardiology and cardiac catheterisation.
Description: Second edition. | Boca Raton, FL : CRC Press, Taylor & Francis Group, [2019] | Preceded by Cardiology and cardiac catheterisation : the essential guide / edited by John Boland and David W.M. Muller. 2001. | Includes bibliographical references and index.
Identifiers: LCCN 2018050505| ISBN 9781138481510 (hardback : alk. paper) | ISBN 9781351060356 (ebook)
Subjects: | MESH: Cardiac Catheterization | Cardiac Surgical Procedures
Classification: LCC RC683.5.C25 | NLM WG 141.5.C2 | DDC 616.1/20754--dc23
LC record available at https://lccn.loc.gov/2018050505

Visit the Taylor & Francis Web site at
http://www.taylorandfrancis.com

and the CRC Press Web site at
http://www.crcpress.com

To all scholars, teachers and researchers everywhere.

Contents

Foreword

The collective knowledge and expertise contained within a major clinical, teaching and research institute such as St Vincent's Hospital, Sydney, is truly impressive and would fill several books of encyclopaedic proportions. This textbook is an attempt to tap into a small part of that immense knowledge by documenting information from one specific area of medicine: the cardiac catheterisation laboratory. To this end, much of the information provided in this textbook forms part of the coursework for the Bachelor of Echocardiography (Cardiac Physiology), Graduate Diploma of Echocardiography provided by Central Queensland University, Australia, and we proudly acknowledge this collaboration between St Vincent's Hospital and CQ University.

A publication of this type would not be possible without collaboration from many individuals and organisations. We are deeply grateful to our publisher, Taylor & Francis Group for accepting what was initially a tenuous project depending on the dedication and goodwill of so many people, and to all our contributors for their willingness to participate in this production. We believe the final product justifies their commitment and reflects the highest standards of academia.

We are also indebted to all our reviewers and assistant editors, all of whom devoted countless hours of work in editing, proofing and re-proofing all material. In particular, we wish to thank Pow-Li Chia, Dennis Kuchar, David W. Baron, Lawrence Schneider, Krishna Kathir, Christopher Anthony, Gary Gazibarich, Matthew Cameron, Julie Parkinson, Steven Faddy and Roslyn Prichard for editorial assistance, and Medici Graphics and Imagination Graphics for their graphics artwork, as well as Quok Ngo and Julie Williams, our librarians at St Vincent's Hospital, for invaluable assistance with documenting references.

Our gratitude extends to Medtronic and Edwards Lifesciences for initial seed funding and material for a draft copy, and to Boston Scientific, Abbott, Terumo, Edwards Lifesciences and other corporations for providing educational material reproduced herein.

Finally, to our families and colleagues who supported us in so many undefinable ways during a difficult period, we thank you all for your patience and understanding.

John Edward Boland

David W. M. Muller

Preface

The new entrant into the world of the cardiac catheterisation laboratory faces a highly complex environment with many layers of practice, including an arcane language of pressure measurement, haemodynamic assessment, imaging and radiation use and safety, plus a myriad of unique diagnostic and therapeutic procedures. For many beginners, it is a completely overwhelming and often bewildering experience.

To make catheterisation comprehensible, it is natural to turn to a comprehensive text for information. The last decade has seen a cascade of books on advanced techniques, specialised technologies, and the many sub-specialties that have developed within the international community. There are also now a growing number of case-based compendiums on advanced interventional procedures and the newest devices. These texts, however, add to the subspecialist's need to know more and more about less and less, leaving a void for the professional seeking something more general or basic.

What is needed is a complete source that addresses the basics and makes the fundamentals of cardiac catheterisation more accessible. *Interventional Cardiology and Cardiac Catheterisation: The Essential Guide* fills this void, presenting the basics in a current, up-to-date manner. As an example, this spirit is captured in the introduction in Chapter 9, which notes that the chapter 'highlights recent changes in nursing practice'. The same spirit is evident in chapters on more advanced subjects, such as Chapter 40 where discussion of background information makes the details of the newest therapies eminently understandable.

The first chapters detail the fundamentals of imaging, monitoring systems, and basic cardiac physiology from the laboratory perspective, followed by the fundamentals of thrombosis, anticoagulation, vascular access and haemostasis. Basic clinical and interventional pharmacology are addressed by experts in the field. The basics of the broad topics of patient management, nursing perspective, coronary and peripheral vascular intervention, intervention for myocardial infarction, pulmonary hypertension, transplantation, and therapies for structural and congenital disease are all covered by experienced authors with many decades of cumulative experience.

The breadth of material covered helps this text exceed the expectations defined by the title 'essential guide', and is well targeted to the health care professional who is new to the catheterisation laboratory. It also true that even the most experienced providers sometimes need to revise the basics, and this book addresses that need as well. The uneasy feeling that most people have on first exposure to a cardiac catheterisation laboratory, 'How can I ever learn all of this?!' is best treated with knowledge and experience. This textbook provides the essential knowledge that is the first part of the knowledge and experience equation.

Ted Feldman
Cardiac Catheterization Laboratory
Interventional Cardiology
NorthShore University Health System
Evanston Hospital
Clinical Medicine
University of Chicago Pritzker School of Medicine

Editors

John Edward Boland is a Science graduate with a background in research and education and has participated as convenor, presenter or invited speaker at numerous local and international scientific and educational meetings. With a particular interest in instrumentation and technology, he has worked as Physiologist/Senior Hospital Scientist for over 30 years as part of the clinical team in the cardiac catheterisation laboratories at St Vincent's Hospital, Sydney, and has a conjoint appointment as Senior Lecturer with Central Queensland University. He is an associate member of the Cardiac Society of Australia and New Zealand and the New South Wales Diagnostic and Interventional Cardiology Nurses Group.

David W. M. Muller is director, Cardiac Catheterisation Laboratories at St Vincent's Hospital, Sydney, and St Vincent's Private Hospital, and is associate professor of medicine at the University of New South Wales. His major interests include optimising the outcomes of complex coronary and peripheral vascular interventions, and the percutaneous management of structural heart disease. He is Principal Investigator for numerous international clinical trials including several first-in-man trials of new devices. He has authored or co-authored multiple peer-reviewed papers, book chapters and abstracts, and has served as an editorial consultant to all the major cardiology journals.

Foreword to the first edition

Cardiac catheterisation began in 1929, when Werner Forsmann exposed a vein in his left arm, introduced a ureteric catheter under local anaesthetic, walked to the X-ray department and advanced it under fluoroscopic guidance into the right atrium. This was lost in the world literature until a Frenchman, A. F. Cournard, and an American, D. W. Richards, in 1914 used the technique to measure cardiac output and pulmonary artery pressures. In 1947 Lewis Dexter and his colleagues used cardiac catheterisation to study and diagnose congenital heart disease.

In Australia, catheterisation of the right heart began at Royal Prince Alfred Hospital in 1947 and at St Vincent's Hospital, both in Sydney, in 1954. At St Vincent's Hospital, the studies were carried out in a small room in the X-ray department under fluoroscopic control. There was no image intensification and no check or control of radiation safety. Pressures were recorded using cumbersome equipment that often took an hour or more to calibrate, and pressure waveforms were recorded using either direct writing pens or photographic equipment. There were no display screens or computers. Catheters were re-used and were sterilised by boiling in water. It was not unusual for the patient to experience rigors after the procedure as a result of pyrogens within the catheter. There were 104 cases performed in the first year.

The senior doctors had learned the techniques in Great Britain and America but were largely self-taught. They instructed the assisting nurses and later the medical registrars, science graduates and technicians. Collective knowledge and expertise were passed down by word and example. There was no course and no textbook to introduce the newcomer to the mysteries of cardiac output, the Fick principle, or the changes in waveform in the different cardiac chambers.

In 1957, catheterisation of the left heart began, and Dr George Benness performed the first coronary arteriogram in Australia at St Vincent's Hospital in 1962.

Since then, image intensification, display screens, computers, sophisticated catheters and percutaneous techniques have revolutionised the cardiac catheterisation laboratory. The laboratory has become a relatively insulated section of the hospital where several disciplines interact in a very sophisticated environment to provide high-class patient care. Despite these advances there has until now been no textbook to which the newcomer could turn to for appropriate information.

John E. Boland and David W. M. Muller have now filled this void by editing a valuable contribution covering all aspects of the techniques and problems encountered in both the cardiac diagnostic and research laboratories. Their co-authors are experienced cardiologists and scientists from Australia and overseas.

I hope that this excellent monograph will be widely read and prove of great help to the many medical, nursing and health professional support staff without whom modern procedural cardiology would not be possible.

John B. Hickie
Emeritus Professor

Preface to the first edition

The field of cardiovascular medicine has catapulted forward in the past few years, owing to significant changes in our approach to patients with acute ischemic heart disease, valvular abnormalities, and prevention of serious arrhythmias. Back in the 1980s, cardiology was revolutionised by an aggressive approach to restoring coronary blood flow in acute myocardial infarction. This took several years to become standard practice, but the spirit of more aggressive management has been transmitted to virtually all diagnoses and treatments in cardiology and cardiac surgery. Of note, these changes have only come about as an outgrowth of intensive clinical investigation, with rigorous, large-scale randomised trials and insightful mechanistic studies. The buzz word of 'evidence-based medicine' has been a cornerstone for accepting many of the newer and more active strategies.

It is hard to find a reference source that captures the latest developments in a comprehensive way. But this book, carefully edited by John E. Boland and David W. M. Muller, is a superb contribution to our field. This monograph covers core clinical areas such as the electrocardiogram, pressure wave forms, and physiological monitoring. Building on this theme, there is heavy emphasis on the physiologic approach to the patient, with chapters on cardiac output and shunts, determination of oxygen status, use of pressure-volume loops for assessing left ventricular function, and two chapters dedicated to interpreting pressure waveforms. With fundamental reviews of atherosclerosis, coagulation, and cardiovascular pharmacology, all of the latest therapies are reviewed including anticoagulants, new anti-platelet agents, and reperfusion therapy. Not just the pharmacology is reviewed, but also device therapies including stenting, vascular closure devices, catheter-based reperfusion of acute myocardial infarction, endovascular therapy of the carotid and peripheral vasculature, approach to valvular diseases, and the potential for angiogenesis and gene therapy. Some particularly useful and hard to find chapters are included on radiation safety, nursing considerations, infection control, haemodynamic monitoring in transplant patients, and evidence-based cardiac catheterisation.

In aggregate, this book is a unique monograph which covers many vital aspects of cardiovascular medicine and surgery in a thorough, refreshing, and highly pragmatic fashion. It will undoubtedly be well received by the cardiology physician, trainee, and nurse community. John E. Boland and David W. M. Muller, together with their superb expert contributors, deserve kudos for their fine work.

Eric J. Topol
Department of Cardiology
Cleveland Clinic Foundation
Cleveland, Ohio

Contributors

Usaid Allahwala
Department of Cardiology
Royal North Shore Hospital
and
University of Sydney
Sydney, Australia

Taraneh Amir-Nezami
Department of Vascular Surgery
St Vincent's Hospital
Sydney, Australia

David Andresen
Infectious Diseases
St Vincent's Hospital
Sydney, Australia

Alberto P. Avolio
Department of Biomedical Sciences
Faculty of Medicine and Health Sciences
Macquarie University
Sydney, Australia

Edward Barin
MQ Health: Cardiology, Macquarie University
Health Sciences Centre
and
Department of Clinical Science
Faculty of Medicine and Health Sciences
Macquarie University
Sydney, Australia

David W. Baron
Cardiac Catheterisation Laboratories
St Vincent's Hospital
Sydney, Australia

Paul Bhamra-Ariza
Frimley Health NHS Trust
London, United Kingdom

Ravinay Bhindi
Department of Cardiology
Royal North Shore Hospital
and
University of Sydney
Sydney, Australia

John Edward Boland
School of Medical and Applied Sciences
Central Queensland University
and
Cardiac Catheterisation Laboratories
St Vincent's Hospital
Sydney, Australia

Richard Brogan
School of Medicine
Flinders University of South Australia
Adelaide, Australia

Mark Butlin
Department of Biomedical Sciences
Faculty of Medicine and Health Sciences
Macquarie University
Sydney, Australia

Terence J. Campbell
Professorial Unit
St Vincent's Hospital
Sydney, Australia

Gerard Carroll
University of New South Wales
and
The Mater Hospital
Sydney, Australia

and

Riverina Cardiology
and
Wagga Wagga Rural Referral Hospital
Wagga Wagga, Australia

Derek P. Chew
School of Medicine
Flinders University
and
Department of Cardiovascular Medicine
Southern Adelaide Local Health
    Network
Adelaide, Australia

Ming-Yu (Anthony) Chuang
Flinders Medical Centre
Flinders University School of Medicine
and
Department of Cardiovascular Medicine
Southern Adelaide Local Health
    Network
Adelaide, Australia

David E. Connor
School of Medical and Applied Science
and
St Vincent's Centre for Applied Medical
    Research
St Vincent's Hospital
and
University of New South Wales
Sydney, Australia

Steven Faddy
Clinical Services
NSW Ambulance Service
Rozelle, Australia

Michael P. Feneley
Department of Cardiology
St Vincent's Hospital
Sydney, Australia

Andrew Fenning
Medical and Applied Physiology
    Metabolic & Physiological Health
    Medical Sciences & Pharmacology
School of Medical and Applied Sciences
CQ University
North Rockhampton, Australia

Tom Gavaghan
Sydney Adventist Hospital
Wahroonga, Australia

Gary J. Gazibarich
Department of Thoracic Medicine
St Vincent's Hospital
Sydney, Australia

Anthony Grabs
Department of Vascular Surgery
St Vincent's Hospital
Sydney, Australia

Brendan Gunalingam
Cardiac Catheterisation Laboratories
St Vincent's Hospital
Sydney, Australia

and

Gosford Public and Private Hospitals
Gosford, Australia

Peter Hadjipetrou
Interventional Cardiologist
St Andrews Hospital Heart Institute
Brisbane, Australia

Christopher S. Hayward
Department of Cardiology
St Vincent's Hospital
and
University of New South Wales
and
Victor Chang Cardiac Research Institute
Sydney, Australia

Sara Hungerford
St Vincent's Hospital Sydney
and
University of New South Wales
and
The Mater Hospital
Sydney, Australia

Arjun Iyer
Cardiothoracic Surgery and Transplantation
St Vincent's Hospital
Sydney, Australia

Andrew Jabbour
University of New South Wales
and
Cardiovascular Imaging
St Vincent's Hospital
and
Victor Chang Cardiac Research Institute
Sydney, Australia

Pankaj Jain
Department of Cardiology
St Vincent's Hospital
and
University of New South Wales
Sydney, Australia

Paul Jansz
Cardiothoracic Surgery and Transplantation
St Vincent's Hospital
Sydney, Australia

Cameron Jeffries
South Australian Medical Imaging
Flinders Medical Centre
Adelaide, Australia

Fuyue Jiang
Cardiac Catheterisation Laboratories
St Vincent's Hospital
Sydney, Australia

Marcus Juul
Department of Thoracic Medicine
St Vincent's Hospital
Sydney, Australia

Steven Kelly
Cardiac Catheterisation Laboratories
St Vincent's Hospital
Sydney, Australia

Anne Keogh
Pulmonary Hypertension Unit
St Vincent's Hospital
and
University of New South Wales
Sydney, Australia

Nicholas P. Kerr
Cardiac Electrophysiology and Pacing
St Vincent's Hospital
Sydney, Australia

Eva Kline-Rogers
Cardiovascular Nurse Practitioner
University of Michigan Medical Center
Ann Arbor, Michigan

Eugene Kotlyar
Department of Cardiology
St Vincent's Hospital
and
University of New South Wales
and
University of Notre Dame
Sydney, Australia

Dennis L. Kuchar
Cardiac Electrophysiology and Pacing
St Vincent's Hospital
and
Faculty of Medicine
University of New South Wales
and
Victor Chang Cardiac Research Institute
Sydney, Australia

William Lee
Cardiac Electrophysiology and Pacing
St Vincent's Hospital
and
Victor Chang Cardiac Research Institute
and
University of New South Wales
Sydney, Australia

Harry C. Lowe
Cardiac Catheterisation Laboratories
Concord Repatriation General Hospital
and
Centre for Thrombosis and Vascular Research
Faculty of Medicine
University of New South Wales
Sydney, Australia

Jeffrey Lui
Philips Healthcare Australia and New Zealand
Sydney, Australia

Peter Macdonald
Cardiac Transplant Unit
St Vincent's Hospital
Sydney, Australia

David W. M. Muller
Cardiac Catheterisation Laboratories
St Vincent's Hospital
University of New South Wales
Victor Chang Cardiac Research Institute
Sydney, Australia

Kavitha Muthiah
Department of Cardiology
St Vincent's Hospital
Sydney, Australia

Mayooran Namasivayam
Department of Cardiology
St Vincent's Hospital
and
Faculty of Medicine
University of New South Wales
and
Victor Chang Cardiac Research Institute
Sydney, Australia

Brian J. Nankivell
Department of Medicine
University of Sydney
Westmead Hospital
Westmead, Australia

Anthony Nicholson
School of Animal and Veterinary Sciences
University of Adelaide
Roseworthy, Australia

Geoffrey S. Oldfield
John Hunter Hospital
and
CCU, Catheterisation & Angioplasty
   Laboratory
Lake Macquarie and Lingard Private
   Hospitals
Newcastle, Australia

James Otton
Department of Cardiology
Liverpool Hospital
and
Victor Chang Cardiac Research Institute
Sydney, Australia

Julie Parkinson
Cardiac Angiography Unit
Gosford Hospital
Gosford, Australia

Patrick Pender
Department of Cardiology
Liverpool Hospital
Sydney, Australia

Giulietta Pontevivo
Infection Prevention Management and
   Staff Health Services
St Vincent's Hospital
Sydney, Australia

David A. Roy
Cardiac Catheterisation Laboratories
St Vincent's Hospital
Sydney, Australia

Paul Roy
Cardiac Catheterisation Laboratories
St Vincent's Hospital
Sydney, Australia

Peter Ruchin
University of New South Wales
and
The Mater Hospital
Sydney, Australia

and

Riverina Cardiology
and
Wagga Wagga Rural Referral Hospital
Wagga Wagga, Australia

Neville Sammel
Department of Cardiology
St Vincent's Hospital
Sydney, Australia

Smriti Saraf
The Manchester Foundation Trust
Manchester, United Kingdom

Martin Shaw
Department of Anesthetics
St Vincent's Hospital
Sydney, Australia

David Smythe
Cardiology Department
Christchurch Hospital
Christchurch, New Zealand

Roberto Spina
New York Presbyterian Hospital
Columbia University Medical Center
New York, New York

and

Cardiac Catheterisation Laboratories
St Vincent's Hospital
Sydney, Australia

Rajesh N. Subbiah
Cardiac Electrophysiology and Pacing
St Vincent's Hospital
and
Victor Chang Cardiac Research Institute
and
University of New South Wales
Sydney, Australia

Isabella Tan
Department of Biomedical Sciences
Faculty of Medicine and Health Sciences
Macquarie University
Sydney, Australia

Bruce Toben
Senior Director of Scientific Affairs
Instrumentation Laboratory
San Diego, California

Siddharth J. Trivedi
Department of Cardiology
Westmead Hospital
Sydney, Australia

Jo-Anne M. Vidal
Cardiac Catheterisation Laboratories
St Vincent's Hospital
Sydney, Australia

Bruce Walker
Cardiac Electrophysiology and Pacing
St Vincent's Hospital
and
Victor Chang Cardiac Research Institute
and
University of New South Wales
Sydney, Australia

Louis W. Wang
St Vincent's Clinical School
University of New South Wales
Sydney, Australia

Edwina Wing-Lun
University of Notre Dame
and
University of New South Wales
and
Cardiac Catheterisation Laboratories
St Vincent's Hospital
Sydney, Australia

Christopher Yu
Concord Repatriation General Hospital
Sydney, Australia

PART 1

Instrumentation and technology

1

The cardiac imaging and monitoring systems

STEVEN KELLY AND JEFFREY LUI

INTRODUCTION: HISTORY

In November 1895 Wilhelm Conrad Roentgen, a physicist at the University of Wurtzburg in Germany, saw a weak, flickering greenish light on a piece of cardboard coated with a fluorescent chemical preparation while experimenting with a cathode ray tube. Roentgen later verified that the cathode ray tube was the source of invisible rays with an unexpected power of penetration.

A month later the first image of human anatomy, the hand of Roentgen's wife, was obtained using an exposure time of 30 minutes. He reportedly told his wife, 'I am doing something that will cause people to say, "Roentgen has gone mad."' Whether this quote can be attributed to Roentgen or not, the statement well describes the ensuing furor that 'he expected' following the presentation of his paper 'A New Type of Rays.'

Today, over 120 years later, the ability to see into the living body without need for surgical invasion is perhaps the most historically significant advancement in medical diagnostics, having far-reaching implications for medical therapy, specifically in cardiovascular disease.

In 1929 Werner Forssmann introduced a catheter into his own right atrium via the antecubital vein, with the intent to develop a method of rapid delivery for medications. This event, as reported, involved a nurse tricked into assisting in the procedure and a stroll to the Radiology Department to image the advancement of the ureteric catheter under fluoroscopy to the right atrium. That year, the first X-ray tube featuring a rotating anode disc was released.

Over the next 30 years, cardiac catheterisation developed from a method by which cardiac physiology could be studied experimentally, to an established clinical investigational technique used in the diagnosis of congenital and valvular heart disease. In 1959 cardiac catheterisation became the preferred method for investigation of coronary artery disease.

Advances in radiological and cardiac imaging techniques over the same period included development of the mechanical cassette changer, the serial cut film changer, the image intensifier (1952) and acceptance of 35 mm cine film to capture rapid sequence X-ray images. These developments formed a technical framework on which early imaging systems in the cardiac laboratory were based. In the 1960s television provided an interactive means of obtaining clinical information from an X-ray source.

Cardiologists of the early 1970s, in collaboration with various imaging companies, helped to develop the first dedicated cardiac stand using 35 mm cine film as the recording medium. The first dedicated cardiac stands of this period were based on a parallelogram or U-arm using conventional X-ray generators and featured the image intensifier above the patient.

In 1976 the Optimus Modular 200 X-ray generator and Polydiagnost C (parallelogram based) gantry were introduced. The combination of this generator and gantry formed the backbone in many of the cardiac centres worldwide for the next 20 years. This generator, with its tetrode switching of high-tension voltages, was the first to incorporate the 'measuring shot' technique, negating the need to pre-determine the exposure parameters of voltage, current and time.

Advances in cardiac surgery during the 1970s led to coronary artery bypass surgery becoming a viable clinical option for patients suffering coronary artery disease. During this period, significant technological refinements in both surgery and cardiac catheterisation techniques promoted a need for an increased diagnostic yield from cardiac imaging, resulting in the first digital cardiac imaging systems in late 1985.

The enormous demand placed on imaging equipment by routine diagnostic procedures, and more so by prolonged interventional procedures, saw further technical advances in imaging equipment. In 1989, again an advancement specifically tailored to the needs of cardiac imaging, saw the development of the Maximus Rotalix Ceramic (MRC) X-ray tube featuring a continuously rotating anode with liquid metal spiral grove bearing technology. This X-ray tube provided a mechanism by which the enormous heat loadings produced by cardiac procedures could be effectively dissipated, and just as importantly, provided a significant reduction in radiation dose.

Since the initial use of 35 mm cine film as a recording medium, several alternatives have been used, all essentially for cost saving purposes and all in an analogue format of lesser quality than images obtained digitally. In early 1995 this problem was overcome by digital systems using compact disc technology as an archive medium.

CURRENT TECHNOLOGY

The modern cardiac catheterisation laboratory is no longer an X-ray imaging system based on or modified from angiography equipment used in Radiology and demands the highest quality in equipment design and performance. Today's cardiac laboratory consists of:

1. X-ray generator capable of pulsed fluoroscopy at rates equal to standard acquisition rates of 12.5/15 frames per second (fps) and allowing digital acquisition at rates up to 25/30 fps. An achievable current of 1000 milliamperes (mA) at 100 kilovolts (kV) is essential.
2. X-ray tube incorporating a continuously rotating anode and using liquid metal lubricated spiral groove bearing technology and an oil heat exchanger.
3. High-definition digital dynamic Flat Detector with configurations being either a 12-inch (20 × 20 cm) detector size or a 20-inch (30 × 40 cm) detector size.
4. A large-format, configurable monitor capable of multiple inputs.
5. Digital storage device.
6. Archive device ± review station(s).
7. Networking capabilities for multi-laboratory/multi-centre archive and review.
8. Haemodynamic monitoring system.

Specifications and instrumentation

A typical cardiac catheterisation laboratory is shown in Figure 1.1a.

WHERE DOES IT ALL BEGIN?

X-rays are produced within an X-ray tube when electrons from the cathode filament bombard and interact with a rotating disc of metal, the anode. The anode and cathode are mounted a short distance apart. A high voltage is applied between the anode (positive terminal) and the source of electrons, the cathode filament (negative terminal). A high voltage is required to

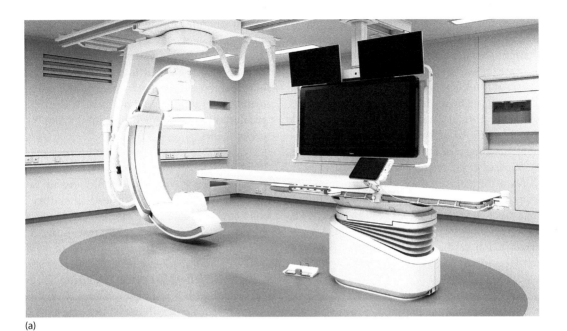

(a)

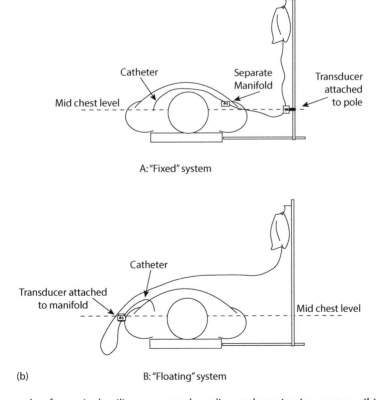

(b)

Figure 1.1 (a) Example of a typical ceiling-mounted cardiac catheterisation system. (b) Difference between a transducer system attached to a pole at mid-chest level ('Fixed') and one attached to a moveable manifold ('Floating'). ([a] Courtesy of Philips Healthcare Australia & New Zealand.)

accelerate electrons from the cathode filament and is obtained from a transformer that converts mains voltages (415 V) to the voltages required for diagnostic imaging, 40–130 kilovolts (kV). This transformer and other components form the basis of the X-ray generator. Bombardment of electrons on the heavy metal of the anode results in the generation of X-rays. The anode contains a high proportion of a heavy metal such as molybdenum or tungsten, as heavy metals maximise generation of X-ray energy.

X-ray generators used in cardiac imaging are microprocessor-controlled and contain medium- to high-frequency converters. The kilowatt (kW) is the unit used to describe the power output of X-ray generators. For cardiac imaging up to 100 kW of power is required.

WHAT IS IMAGE QUALITY?

The clinical information obtained in cardiac imaging is a function of spatial resolution and the dynamic contrast range displayed. Image contrast is affected by high voltage. A high kV results in increased penetration and consequently in reduced image contrast. Due to the inherent properties of the iodine-based contrast medium used in cardiac imaging, subtle differences in image contrast are most evident when images are acquired at approximately 70 kV. The high-frequency generators used in cardiac imaging require high output power to allow acquisition of images to occur around this value.

Because cardiac structures move during acquisition, requiring a short generator switching time ('exposure time') is required, this value being fixed at approximately 8 milliseconds (ms). To then be able to acquire images without motion artefact and at voltages best suited to iodine based contrast (70 kV), the X-ray generator must operate at currents of at least 500–600 mA, and typically at values up to 1000 mA. This is required to maximise contrast resolution.

The high voltage supply from the X-ray tube accelerates electrons from the cathode. If this voltage varies over time, the X-ray output will change during an exposure, thus influencing image quality. Modern X-ray generators are therefore designed to have very low variation in the higher voltages. The control unit of a generator controls tube current and exposure time, controls anode rotation and has other additional functions.

Much development in recent times has been focused on minimising radiation dosage to the patient, clinician and staff, while still maintaining a medical diagnostic level of image quality to cater for diagnostic and interventional purposes. Today's technologies better manage the diagnostic and interventional environment with the core consideration of dose management driving recent developments.

'THE BIT UNDER THE TABLE'

The X-ray tube is contained within a metal housing lined on the inside with lead shielding. The tube housing provides the mechanical connection between the X-ray tube and the rest of the X-ray system and is filled with circulating oil to conduct heat away from the X-ray tube. X-rays are emitted through an opening in the metal housing. The tube is provided with a window made of a very light material such as beryllium or thin glass to permit unrestricted outflow of X-rays in the chosen direction.

A collimator (a mechanism to attenuate, or focus, or restrict a beam of energy into a narrow field or column) is mounted on the X-ray tube housing. The collimator limits the X-ray beam to the minimum area needed for the diagnostic procedure. This protects the patient and operator from unnecessary radiation and improves image quality by reducing the amount of scattered radiation. In some systems an iris diaphragm located within the collimator produces a circular field of irradiation focused to the digital detector. The collimator also contains two pairs of lead shutters that can be adjusted to limit the beam area through a rectangular field. A single or double semi-transparent wedge-shaped filter(s) is incorporated within the collimator to overcome attenuation differences between different anatomical areas.

The rotating anode of the X-ray tube is coupled to the static part of the tube by liquid metal, lubricated spiral groove bearings that have replaced ball bearings in the anode support construction. Unlike conventional X-ray tubes, the anode in X-ray tubes of dedicated cardiac imaging equipment rotates continuously. This produces an instantaneous response from the X-ray tube when fluoroscopy or digital acquisition of X-ray images is required. Added benefits of this technology include silent operation and an extended X-ray tube lifetime due to wear-free operation.

When electrons strike the anode target disc, approximately 1% of the total energy generated is converted into actual X-rays. The other 99% of the electron beam energy generates heat. In conventional X-ray tubes this excess heat is stored in the anode, then transmitted outwards from the anode through the tube envelope by heat radiation and convection. Only a small amount of heat is transmitted by point heat conduction due to the limited area provided by conventional X-ray tubes equipped with ball bearing construction.

The cathode contains one or more filaments that are heated to release electrons. The cathode cup is shaped to focus the electrons onto a specific point on the anode known as the focal spot. When a high voltage is applied between the anode and cathode, electrons flow with increasing velocity towards the anode. The filament current determines the quantity of electrons emitted at a given voltage and hence the number of X-rays produced by the X-ray tube. The total flow of electrons is the tube current. This quantity is expressed in mA. Most X-ray tubes are equipped with two filaments, producing two focal spots of different sizes.

The X-ray tube load is defined as the amount of energy absorbed by the tube during an exposure and is expressed in kilowatt-seconds or kilojoules. This measure is a function of tube current, exposure time, and voltage. Electrons hitting other parts of the X-ray tube rather than the focal spot also produce X-rays. These are referred to as extrafocal or off-focus radiation and affect the contrast resolution of the image and can be reduced by appropriate collimation.

WHAT IS THE 'I.I.'?

Images were previously formed in an Image Intensifier (I.I.) that received X-rays that had passed through the patient, and converted and amplified these 'signals' into an electrical interaction that was received as an image. The term 'I.I.' is still used today to describe the digital detector above the patient, and in some instances the entire imaging gantry. Like the use of the term 'cine' to describe a digital acquisition run or the acquisition foot pedal, both terms continue to be used incorrectly as a consequence of 'old habits' not necessarily 'dying hard'.

The image intensifier was developed to replace the fluorescent screen of earlier X-ray imaging systems. The latest cardiac laboratory systems feature a flat-panel detector. This detector in combination with advanced imaging chains generates an image resolution of up to 1344 × 1344 pixels at 16 bits depth for a 12 inch detector, and 2480 × 1920 pixels at 16 bits depth for a 20 inch detector.

A flat-panel detector offers a wider range of zoom and field of view (FOV) options as well. With a 12-inch (20 × 20 cm) dynamic flat panel detector, the clinician is able to capture in one FOV the apex of the heart and the outflow tracts. Field sizes available on a 12-inch detector are 30, 27, 22, 19, 15 cm (12, 11, 8, 7, 6 inch) diagonal square formats, while a 20-inch (30 × 40 cm) dynamic flat panel detector has 48, 42, 37, 31, 27, 22, 19, 15 cm (19, 17, 15, 12, 11, 9, 7.5, 6 inch) diagonal square formats. As before, the lower the magnification, the greater the FOV and the lower the radiation dose generated.

WHAT EVER HAPPENED TO CINE FILM?

Digital imaging offers enhanced image quality and new diagnostic and analytical possibilities.

Quantitative analysis of coronary vessel profile and densitometric flow, as well as ventricular functionality, can be derived from the digital image data. A digital image consists of a set of numbers that can be displayed by assigning a grey level to each number. The maximum number of different grey levels that can be distinguished by the human eye is about 64. Assigning the full range of numbers to the total number of grey levels provides a display of the total brightness range in the image. However, it is also possible to assign a smaller range of numbers to the total number of grey levels, in which case an average level and a smaller window width are used so that numbers outside this window are displayed either in white or black. This technique is used for optimum display of a smaller attenuation range, such as that in cardiac imaging.

PHYSIOLOGICAL AND HAEMODYNAMIC MONITORING

Accurate haemodynamic monitoring is an essential requirement for a cardiac catheterisation laboratory. Most modern imaging systems can integrate with systems responsible for monitoring cardiac and haemodynamic physiology, with specific requirements for accuracy, safety, and reliability inherent in invasive cardiovascular investigations.

The monitoring system plays a primary role in detecting alterations in patient status and quantifying physiological measurements. There are unique requirements in areas such as equipment mounting, cabling, and display screens. There are also specific regulations regarding power reticulation and earth leakage. It is recommended that an emergency power supply be installed, particularly if the haemodynamic system is used as a vital signs monitor.

Physiological signals such as pressure waveforms are sampled by the haemodynamic system, and signal analysis algorithms are automatically applied to obtain the required data that are presented as customised windows on the same large, high-resolution displays as the angiographic images for the physician and system operator, enabling all parameters to be easily observed and monitored by staff. Displayed on the operator screen are various control windows and menus permitting system functions to be accessed. Controls are also provided via the keyboard and protocol-based command sequences that are available both in the viewing room and at the patient table. The protocols are similar to short programs that when executed perform a series of functions that would otherwise require many specific operator actions, and may be customised for many specific procedure types. In addition, if specific groups of measurements are made during a procedure, then certain derived parameters are automatically calculated and are made available immediately. The immediate availability of such calculated determinates as vascular resistance or valve areas is invaluable during an interventional study.

As a result, computerised instrumentation has revolutionised patient monitoring, operator access, data analysis and reporting, particularly with the introduction of more advanced minimally invasive cardiac procedures that require integration with technologies such as intravascular ultrasound (IVUS), optical coherence tomography (OCT), fractional flow reserve (FFR/iFR), and electrophysiology and structural heart and haemodynamic software to improve workflow and optimise patient care.

HAEMODYNAMIC PRESSURE MEASUREMENT

Pressure measurement depends on correct use of the transducer system. Modern transducers are available as sterile, disposable, pre-calibrated, single-use units and may be either 'fixed' to a bedside pole at mid-chest level, or 'floating' (Figure 1.1b) attached to a manifold. In either case, all transducers must be balanced ('zeroed') to atmospheric pressure at mid-chest level immediately prior to use to avoid false high or low pressure signal bias. Balancing compensates for the effect of atmospheric pressure (760 mmHg at sea level), making atmospheric pressure equivalent to zero mmHg in relation to internal body measurements. Mid-chest level is normally taken as half the height of the patient's chest from the table top, along the mid-axillary line.

With a 'fixed' transducer independent of a manifold, pressures are accurate irrespective of manifold level. With a 'floating' transducer attached to a manifold, the manifold unit must be positioned at mid-chest level whenever a pressure is measured. Otherwise, variations in hydrostatic pressure exerted by the column of fluid in the flush line may affect readings. Raising a transducer 1.34 cm above mid-chest level induces an artefactual drop of 1 mmHg in recorded pressure; conversely, lowering the transducer 1.34 cm raises recorded pressure by 1 mmHg. Such differences may become critical in evaluating right heart pressures and valve gradients.

Most haemodynamic systems are modular in design, permitting a high degree of versatility in application. Multi-parameter data acquisition modules with ward monitor compatibility make the patient interface simple and highly flexible, allowing parameters such as electrocardiogram, pulse oxymetry, respiration, non-invasive blood pressure, and thermodilution cardiac output to be directly available. All physiological information is usually recorded in real time onto the system hard drive and may be recalled at any time during the case for review. Controls of a haemodynamic system must permit detailed access to all functions and there must be provision for institutional details, display setup, automatic data logging, hardware settings, and a means of data backup.

CURRENT TRENDS

The 'Cath Lab' is now a department shared between cardiologists, vascular surgeons, cardio-thoracic surgeons, and other specialists who require a theatre-like environment that is flexible, easily accessible, and has the ability to undertake imaging when needed. This evolution, combined with the increasing complexity of invasive procedures currently being undertaken, has enabled the fusion of imaging modalities into enhanced diagnostic and interventional necessities.

For example, procedures such as endovascular treatment of an abdominal aortic aneurysm involve calculations and device planning using computed tomography (CT), and the ready availability of this CT information prior to and during the procedure provides an anatomical understanding that enhances and optimises procedural outcomes. These data can be overlaid or 'fused' with live fluoroscopy during the procedure to determine correct device placement.

Similarly, multi-modality image fusion in procedures such as radiofrequency or thermal ablation to treat atrial fibrillation and left atrial appendage closure offers a dimension of understanding and reassurance in therapy delivery not previously available.

The long-awaited use of large format display devices in the control room is a welcome addition. The control room may be finally rid of multiple workstations and multiple monitors, and all aspects of imaging, monitoring and data archival may be managed at a single, interactive and configurable workplace.

It is expected that cardiac catheterisation laboratories will continue to evolve through developments in workflow enhancements, radiation dose management, and clinically-driven outcomes.

Workflow enhancements

As the dynamics in the healthcare environment change, so do requirements within the cardiac catheterisation laboratory. With a growing number of patients and an increasing trend towards more complex procedures, cardiac imaging systems will be required to streamline workflows via third-party technologies, and to seamlessly integrate, retrieve and interact with external imaging/analysis modalities (CT, IVUS, FFR, and magnetic resonance imaging [MRI]) and other advanced interventional tools to provide the clinician with all possible information to perform the procedure most effectively and most efficiently. Multi-modality hybrid rooms with combined angiography and CT/MRI exist today, and the cost-effectiveness and clinical wealth of these concepts are now better understood.

Radiation dose management

Patient and operator radiation exposure has previously been considered an unavoidable procedural and occupational risk, and is still evolving. Our understanding of what to better protect (e.g. eyes) and how to do this is paramount. Currently available technologies such as X-ray tubes equipped with spiral groove bearings, and the associated benefits of X-ray spectral beam filtration, combined with integrated radiation dose reports, real-time dose read-out, and accumulated dose warnings have caused significant changes in occupational exposure and procedural practice.

The radiation dose-saving benefits derived from spiral groove bearing X-ray tubes is a consequence of the enormous heat dissipation properties of these devices and the ability of these X-ray tubes to function under the extra stress of additional copper and aluminium filtration. The resultant reductions in radiation dose are essential considerations in today's climate of occupational health and safety. Patient or staff litigation because of not providing the safest possible work and clinical environment remains a major concern.

Clinical case studies demonstrating radiation injuries caused by cardiac procedures continue to be presented. High radiation dose procedures may include those involving chronic total occlusion of the coronary vessel, pulmonary vein isolation to treat atrial fibrillation, and biventricular device implantation. All technologies and dose-saving applications must be employed by all staff with active discussion and revision during the procedure regarding ways to minimise radiation dose and still provide optimal patient outcomes.

Clinically driven outcomes

As data-driven medicine becomes standard practice, as is especially evident with new medical devices, it becomes important for all necessary information during the procedure to be easily archived and retrievable. Hospital information technology networks and infrastructure will be a key focus in this area in order to manage these data requirements. Capturing all data throughout a patient's healthcare continuum will become a focus on improving patient outcomes and cardiac laboratory performance. Monitoring systems and collating data remotely can be foreseen as trends for the future.

SUMMARY

The modern cardiac catheterisation laboratory has a need for rapid patient turnover in the safest possible environment for patients and staff. To facilitate this, imaging and monitoring systems must have a well-designed, clear and logical user interface, producing efficiencies and a reduction in the amount of operator time required to obtain the required information. As the complexity of procedures being undertaken increases, so too must the ability to integrate laboratory information and functionality with other imaging tools and analytical devices to maximise efficiency, to increase functionality, and to maximise diagnostic yield and interventional outcomes.

ACKNOWLEDGEMENT

The authors acknowledge the input from Chris Lee, who contributed to development of this chapter.

FURTHER READING

Balter S, Moses J. Managing patient dose in interventional cardiology. *Catheter Cardiovasc Interv.* 2007;70(2):244–249.

Bartal G, Vano E, Paulo G, Miller DL. Management of patient and staff radiation dose in interventional radiology: Current concepts. *Cardiovasc InterventRadiol.* 2014;37(2):289–298.

Boland JE, Wang LW, Love BJ, Christofi M, Muller DW. Impact of new-generation hybrid imaging technology on radiation dose during percutaneous coronary interventions and trans-femoral aortic valve implantations: A comparison with conventional flat-plate angiography. *Heart Lung Circ.* 2016;25(7):668–675.

Boland JE, Wang LW, Love BJ, Wynne DG, Muller DW. Radiation dose during percutaneous treatment of structural heart disease. *Heart Lung Circ.* 2014;23(11):1075–1083.

Chenier M, Tuzcu EM, Kapadia SR, Krishnaswamy A. Multimodality imaging in the cardiac catheterization laboratory: A new era in sight. *Intervent Cardiol.* 2013;5(3):335.

Christopoulos G, Christakopoulos GE, Rangan BV, Layne R, Grabarkewitz R, Haagen D, et al. Comparison of radiation dose between different fluoroscopy systems in the modern catheterization laboratory: Results from bench testing using an anthropomorphic phantom. *Catheter Cardiovasc Interv.* 2015;86(5):927–932.

Fetterly KA, Mathew V, Lennon R, Bell MR, Holmes Jr DR, Rihal CS. Radiation dose reduction in the invasive cardiovascular laboratory: Implementing a culture and philosophy of radiation safety. *JACC: Cardiovasc Interv.* 2012;5(8):866–873.

Gislason-Lee AJ, McMillan C, Cowen AR, Davies AG. Dose optimization in cardiac x-ray imaging. *Med Phys.* 2013;40(9):091911.

Miller DL, Balter S, Schueler BA, Wagner LK, Strauss KJ, Vañó E. Clinical radiation management for fluoroscopically guided interventional procedures. *Radiology.* 2010;257(2):321–332.

2

Non-invasive physiological monitoring

MARK BUTLIN, ISABELLA TAN, EDWARD BARIN AND ALBERTO P. AVOLIO

INTRODUCTION

Physiological monitoring broadly encompasses the measurement of a biological signal over time and referencing this against the expected value of the parameter in order to make a decision about what action, if any, needs to be taken to bring that biological parameter back to a normal range. This could be weight or waist and hip circumference measured over months or years, with an interest in keeping a healthy body mass index or hip-waist ratio. It could also be the minute-to-minute tracking of body temperature for monitoring of fever. In the field of cardiology, the most commonly monitored parameter is brachial blood pressure over the course of years for management of hypertension. Specific conditions of the heart are commonly diagnosed using the electrocardiogram and echocardiography. The electrocardiogram is treated as a sole topic in other text books and is addressed

with specific attention to ischaemic heart disease in Chapter 19 of this book. Echocardiography is also addressed in many textbooks from a technical standpoint and is discussed in the context of pre-procedural diagnosis in Chapter 27, and as imaging support in structural heart interventions in Chapter 36.

This chapter addresses other broader diagnostic and monitoring tools in interventional cardiology. The coupling of the heart with the systemic and pulmonary vasculature results in the functional distribution of blood to all organs of the body. If blood pressure and blood flow are not optimal, risk of cardiovascular events and end-organ damage increases. By measuring blood pressure and flow both peripherally and centrally and comparing the measured values against the expected healthy, normal values, a picture of cardiovascular health can be developed to inform treatment options.

PERIPHERAL BLOOD PRESSURE AND FLOW

Gaining quantification of the vitality of the arterial pulse from a site peripheral to the heart, such as the neck (e.g. carotid artery) or arm (e.g. radial artery), is a medical method that has been in use since antiquity. As medical methods become more advanced, the most routinely used physiological signals are still the pulse rate measured from an electrocardiogram, finger blood volume pulse (plethysmography) or manual radial pulse palpation, along with brachial artery blood pressure measured with a cuff around the upper arm.

Brachial artery blood pressure measurement

The main predictor of general cardiovascular risk remains systemic arterial blood pressure, with the specific diagnosis being the category of hypertension measured against current guidelines[1] using non-invasive assessment of brachial arterial pressure. This is done with an inflatable cuff placed around the upper arm. As the cuff is deflated through the range of physiologically possible arterial pressures, a signal associated with the pressure in the artery is used to estimate the peak (systolic pressure) and minima (diastolic pressure) of the arterial pulse. Riva-Rocci first described the technique in 1896 with systolic pressure associated with the first palpation of the radial artery pulse on cuff deflation. In 1905, Korotkoff, at a time of expanded use of the stethoscope, described the use of characteristic sounds associated with the movement of the brachial artery and the blood within it to estimate both systolic and diastolic brachial artery pressure.[2] The twentieth century saw development and validation of automatic methods for measuring brachial artery blood pressure using either Korotkoff's auscultatory technique and computer-based analysis, or more commonly techniques using the magnitude of oscillation in cuff pressure associated with the arterial pulse (oscillometry).

Cuff size is highly important, as the pressure in the cuff needs to be transmitted to the brachial artery. A small cuff tends to lead to overestimation of blood pressure and is seen where a standard adult-sized cuff is used on obese individuals or people with larger arm diameters. Conversely, an overly large cuff can lead to underestimation of blood pressure, as occurs with use of a standard adult cuff in individuals with a small arm diameter or in children. The relationship of the systemic vasculature and the heart is generally assessed through use of these two numbers (brachial systolic and diastolic blood pressure), as it has for over one hundred years. Medical research widens assessment to include the quantification of other fiducial points of the arterial blood pressure waveform (Figure 2.1), also allowing assessment

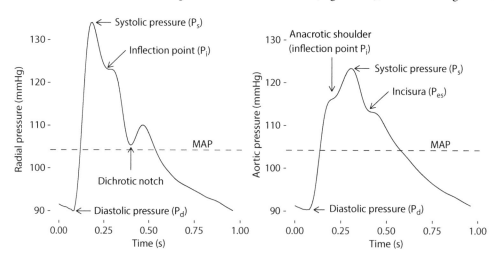

Figure 2.1 Features of the blood pressure waveform as observed at the aorta and the periphery (radial artery). Due to pulse pressure amplification, the peripheral (e.g. brachial) systolic pressure is always *greater* than aortic systolic pressure, even though the total power in the waveform at the peripheral site is less (*Abbreviation*: MAP, mean aortic pressure).

of derived parameters such as the augmentation index and form factor.[3] Some parameters associated with the stiffness of the large arteries, such as the pulse wave velocity between the carotid and femoral artery sites, have added value in predicting cardiovascular risk above and beyond brachial blood pressure alone,[4] and are adopted in current guidelines for assessment of cardiovascular risk.[5] As for brachial blood pressure, these additional measures for quantifying the function of the systemic arteries do not offer diagnosis for specific cardiac conditions. However, they are valuable in quantifying a patient's cumulative cardiovascular risk to guide treatment and success of interventions.

Due to the highly dynamic nature of blood pressure, the diagnosis of hypertension can be problematic with the use of single measures. Notwithstanding issues around measurement technique (e.g. body position, arm position, cuff deflation rate, and operator digit-preference), the effect of the environment and diurnal variation means that a single measure of blood pressure rarely reflects the true nature of a person's blood pressure. Home measurement of blood pressure with a reliable, validated automatic blood pressure device can be used to rule out cases of white-coat hypertension or masked hypertension. However, only 24-hour, ambulatory measures of brachial artery blood pressure provide the information required to assess whether the day time variability in blood pressure is within the expected normotensive range, and whether night time blood pressure dips in the expected fashion. In taking out-of-clinic values of blood pressure, it is important to note that the cut-offs for hypertension are lower in the day and even lower at night, reflecting the effect of the clinic environment on blood pressure and the expected nocturnal dip in blood pressure.[6]

Thresholds for the diagnosis of hypertension are based on risk-prediction using the cuff-based measure of brachial artery pressure. However, all cuff-based methods of measuring brachial arterial pressure underestimate true systolic pressure as assessed by invasive means, and overestimate true diastolic pressure. Additionally, arterial pressure varies throughout the systemic vasculature, with systolic pressure at the arm being higher than the systolic pressure in the aorta, due to pulse pressure amplification through increased local vascular stiffness.

Continuous measurement of peripheral blood pressure

Cuff-based assessment of blood pressure captures the systolic and diastolic blood pressure at a point in time. It does not and cannot provide continuous measurement of blood pressure. Continuous blood pressure measurement is critical in physiological monitoring situations presented in intensive care and during administration of anaesthesia. This type of monitoring is provided by connecting a pressure sensor to the artery by either placing a solid-state pressure sensor-tipped catheter within the artery via percutaneous access, or by connecting an external pressure sensor to a fluid line that is fed into the artery. In 1967, the Czech physiologist Jan Peňàz described a non-invasive technique for continuous blood pressure monitoring, based on a servo-nulling technique to keep blood volume in the finger constant by constantly changing the pressure applied to that finger, otherwise known as vascular unloading (Figure 2.2a). Volume in the finger is monitored using photoplethysmography, a technique that is detailed later in this chapter. The instantaneous pressure in the cuff required to maintain the finger blood volume reflects the instantaneous arterial pressure in the finger.

The two main disadvantages of this device are comfort and accuracy in terms of absolute arterial pressure. As the cuff is constantly at a pressure above venous pressure, there is no venous return from the finger while the device is in operation. This has been overcome in some commercial systems with use of two finger cuffs used sequentially to limit the period of time one finger is exposed to supra-venous pressures.

While the method is very good for tracking changes in blood pressure, the measure of blood pressure in absolute terms is less accurate. Some commercial devices build in mathematical estimates of the relative brachial artery pressure or calibrate the finger blood pressure to blood pressure measured in the upper arm using conventional cuff-based oscillometric techniques. However, while the accuracy and tracking of changes in blood pressure are useful for clinical tests such as autonomic function testing, the technique is not of a suitable accuracy to replace invasive blood pressure measurement in critical care situations.

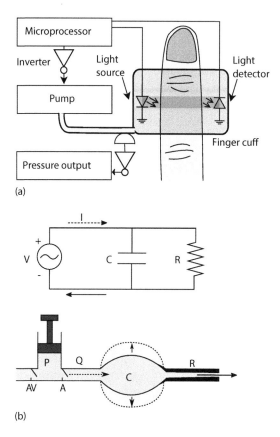

(a)

(b)

Figure 2.2 **(a)** The Peňàz or servonulling, vascular unloading technique for continuous, non-invasive monitoring of blood pressure. The volume (measured by light source and detector) is kept constant by inversely adjusting pressure in a cuff around the finger. The pressure in the cuff is approximately equal to the blood pressure in the finger. **(b)** *Windkessel* simplification of the systemic arterial system in representation of electrical and fluid dynamic analogues. Estimation of the total peripheral resistance (R) and total compliance (C) and measurement of arterial pressure (P, or voltage V in the electrical analogue) allows for calculation of blood flow (cardiac output, Q, or current I in the electrical analogue). AV and A represent the schematic position of the atrioventricular and aortic valves of the left ventricle.

Ultrasound for measurement of peripheral blood flow

Doppler ultrasound insonation of vessels can be used to quantify relative blood flow in the more superficial, but still large, blood vessels of the body. It can be used to quantify venous blood flow in detecting disorders such as deep vein thrombosis. Clinically, this is not routinely used in the peripheral arterial vasculature except for use in blood pressure measurement in the ankle in conjunction with an occlusive cuff to assist in the diagnosis of peripheral vascular disease and significant atherosclerosis in peripheral vessels.

Pulse oximetry and the photoplethysmogram

The most commonly measured physiological variables following height and weight are heart rate and blood pressure. In the hospital environment, this is closely followed by pulse oximetry. This is valuable in the critical care environment, as pulse oximetry is a very accurate method for estimation of arterial haemoglobin oxygen saturation. When a strong signal is received, a local blood volume waveform that oscillates with the cardiac cycle can be measured (plethysmography), giving a quick and easy method for continuous monitoring of heart rate.

Plethysmography (derived from the Greek word, *plethys*, meaning fullness, or *plethysmos*, meaning enlargement) is the transduction of tissue volume, including the transiently changing volume of blood within that tissue. The concept was first proposed by physiologist Angelo Mosso during his studies in Leipzig in 1873–1874, with Mosso's plethysmograph reported in *Scientific American* in 1876.[7] The mechanics of plethysmography can take many forms, but the most simplistic to use is photoplethysmography, a method first presented by Alrick Hertzman and Clair Spealman at the 49th Annual Meeting of the American Physiological Society in Memphis, Tennessee in 1937.[8]

Photoplethysmography devices use a probe that transmits and receives light. Light transmission is most commonly through the tip of a finger, but can also be through the ear lobe, toe or bridge of the nose. These light transmission probes require a relatively small volume of tissue through which light can be transmitted without significant obstruction. Other devices use reflectance of light, with the light emitting and receiving diodes on the same plane. These devices can be placed on any area of well-perfused skin and are commonly used in a flexible adhesive probe for placement on the skin of neonates and infants for monitoring blood oxygen and heart rate.

Regardless of the probe configuration, a photoplethysmography device can measure the short-term time-varying changes in the absorption of light, which is associated with blood volume in the tissue, and changes in the wavelength of light absorbed, which is associated with the oxygen saturation of haemoglobin. By shining light of two wavelengths (red light at approximately 660 nm and near-infrared at approximately 940 nm) into the tissue, the arterial oxygen saturation (SpO_2) can be estimated, as light intensity in these two wavelength ranges differ between oxyhaemoglobin (HbO_2) and haemoglobin (Hb). While this is a well-validated technique and in common usage in clinical monitoring, the use of the photoplethysmogram (the short-term time-varying signal associated with blood volume changes at the frequency of the cardiac cycle) has no standard for clinical measurement. However, it is commonly used for measurement of heart rate, as it is observed to be reliably in phase with a simultaneously-recorded electrocardiogram. The photoplethysmogram has been used experimentally for derivation of cardiac output, respiration, arterial compliance, endothelial

function, Raynaud's disease, and autonomic function assessment.[9] However, these have not yet had an uptake in common clinical usage.

CARDIAC OUTPUT AND AORTIC BLOOD PRESSURE

Peripheral measures characterising the dynamics of the systemic arterial vasculature often correlate with measures of blood pressure and flow dynamics of the aorta and are in many cases statistically predictive of risk of cardiovascular events. Theoretically, a measure anatomically closer to the organ of interest (heart, brain, kidney) would be more highly predictive and more clinically useful.[10] As anatomically deeper regions are more difficult to interrogate non-invasively, methods have been developed to derive measures such as cardiac output and aortic blood pressure using related cardiovascular signals that can be measured transcutaneously.

Measurement of cardiac output necessitates access to a point in the vasculature where the total blood flow passes, such as the ascending aorta or pulmonary artery. Due to the position of these sites, methods of cardiac output measurement are generally invasive, along with risks and inconvenience that are associated with such invasive measures. The gold standard, and most accurate method of measuring cardiac output, is to use aortic electromagnetic or ultrasonic flow sensors placed on the ascending aorta or pulmonary artery – a highly invasive method that is not practicable in all but the most invasive of surgeries.

In cardiac catheterisation procedures, an average cardiac output can be obtained using indicator dilution techniques, most commonly thermodilution in the pulmonary artery via right heart catheterisation. Given the invasiveness of direct flow measurement, thermodilution is often used as the reference value despite having limitations in both technical aspects[11] and accuracy,[12] and not providing a continuous measurement of cardiac output.

A number of non-invasive techniques exist for estimation of cardiac output, with varying accuracy and convenience of measurement. While absolute accuracy of these techniques varies, non-invasive techniques have a clear advantage over invasive thermodilution techniques in that continuous tracking of changes in cardiac output can be achieved. Therefore, many non-invasive cardiac output assessment techniques allow for continuous monitoring of cardiovascular dynamics in situations of critical care.

Ultrasound-based methods for estimation of cardiac output

Transoesophageal Doppler is a technically non-invasive but intrusive method of placing an ultrasound probe at a relatively defined angle to the ascending aorta. The placement of the Doppler probe in the oesophagus aligns (in normal anatomy) the probe parallel and proximal to the descending aorta. This means the angle of insonation is known and the absolute velocity of blood can be calculated by the Doppler shift in frequency. Cardiac output can then be estimated by assuming an average aortic diameter to calculate flow (L/min) from velocity (m/s). As measurement is in the descending aorta, assumptions must be made about flow of blood through the common carotid and brachiocephalic branches of the aortic arch that also comprise the cardiac output as would be viewed at the left ventricular outflow tract.

The ascending aorta can also be examined using transthoracic Doppler. However, the angle of insonation of the aorta is more difficult to estimate from the skin surface and therefore the estimation of cardiac output using transthoracic Doppler tends to be less accurate. Despite the theoretical advantages of using transoesophageal Doppler for cardiac output measurement, the absolute accuracy is relatively low, with a meta-analysis in 2010 putting the correlation with invasive thermodilution technique at r = 0.69, and a percentage error of 42%.[13] However, due to the anatomical position of the ultrasound probe, the technique is very useful for continuous tracking of short-term changes in cardiac output.

Cardiac output is also a standard parameter estimated in echocardiography. By capturing the systolic and diastolic left ventricular area in an imaged 2-dimensional (2D) cross-section, the difference in these areas is multiplied by a factor to arrive at an estimation of the volume of blood ejected (stroke volume). Multiplication of the estimated stroke volume with the measured heart rate gives cardiac output. As there are necessary assumptions made about the 3D geometry of the ventricle, there is a limit to the accuracy of this method. Furthermore, as the method uses echocardiography, often with manual input in the analysis steps, this method is not useful for continuous monitoring of cardiac output, but is useful for routine non-invasive estimation of left ventricular function in terms of stroke volume.

Bio-impedance-based methods for estimation of cardiac output

Bio-impedance is the measurement of the resistance of a region of body tissue to an oscillatory electrical voltage. The bio-impedance changes with the type and density of material (e.g. bone, skeletal muscle and blood all have different bio-impedance) and with the volume of tissue. Therefore, bio-impedance measured across the chest gives a signal that can vary with changes in lung volume and in blood volume. If an alternating current in the frequency range of 20 kHz–100 kHz is passed through the chest, the approximate resistivity of blood is 150 Ω/cm, the resistivity of cardiac muscle is 750 Ω/cm, the resistivity of the lungs is 1275 Ω/cm, and the resistivity of fat is 2500 Ω/cm.[14] As electricity will take the path of least resistance (impedance), the charge across the chest is primarily conducted by blood, and any change in impedance is primarily a change in the volume of blood. Careful anatomical placement of the electrodes attempts to isolate blood volume changes in the heart and arrive at a measure of stroke volume through these changes in impedance. A 2017 meta-analysis placed the mean bias of cardiac output measurement by thoracic bio-impedance against invasive techniques at −0.22 L/min with a percentage error of 42%.[15] Despite this relatively large percentage error, the bio-impedance technique is very readily applied for continuous tracking of stroke volume as the technique requires only electrode stickers placed accurately on the chest.

Cardiac output estimation using the Fick principle

Physiologist Adolf Eugen Fick described the principles of gas diffusion into fluid through a membrane, and using this knowledge proposed a measure of cardiac output (CO) by using the logical equating of the amount of oxygen taken up by the lungs (VO_2) with the difference of the oxygen content between the pulmonary artery ($CO \times C_a$) and the pulmonary vein ($CO \times C_v$).

$$VO_2 = \left(CO \times C_a\right) - \left(CO \times C_v\right) \quad (2.1)$$

$$CO = VO_2 / \left(C_a - C_v\right) \quad (2.2)$$

Arterial and venous blood sampling and blood oxygen quantification can provide C_a and C_v. VO_2 can be measured as the difference of inspired and expired oxygen (see Chapters 16 and 17). The Fick principle can be applied to any gas that diffuses easily in blood. Various devices use gas rebreathing to estimate arterial and venous levels of the gas. Measurement of inspired and expired carbon dioxide can provide cardiac output estimation without blood sampling,[16] but this technique suffers from accuracy problems at higher pulmonary shunt levels.[17] Rebreathing a combination of two inert gases (nitrous oxide, soluble in blood, and sulphur hexafluoride, insoluble in blood) allows for correction for pulmonary shunt and has good agreement with other estimates of cardiac output such as thermodilution, the Fick principle by oxygen measurement and cardiac magnetic resonance imaging.[18] Measurements of cardiac output using the Fick principle are not useful for continuous monitoring purposes, but it is a relatively easy, if demanding, non-invasive method to estimate cardiac output at a single point in time.

Pulse transit time and pulse contour analysis for cardiac output estimation

The shape of the arterial pressure waveform is a result of the time-dependent ejection of blood from the left ventricle and the resistance and compliance of the systemic arterial vasculature. The contour of the arterial waveform therefore carries information relating to the stroke volume of the left ventricle. However, to extract this information, assumptions about the state of the systemic vasculature, and the dynamics of the heart need to be made. Addition of other cardiovascular measurements, such as stiffness of the arteries, does not remove all assumptions, but reduces the number of unknowns, and potentially increases the accuracy of stroke volume and cardiac output estimation using the arterial pulse.

The concept of pulse contour analysis for stroke volume estimation has been accredited to work of J. Erlanger and D.R. Hooker of Johns Hopkins Hospital conducted in 1904.[19] Many models have been proposed using similar methods, generally relying on techniques to estimate parameters of the *Windkessel* representation of the systemic vasculature (Figure 2.2b).

Total peripheral resistance, arterial compliance and vascular impedance cannot be measured directly using non-invasive techniques. However, information on vascular model parameters can be gained from the pulse contour,[20] and from the

stiffness of arteries as assessed by the pulse transit time.[21,22] In addition, or alternatively, the model parameters can be drawn from a population morphometric table assigning average population values based on the patient's gender, age, height and weight.

While devices show good ability to track change in cardiac output, accuracy in absolute cardiac output often relies on initial calibration using invasive techniques such as thermodilution. Although these devices require invasive calibration, they have the advantage that once calibrated they provide relatively good, continuous tracking of cardiac output.

A move toward devices that do not require initial calibration using invasive measures is reliant upon measurement of both pulse transit time and analysis of the arterial pulse waveform contour.[23] The arterial pulse can be taken from an intra-arterial line if in place, a radial waveform measured non-invasively using a technique such as tonometry, or the finger blood pressure waveform measured using the Peñàz technique previously described. Commercial application of this technique initially had relatively poor agreement with measured cardiac output,[24] but various developments in the derivation of cardiac output (proprietary information) have seen incremental improvement in cardiac output estimation. While tracking of changes in cardiac output is very good, absolute values of cardiac output are not acceptable for interventional procedures.[25] These systems do offer the advantage of providing an accurate, real-time, *continuous* measure of cardiac output, but only with initial calibration using a standard invasive technique.

Arterial pulse contour analysis for non-invasive calculation of aortic pressure

The total power in the pressure waveform near the heart is greater than in peripheral sites such as the brachial artery. However, due to wave reflection from impedance mismatches such as arterial branching and decreasing arterial diameters, the systolic pressure at the brachial artery is greater than the systolic pressure at the aorta (Figure 2.1). Diastolic and mean pressure remain relatively constant throughout the large arteries. The difference between aortic and brachial systolic (and pulse) pressure is not the same for all people.

Although aortic blood pressure can be measured during cardiac catheterisation procedures, methods also exist for non-invasive calculation of the aortic pressure using peripheral arterial waveforms calibrated to brachial blood pressure. This allows use of aortic pressure in clinical workup for patients. The technique of non-invasive estimation of aortic blood pressure relies on there being an intransient relationship between the radial (or brachial) blood pressure waveform and the blood pressure waveform of the aorta that is relatively consistent across adult age and gender.[26] Several commercial devices now exist that estimate aortic blood pressure using the volume displacement waveform measured from a brachial cuff, making measurement of aortic blood pressure no more difficult than measurement of brachial blood pressure.

These devices show good accuracy, but two conventions of reporting calculated aortic blood pressure exist.[27] The first systems reported aortic blood pressure relative to *non-invasively measured* brachial blood pressure. As already mentioned, cuff-based assessment of brachial blood pressure underestimates systolic pressure, and these devices report aortic systolic pressure that is proportionally lower than the reported non-invasively measured brachial blood pressure. A second convention is to report aortic blood pressure relative to the *invasively measured* brachial blood pressure. The second convention results in an aortic systolic blood pressure lower than the invasively measured brachial blood pressure but sometimes higher than the non-invasively measured brachial blood pressure. The first convention offers the advantage of a relative blood pressure that makes sense physiologically compared to the reported cuff-based brachial pressure measure. The second convention offers the advantage of being closer to the measured aortic blood pressure, and so may be of greater utility when used in calculations with intra-ventricular blood pressure measures.

Non-invasive calculation of the aortic blood pressure waveform allows not just quantification of aortic systolic pressure, but other waveform features. The blood pressure waveform has consistent features that allow quantification beyond the peak (systolic) and minima (diastolic) points. The inflection point (P_i Figure 2.3) of the waveform is associated with wave reflection and the stiffness of the arteries. The augmentation index ($AIx = [P_s − P_i]/[P_s − P_d]$) uses the inflection point to indicate the degree to which the forward travelling wave is augmented by the reflected, backward travelling pressure wave. This index tends to increase (due to increasing stiffness of arteries) in the first three decades of adult life.

The sub-endocardial viability ratio (SEVR, Figure 2.3), or Buckberg index, uses the ratio of the

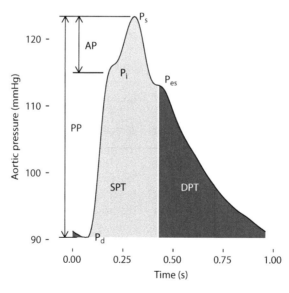

Figure 2.3 Waveform features of the aortic blood pressure waveform allows calculation of the augmentation index (AIx, the ratio of the augmentation pressure [AP] to the pulse pressure [PP]) and the sub-endocardial viability ratio (SEVR, the ratio of the area of the diastolic pressure time [DPT] to the systolic pressure time [SPT]). Augmentation pressure is calculated as the difference between the systolic pressure (P_s) and the inflection point (P_i). Pulse pressure is the systolic (P_s) diastolic (P_d) pressure difference. The systolic pressure time commences at the diastolic point (P_d) and finishes at the inflection that is non-causally, approximately coincidental with the closing of the aortic valve and end of systole (P_{es}).

diastolic and systolic areas of the blood pressure waveform as an estimate of the myocardial supply to demand ratio.[28,29] Prognostic significance of the marker for cases of angina was shown in 1976[30] and more recently has been shown to be an independent predictor of cardiovascular mortality in chronic kidney disease.[31]

CONCLUSION

Non-invasive cardiovascular measurements have proven useful in the diagnosis and management of cardiovascular disease. The electrocardiogram and echocardiography allow non-invasive estimation of function of the heart. A number of other non-invasive tools, both historic and developing, allow a more complete characterisation of the interaction of the heart with the systemic vasculature. Both peripheral and central aortic blood pressure and flow can be interrogated with varying accuracy and utility in both diagnosis and monitoring in cardiovascular health.

REFERENCES

1. Whelton PK, Carey RM, Aronow WS, Casey DE, Collins KJ, Dennison Himmelfarb C, et al. 2017ACC/AHA/AAPA/ABC/ACPM/AGS/APhA/ASH/ASPC/NMA/PCNA Guideline for the prevention, detection, evaluation, and management of high blood pressure in adults: A report of the American college of cardiology/American heart association task force on clinical practice guidelines. *Hypertension*. 2018;71(6):e13–e115.
2. Korotkoff NS. A contribution to the problem of methods for the determination of blood pressure. *Rep Imp Mil Med Acad St Petersburg*. 1905;11:365–367.
3. Avolio AP, Butlin M, Walsh A. Arterial blood pressure measurement and pulse wave analysis: Their role in enhancing cardiovascular assessment. *Physiol Meas*. 2010;31(1):R1–R47.
4. Willum-Hansen T, Staessen JAAJA, Torp-Pedersen C, Rasmussen S, Thijs L, Ibsen H, et al. Prognostic value of aortic pulse wave velocity as index of arterial stiffness in the general population. *Circulation*. 2006;113(5):664.
5. Mancia G, Fagard R, Narkiewicz K, Redon J, Zanchetti A, Böhm M, et al. 2013 ESH/ESC Guidelines for the management of arterial hypertension: The task force for the management of arterial hypertension of the European Society of Hypertension (ESH) and of the European Society of Cardiology (ESC). *Eur Heart J*. 2013;34(28):2159–2219.
6. O'Brien E, Parati G, Stergiou G, Asmar R, Beilin L, Bilo G, et al. European society of hypertension position paper on ambulatory blood pressure monitoring. *J Hypertens*. 2013;31(9):1731–1768.
7. Anonymous. The Plethysmograph. *Sci Am*. 1876;34(26):403–404.
8. Hertzman AB, Spealman CR. Observations on the finger volume pulse recorded photo-electrically (*Am J Physiol*). In: *Proceedings of the American Physiological Society – Forty-Ninth Annual Meeting*. 1937;334.
9. Allen J. Photoplethysmography and its application in clinical physiological measurement. *Physiol Meas*. 2007;28:R1–R39.
10. Avolio AP, Butlin M. Indices of central aortic pressure waveform and ventricular function: An intimate conversation changing direction with age. *J Hypertens*. 2016;34(4):634–636.
11. Cholley BP. Benefits, risks and alternatives of pulmonary artery catheterization. *Curr Opin Anaesthesiol*. 1998;11(6):645–650.
12. Gawlikowski M, Pustelny T. Analysis of actual accuracy in cardiac output measurements by means of thermodilution. *Bull Pol Acad Sci*. 2012;60(3):581–587.
13. Peyton PJ, Chong SW. Minimally invasive measurement of cardiac output during surgery and critical care: A meta-analysis of accuracy and precision. *Anesthesiology*. 2010;113:1220–1235.
14. Baker LE. Principles of the impedance technique. *IEEE Eng Med Biol Mag Q Mag Eng Med Biol Soc*. 1989;8:11–15.
15. Joosten A, Desebbe O, Suehiro K, Murphy L-L, Essiet M, Alexander B, et al. Accuracy and precision of non-invasive cardiac output monitoring devices in perioperative medicine: A systematic review and meta-analysis. *BJA Br J Anaesth*. 2017;118(3):298–310.
16. Young BP, Low LL. Noninvasivemonitoring cardiac output using partial CO_2 rebreathing. *Crit Care Clin*. 2010;26(2):383–392.

17. Rocco M, Spadetta G, Morelli A, Dell'Utri D, Porzi P, Conti G, et al. A comparative evaluation of thermodilution and partial CO_2 rebreathing techniques for cardiac output assessment in critically ill patients during assisted ventilation. *Intensive Care Med.* 2004;30(1):82–87.

18. Saur J, Fluechter S, Trinkmann F, Papavassiliu T, Schoenberg S, Weissmann J, et al. Noninvasive determination of cardiac output by the inert-gas-rebreathing method – comparison with cardiovascular magnetic resonance imaging. *Cardiology.* 2009;114(4):247–254.

19. Berton C, Cholley B. Equipment review: New techniques for cardiac output measurement – oesophageal doppler, fick principle using carbon dioxide, and pulse contour analysis. *Crit Care Lond Engl.* 2002;6:216–221.

20. Wesseling KH, de Wit B, Beneken JE. Arterial haemodynamic parameters derived from noninvasively recorded pulsewaves, using parameter estimation. *Med Biol Eng.* 1973;11:724–731.

21. Keyt AT. Cardiographic and sphygmographic studies. *N Y Med J.* 1878;27:126–140.

22. Bramwell JC, Hill AV. Velocity of transmission of the pulse-wave and elasticity of arteries. *The Lancet.* 1922;199(5149):891–892.

23. Ishihara H, Okawa H, Tanabe K, Tsubo T, Sugo Y, Akiyama T, et al. A new non-invasive continuous cardiac output trend solely utilizing routine cardiovascular monitors. *J Clin MonitComput.* 2004;18:313–320.

24. Zimmermann A, Kufner C, Hofbauer S, Steinwendner J, Hitzl W, Fritsch G, et al. The accuracy of the vigileo/floTrac continuous cardiac output monitor. *J Cardiothorac Vasc Anesth.* 2008;22(3):388–393.

25. Lin S-Y, Chou A-H, Tsai Y-F, Chang S-W, Yang M-W, Ting P-C, et al. Evaluation of the use of the fourth version FloTrac system in cardiac output measurement before and after cardiopulmonary bypass. *J Clin MonitComput [Internet].* 2017 [cited 2018 February 25]; Available from: http://link.springer.com/10.1007/s10877-017-0071-6.

26. Chen CH, Nevo E, Fetics B, Pak PH, Yin FC, Maughan WL, et al. Estimation of central aortic pressure waveform by mathematical transformation of radial tonometry pressure. Validation of generalized transfer function. *Circulation.* 1997;95(7):1827–1836.

27. Ding F- Buckberg GD, Fixler DE, Archie JP, Hoffman JI. Experimental subendocardial ischemia in dogs with normal coronary arteries. *Circ Res.* 1972;30(1):67H–81H.

28. Buckberg GD, Fixler DE, Archie JP, Hoffman JI. Experimental subendocardial ischemia in dogs with normal coronary arteries. *Circ Res.* 1972;30(1):67–81.

29. Hoffman JI, Buckberg GD. The myocardial supply: Demand ratio—A critical review. *Am J Cardiol.* 1978;41(2):327–332.

30. Gunstensen J, Scully HE, Kelly T, Adelman AG, Williams WG, Wigle ED, et al. Prognostic significance of endo-cardial viability ratio in aortocoronary bypass surgery. *Can J Surg J Can Chir.* 1976;19(2):93–96.

31. Di Micco L, Salvi P, Bellasi A, Sirico ML, Di Iorio B. Subendocardial viability ratio predicts cardiovascular mortality in chronic kidney disease patients. *Blood Purif.* 2013;36(1):26–28.

3

Determination of oxygen status in human blood

MARCUS JUUL

INTRODUCTION

Assessment of cardiac, pulmonary and circulatory function are enhanced by knowledge of the blood oxygen status. For example, oxygen saturation analysis from multiple sites allows intracardiac shunts to be localised and quantified. The ability to measure all components of oxygen status as well as a knowledge of their interaction and variabilities provides important information on the integrity of the cardiopulmonary system.

Approximately 80% of total oxygen consumption occurs within mitochondria by oxidative phosphorylation. Oxygen combines with electrons to produce free energy which in turn is used to pump hydrogen ions (H$^+$) from within the mitochondrion to the cytoplasm against an electrochemical gradient. The H$^+$ then diffuses back along its gradient, releasing free energy that is used to produce ATP from ADP. ATP provides energy for most biological processes. A moderate to severe reduction in oxygen supply causes an increase in the rate of glycolysis (ATP production from cytoplasmic anaerobic fermentation) in order to maintain cellular energy supply.[1] However, glycolysis, unlike oxidative phosphorylation, does not provide sustained energy supply because the lactate product of glycolysis leads to acidosis, which compromises optimal cellular function. The remaining 20% of oxygen consumption occurs in subcellular organelles that are involved in biosynthetic, biodegradative and detoxification oxidations. Some of the enzymes reacting with oxygen in these processes are sensitive to only moderate decreases in oxygen supply as a result of their low oxygen affinity (e.g. metabolic processes involved in neurotransmitter production), unlike mitochondrial enzyme activity, which has a high oxygen affinity.[1] Measurement and maintenance of oxygen status is therefore essential if biochemical disorders resulting from poor oxygen supply are to be minimised.

Oxygen status of blood is defined by the following parameters: oxygen concentration (content) $ctO_2(B)$, oxygen saturation $SO_2(B)$, oxygen tension $pO_2(B)$ and haemoglobin concentration $ctHb(B)$. (The IFCC/IUPAC system of nomenclature is used throughout this text. 'B' means 'in blood'.)

Oxygen concentration refers to the total amount of oxygen contained within a unit volume of blood and is commonly expressed as mmol/L, Vol% or mls oxygen per dL of whole blood. Oxygen is carried in blood in two states:

1. *Dissolved oxygen in blood:* The amount of dissolved oxygen in the blood depends upon the $pO_2(B)$ (it also varies slightly with ctHb) and is 0.003 mL/dL blood/mmHg $pO_2(B)$ (concentrational solubility coefficient for oxygen in blood, called α).[2,3]
2. *Oxygen bound to haemoglobin*, of which oxygen saturation [$SO_2(B)$] is the percentage that oxygen-bound haemoglobin constitutes of the total haemoglobin capable of carrying oxygen.[4,5] Oxygen bound to haemoglobin constitutes approximately 99% of the oxygen content of blood. Ideally, when fully saturated with oxygen, each gram of normal haemoglobin holds 1.39 mL of oxygen. However, due to the presence of dyshaemoglobins, the in vivo value for fully saturated haemoglobin is 1.36 mL of oxygen/gm haemoglobin.

OXYHAEMOGLOBIN DISSOCIATION CURVE

The association between $pO_2(B)$ and oxygen saturation is governed by the shape of the oxyhaemoglobin dissociation curve (Figure 3.1a). This curve shows how oxygen tension [$pO_2(B)$] (abscissa) affects the reaction between oxygen and haemoglobin, $SO_2(B)$ (ordinate). The S-shaped curve is due to the haemoglobin molecule having four oxygen binding subunits each of which binds one oxygen molecule sequentially in four steps. The affinity for haemoglobin is increased as oxygen binds to haemoglobin (i.e. each successive subunit combination with oxygen facilitates the next subunit combination with oxygen). Conversely, each oxygen dissociation from a subunit facilitates

further dissociations. This accounts for the steepness of middle portion of the curve when the haemoglobin is partially saturated. However, at either limit of the curve, the propensity of oxygen to either associate or disassociate from haemoglobin decreases when the subunits are almost saturated or desaturated with oxygen. This accounts for the curve being flatter at its limits.[4]

The steepness of the middle portion of the curve facilitates oxygen unloading to the tissues because a small decrease in $pO_2(B)$ results in significant dissociation of oxygen from haemoglobin, providing more oxygen for use by tissues. Unloading of oxygen is dependent on factors that can alter the shape and position of the curve on the abscissa. These factors are pH(B), $pCO_2(B)$, blood temperature, 2,3-diphosphoglycerate (2,3-DPG), anaemia, and various substances causing the formation of dyshaemoglobins (haemoglobin derivatives incapable of reversibly binding with oxygen molecules). These shifts in the oxyhaemoglobin dissociation curve can be represented by the value p50, which represents the $pO_2(B)$ at which 50% of the effective blood haemoglobin is in the deoxyhaemoglobin state and thus represents the haemoglobin-oxygen affinity.[4]

When peripheral factors such as vascular disease, anaemia, heavy exercise and cardiac output are the main limitations to oxygen transport, the p50 increases to facilitate oxygen unloading. When the limitation to oxygen transport is due to poor oxygen diffusion in the lungs, the p50 decreases to reduce oxygen unloading. Chemoreceptor control of ventilation, allosteric control of p50 and the diffusing capacities of the lungs and tissues regulate loading and unloading so that the resultant p50 provides the best level of oxygen transport for all conditions.[6]

The influence that pH(B) and $pCO_2(B)$ have on the oxyhaemoglobin dissociation curve is called the Bohr effect and occurs because deoxyhaemoglobin is a weaker acid than oxyhaemoglobin. In tissue, deoxyhaemoglobin accepts H^+ (produced by dissociation of carbonic acid that results from the reaction between water and carbon dioxide) under low $pO_2(B)$/high $pCO_2(B)$ conditions. This decreases haemoglobin affinity for oxygen. In the lung, the high $pO_2(B)$/low $pCO_2(B)$ causes oxygen to combine with haemoglobin. This releases H^+ to

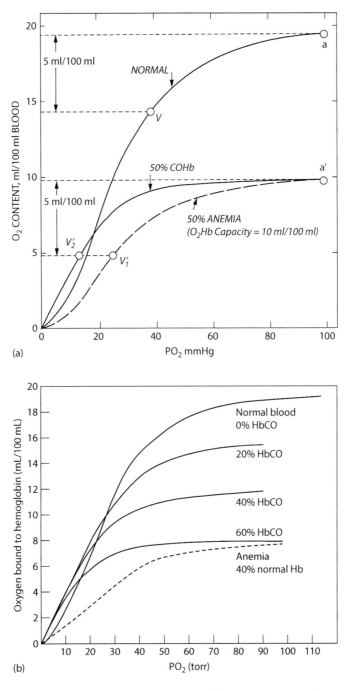

(a)

(b)

Figure 3.1 (a) Effects of carbon monoxide on the oxygen dissociation curve. (b) Oxyhaemoglobin dissociation curves of normal human blood, of blood containing 50% carboxyhaemoglobin and of blood with a 50% normal haemoglobin concentration due to anaemia. ([a] Modified from Roughton, F.J.W. and Darling, R.C., *Am. J. Physiol.*, 141, 17–31, 1944; Reproduced from Comroe, J.H. Jr. *Physiology of Respiration*, 2nd ed., Year Book Medical Publishers, Chicago, IL, 1974. With permission; [b] Reproduced from *Environmental Health Criteria 213 Carbon Monoxide*, 2nd ed., p. 137. World Health Organization, Geneva, Switzerland, 1999. With permission.)

combine with carbonic acid to form bicarbonate that liberates carbon dioxide and water. The high pH(B) (low acidity/low pCO$_2$(B)) increases haemoglobin affinity for oxygen.[4]

2,3-DPG is an important regulator of oxygen release by haemoglobin in adults.[4] It is a product of anaerobic glycolysis in erythrocytes and causes a decrease in haemoglobin affinity for oxygen. Anaemia triggers an adaptive mechanism causing a decrease in haemoglobin affinity for oxygen. This results from an increase in the 2,3-DPG levels in erythrocytes during chronic anaemia.[7]

HAEMOGLOBIN

The haemoglobin complex has four iron-containing haem groups, i.e. four haemoglobin monomer molecules. The haemoglobin molecule has four symmetrically arranged pyrroles with a ferrous iron (Fe^{2+}) at its centre and is also combined with the protein globin.[8,4] The globin molecule has four polypeptide chains. Normal adult haemoglobin (HbA) has two alpha and two beta chains. The alpha polypeptide chains have 141 amino acids and the beta chains have 146 amino acids. Fetal haemoglobin (HbF), with two alpha chains and two gamma chains, has a greater affinity for oxygen than does adult haemoglobin, fetal pO$_2$(B) being lower than adult pO$_2$(B)(4). The greater affinity is due to poor binding of 2,3-DPG by the gamma chains.[2]

The iron is bound to each of the pyrroles and to one of the four polypeptides and allows for reversible Hb-O$_2$ combinations. Oxygen or carbon monoxide can bind with the sixth binding site on the ferrous iron.[4] One molecule of Fe^{2+} can combine with one molecule of oxygen.[8] By changing the relationship of the polypeptide chains to each other, the haemoglobin molecule assumes either a relaxed state that favours oxygen binding or a tense state that decreases oxygen binding. This is achieved by breaking or forming salt-bridges between the polypeptide chains. The two beta chains lie closer to each other when oxygen is bound to haemoglobin. This alters oxygen affinity.[2]

The most frequently occurring haemoglobins are:

Deoxygenated (Reduced) haemoglobin (HHb). This is unassociated with oxygen and is bound to H$^+$ (the term 'deoxygenated' is recommended over 'reduced', as in a chemical sense no reduction has taken place).

Oxyhaemoglobin (O$_2$Hb) is the haemoglobin (monomer) molecule with one oxygen molecule reversibly bound to the ferrous ion.

Carbaminohaemoglobin (HHbCO$_2$). This bond causes structural changes in the haemoglobin molecule, decreasing its affinity for oxygen. The haemoglobin-carbon dioxide bond does not occur on the same location on the haemoglobin molecule as the haemoglobin-oxygen covalent bond.[9] Carbon dioxide is not attached to the haem, but to the amino groups.[8]

Dyshaemoglobins (DysHb) are normal haemoglobins that have temporarily or permanently lost the ability at physiological pO$_2$ to reversibly bind with oxygen. Dyshaemoglobins should be distinguished from **abnormal haemoglobins** which have genetically determined alterations in the globin moiety. Only a few of these haemoglobins have significantly different oxygen affinity.[10] Abnormal haemoglobins can be produced rarely by alterations of the structure in the haem groups or more commonly by genetic substitution of a single incompatible amino acid for a normal amino acid in an alpha or beta chain.[2]

Common dyshaemoglobins are:

Methaemoglobin (MetHb), sometimes referred to as hemiglobin (Hi), is not useful for carrying oxygen and is normally present in blood in amounts that are typically below the detection capacity of commercial multiwavelength haemoximeters. Methaemoglobin can be formed by the action of oxidants. This can result from the action of certain substances such as local anaesthetics, cyano compounds, nitrates and nitrites or even via the action of the superoxide anion (O$_2^-$) that dissociates from the iron instead of O$_2$, leaving the iron in the ferric state (auto-oxidation). In the ferric state the haem iron does not bind to oxygen. Methaemoglobinaemia can occur via excess formation of methaemoglobin (endogenous or exogenous), limited reduction capacity of methaemoglobin to haemoglobin by erythrocytes from genetic deficiency of the methaemoglobin reductase, or the increased tendency of the haemoglobin iron to oxidation (found in rare haemoglobinopathies).

In some instances, oxidants can inhibit metabolic pathways such as oxidative phosphorylation by diffusing into tissues. This inhibits oxygen utilisation.[10,11]

Carboxyhaemoglobin (COHb) occurs normally in amounts of less than 3% in non-smokers living in an urban environment. The increase in haemoglobin-oxygen affinity with carboxyhaemoglobin arises from the influence of the single carbon monoxide molecule in the haemoglobin tetramer on oxygen binding by the other haem groups. As with methaemoglobin, there is a decrease in oxygen capacity with a resultant increase in haemoglobin-oxygen affinity and thus a shift in the oxyhaemoglobin curve to the left. The affinity of carbon monoxide for haemoglobin is approximately 200 times that of oxygen. As well as displacing oxygen, carbon monoxide can enter the cell and inhibit oxidative phosphorylation. The combined effects of carbon monoxide can cause tissue hypoxia, acidosis and central nervous system depression.[10,11] Other haemoglobin derivatives such as Sulfhaemoglobin (SHb), carboxysulfhaemoglobin (SHbCO) and Cyanmethaemoglobin (HiCNHb) are not usually found in significant amounts and account for less than 1% of total haemoglobin.[11]

DETERMINANTS OF OXYGEN STATUS

Currently, for determination of blood gas status, the most commonly used blood gas instruments measure pH, pCO_2, and pO_2. These instruments are used in conjunction with a haemoximeter which calculates total haemoglobin concentration (ctHb), measures oxygen saturation, and, with many, the percentage carboxyhaemoglobin (%COHb, i.e. the carboxyhaemoglobin fraction, $FCOHb$, expressed as a percentage) and percentage methaemoglobin (%MetHb, i.e. the methaemoglobin fraction, $FMetHb$, expressed as a percentage) of the total haemoglobin concentration. This arrangement allows derivation of bicarbonate concentration, base excess, oxygen content, concentration of active haemoglobin and the haemoglobin-oxygen affinity determined by p50.[12]

The single most important parameter in the arterial oxygen status is **oxygen content**. The most important component of oxygen content is the **total haemoglobin concentration,** as haemoglobin controls oxygen transport via the **oxyhaemoglobin dissociation curve** (Figure 3.1a).

In the path from alveoli to tissue cells:

The $pO_2(aB)$ (i.e. the oxygen tension of arterial blood) is a measure of diffusion of oxygen into blood from the lungs but gives no indication of oxygen content.[13] However, $pO_2(aB)$ is a more sensitive diagnostic indicator of respiratory status than oxygen content. This is because the oxyhaemoglobin dissociation curve is flat at normal physiological $pO_2(aB)$ above 70 mmHg. If a patient's $pO_2(aB)$ falls from 90 to 70 mmHg the proportionate fall of $pO_2(aB)$ will be significant (>20%). The proportionate fall of oxygen content will be insignificant (typically 3%–4% for a normal ctHb level).

Oxygen content, cardiac output and/or organ perfusion together determine delivery of oxygen to tissues, where:

- DO_2 (Oxygen Delivery to the Tissues) = Oxygen Content × Cardiac Output, or,
- DO_2 (Oxygen Delivery to an Organ) = Oxygen Content × Organ Perfusion.[13]

Tissue end-capillary oxygen tension, $pO_2(cB)$ (i.e. the oxygen tension of capillary blood) reflects tissue oxygen supply under normal conditions; however, since cardiac output and $pO_2(cB)$ are more difficult to measure, oxygen availability is based on the p50 of arterial blood alone (where oxyhaemoglobin affinity is the p50). Therefore, oxygen content and particularly the oxygen content curve (the graphical relationship between oxygen content (ordinate axis) and $pO_2(B)$ [abscissa]) are predictors of $pO_2(cB)$. In order for oxygen content to be normal, the $pO_2(aB)$, $SO_2(aB)$ and total haemoglobin concentration must be normal.[13] Maintaining a normal $pO_2(cB)$ is crucial because it is the vital parameter in oxygen supply to tissues and is dependent on perfusion parameters, the distribution of capillaries, $pO_2(aB)$ and blood transport properties.[14]

OXYHAEMOGLOBIN DISSOCIATION VS OXYGEN CONTENT CURVES

In order to understand these curves it is important to understand oxygen saturation and oxygen concentration of blood. **Oxygen saturation of haemoglobin**, $SO_2(B)$, is the oxyhaemoglobin fraction of active haemoglobin expressed as a percentage, i.e. $SO_2 = nO_2Hb/(nHHb + nO_2Hb)$ where n refers to the amount of substance of the relevant component. It can also be expressed as $SO_2 = cO_2Hb/(cHb + cO_2Hb)$ where c refers to substance concentration of the relevant component. Concentration of active (effective) haemoglobin is defined by $ceHb = ctHb-cCOHb-c$ $MetHb-cSHb-cXHb$ (i.e. the concentration of unidentified inactive haemoglobin). Oxygen concentration (i.e. content) in blood is defined by: $ctO_2(B) = cO_2Hb(B) + cO_2(B)$ (i.e. the concentration of dissolved oxygen in blood).[3]

Oxygen saturation is a derivative that reflects the $pO_2(B)$ via their relationship in the oxyhaemoglobin dissociation curve. Fractional oxygen saturation of haemoglobin (FO_2Hb) is a derivative calculated by haemoximeters capable of measuring the percentage dyshaemoglobins and on its own is not a useful measurement. This is because a decrease in fractional oxygen saturation could be due to several reasons, e.g. a fall in $pO_2(B)$ and/or an increase in dyshaemoglobins, or a decrease in $Hb-O_2$ affinity.[5] If the plot of oxygen content versus $pO_2(B)$ via the oxygen content curve is displayed (Figure 3.1b), the effects of all factors influencing oxygen availability can be seen more clearly than the oxyhaemoglobin dissociation curve. The oxygen content curve for anaemic blood and blood containing significant carboxyhaemoglobin both show a smaller rise in oxygen content as $pO_2(B)$ rises compared to normal adult blood. The differences between the two graphs, which both illustrate the effects from haemoglobin derivatives, occurs because the oxygen content curve relies on the total amount of haemoglobin available for oxygen transport. The oxyhaemoglobin dissociation curve does not show the effect that changes in haemoglobin concentration have on oxygen carrying capacity. It is therefore limited to illustrating only the differences between haemoglobin-oxygen affinities and not the effects from variations in the amount of haemoglobin available for oxygen transport, as illustrated by the oxygen content curve. The oxygen content curve illustrates and quantifies the ability of blood to release oxygen under different conditions.

NEW PARAMETERS

Apart from the commonly measured and derived parameters already mentioned, new oxygen parameters have been proposed to determine oxygen availability. These are not universally accepted but may provide clinical information for early prophylactic maintenance of oxygen status in critically ill patients, without pulmonary artery catheterisation. These parameters are:

Oxygen Extraction Tension (px). This is the oxygen tension in arterial blood after extraction of 2.3 mmol of oxygen per litre of blood (5.1 mL O_2/dL blood) at constant pH(B) and $pCO_2(B)$. The normal arterio-venous difference in oxygen concentration is 2.3 mmol/L. A px value at or above the normal mixed venous $pO_2(B)$ [i.e. $pO_2(vB)$] thus indicates that the arterial blood is capable of releasing the normal amount of oxygen at or above the normal mixed venous oxygen tension. Px includes the effects of all parameters influencing $ctO_2(B)$. It therefore represents the maximum information on oxygen and is available from one arterial sample.[12]

Extractable Oxygen Concentration of Arterial Blood (Cx). This is the concentration of oxygen that can be extracted from arterial blood at a $pO_2(aB)$ of 38 mmHg. It approximates $pO_2(vB)$ (e.g. a Cx below 1.8 mmol/L suggests cardiac output would need to increase to provide sufficient oxygen to the tissues).[12]

Oxygen Compensation Factor (Qx). This is the standard arterio-venous oxygen content difference (2.3 mmol/L) divided by Cx. Therefore, it is the factor by which cardiac output should rise to maintain a $pO_2(vB)$ of 38 mmHg.[12]

MIXED VENOUS OXYGEN SATURATION

Traditional concepts based on oxygen delivery and a standard level of oxygen extraction do not account for differences in metabolic oxygen requirements. It has been shown that oxygen delivery to tissues can be increased, resulting in significant increases in oxygen consumption until oxygen demands are met and oxygen consumption no longer increases. For critically ill patients whose oxygen demands are different, assessment of this endpoint would be useful.[15] These patients have a higher dependency of oxygen consumption on oxygen delivery levels that would under normal circumstances be considered adequate.[14] **Mixed venous oxygen saturation**, $SO_2(vB)$, is a component in this determination. Increased oxygen demands are usually met by increased oxygen supply. This is achieved by increasing cardiac output so that mixed venous oxygen saturation is maintained to provide a reserve of oxygen. Continuous mixed venous oxygen saturation measurements can be made using invasive fibre-optic probes.[13]

Measurements are based on reflectance of specific light intensities from blood back to the probes. However, if changes in oxygen consumption are confined to a single organ, the mixed venous oxygen saturation does not change significantly and therefore the benefit of measuring it under these circumstances is questionable.[13] Mixed venous oxygen saturation does provide the ability to determine the matching of tissue oxygen delivery and oxygen consumption as well as the point at which oxygen consumption becomes dependent on tissue oxygen delivery. Mixed venous oxygen saturation monitoring indicates when changes in $PO_2(aB)$ result from changes in mixed venous oxygen saturation and not intrapulmonary shunting. It also provides the means to calculate cardiac output, oxygen consumption, and intrapulmonary shunts, and is an indicator of significant problems in overall oxygenation rather than single component problems because the latter are normally compensated for by changes in other related components.[16] A normal arterial oxygen saturation means that if the cardiac output is also normal then oxygen supply to the microvascular bed is normal, whilst analysis of mixed venous oxygen saturation indicates whether oxygen is actually delivered to the tissues. The determination of oxygen affinity of blood provides an even greater ability to ensure that supplied oxygen is properly delivered to tissues, and this involves determination of a complete oxyhaemoglobin dissociation curve using the p50, pH(B) and $pCO_2(B)$.[10]

HAEMOXIMETRY (CO-OXIMETRY)

The most commonly used instruments for measuring the most important parameters in oxygen content [ctHb(B) and $SO_2(B)$] are the haemoximeters® (CO-oximeters). Their efficiency is gauged by their ability to measure different derivatives of haemoglobin accurately.

The haemoglobin percentages and oxygen saturations measured by haemoximeters use the same principles. They use a colour photometry method for measuring total haemoglobin [ctHb(B)] and concentrations of certain haemoglobin derivatives. Light intensities at specific wavelength channels are measured. The intensities are converted to absorbances from which the concentrations of derivatives are based. From this, the various fractions of haemoglobin are derived. The light intensities are the raw input data used in the algorithms for the instrument. Absorbance 'A' at wavelength λ is defined by:

$A = \log (I_0/I_s)$, where I_0 = measured reference light intensity with a clear cuvette sample (i.e. water), I_S = measured intensity with the blood cuvette sample. Subsequent calculations of saturations are based on the Lambert-Beers Law: $Ay^\lambda = E\ y^\lambda \times Cy^\lambda \times L$, where E = proportionality constant (termed molar absorptivity, or the molar extinction coefficient of the particular derivative compound), A = absorbance, L = light path (thickness of cuvette), y = compound derivative, λ = wavelength, C = molar concentration of the compound derivative.[17,18] Thus, the calculation involves measuring the absorbance of both an unknown sample containing haemoglobin and a sample containing a known amount of haemoglobin, and with algebraic rearrangement, calculating the amount of unknown haemoglobin.[19]

Measurement of percentage oxygenated haemoglobin and percentage deoxygenated haemoglobin requires measurement of the total absorbance at only two wavelengths, e.g. the OSM2 (Radiometer Copenhagen) using 506.5 and 600.0 nm.[17] Measurement of other derivatives requires that the total absorbance must be measured at each of several wavelengths so that the minimum number of total absorbance measurements must equal the number of substances being measured,[19] i.e. in order to obtain solutions for n unknowns, there must be n independent equations. Therefore to measure deoxygenated, carboxy, oxy and methaemoglobins, a haemoximeter must use at least 4 wavelengths of light to produce 4 absorbance equations. The set of equations is called a determined matrix. Additional wavelengths can account for sulfhaemoglobin, interfering effects of fetal haemoglobin, and effects of such factors as thermal changes, turbidity and dyes such bilirubin and Methylene Blue. Systems adopting extra wavelengths are referred to as 'overdetermined'. These 'extra' wavelengths, however, do not refer to those needed to compensate for bilirubin, etc., but refer to systems with more wavelengths than light-absorbing components in the sample.[11,19]

The direct photometric measurement of concentration of haemoglobin derivatives requires discrete, narrow bands of light so that the small differences of light absorbed by the derivatives can be differentiated. Photometric measurement of the derivatives relies on the specific light absorption characteristics of each haemoglobin derivative at the selected wavelengths (which in turn requires the concentrations of each entity in reference materials to be known by the manufacturer).[19]

Haemoximeter accuracy is determined by the availability of pure reference materials and the accuracy to which the extinction co-efficients (light absorption characteristics) are known for each component and each of the selected wavelengths. When the fractional amounts of haemoglobin derivatives are low, the haemoximeters may not be ideal for differentiating between subjects and populations that have small differences between them, i.e. <2%–2.5%. This is because haemoximeters are designed to measure haemoglobin fractions over a broad analytical range. An additional problem occurs due to dyshaemoglobins being such a small portion of the whole that any small variability in the background chromophores can result in large but not clinically significant differences between those dyshaemoglobin quantities. Abnormal haemoglobins can also produce altered absorbance characteristics. Wavelength selection can minimise sensitivity to interfering substances such as bilirubin and turbidity.[19] Interfering compounds absorb light in the same wavelength range as the derivative being measured.[18]

Measurement methods are standard for all haemoximeters. There are two types of light sources used by these instruments. The OSM3 (Radiometer Copenhagen) was an example of one where a white or incandescent light source, such as tungsten (maintained at constant intensity) illuminates the haemolysed sample (haemolysed to eliminate light scattering caused by red blood cells). Ultraviolet and infrared blocking filters eliminate high and low wavelength light. The visible light passes through the sample after which it passes through a diffraction grating where the spectrum is separated into individual wavelengths that pass to the photodiodes. The light that some haemoximeters use is referred to as spectral. They use a lamp, neon or thallium hollow-cathode (maintained at constant intensity), that produces multiple precise narrow-band-pass wavelengths called 'lines'. These lines have fixed wavelengths with the bandwidths being sufficiently narrow that differences to the actual bandwidth characteristics of the entire optical path are insignificant. The spectral lines are selected for analysis by blocking undesired light bands with interference filters. Each wavelength requires a separate filter. The light then passes through the sample and is collected by a single photodiode. The disadvantages of this system are that the wavelengths available may not be optimal for determination of a certain derivative and may allow other absorbing materials apart from haemoglobin derivatives to be measured. Both systems use the reference light intensity measured from water in the cuvette and compare it to the detected light (from the sample) at the photodiode. Absorption can thus be determined.[19]

With the advent of discrete multiwavelength spectrophotometers such as the CO-oximeter 2500 and 270 (Ciba-Corning) using 7 wavelengths, OSM3 (6 wavelengths) and the IL482 (Instrument Laboratories), direct measurement of percentage methaemoglobin, percentage carboxyhaemoglobin and more accurate oxygen saturation readings were possible.[20] Even multiwavelength analysers can be affected by dyshaemoglobins. Percentage of sulfhaemoglobin in blood rarely exceeds 1%, but if a sample were to contains as much as 10% sulfhaemoglobin, it has been reported that the OSM3 (discrete wavelength haemoximeter) would measure percentage of methaemoglobin as being 3.5% less than actual and the percentage carboxyhaemoglobin as being 2.5% higher than actual. However, the OSM3 would display a warning that the percentage sulfhaemoglobin is high.[21] Sulfhaemoglobin has different absorption spectra than deoxyhaemoglobin and has a low oxygen affinity. It is capable of reversibly binding with oxygen, although the Sulf-Hb bond is irreversible and its p50 is more than two orders of magnitude (i.e. >100 times) greater than that of normal haemoglobin.[10] Similarly, fetal haemoglobin, which can constitute as much as 90% of the total haemoglobin in newborns can affect discrete wavelength haemoximeters. A fetal haemoglobin level of 80% in a fully oxygenated sample can cause an error of up to 4% in the SO_2 determination[18] unless compensated for.

The ABL 900 series (Radiometer Copenhagen) is an example of the current generation of instruments using full spectrum (visual range), which makes it an overdetermined system. It has a concave holographic grating and employs 256 photodiodes constituting a self-scanning integrated photodiode array. It is capable of measuring a continuous absorption spectrum with a wavelength range of 478–672 nm in 128 channels. It has a spectral resolution of 1.5 nm and a bandwidth of 2 nm. The discrete wavelengths offered by traditional haemoximeters only allow measurement of the spectra for deoxygenated, oxy, carboxy, met and sulf haemoglobins and intralipid, whereas the multiwavelength instruments using the continuous spectrum allow measurement of spectra from conjugated and unconjugated bilirubin and oxy-fetal haemoglobin (O_2HbF).[18]

OXYGEN TENSION (pO₂)

The remaining component of oxygen concentration, pO_2(B), is commonly measured using a Clark electrochemical cell. A platinum cathode is maintained at a negative potential relative to a silver/silver chloride reference electrode (anode), both immersed in electrolyte solution (potassium chloride). Oxygen is reduced at the platinum cathode producing a current proportional to the pO_2(B). It is therefore an amperometric sensor.[22] In order to recognise the analyte, most sensors for blood analytes have a receptor or recognition element that binds with the analyte, and a transduction element that converts the process into a signal which can be electrochemical or optical (optodes). Thus, the Clark electrochemical cell, by measuring the current produced by direct reduction of oxygen, has no recognition element that binds to oxygen and instead uses a recognition system.[23]

Apart from the in vitro methods, intravascular methods have been developed using optical sensors. Light of certain wavelengths illuminates a sample chamber containing dye on a fibreoptic probe. The amount of incident light absorbed by the dye depends on the amount of analyte, or, by another method, the intensity of re-emitted radiation at modified wavelengths is determined by the amount of analyte. These instruments can be affected by thrombosis, reduced blood flow and vessel wall effect, i.e. measurement of tissue gas exchange if forced against the vessel wall.[22]

In 1994 in vitro measurement of pO_2(B) was introduced by AVL Scientific Corporation based in Graz, Austria and Roswell, GA, USA, manufacturing the OPTI line of portable in vitrodiagnostics tests that employed fluorescent optical chemosensors. Specific compounds can emit light when they descend back to a ground state after being excited to a higher electronic state. This is termed luminescence. When the excitation energy is provided by light (instead of chemicals or electricity), it is termed fluorescence. When oxygen is present, the oxygen quenches or reduces the fluorescence of the immobilised oxygen-specific dye or indicator molecules (with a long excited-state lifetime). The amount of quenching is proportional to the amount of oxygen present in the sample. If a long-lived fluorophore is put into a molecular substance with high oxygen solubility, e.g. polydimethylsiloxane, the sensor can be adapted for measurement at very low partial pressures of oxygen. The Stern–Volmer equation describes the relationship between the partial pressure of oxygen pO_2(B) and fluorescence intensity: ($I_0/I = 1 + kPO_2$), where I_0 is the maximum intensity at 0 mmHg oxygen, I is the fluorescence intensity in the presence of pO_2(B) and k is the (inverse) Stern–Volmer quenching constant related to the oxygen diffusion rate and quenching cross-section.[23]

Biosensor electrodes using enzymes, antibodies and nucleic acids have been used for in vivo blood gas monitoring.[14] Transcutaneous monitoring using heated Clark electrodes placed on the skin are used widely in neonatology for pO_2(B) measurements. Their accuracy is dependent on adequate skin circulation. Another non-invasive method of (oxygen only) blood gas analysis is pulse oximetry (see Chapter 2); however, this method presumes, as do the two wavelength haemoximeters, that only oxygenated and deoxygenated haemoglobin are present in blood.[14]

Determination of oxygen status in human blood is essential in evaluating the severity of conditions that produce oxygen depletion. Oxygen depletion ultimately leads to abnormalities in cellular oxygen metabolism, resulting in organ and whole-body functional abnormalities[1]. The evolution of instruments capable of accurately measuring the related components of oxygen status allows for greater scope in patient management.

REFERENCES

1. Robin EB. Tissue O2 utilization. In: Loeppky JA, Riedesel ML, editors. *Oxygen Transport to Human Tissues*. New York: Elsevier/North Holland; 1982:179–186.
2. Ganong WF. Gas Transport between the lung and the tissues. *Rev Med Physiol*. New York: McGraw-Hill; 2001:336–355.
3. Wimberley PD, Siggaard-Andersen O, Fogh-Andersen N, Zijlstra WG, Severinghaus JW. Haemoglobin oxygen saturation and related quantities: Definitions, symbols and clinical use. *Scand J Clin Lab Invest*. 1990; 50(4):455–459.
4. Levitzky MG. *Pulmonary Physiology*. 3rd ed. New York: McGraw-Hill. 1991.
5. Oesburg B, Rolfe P, Siggaard Andersen O, Zijlstra WG. Definition and measurement of quantities pertaining to oxygen in blood. In: Voupel, P, Zander, R, Bruley, DF, editors. *Oxygen Transport to Tissue XV. Advances in Experimental Medicine and Biology*, 345, pp. 925–930, 1994.
6. Hsia CC. Respiratory function of hemoglobin. *N Engl J Med*. 1998; 338(4):239–248.
7. Zschiedrich H. Therapeutic threshold values for chronic alterations in hemoglobin concentration. In: Zander R, Mertzlufft F, editors. *The Oxygen Status of Arterial Blood. Basel*. New York: Karger; 1991:174–183.
8. Ross G. *Essentials of Human Physiology*. Year Book Medical Publishers, Incorporated; 1978.
9. Reeder GD. The Biochemistry and physiology of hemoglobin: A self study module. *Am Soc Extra-Corporeal Technoll*. Reston, VA; 1986:250.
10. Zijlstra WG, Maas AH, Moran RF. Definition, significance and measurement of quantities pertaining to the oxygen carrying properties of human blood. *Scand J Clin Lab Invest Suppl*. 1996; 224:27–45.
11. Moran RF. Application of hemoglobin derivatives in STAT analysis. *Blood Gas News*. 1999; 8(1):4–11.
12. Siggaard-Andersen O, Wimberley PD, Fogh-Andersen N, Gothgen IH. Arterial oxygen status determined with routine pH/blood gas equipment and multi-wavelength hemoximetry: Reference values, precision, and accuracy. *Scand J Clin Lab Invest Suppl*. 1990; 203:57–66.
13. Zander R, Mertzlufft F. *The Oxygen Status of Arterial blood*. S Karger publication. 1991.
14. Waldau T. Blood gases-measurement methods and interpretation of results. *Blood Gas News*. 1995; 4(7–12):7.
15. Shapiro B. Assessment of oxygenation: Today and tomorrow. *Scand J Clin Lab Invest*. 1990; 50(sup203):197–202.
16. Ahrens T, Rutherford K, Basham KAR. *Essentials of Oxygenation: Implication for Clinical Practice*. Jones & Bartlett Learning. 1993.
17. *OSM2Hemoximeter User's Handbook*. P ed. Copenhagen: Radiometer; 1988.
18. Singer P, Hansen H. Supression of fetal hemoglobin and bilirubin on oximetry measurement. *Blood Gas News*. 1999; 8:12–17.
19. Brunelle JA, Degtiarov AM, Moran RF, Race LA. Simultaneous measurement of total hemoglobin and its derivatives in blood using CO-oximeters: Analytical principles; their application in selecting analytical wavelengths and reference methods; A comparison of the results of the choices made. *Scand J Clin Lab Invest*. 1996; 56(sup224):47–69.
20. Mertzlufft F. *Determination of Arterial O2 Saturation: Oxymetry. The Oxygen Status of Arterial Blood*. Karger Publishers. 1991; 88–97.
21. Wu C, Kenny MA. A case of sulfhemoglobinemia and emergency Measurement of sulfhemoglobin with an OSM3 CO-oximeter. *Clin Chem*. 1997; 43(1):162–166.

22. Mahutte CK. On-line arterial blood gas analysis with optodes: Current status. *Clin Biochem.* 1998; 31(3):119–130.

23. Tusa JK, He H. Critical care analyzer with fluorescent optical chemosensors for blood analytes. *J Mater Chem.* 2005; 15(27–28):2640–2647.

24. Roughton, FJW, Darling, RC. The effect of carbon monoxide on the oxyhemoglobin dissociation curve. *Am J Physiol.* 1994; 141:17–31.

25. Comroe, JH. Jr. *Physiology of Respiration*, 2nd ed, Chicago: Year Book Medical Publishers. 1974.

26. Raub, J. *Environmental Health Criteria 213 Carbon Monoxide*, 2nd ed., Geneva, Switzerland: World Health Organization. 1999; p.137.

4

Coagulation and the coagulation cascade

JOHN EDWARD BOLAND AND DAVID E. CONNOR

INTRODUCTION

The process of haemostasis and coagulation depends on interaction between platelets and the many circulating plasma proteins involved in thrombus formation, as illustrated by the various complex mechanisms of the coagulation cascade. This chapter outlines the theory of coagulation and describes the vascular, cellular, biochemical and pharmacological sequence of events that comprise the coagulation cascade and regulate haemostasis and coagulation.

HAEMOSTASIS

Haemostasis is the body's mechanism for preventing blood loss following vascular injury. Primary haemostasis includes mechanisms such as vasoconstriction, adhesion of opposing vessel surfaces and formation of a primary platelet plug at sites of injury. These mechanisms alone may be sufficient to staunch blood loss from very small vessels such as capillaries. More severe damage requires secondary haemostasis, with aggregation of platelets and activation of the coagulation system, leading to blood clot formation.

Coagulation is an extension of haemostasis and results from interaction between blood vessels and platelets with various circulating plasma proteins, or coagulation factors. There have been many excellent reviews and detailed monographs on the pharmacology, biochemistry and physiological activity of platelets and coagulation factors and will not be repeated here. This presentation briefly reviews the coagulation process and describes current concepts in the coagulation cascade.

PLATELETS

Platelets are small, anuclear discoid-shaped cells that circulate in a quiescent (resting) state. In adults, platelets exist in the circulation for approximately 7–10 days in the order of 150–400 platelets per litre of blood. Platelets are derived from bone marrow megakaryocytes, with each megakaryocyte responsible for the generation of 1,000 platelets.

Vascular injury to the sub-endothelium results in exposure of collagen to the circulation. Immediately following injury and directly as a result of contact with exposed sub-endothelial collagen, platelets enlarge, change shape to become rounded, extend pseudopodia, adhere to vessel walls at the site of injury, release their granular contents, and aggregate to form a haemostatic plug (a sequence of events referred to as platelet activation, adhesion, release, aggregation, and agglutination stages). A flow chart indicating platelet activity and its role in haemostasis and subsequent coagulation is illustrated in Figure 4.1.

Quiescent platelets maintain an asymmetric distribution of phospholipids such as the negatively charged phosphatidylserine and phosphatidylethanolamine predominantly confined to the internal leaflet, while the remaining phospholipids, such as sphingomyelin and phosphatidylcholine are confined to the outer leaflet. Upon activation, the ability to maintain this asymmetric distribution is lost, with the platelet membrane selectively binding coagulation factors XI, IX, VIII, V and X, providing a catalytic surface for many reactions in the coagulation cascade. This helps restrict coagulation activity to a specific location and to enormously accelerate and amplify the entire process. Other platelet activators include adenosine diphosphate (ADP), thrombin, and adrenalin.

Platelets contain granules with various biologically active agents. The internal structure of platelets consist of organelles such as alpha granules, dense granules, mitochondria, lysosomes, and peroxisomes. The more numerous alpha granules

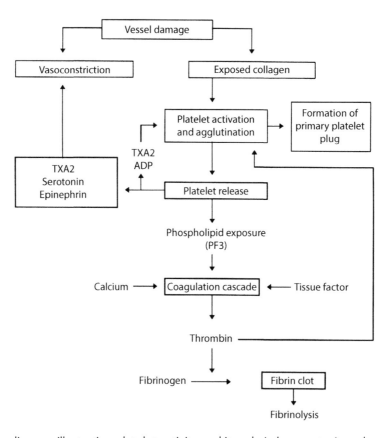

Figure 4.1 Flow diagram illustrating platelet activity and its role in haemostasis and coagulation.

contain proteins (including platelet factor 4), coagulation factors (fibrinogen, factors V and VIII) and glycoproteins. Dense granules contain nucleotides (but not DNA), calcium, and serotonin. Upon activation, platelets release their granular contents, including ADP and thromboxane A2 (TXA2), both of which promote platelet aggregation in positive feedback mechanisms (as in Figure 4.1). Antiplatelet drugs such as clopidogrel, prasugrel, and ticlopidine exert their antiplatelet effects by inhibiting the binding of ADP to its platelet receptor, thereby specifically inhibiting ADP-induced platelet aggregation.

Cyclooxygenase is an enzyme that triggers two pathways of arachidonic acid metabolism, one in platelets, the other in endothelial cells. In platelets, enzymatic activity of cyclooxygenase metabolises arachidonic acid (a polyunsaturated fatty acid and component of the platelet phospholipid membrane) into the prostaglandins PGG and PGH2, which are in turn converted by thromboxane synthetase into TXA2. Like serotonin and epinephrine, which are also released from platelets during haemostasis, TXA2 is a potent vasoconstrictor as well as a potent platelet agonist.

Counter to the effects of TXA2, the second pathway of arachidonic acid metabolism in endothelial cells produces prostacyclin, a potent vasodilator and inhibitor of platelet aggregation. Prostaglandins can inhibit platelet function by blocking platelet surface receptors. Like TXA2, prostacyclin is produced by the action of cyclooxygenase on arachidonic acid but is synthesised by vascular endothelium and smooth muscle cells, not platelets; it acts by increasing intracellular cyclic AMP levels. Cyclooxygenase is therefore instrumental in generating both prostacyclin from endothelium (platelet inhibition) and TXA2 from platelets (platelet stimulation). These opposing physiological effects of TXA2 and prostacyclin (along with other physiological and biochemical interactions) serve to regulate and restrict the procoagulant effect of platelets, thus limiting coagulation activity to a specific location.

ASPIRIN AND PLATELET ACTIVITY

Aspirin, a powerful platelet antagonist, exerts its anticoagulant effect by blocking activity of cyclooxygenase (by the irreversible acetylation of cyclooxygenase), thus inhibiting production of TXA2 and suppressing a promoter of platelet aggregation. In blocking cyclooxygenase, however, aspirin (and related compounds) also suppress production of prostacyclin, a platelet inhibitor. This dual effect of aspirin, influencing production of both prostacyclin and TXA2, has no effect on other activators of platelet aggregation such as thrombin, collagen, or ADP. Its potential anticoagulant effect as a platelet antagonist is therefore limited. The introduction of low-dose aspirin therapy is an effort to balance the effects of aspirin on platelets and endothelium without comprising its benefits as an anticoagulant.

ASPIRIN AND PAIN RELIEF

Prostaglandins also trigger pain and inflammation as part of the inflammatory response. Aspirin, like other non-steroidal anti-inflammatory drugs, reduces pain and inflammation by lowering prostaglandin levels, which it does by blocking cyclooxygenase (used to produce prostaglandins). There are two known types of cyclooxygenase, called COX-1 and COX-2. COX-1 stimulates platelets and protects the stomach lining by producing a protective layer of mucous. COX-2 triggers pain and inflammation. Aspirin blocks both COX-1 and COX-2. In doing so, prolonged use of aspirin can cause ulcers and internal bleeding. The search for new types of analgesic has resulted in a new family of non-steroidal anti-inflammatory drugs called COX-2 inhibitors, which selectively block COX-2 but not COX-1. COX-2 inhibitors can therefore reduce pain and inflammation without affecting platelet activity.

GP IIB/IIIA ANTIBODIES AND COAGULATION

Platelets also have glycoproteins on their surface that act as receptors for several adhesive proteins that enable platelets to bind selectively to vessel walls and each other. There are nine major platelet glycoproteins, numbered I to IX. Glycoprotein Ia (GP Ia) binds platelets directly to collagen, while glycoproteins Ib, IIb, and IIIa (GP Ib, GP IIb, GP IIIa) bind to Von Willebrand factor (VWF, a component of factor VIII plasma protein), which itself has receptors that bind to myofibrils in smooth muscle cells. Glycoproteins fibronectin and vitronectin are also involved in platelet binding.

The platelet glycoproteins GP IIb and GP IIIa are also essential for platelet aggregation. During platelet activation, the GP IIb/IIIa complex undergoes a conformational change that allows the binding of fibrinogen. This then facilitates the binding to other activated platelets, resulting in the formation of platelet aggregates. The monoclonal antibody abciximab (Eli Lilly Australia) exerts its antiplatelet effect by selectively and irreversibly blocking the GP IIb/IIIa receptor site, thus preventing fibrinogen binding to platelets and inhibiting fibrin formation. Failure of activated platelets to aggregate and bind with fibrinogen via GP IIb/IIIa prevents continuation of the coagulation sequence and is therefore considered the final common pathway for platelet aggregation and eventual fibrin formation. This mechanism is also exploited by other oral Gp IIb/IIIa antagonists currently under investigation for their effectiveness in preventing primary and secondary thrombosis following coronary interventions.

THE COAGULATION CASCADE

Once platelets are activated to aggregation and release stages, coagulation proceeds to completion. The coagulation cascade theory, originally proposed by McFarlane in 1964, is now universally accepted as representing the mechanism of coagulation. It may be defined as a complex series of biochemical reactions, each step of which results in the activation of the next step in the sequence, in a 'cascade' or waterfall effect. More recently, a cell-based model of haemostasis has been proposed that further accommodates the role of platelets and thrombin in the amplification of the procoagulant response. Both models begin in response to vessel injury and culminate in the conversion of fibrinogen to fibrin, with cross-linked fibrin monomers comprising the proteinaceous element of a clot.

THE COAGULATION FACTORS

Thirteen factors were originally identified and numbered accordingly, with the exception of factor VI (accelerin, or activated factor V) which is not recognised. Table 4.1 lists these and other coagulation components along with molecular weights and concentrations in blood. By convention, certain factors are usually referred to by name rather than number (tissue factor, prothrombin, fibrinogen, calcium). With the exception of factor III (tissue factor or thromboplastin), coagulation factors normally circulate in plasma in a dormant or inactive state until activated. Activation of circulating factors in the cascade results by specific proteolytic cleavage of polypeptide molecules from the parent plasma protein.

BIOCHEMISTRY OF COAGULATION FACTORS

All the factors have been identified as enzyme precursors or cofactors, except for calcium (factor IV), platelet phosphatidylserine (platelet factor III) and fibrinogen (factor I), which is basically a substrate with no enzymatic activity. All enzymes in the cascade are serine proteases (proteins with the amino acid serine at the active site), except for factor XIII which is a transglutaminase. Tissue factor, high molecular weight kininogen (HMWK) and factors VIII and V have been designated as cofactors, meaning they participate in reactions, not as enzyme precursors but as catalysts, selecting and localising relevant substrate sites and increasing the catalytic efficiency of their respective activated enzymes. The biochemical properties of coagulation factors permit their classification into three major groups: The fibrinogen, prothrombin, and contact groups.

The **fibrinogen group** consists of factors I, V, VIII, and XIII. They all interact with thrombin, are present in plasma but not serum (meaning they are used up during coagulation), they increase during inflammation and pregnancy, and do not depend on vitamin K for their synthesis; factors V and VIII lose activity in stored plasma.

The **prothrombin group** includes factors II, VII, IX, and X, and depends on vitamin K for synthesis. Vitamin K activity permits binding of calcium and phospholipid to form reactive complexes with these factors, an essential process in coagulation. Absence of vitamin K seriously curtails production of thrombin, the crucial element in converting fibrinogen to fibrin. Warfarin exerts its anticoagulant effect by inhibiting manufacture of vitamin K, thus interfering with production of the prothrombin group of factors and indirectly inhibiting production of thrombin. Without thrombin, coagulation cannot proceed to completion. Warfarin does not influence the activity of

Table 4.1 Basic properties of the major coagulation factors

Component	Factor no	Active form	Molecular weight	Plasma concentration μg/mL	Plasma concentration μm
Fibrinogen	I	Fibrin subunit	330,000	3000	9.09
Prothrombin Prethrombin	II	Serine protease	72,000	100	1.388
Tissue factor Thromboplastin	III	Cofactor			
Calcium	IV		20		
Proaccelerin Labile factor Thrombogen A globulin accelerator (ACG)	V	Cofactor	330,000	10	0.03
Proconvertin Stable factor SPCA Autoprothrombin 1	VII	Serine protease	50,000	0.5	0.01
VWF Antihaemophilic A factor (AHF) Antihaemophilic globulin (AHG) Antihaemophilic factor A Platelet cofactor 1 Thromboplastinogen	VIII	Cofactor	330,000	0.1	0.0003
Christmas factor Plasma thromboplastin component (PTC) Antihaemopholic factor B (AHB) Autoprothrombin II Platelet cofactor II	IX	Serine protease	56,000	5	0.08928
Stuart factor Stuart-Power factor Autothrombin III Thrombokinase	X	Serine protease	58,800	8	0.13605
Plasma thromboplastin antecedent (PTA) Antihaemophilic factor C	XI	Serine protease	160,000	5	0.031

(Continued)

Table 4.1 (*Continued*) Basic properties of the major coagulation factors

Component	Factor no	Active form	Molecular weight	Plasma concentration μg/mL	Plasma concentration μm
Hageman factor Contact factor	XII	Serine protease	80,000	30	0.375
Fibrin stabilising factor Fibrinase Fibrinoligase Laki-Lorand factor	XIII	Transglutaminase	320,000	10	0.03125
Prekallikrein Fletcher factor		Serine protease	86,000	50	0.5814
HMWK Fitzgerald factor		Cofactor	110,000	70	0.6363
Protein C		Inhibitor	62,000	4	0.0645
Protein S		Inhibitor	69,000	10 (free)	0.1449
Protein Z		Inhibitor	62,000	2.2	0.0355
Fibronectin		Receptor	450,000	300	0.6667
Antithrombin III		Inhibitor	58,000	290	5
Plasminogen			90,000	216	2.4
Urokinase			53,000	0.1	0.001887
Heparin cofactor II		Cofactor	66,000	90	1.3636
Alpha2-Antiplasmin		Inhibitor	63,000	60	0.9524
Protein C inhibitor		Inhibitor	57,000	4	0.0702
Alpha-2 Macroglobulin			725,000	2100	2.8966

Source: Modified, courtesy of R² Diagnostics, Inc. 412 S. LaFayette Blvd, South Bend, IN.
Note: For historical interest the original outdated names of factors I to XIII are included.

already-activated factors. It therefore requires a few days to demonstrate its effects and is initially administered in conjunction with heparin. This group also requires calcium for activation, is present in both plasma and serum (except for prothrombin) and remains stable in stored plasma.

- The **contact group** consists of factors XI, XII, prekallikrein, and HMWK; they are not dependent on vitamin K or calcium and remain stable in stored plasma.

COAGULATION PATHWAYS

The traditional model of coagulation is separated into two different pathways: intrinsic and extrinsic. Both pathways follow their own independent sequence of events, then meet at a common point and form a common pathway. The intrinsic pathway is so called because all required factors are contained within the blood. The intrinsic pathway is slower than the extrinsic, taking two to three minutes to induce thrombin formation. Factors unique to this pathway are factors XII, XI, IX, and VIII. The extrinsic pathway requires a substance outside the blood, tissue factor, for activation and is faster than the intrinsic. Coagulation time for the extrinsic pathway is 10 to 20 seconds. Factor VII is unique to this pathway.

The common pathway includes final stages of the coagulation cascade and is shared by both extrinsic and intrinsic pathways. Factors that form the shared common pathway are factors X, prothrombin and fibrinogen (and consequently include thrombin, fibrin, and factors VIII, V, and XIII). The cascade sequence is shown diagrammatically in simplified form in Figure 4.2.

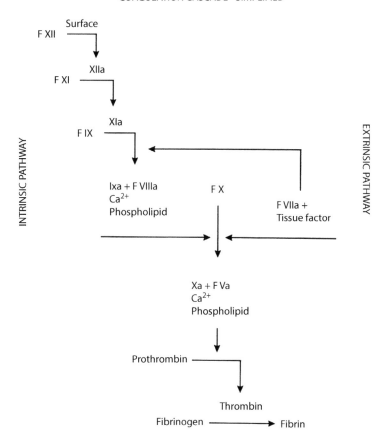

COAGULATION CASCADE - SIMPLIFIED

Figure 4.2 Simplified representation of the coagulation cascade.

INTRINSIC PATHWAY

In vitro experiments have demonstrated that the intrinsic pathway can be activated by contact with glass, kaolin, Celite®, or in general by a negatively charged surface. The process begins by interaction between small amounts of activated factor XII with high molecular weight kininogen (HMWK), which converts the coagulation factor prekallikrein into kallikrein in a positive feedback mechanism. Kallikrein then interacts with HMWK to further activate increasing amounts of factor XII. This reaction is not known to occur in vivo, where the initial activation stimulus for factors XII and XI remains unclear, although thrombin can activate factor XII. The physiologic significance of the intrinsic pathway in vivo is therefore in doubt.

The first step in the classic coagulation pathway is initiated by a contact factor, specifically contact of platelets with exposed collagen in damaged vessels. Activation of platelets then stimulates activity of coagulation factors. A change in molecular configuration stimulates conversion of factor XII into its activated form, designated as XIIa, which then activates factor XI into XIa, which then interacts with factor IX to form IXa, which in turn forms a complex (tenase complex) with cofactor VIII, calcium and phospholipid to activate factor X and start the common pathway. Thrombin accelerates this process by stimulating increased production of factors V and VIII in a positive feedback effect.

EXTRINSIC PATHWAY

Tissue factor is expressed on the surface of adventitial cells, which are normally insulated from the circulation. Tissue factor (also known as thromboplastin, thrombokinase, protozyme, or CD142) is a 47 kDa glycoprotein expressed by a number of cell types including monocytes, endothelial cells and to a lesser extent fibroblasts and smooth muscle cells. Although controversial, there is limited information that platelets may also express tissue factor.

When a vessel is damaged, exposed tissue factor comes into contact with blood. Independently of the intrinsic system, activation of the extrinsic pathway starts by interaction of factor VII with tissue factor which together with calcium form a complex to activate factor X. This also begins the common pathway.

COMMON PATHWAY

Once begun, the common pathway proceeds by interaction between factor Xa and cofactor V, which together with calcium, platelet phospholipid and prothrombin form a complex (prothrombinase complex) to stimulate conversion of prothrombin into thrombin, which then converts fibrinogen into fibrin. Thus, conversion of prothrombin to thrombin by factor Xa can be mediated by either the intrinsic or extrinsic pathways.

FIBRIN FORMATION

Following conversion of prothrombin into thrombin by factor Xa, fibrin formation occurs by hydrolysis of negatively charged fibrinopeptides A and B from the soluble fibrinogen molecule in plasma. The remaining like-charged monomers of fibrin form weak hydrogen bonds to build a polymer of fibrin sub-units. Thrombin activates factor XIII which, together with calcium, stabilises the growing complex by covalent bonding to form a stable clot, strengthened by trapped inclusions such as platelets and other cells. Clot retraction follows, which further compacts the clot.

FIBRINOLYSIS

Following coagulation, fibrinolysis begins by conversion of circulating plasminogen into plasmin, notably by release of tissue plasminogen activator (tPA) from endothelium. Plasmin induces fibrinolysis by proteolysis of fibrinogen and other proteins into fibrin degradation products. Fibrinolysis is regulated by inhibitors such as $\alpha2$-antiplasmin and $\alpha2$-macroglobulin, which inactivate plasmin, plasminogen activator inhibitor-1 (PAI-1), which inactivates tPA, and activated protein C, which promotes fibrinolysis by targeting inhibitors of tPA.

THROMBIN

Thrombin plays a central role in coagulation (Figure 4.3) as well as participating in other physiological activities such as leucocyte activation. It is a potent platelet agonist, directly promotes fibrin formation and stabilises the fibrin clot by activating factor XIII. It also regulates its own production by a positive feedback effect in generating factors V and VIII in the coagulation cascade. Thrombin also activates protein C, which, together with thrombomodulin (a product of endothelium) and protein S, indirectly inhibits thrombin formation by inactivating factors Va and VIIIa. It activates factor XII and is known to activate factor XI in vivo. Thrombin also both promotes and inhibits fibrinolysis by promoting release of tPA from endothelial cells, as well as stimulating activity of the tPA inhibitor PAI-1. The antithrombotic/anticoagulant drug enoxaparin (a low molecular weight heparin, LMWH) has a double effect on coagulation, inactivating thrombin and inhibiting the activity of prothrombinase (a complex of factor Xa, cofactor V, calcium, phospholipid and prothrombin).

HEPARIN

Heparin is a naturally occurring anticoagulant and is considered the most effective anticoagulant known. Heparin exerts its anticoagulant effect primarily by potentiating the effect of antithrombin (which inhibits thrombin, factors XIIa, XIa, Xa, IXa, and Va) and heparin cofactor-II which inhibits thrombin. Although an effective anticoagulant in depressing thrombin activity, efficacy of heparin is limited, partly by its inability to inhibit thrombin already bound to fibrin, and because of circulating inhibitors such as Heparinase and PF4.

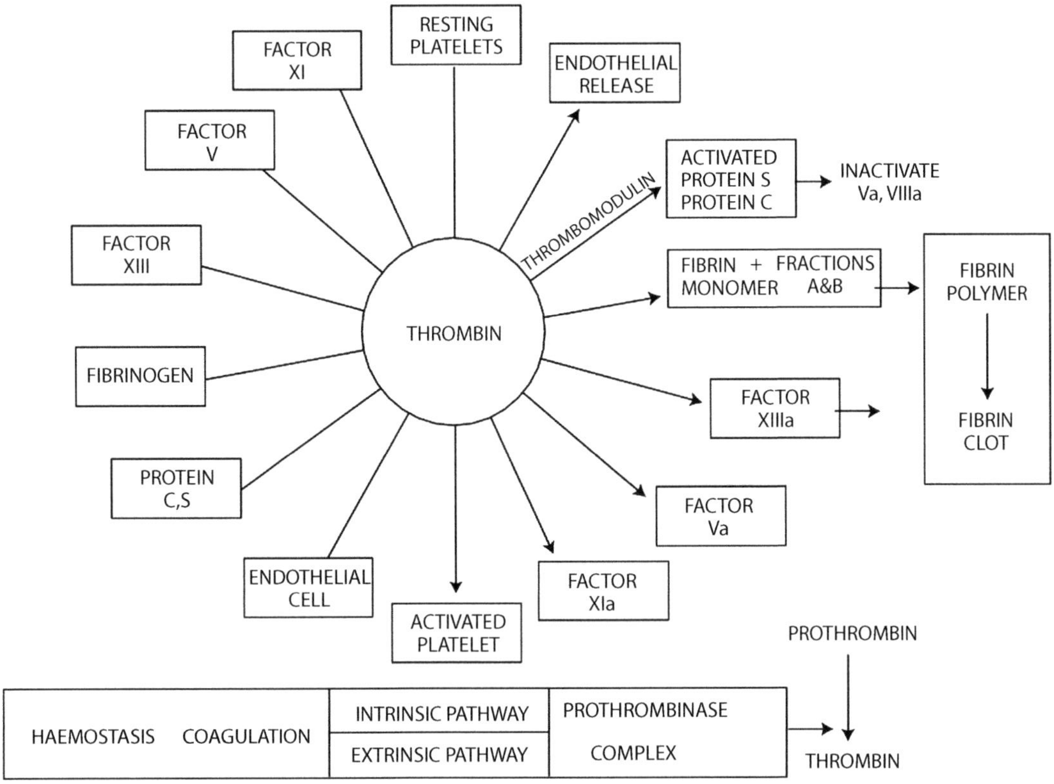

Figure 4.3 Central role of thrombin in coagulation as an activator of platelets, coagulation proteins and endothelial cells, and in fibrin formation.

ALTERNATIVE PATHWAY

Because the coagulation cascade was derived largely from in vitro experiments, it was originally considered that the intrinsic and extrinsic pathways operated as separate, unrelated events. This model has now been refined into a 'Cell-based Model of Haemostasis' that is split into three different phases involving initiation, amplification, and propagation. The cell-based model of haemostasis has developed into a model that encompasses the capacity of not only circulating proteins to contribute to coagulation, but also the capacity of cells such as platelets to support coagulation by acting as a source of phosphatidylserine to act as the catalytic site for the cleavage of many of these circulating proteins. This model is a thrombin-centric model that accommodates the role of thrombin in amplifying the platelet response to vascular injury and the role of thrombin in activating multiple coagulation factors.

The initiation phase follows vascular insult and commences following release of tissue factor into the circulation, leading to activation of factor X and the subsequent formation of a trace amount of thrombin. The amplification phase commences following adherence of platelets to exposed von Willebrand factor (factor VIII) at the site of vascular injury and involves the activation of platelets, factor VIII, and factor XI by these trace amounts of thrombin. Factor XIa is responsible for factor IX activation, which combines with factor XIIIa to stimulate further factor X activation. Factor Xa then combines with factor Va on the activated platelet surface to stimulate further Thrombin formation. The propagation phase then occurs, whereby thrombin formation leads to the formation of long fibrin monomers that spontaneously form a fibrin clot. When these and other components are included, a diagrammatic representation of the cascade becomes more complex, as shown in Figure 4.4.

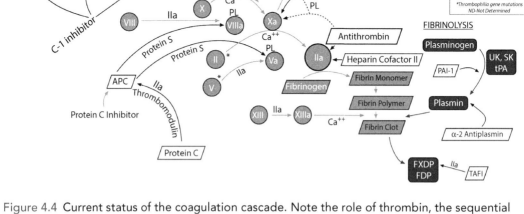

Figure 4.4 Current status of the coagulation cascade. Note the role of thrombin, the sequential activation of coagulation factors via the two major pathways, and the action of inhibitors (dotted lines). (Courtesy of R² Diagnostics, Inc., South Bend, IN.)

INHIBITORS AND COAGULATION

Inhibitors play a crucial role in regulation. They may either inhibit coagulation by inhibiting pro-coagulant activity, or promote coagulation by restricting activity of anti-coagulants. In the latter sense they can even inhibit other inhibitors (see Figure 4.4). Inhibitors of coagulation include antithrombin, heparin, heparin cofactor-2, proteins C and S, α2 macroglobulin, α2-antitrypsin, C-I inhibitor, and tissue factor pathway inhibitor (TFPI-1). Some (e.g. thrombin, protein C) have multiple roles in regulation and can enhance activators or inhibitors.

PHYSIOLOGICAL REGULATION

Uncontrolled coagulation, such as occurs in disseminated intravascular coagulation (DIC), is as physiologically untenable as uncontrolled bleeding. The coagulation process is therefore finely regulated by a balance of activators and inhibitors, which, together with vascular responses such as vasodilation or vasoconstriction, act in concert to either disperse or restrict the activity of coagulation factors to specific sites. Additional mechanical factors such as differences in shear stress from variations in blood flow between arteries and veins can also influence platelet binding activity. Blood flow itself, regulated partly by vessel diameter, is also effective in restricting or removing activated factors from a local area of injury.

Another example of balanced coagulation activity, the antagonistic effect of TXA2 and prostacyclin, has already been described, as have examples of positive feedback effects (ADP, TXA2, HMWK, and factor XII, thrombin). Indeed, positive feedback mechanisms have widespread application in regulating many biological systems and are well represented in the coagulation cascade.

Failure of this system of physiological control can lead to an imbalance in the regulation of coagulation, possibly leading to a variety of potential disease states.

COAGULATION AS A SINGLE PROCESS

Instead of considering coagulation as a rigid system of discrete pathways with the traditional step-wise conversion of zymogens (inactive precursor plasma proteins) to their derivative enzymes, it has been suggested that the coagulation cascade can be reinterpreted as consisting of only three separable groups of reactions: (1) contact factor activation of factor XIa, (2) conversion of factor X to Xa via factors IX and VIII, and (3) conversion of prothrombin to thrombin with resultant fibrin formation (a fourth reaction, activation of factors IX and X by factor VII may also be included).

The merit of this proposal lies in its consideration of coagulation as an interrelated sequence of simultaneous events that operate in vivo to regulate activity of circulating plasma proteins, rather than the somewhat artificial separation into a step-wise sequence of individual reactions. The concept of a cascade, however, is still a useful and simple way of presenting what may otherwise be considered an incomprehensible biochemical process.

Another way of demonstrating coagulation is to illustrate reactions in diagrammatic form, as in Figure 4.5. This has the additional benefit of consolidating apparently unrelated events into a unified structure, graphically displaying the interaction of various components. In this illustration the cascade itself is presented as being secondary to the main protagonists of coagulation, which are platelets, endothelium, and thrombin.

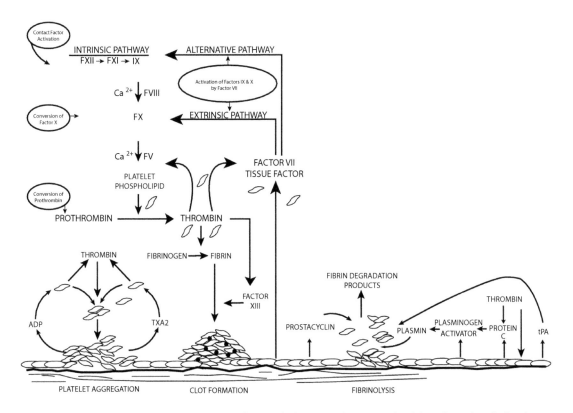

Figure 4.5 Diagrammatic representation of coagulation reactions, emphasising the role of platelets, thrombin, and endothelium.

FURTHER READING

Bayer. The coagulation cascade 2017. Available
    from: https://www.thrombosisadviser.com/
    the-coagulation-cascade.
Crampton L. How blood clots: Platelets and
    the coagulation cascade: Owlcation;
    2017 [Available from: https://owlcation.com/
    stem/How-Does-Blood-Clot-and-What-
    Causes-Coagulation.
Dahlbäck B, Villoutreix BO. The anticoagulant
    protein C pathway. *FEBS letters*. 2005;
    579(15):3310–3316.
Gailani D, Renné T. Intrinsic pathway of coagu-
    lation and arterial thrombosis. *Arterioscler
    Thromb Vasc Biol*. 2007; 27(12):2507–2513.
Gale AJ. Continuing education course# 2: Current
    understanding of hemostasis. *Toxicol Pathol*.
    2011; 39(1):273–280.
Hoffman M, Monroe III DM. A cell-based model
    of hemostasis. *Thromb Haemost*. 2001;
    85(06):958–965.
Moake JL. Overview of Hemostasis: Merck;
    2017 [Available from: https://www.scribd.
    com/document/360233415/Overview-of-
    Hemostasis-Hematology-and-Oncology-
    Merck-Manuals-Professional-Edition-1.
Nieuwenhuizen PV. Coagulation cascade:
    The Khan Academy; 2018 [Available from:
    https://www.khanacademy.org/science/
    health-and-medicine/advanced-hematologic-
    system/hematologic-system-introduction/v/
    coagulation-cascade.
Palta S, Saroa R, Palta A. Overview of the coagulation
    system. *Indian J Anaesth*. 2014; 58(5):515.
Smith SA, Travers RJ, Morrissey JH. How it all
    starts: Initiation of the clotting cascade. *Crit
    Rev Biochem Molec Biol*. 2015; 50(4):326–336.

5

Thrombosis, heparin and laboratory monitoring of heparin therapy

STEVEN FADDY

INTRODUCTION: THROMBOSIS

Thrombosis has been described as the pathologic process resulting from the inappropriate initiation and propagation of the coagulation system. Thrombosis occurs as the result of endothelial damage or alteration of blood flow characteristics. Once a thrombus forms in a blood vessel, a series of positive feedback mechanisms may assist in continued growth of the clot until it completely occludes the vessel. In the case of the coronary arteries, this can have dire consequences. Acute coronary conditions such as myocardial infarction and unstable angina are usually the result of thrombosis secondary to rupture of atherosclerotic plaque.

Normal endothelium has a number of properties that inhibit thrombus formation (antithrombotic properties) or which promote thrombus formation in response to injury (prothrombotic properties). Normal haemostasis is a delicate balance between these properties, maintaining uninterrupted blood flow under normal circumstances and promoting clot formation in response to injury. Pathologic thrombus formation can result either from inhibition of antithrombotic properties or induction of prothrombotic properties.

The pathology giving rise to thrombosis can be broadly grouped into three categories: abnormalities in endothelial function, changes in blood flow characteristics and abnormalities in blood components (including platelet function and anomalies in the coagulation and fibrinolytic systems). Abnormalities in one or more of these groups can initiate and propagate thrombus formation.

Endothelial function

The common antithrombotic and prothrombotic properties of normal vascular endothelium are listed in Table 5.1. Normal endothelium inhibits thrombus formation by a number of mechanisms. Prostacyclin (Prostaglandin I_2) is produced by endothelial cells and released into the blood stream, causing inhibition of platelet activation and inducing vasodilation via an increase of cyclic AMP. Endothelium-derived relaxing factor (EDRF, nitric oxide) is another molecule produced and secreted by endothelium, and inhibits

Table 5.1 Common antithrombotic and prothrombotic properties of normal vascular endothelium

Antithrombotic properties	
Prostacyclin (Prostaglandin I$_2$)	Inhibits platelet activation, promotes vasodilation
Endothelium-derived relaxing factor (EDRF, NO)	Inhibits platelet activation, promotes vasodilation
Thrombomodulin	Binds thrombin, activates Protein C
Glycosaminoglycans	Bind ATIII and heparin co-factor II to thrombin
Tissue plasminogen activator (t-PA)	Promotes fibrinolysis
Tissue factor pathway inhibitor (TFPI)	Inactivates factors VIIa and Xa
Receptors for t-PA and u-PA	
Ecto-ADPase	
Prothrombotic properties	
von Willebrand factor	Activates platelets, assists coagulation cascade
Factor V	Promotes thrombin generation
Tissue factor	Activates extrinsic pathway
Plasminogen activator inhibitor-1 (PAI-1)	Inhibits fibrinolysis

platelet activation and induces vasodilation by increasing cyclic GMP. Other antithrombotic agents such as Ecto-ADPase and thrombomodulin are not released into the blood but are expressed on the surface membrane of the endothelial cell. Thrombomodulin is a protein that, in response to binding with thrombin, activates the naturally occurring anticoagulant Protein C. Heparin sulfate glycosaminoglycans are expressed on the cell surface and catalyse binding of antithrombin III and heparin cofactor II to thrombin and other coagulation proteins, inactivating them and arresting propagation of the coagulation response. Plasminogen activators such as tissue plasminogen activator (tPA) and urokinase (uPA) are produced and released by endothelium in response to a range of stimuli. These molecules bind to fibrin, which allows them to form complexes with circulating or membrane-bound plasminogen. Formation of plasmin results, facilitating fibrinolysis. Tissue factor pathway inhibitor (TFPI) is a membrane-bound protein that inactivates factors VIIa and Xa.

Thrombosis can be promoted in response to disease or injury by the loss (or masking) of the antithrombotic properties of endothelium, or by expression of the prothrombotic properties. A number of pathological states can lead to alterations in antithrombotic capabilities of endothelium. Atherosclerosis leads to a localised decrease in production of prostacyclin and tPA, while EDRF production is inhibited in patients with hypercholesterolaemia or hypertension. Reduced expression of thrombomodulin and decreased EDRF production

have been noted in patients with hyperhomocyst(e) inaemia, which has been identified as a risk factor for atherosclerotic disease in young individuals with a strong family history of coronary artery disease.

In addition to loss of antithrombotic properties, diseased or damaged endothelium can also express a number of prothrombotic properties to promote thrombosis. Tissue factor (factor III) is produced and expressed on the surface of endothelial cells in response to a number of plasma proteins including interleukin-1, tumour necrosis factor, and some endotoxins. Expression of tissue factor induces activation of the extrinsic coagulation pathway. Dysfunctional endothelial cells can express factor V on their cell surface and, in response to hypoxia, can express a molecule capable of activating factor X. On exposure to thrombin, endothelial cells produce and secrete von Willebrand factor and plasminogen activator inhibitor-1 into the blood. The action of coagulation factors is described in Chapter 4.

Blood flow

Blood flow patterns within arteries also play a part in maintaining fluidity of blood. Blood flows through arteries in concentric layers called laminae. Layers at the centre of the arterial lumen circulate at a higher velocity and carry heavier particles such as red and white blood cells. Platelets are displaced to the outer layers which flow with less velocity and approach stasis near the vessel wall. Platelets become trapped in the outer layers and are inhibited from moving into the more central laminae by the relative differences in flow rates. This phenomenon benefits the clotting process by providing a concentration of platelets close to the site of any vessel injury. Low velocity blood flow near the vessel wall prevents the weak platelet plug from being dislodged before reinforcement by the secondary coagulation pathways.

The difference in flow velocity from its maximum at the centre of the artery to the almost static flow rate near the wall of the artery is known as the **velocity gradient**. The steepness of the velocity gradient is directly related to the **shear rate**. The shear rate has been described as the rate at which one layer of fluid moves with respect to the adjacent layers. An increase in shear tends to increase the number of platelets deposited in response to vessel injury. Such increases are typically seen in response to injury in the microvasculature. Decreased shear rates tend to increase the amount of fibrin deposited and are more common in larger veins and vascular pockets. In the heart, such pockets include aneurysms in vessels or the ventricle, and the left atrial appendage of patients with atrial fibrillation.

Arterial thrombosis is brought about by increased flow and high shear and is characterised by a predominance of platelets in the thrombus. Vessel bifurcations are at particular risk of thrombosis because they divide flow patterns. Endothelium at the inner junction is exposed to high flow velocities and the potential for turbulent flow, which dramatically increase local shear forces. Normal endothelium is adapted to withstand these highly prothrombotic effects. Continued exposure and other factors such as hypertension, however, reduce the resistance of endothelium and increase the risk of thrombosis.

Once a clot forms it is prevented from growing larger by the antithrombotic properties of the surrounding endothelium. Yet, formation of even the smallest clot will disturb blood flow properties within the artery, leading to turbulent flow patterns and increased shear forces. Endothelial damage is initiated or worsened, and platelet activation and adhesion increase by virtue of increased collision frequency between platelets. The thrombus grows in size and intrudes further into the vascular lumen, worsening the turbulent flow patterns and leading to further growth of the thrombus. This 'snowballing' effect has the potential to continue to enlarge the size of the thrombus until the entire lumen of the artery is occluded.

Clots formed in response to vessel injury are not alone in altering blood flow properties in this manner. Any obstruction, including atherosclerosis, will alter blood flow properties within the artery and promote formation and propagation of a thrombus (see Figure 5.1).

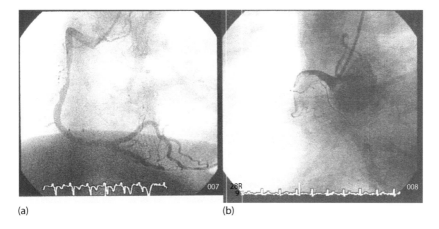

(a) (b)

Figure 5.1 Case study of a 60-year-old male who underwent cardiac catheterisation for investigation of recent-onset exertional chest pain. His history included coronary angioplasty to the left circumflex and second obtuse marginal arteries two years previously, and both were found to be free of obstructive disease. The angiogram showed a 70% narrowing in the mid right coronary artery (a). The patient was discharged to be treated medically and placed on the non-urgent waiting list for angioplasty of this lesion. Six weeks later, he began experiencing episodes of unstable angina and was readmitted for angioplasty of the RCA lesion. Initial angiography showed the vessel was occluded proximally by thrombosis (b), with retrograde flow from the left system only reaching the crux. The patient was treated with thrombolytic therapy before angioplasty was attempted.

Venous thrombosis is the result of decreased flow and, in some cases, complete stasis of blood. Low rate of blood flow increases venous pressure and causes dilatation of the vessel, the distension inducing endothelial dysfunction. Prothrombotic substances are released and the decreased flow inhibits dilution of these substances, facilitating the initiation and growth of the thrombus. Due to low flow rates, the thrombus is typically rich in red blood cells and fibrin.

This type of peripheral thrombus formation is brought about by several conditions such as immobilised post-operative states and low-output congestive heart failure. In the heart, this process can manifest as thrombus in an arterial aneurysm (Figure 5.2a), thrombus in an aneurysm of the ventricle (Figure 5.2b) or thrombus in the left atrial appendage in patients with atrial fibrillation (Figure 5.2c).

The same mechanism is responsible for clot formation in catheters and sheaths during cardiac catheterisation. Anticoagulants such as heparin are given during the procedure primarily to reduce the risk of thrombosis in environments of low shear stress.

Blood constituents

As previously discussed, the coagulation process is a complex and delicately balanced interaction among platelets, vascular endothelium coagulation factors, fibrinolytic proteins, and naturally occurring anticoagulants. The pathological process of thrombosis can result from abnormalities in one or more of these groups. Such abnormalities are referred to as prothrombotic or hypercoagulable states. It should be noted that prothrombotic states not only result from excesses or deficiencies of these factors (primary prothrombotic states) but also as the result of abnormalities brought about by a number of disease states (secondary prothrombotic states).

Spontaneous lysis of a thrombus occurs via a variety of mechanisms outlined above. Whether

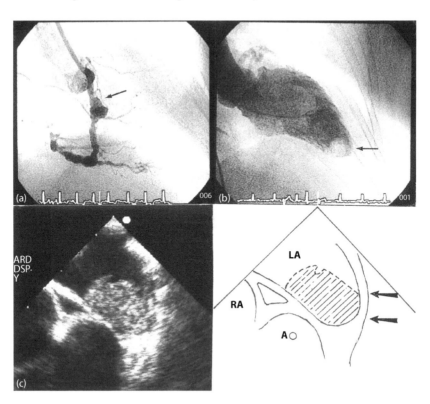

Figure 5.2 Venous thrombosis in the heart: **(a)** a partly thrombosed (arrow) aneurysm of the right coronary artery; **(b)** thrombus (arrow) in an akinetic left ventricular apex; **(c)** transoesophageal echocardiogram of a thrombus (arrow) in the left atrial appendage of a patient with atrial fibrillation and severe spontaneous echo contrast. (*Abbreviation:* LA, left atrium; RA, right atrium; Ao, aortic root.)

spontaneous or resulting from thrombolytic therapy, presence of residual thrombus predisposes the patient to recurrent thrombotic occlusion. The presence of fragmented thrombus appears to be one of the most powerful thrombogenic risk factors. Platelet deposition has been shown to be two to four times higher on residual thrombus compared to a severely injured arterial wall.

THROMBOSIS AND ATHEROSCLEROSIS

Atherosclerosis alone is rarely fatal. Acute coronary and cerebrovascular conditions are usually the result of thrombosis formed secondary to rupture or fissure of the surface of an atherosclerotic plaque. Thrombosis at the site of a plaque rupture is an important mechanism in the progression of atherosclerosis but not all plaque ruptures lead to thrombotic occlusion or plaque progression.

Patients with ischaemic heart disease usually have numerous plaques in their coronary arteries. Although only a small number may be identified angiographically, many more can be seen by intravascular ultrasound (IVUS). The reason for this is that most plaques do not encroach into the vascular lumen, they undergo compensatory abluminal vascular enlargement or 'remodelling'. Hence, the lumen may remain unobstructed despite the presence of large amounts of atherosclerotic plaque.

Composition of plaque is a greater determinant of the risk of rupture and thrombosis than severity of stenosis. Atherosclerotic plaque contains two distinct components. The atheromatous component forms the core of the plaque and is soft and rich in lipids. The outer sclerotic plaque is collagen-rich and hard. Rupture occurs more frequently in plaques with a large, soft atheromatous component. When spontaneous or mechanically-induced rupture of atherosclerotic plaque occurs the atheromatous core of the plaque is exposed. The atheromatous core is the most thrombogenic component of human atheromatous plaque. Thus, plaques with a large core content are at high risk of leading to acute coronary conditions if rupture occurs.

Chapter 21 discusses diagnostic methods for determining the composition of atherosclerotic plaques in vivo.

In most plaques, the sclerotic component accounts for the majority of plaque volume. The collagen contained therein is produced by adjacent smooth muscle cells and is responsible for the mechanical strength of the plaque. Smooth muscle cell proliferation may protect plaques against rupture and these cells are often missing from sites of plaque rupture. Inflammation and macrophage infiltration may weaken the fibrous sclerotic cap, reducing tensile strength of the plaque, predisposing to rupture, and leading to thrombosis. In eccentric plaque lesions, the shoulders are at particular risk for active inflammation, concentration of biomechanical and haemodynamic forces, and rupture.

CORONARY THROMBOSIS

There appear to be three main factors that determine whether a thrombus will form at the site of plaque rupture and how severely the process will affect the coronary circulation. First, severity of stenosis plays a part by altering blood flow characteristics and increasing local shear forces. The second and perhaps the major determinant is the composition of exposed plaque, with the soft atheromatous core more likely to evoke a prothrombotic response. Third, the delicate balance between the antithrombotic and prothrombotic properties of endothelium and blood may promote or impede a thrombotic response to plaque rupture.

Other factors play a role in coronary thrombosis. The apparently non-random onset of acute coronary syndromes (unstable angina, myocardial infarction) have led some to suggest that catecholamines may play a part in platelet activation and thrombin generation. Increased frequency of these conditions is associated with early mornings (particularly the first half hour after waking), Mondays, winter months and cold days, emotional stress, vigorous exercise, and eating. There is increasing evidence of enhanced platelet reactivity in smokers. It has been suggested that this too is due to catecholamine stimulus, since cessation of smoking results in a sharp decrease in acute vascular events. The pathophysiology behind this relationship is unclear, but it may be due to plaque disruption (surges in sympathetic tone produce sudden increases in blood pressure, heart rate, contraction, and coronary flow), thrombosis (platelet aggregation and thrombin generation promoted by circulating catecholamines) and vasoconstriction (occurring locally around plaque lesion).

Other studies are showing increasing evidence of relationships such as hypercoagulability in patients with progressive coronary disease, enhanced platelet reactivity at the site of vascular damage in experimental hypercholesterolaemia and enhanced platelet reactivity in young patients with a strong family history of coronary artery disease.

HEPARIN

Heparin molecules are heterogenous mixtures of sulphated simple chain polysaccharides of variable length that bond covalently to a polypeptide matrix to form the macromolecule heparin proteoglycan. The functional domain of the heparin molecule consists of regular segments of trisulphated disaccharide units interspersed between variable lengths of saccharide chains. Variations in the saccharide sequence of the functional domain determine the biological activity of the molecule. The various biological functions of heparin include suppression of aldosterone secretion, activation of lipoprotein lipase and inhibition of smooth muscle hyperplasia.

Heparin is not absorbed well by the gastrointestinal tract, so it must be given by either intravenous or intramuscular injection. It is inactivated by the liver and excreted by the kidneys in urine. The half life has been reported to be approximately one hour, but others have shown that the half life increases with increasing dose.

Heparin does not possess any anticoagulant properties, it acts as a co-factor. The anticoagulant and antithrombotic properties of heparin result from binding with a naturally occurring plasma protein, antithrombin III (ATIII). This is achieved when the functional domain of the heparin molecule is made up of a unique pentasaccharide (known as the ATIII binding site). When heparin binds to ATIII it induces a conformational change in the ATIII molecule, exposing an arginine molecule that is essential in the binding of thrombin. ATIII in its native form is capable of binding thrombin but when bound to heparin becomes about 1,000 times more efficient at binding thrombin.

The heparin molecule 'snares' thrombin by electrostatic binding at some point along the saccharide chain. The captured heparin molecule then migrates along the heparin chain until it is bound by antithrombin III. The ATIII-thrombin complex dissociates from the heparin chain and is cleared by the reticuloendothelial system. The heparin chain is left to bind another ATIII molecule and be re-used.

The heparin-ATIII complex has both antithrombotic and anticoagulant activity. The anticoagulant effect results from its direct scavenging effect on thrombin described above, and is more readily seen when full therapeutic doses of heparin are given to treat ongoing thrombosis. At low prophylactic doses given to prevent thrombosis, the antithrombotic effect of heparin appears to be more important. Heparin prevents generation of thrombin, and hence coagulation, by inhibiting activated factors XI, IX and more importantly, factor X, thereby slowing a large part of the coagulation cascade responsible for thrombin production.

Activated factor II (thrombin) is an appropriate molecule to target in attempting to prevent or reverse thrombus formation. It is responsible for activating the final step in the coagulation cascade, conversion of fibrinogen to fibrin. If thrombin is removed, activation of any part of the coagulation cascade will not result in clot formation. As discussed earlier, thrombin has a number of positive feedback mechanisms for its own production. It is able to activate factors V and VIII and can activate platelets, which facilitate activation of the coagulation system and, ultimately, generation of thrombin. Inhibition of this enzyme inhibits these positive feedback mechanisms and prevents further clot formation.

Following spontaneous or chemically induced lysis of a thrombus, thrombin may become exposed to circulating blood, leading to activation of platelets and coagulation factors and culminating in further thrombosis. The antithrombin activity of heparin is limited for three major reasons. First, residual thrombus contains thrombin bound to fibrin, which is poorly accessible to the heparin-ATIII complex and requires about 20 times more heparin for inactivation compared to unbound thrombin. Second, platelet-rich arterial thrombus releases large amounts of platelet factor 4, which inhibits heparin. Third, the fibrin II monomer, formed by the action of thrombin on fibrinogen, is also an inhibitor of heparin. Hirudin, a naturally occurring compound derived from leech saliva, has antithrombin properties and is at least 10 times smaller than the heparin-ATIII complex. It has no natural inhibitors. As such, it is more accessible to thrombin bound to fibrin, and may prove to have a clinically useful role in this situation.

Heparin is manufactured in two basic forms: unfractionated and low molecular weight heparin (LMWH). Unfractionated heparin chains vary greatly in length, averaging around 50 monosaccharide units per chain (average molecular weight 15,000 daltons). Heparin chains containing the ATIII binding site account for less than one third of all chains in commercially produced preparations made from porcine or bovine intestinal mucosa or bovine lung. Low molecular weight heparins are produced from unfractionated heparin by controlled enzymatic depolymerisation of the unfractionated heparin chain and have a molecular weight of less than 6,000.

Low molecular weight heparin has a half life two to four times longer than unfractionated heparin allowing subcutaneous administration once per day, and has a higher bioavailability than unfractionated heparin, allowing more accurate dosing based on body weight. LMW heparin possesses a lower antithrombin activity than unfractionated heparin as evidenced by its lack of effect on the APTT, but has greater effect on inhibition of factor Xa.

The antithrombin activity of the heparin-ATIII complex is proportional to the mean chain length of the heparin molecule. Anti-Xa activity is not dependent on chain length. Unfractionated heparin and LMW heparin exhibit comparable efficacy in vivo, suggesting that anti-Xa activity may play an important role in the action of LMW heparins. It has also been suggested that LMW heparins contain an abundance of chains without the ATIII binding site, and exert their effect not by binding heparin but by neutralising inhibitors such as platelet factor 4, which otherwise block the ATIII binding sites on heparin chains. LMWH may also stimulate the release of tissue factor pathway inhibitor.

Excretion of heparin varies according to the type of heparin used. The higher molecular weight heparins, which possess the majority of antithrombin activity, bind to endothelial cells and monocytes. Endothelial cells internalise and depolymerise these chains eventually releasing lower molecular weight heparin chains. This may explain the apparent preservation of anti-Xa activity for some time after antithrombin activity begins to diminish. LMW heparins are cleared

mostly by the kidneys and the half-life may be prolonged in patients with underlying renal pathology such as chronic renal failure. Patients with acute pulmonary embolism have been shown to have an enhanced rate of heparin excretion.

An increased prothrombotic potential has been noted in some patients following cessation of intravenous heparin therapy. Thrombin generation has been found to be greatest among patients in whom heparin was ceased abruptly compared to those who were weaned off the infusion over twelve hours, and fibrinopeptide A (FPA), a marker of thrombin activity, can be detected in the coronary circulation of patients following percutaneous interventions. These patients demonstrate a significant increase in FPA levels several hours after cessation of therapy. Although the underlying mechanism of rebound prothrombotic activity is unknown, tissue factor and the extrinsic coagulation pathway have been implicated as likely culprits.

LABORATORY MONITORING OF HEPARIN THERAPY

Heparin has the effect of slowing down the intrinsic pathway of the coagulation cascade. When utilising heparin therapy it is necessary to closely monitor the level of anticoagulation. Although some authors suggest there is no correlation between overheparinisation and risk of bleeding, any detected increase in laboratory tests of clotting times resulting from heparin therapy generally receives prompt medical evaluation. Under-anticoagulation may block the desired therapeutic effect of clot prevention or lysis.

Several laboratory tests exist for monitoring therapeutic heparin administration. Each has relative advantages and disadvantages. Unlike tests for other therapeutic drugs such as digoxin, quinidine or antimicrobials, assays for anticoagulant therapy do not test the direct concentration of drug in the blood but rather the overall effect of the drug on the coagulation system. In doing so, these assays take into account the action of the drug on coagulation factors, the body's response to the drug (such as rate of excretion) and the ability of other factors to antagonise the drug (such as replenishment of coagulation factors by the liver or the amount of ATIII available to bind thrombin). Tests of heparin anticoagulation are only screening tests of the intrinsic pathway, which starts with activation of factor XII and ends with clot formation. An extended test result indicates inhibition of one or more coagulation factors, but does not identify which one(s).

Activated partial thromboplastin time (APTT)

The most commonly used test is the activated partial thromboplastin time (APTT). The closely controlled conditions under which the test is performed, standardisation of reagents and methods, and the frequency with which the assay is requested make this test the gold standard in monitoring of heparin therapy.

The target APTT for a patient on therapeutic heparin should be 1.5–2.5 times the mean of the normal range for the institution.

As the preferred method, the APTT is highly standardised. Each laboratory standardises its normal range with respect to heparin sensitivity and constantly monitors this sensitivity with multiple-level quality control samples. The results are highly reproducible. Regardless of the method, very precise volumes are used. Current instrumentation possesses extremely sensitive clot detection systems, and most institutions run samples in duplicate to avoid reporting erroneous results.

The APTT is not necessarily appropriate to every clinical setting. It is less sensitive at the higher concentrations of heparin used in coronary angioplasty and cardiopulmonary bypass, where the dose-response has been demonstrated to be non-linear. Most laboratories assign an upper limit above which results are reported as 'greater than' the threshold value.

The APTT has very specific collection requirements. Blood cannot be drawn through heparinised catheters or cannulae. A clean, non-traumatic venepuncture is required to avoid activation of the coagulation cascade by prothrombotic mechanisms. Such activation may initiate the coagulation cascade before the anticoagulant can take effect, resulting in a shorter APTT time because the assay has commenced part way through the cascade, or a longer APTT time because some of the available coagulation factors have been used up prior to the assay. The citrate tube must be filled correctly as over- or under-filling will alter the dilution factor of 9 volumes blood to 1 volume citrate and render the result invalid.

Obtaining an APTT result is often a time-consuming process. Specimens must be transported to the pathology laboratory and processed by the central specimen reception department. Once in the haematology department the specimen requires a 10- to 15-minute centrifugation to obtain platelet-poor plasma for analysis. The assay involves an incubation, usually three to five minutes, and the endpoint may not be reached for up to three minutes. Quality control results must be verified prior to reporting of test results.

Activated clotting time (ACT)

In settings such as the cardiac operating room or catheter lab, where such delays may be to the detriment of the patient, results are required more promptly. The activated clotting time (ACT) is one test that provides comparable information to the APTT in a much shorter time. The ACT has no specimen preparation, improving the turnaround time for obtaining results. Whole blood is used and is injected directly into a tube containing an activator. A simple clot detection system times clot formation and the microprocessor-controlled solid-state electronics ensure accuracy of results. The test is designed to be used as a bedside monitoring test (see Chapter 6).

The various ACT tests available are sensitive to different levels of heparin anticoagulation. High levels of heparin are used in coronary artery bypass graft (CABG) surgery and coronary angioplasty, moderate levels in extracorporeal membrane oxygenation (ECMO) and haemodialysis, and low levels are used prophylactically after myocardial infarction and some surgical procedures. The type of activator used may affect the degree of prolongation of the ACT. There are a number of activators to choose from, depending on the particular clinical situation and the individual patient.

Diatomaceous Earth is used for high levels of heparin. Protease inhibitors such as aprotinin are often administered to patients to reduce postoperative bleeding, particularly during coronary bypass surgery. These agents can prolong an ACT activated by diatomaceous earth.

Kaolin is also used to test high heparin levels. This activator is unaffected by protease inhibitors and is an alternative for patients receiving agents such as aprotinin.

Glass particles are used for moderate levels of heparin. The clotting process is initiated whenever blood is exposed to a foreign surface. Glass beads markedly enhance the surface area available to activate the clotting process.

General surgical specimens and those from patients on low dose heparin therapy are often tested without an activator. Low levels of heparin permit clotting in a short period without the enhancement of coagulation activators.

A novel use of the ACT was described by Pitney and associates. They used a heparinase additive to counteract the heparin in the sample and provide a current heparin-free baseline ACT. When performed simultaneously with a standard ACT in a dual-chamber analyser, the difference between the two results, the ACT Differential, was shown to correlate more closely to the APTT than to the standard ACT, and was therefore a better indicator of anticoagulation status than the standard ACT.

Several factors may limit the accuracy and usefulness of the ACT. In a properly maintained and operated instrument, accuracy and precision are largely dependent on quality of the specimen. Collection technique is an important factor. As with the APTT, blood must not be collected through heparinised cannulae. The cannula, catheter, or arterial sheath must be aspirated before specimen collection to ensure that only whole blood is collected and tested. Inadequate mixing of specimen and activator will also lead to erroneous results. Vigorous agitation is often required to completely dissolve the activator. Other common pitfalls include improper storage of test kits (particularly prolonged exposure to heat), haemodilution, contamination by cardioplegic solutions, hypothermia, and platelet dysfunction from a variety of causes.

Comparison of ACT and APTT

Both the APTT and ACT have a clinically useful role in monitoring heparin therapy. The APTT is routinely used for monitoring therapeutic and prophylactic heparinisation, while the ACT is used in special procedures such as angioplasty and coronary artery bypass surgery, which require large doses of heparin. In these procedures the importance of maintaining therapeutic anticoagulation is paramount, and the time delay inherent in processing APTT samples through a central hospital laboratory may not be in the best interest of the patient. The ACT is a bedside test that requires no specimen preparation and provides a faster turnaround of results, allowing a more rapid response to any change in anticoagulation status.

Point-of-care systems are now available for bedside monitoring of APTT. These devices can use plasma or whole blood, but are still limited by the finite linear response of the APTT assay.

The ACT is theoretically a more accurate measurement of anticoagulation status as the patient's own platelets, calcium and phospholipid are used for the clotting process.

The APTT uses standardised concentrations of calcium and phospholipid which may not be representative of the true physiological state of the patient. The APTT is a highly standardised test and subject to strict quality control. Conversely, performance of an ACT is less rigidly structured and, although manufacturers recommend quality control be performed once per shift with dual level controls, quality control is performed on a less regular basis if at all.

Numerous studies have compared the APTT and ACT for monitoring heparin therapy in interventional cardiology procedures. Some report good correlation, while others report a poor correlation. Some studies found the ACT a more useful test while others found the APTT to be more useful. Several studies have reported finding subtherapeutic ACT values in patients with APTT values within therapeutic limits. This has led to suggestions that further study is required to investigate risks associated with prolonged use of heparin at therapeutic ACT levels and even that the ACT should be used as the reference standard.

Bedside APTT assays correlate well with laboratory assays. As with the laboratory assay, some studies have shown that the bedside assay does not correlate well with the ACT while others have shown good correlation.

Given that the ACT gives a more linear response to increasing heparin dose, uses the patient's own calcium, platelets and phospholipid in the assay, and provides a more rapid turnaround of results compared to the APTT, the ACT appears to be the better test for assessment of heparin therapy for interventional cardiology procedures (see Chapter 6).

FURTHER READING

Becker RC, Spencer FA, Li Y, et al. Thrombin generation after the abrupt cessation of intravenous unfractionated heparin among patients with acute coronary syndromes: Potential mechanisms for heightened prothrombotic potential. *JACC* 1999; 34(4):1020–1027.

Casa LD, Deaton DH, Ku DN. Role of high shear rate in thrombosis. *J Vasc Surg.* 2015; 61(4):1068–1080.

Deitcher S. Hypercoaguable states. In: *Disease Management.* Lyndhurst OH: Cleveland Clinic Foundation, 2010. Accessed at: https://www.clevelandclinicmeded.com/medicalpubs/diseasemanagement/hematology-oncology/hypercoagulable-states/ Accessed: 7 May 2018.

Falk E, Fuster V. Atherothrombosis: Disease burden, activity, and vulnerability. In: Fuster V, Walsh R, editors. *Hurst's the Heart.* Vol 2, 13th ed. New York: McGraw-Hill Companies; 2011. p. 2444.

Fuster V, Harrington RA, Narula J, Eapen ZJ, editors. *Hurst's the Heart.* 14th ed. New York: McGraw-Hill Education, 2017.

Kaushansky K, Lichtman MA, Prchal JT, Levi MM, Press OW, Burns LJ, Caligiuri M, editors. *Williams Hematology* 9th ed. New York: McGraw-Hill. 2016. Part XII: Hemost Thrombosis.

Koeppen BM, Stanton BA. *Berne and Levy. Physiology ebook.* 7th ed. Philadelphia, PA: Elsevier; 2018. p. 869.

Moynihan K, Johnson K, Straney L, Stocker C, Anderson B, Venugopal P, Roy J. Coagulation monitoring correlation with heparin dose in pediatric extracorporeal life support. *Perfusion.* 2017; 32(8):675–685.

Smythe MA, Caffee A. Anticoagulation monitoring. *Journal of Pharmacy Practice.* 2004; 17(5):317–326.

Smythe MA, Koerber JM, Nowak SN, Mattson JC, Begle RL, Westley SJ, Balasubramaniam M. Correlation between activated clotting time and activated partial thromboplastin time. *Ann Pharmacother.* 2002; 36(1):7–11.

Watkins MW, Luetmer PA, Schneider DJ, et al. Determinants of rebound thrombin activity after cessation of heparin in patients undergoing coronary interventions. *Cathet Cardiovasc Diagn* 1998; 44(3):257–264.

6

Laboratory coagulation assays

BRUCE TOBEN AND DAVID E. CONNOR

INTRODUCTION

Diagnostic imaging and minimally invasive therapeutic procedures are constantly evolving in parallel with new developments in technology. The population being treated is increasing in age, severity, and comorbidity. The culmination of these factors has resulted in a greater incidence of heparin resistance and a higher risk for administration of subtherapeutic anticoagulation during cardiac catheterisation associated procedures. The use of Point-of-Care (POC) coagulation devices to measure bedside Activated Clotting Time (ACT) tests in a timely manner, guides the administration of unfractionated heparin in this challenging scenario. Over the past few years, POC coagulation systems have advanced, with more manufacturers and an increased variety of ACT test types now commercially available. However, the results of the ACT tests vary from one instrument to another and between different manufacturers, and cannot be interpreted as the same. Not being aware of this lack of test

result uniformity could lead to misinterpretation of results and contribute to an adverse event. To avoid this pitfall, all clinicians and technical staff associated with assuring optimal heparin management must become familiar with the hospital's POC analyser and the unique characteristics of the ACT assay being measured. Methodically evaluating a new ACT system prior to implementation will establish expected results, validate clinical decision-making and develop confidence in heparin protocols.

BACKGROUND

Use of small, self-contained, coagulation analysers has been instrumental in monitoring unfractionated heparin administration at the POC for five decades. With the launch of the first Haemochron series of instruments to measure ACT by International Technidyne Corporation in 1969, the development of protocols for heparin dosing and neutralisation became embedded into cardiopulmonary bypass procedures to ensure unimpeded extracorporeal circulation during surgery. Shortly thereafter, these same POC coagulation analysers were placed in the angiography Suite to assess the effects of heparin during minimally invasive procedures. In the imaging area, these devices were initially used to manage administration of heparin during percutaneous coronary angioplasty and stenting, and then migrated over time to the electrophysiology laboratory for atrial ablation, for use during endovascular and interventional neuroradiology techniques, and now enabling transcatheter aortic and mitral valve implantation. All of these interventions carry risks of developing thromboembolic events during the procedure if optimal anticoagulation is not maintained, and significant localised bleeding with haematoma formation if onboard heparin activity remains elevated at the time of sheath removal. Reliance on POC coagulation devices in the angiography suite is tasked with managing the complexities associated with heparin administration while mitigating adverse events associated with subtherapeutic or supratherapeutic anticoagulation therapy.

MONITORING HEPARIN ADMINISTRATION

The most requested and readily available coagulation test measured with a POC instrument in the angiography suite is the ACT test. Results are used to exclusively monitor the intrinsic coagulation pathway and titrate the effects of unfractionated heparin. The anti-Xa assay may be used to guide heparin therapy as well; however, this laboratory test does not exist in a POC test panel nor can the results be analysed in a timely manner to support catheterisation procedures. Moreover, conducting serial anti-Xa tests on one patient can be cost-prohibitive. Although the activated partial thromboplastin time (APTT or PTT) is also indicated to monitor unfractionated heparin and can be analysed by a POC coagulation device, the sensitivity of this assay is typically centred for heparin concentrations lower than typically administered for most minimally invasive procedures. Consequently, it is essential that those involved in the heparin management of patients undergoing imaging procedures become knowledgeable in all aspects of the ACT test: its technology, indications and limitations.

ACTIVATED CLOTTING TIME TEST

The ACT test is distinctive in the realm of coagulation assays, as it exists exclusively as a POC test, not measured in the laboratory. There are no standardised traceable clot activating reagents and there is no laboratory 'reference' analyser to calibrate against. Each manufacturer of an ACT test uses different chemical compounds and/or concentrations of reagents to accelerate or activate the clotting cascade. Each manufacturer of an ACT test uses a different method to identify when a clot is formed. Some analysers warm the specimen within seconds to 37°C, while others may take minutes. Because of the variations in how the ACT test is measured, results from a single specimen will report different values if analysed in devices by more than one manufacturer or instrument model.

Although it should not be expected for ACT results to match system-to-system, it is anticipated that results show a trend. In general, trending is clinically consistent and relatively predictable. Appreciating that results will be 'similar but different' needs to be understood when comparing one ACT system to another, and it is of paramount importance for patient safety when instituting heparin protocols. Therefore, it is required that prior to implementing a new ACT test system, a series of validation studies be performed to set expectations of system performance and to assess the appropriateness of established procedural target times.

INSTRUMENT VALIDATION TESTING

Good laboratory practice guidelines dictate that all analysers, including POC devices that monitor the effects of heparin be evaluated in the same environment where patient testing will be conducted. Separate ACT evaluations should be performed dedicated to a specific imaging procedure. This will ensure that the data collected will yield the ACT system's expected performance in the same general patient profile and heparin management protocol. For example, separate evaluations should be conducted for patients undergoing angioplasty and stenting, and for atrial ablation procedures, and another for each additional procedure type. Because heparin dosing is significantly different in these procedures, the study should not combine the data, but evaluate ACT results separately for each procedure type. In this example, the system performance may respond differently primarily due to the heparin concentrations administered and the sensitivity range of the reagent. ACT systems may also demonstrate differences in performance when exposed to changes in temperature, which is another reason that evaluations should be conducted in the location of the intended use, especially if ambient temperature is significantly cooler in a room dedicated to a specific procedure.

A familiarisation period is often overlooked as an important step in the implementation of a new system. Laboratory guidelines recommend a five-day period in which the instrument should be handled by new operators and data not collected for statistical analysis. Device training is part of this process as selected personnel learn the analyser's operation, maintenance requirements and advanced functions of the instrument. Commonly, the manufacturer will initially educate operators on-site. Maintaining a detailed roster of training is necessary and needs to be archived within the department. The roster should include date, name/signature of attendee, key components of training, who conducted the class and results of a written test. In addition, proficiency testing is also required to evaluate each operator's performance. New operators should be tested to ensure they can produce analyte results with liquid quality control (LQC) material and produce values within pre-established ranges published by the LQC manufacturer. Documents attesting to satisfactorily completing this practicum must also be filed to demonstrate operator competency.

Among the specific laboratory tests that are required for Methods Validation for coagulation testing are: *Trueness, Precision, Method Correlation*, and development of *Normal Ranges*.

Trueness or Accuracy study

Trueness or *Accuracy* is how close the average measured result approaches the 'true' value. As stated previously, there are no 'reference' or traceable reagents to calibrate an ACT system, hence in its purest sense, an ACT result cannot be graded in terms of true accuracy. However, external LQC materials, specifically designed for a manufacture's ACT system, can be used to evaluate the instrument and the assay's performance. The LQC kits are commonly supplied with two concentrations or levels that simulate the clotting time of blood with and without onboard heparin. ACT values displayed within pre-established ranges as published by the manufacturer indicate that the ACT system is performing within specification and thereby report 'accurate' results.

Precision study

Precision is a measure of reproducibility and is assessed in combination with trueness. Commonly, LQC is used for these purposes since the 'known' range for recovery has been pre-established or assayed. This procedure is performed by analysing multiple tests of both levels of the analyte concentrations over a period of many days. Testing over a span of days may challenge system performance because of changes in ambient temperature, humidity, barometric pressure, but most of all, more than one operator. Acceptable performance criteria are also published by the manufacturer.

Methods Correlation study

A *Methods Correlation* study is a patient-oriented test that demonstrates the analytical performance of the new ACT system when compared to the predicate or existing ACT system. As already stressed, it is expected that a new ACT system will not report the same result as the current or predicate instrument. To ensure heparin management remains unaltered when the new system is implemented for patient management, it is necessary to calculate the average bias between systems (predicate to new) and evaluate whether procedural target times need adjusting. The overall objective of this study is to guard against improper heparin dosing because the ACT results might be misinterpreted.

When conducting a Methods Correlation study, both the predicate ACT system (the instrument being used for patient management) and the new system should be side by side, measuring ACT tests from the same syringe specimen. Data should be collected from baseline (sample taken prior to the first heparin bolus administration) through to sheath removal or completion. A minimum of 20 paired datasets could be used for statistical analysis, but at least 40 datasets for each procedure type are preferred. All data sets must emanate from blood samples obtained during the same procedure, and not be pooled from different procedure types. Donor blood that is spiked with heparin will not be representative of clinical practice and should not be used for the purpose of a Methods Correlation study.

If more than one new ACT system of the same manufacturer and model has been purchased, then one analyser can be selected for evaluation as representative of the new system. Prior to testing, the predicate ACT system should be qualified for performance by running quality control tests, including LQC. Similar to the quality checks performed on the predicate instrument, the new device needs to successfully pass quality control before a Methods Correlation study begins.

After all data has been collected, they should first be reviewed for possible outliers (results inconsistent with expected performance). These outlier results may have been influenced by artefact or sample contamination, improper instrument operational technique or analysis outside the temperature specifications of the system. Data that contains >10% outliers is not statistically appropriate for analysis. From the datasets remaining, the average bias should be calculated that includes results from baseline through to sheath removal. The data should then be assessed separately for baseline, sheath removal and the procedural target time (the ACT result whereby the minimal heparin effect was reached and the imaging procedure was initiated safely, without incident). The bias calculation (positive seconds or negative seconds) reflects how 'on average' the new ACT system will report results different than the predicate system during that imaging procedure. The average bias calculation is also used to adjust both the procedural target time and sheath removal time. Reviewing the procedural target time and sheath removal time separately will fine-tune the areas of clinical importance. Conducting this evaluation will maintain the same heparin management protocols used with the predicate system, when implementing the new ACT system.

Collecting baseline ACT data from the Methods Correlation study can also be used to determine a new 'Patient Baseline Range'. Performing routine baseline measurements can uncover the presence of unsuspected anticoagulants such as warfarin that may elevate ACT results. For those procedures where protamine sulfate is administered to neutralise the heparin effect at the conclusion of the case, performing a baseline ACT is required. Effective heparin neutralisation is achieved if the post protamine ACT is within ±10% of the baseline ACT result.

Normal Range study

Establishing a *Normal Range* or *Reference Interval* for each analyte reported is an absolute requirement of laboratory testing. 'Normal' is defined as a sample collected from a healthy, non-hospitalised individual. Although the manufacturer will publish a normal ACT range, each institution should establish its own. The rationale behind this recommendation is that the population within the geographic area of the healthcare facility may exhibit a different response to the ACT test when compared to the region or population studied by the manufacturer, or the criteria selection of healthy donors may be different than the manufacturer's study group. Therefore, it is good laboratory practice for each facility to develop its unique institutional-based ranges.

GENERAL GUIDELINES OF ACT TESTING

- As with any instrument or device used in patient management, it should only be operated as 'intended'. In respect to ACT testing, each manufacture publishes a list of limitations where the instrument or assay performance may report erroneous or unexpected results. These may include: storage or operating the device/reagents outside recommended temperature conditions, testing a specimen beyond its hematocrit restrictions, testing with onboard anticoagulants other than unfractionated heparin and testing patients with known coagulopathies, such as Lupus or elevated antiphospholipid antibodies.
- Sample collection and handling are key aspects for reliable ACT interpretation. Timing between administering the heparin bolus and obtaining a specimen for ACT measurement must be consistent with the protocol that established the procedural target times. This is typically 5 minutes. Premature or delayed testing could affect an ACT result and lead to an erroneous interpretation, which may contribute to

subtherapeutic or supratherapeutic anticoagulation administration.

- Removing an insufficient waste volume prior to sample collection is the most common source for erroneous results. Most manufactures recommend following the Clinical and Laboratory Standards Institute (CLSI) Guideline POCT14-A: 'For indwelling catheters, the line should be flushed with 5 mL saline; separate, single-use syringes should be used to collect at least 5 mL or 6 dead space volumes of blood (to be discarded) prior to collection of blood specimens for testing, to minimise effects of haemodilution (e.g. crystalloid fluid in line) or heparin in solutions used for flushing indwelling lines. Institutional policies and procedures should be followed.'

- Begin the test sequence immediately after obtaining the sample as a delay may cause lower than expected results. Mix the sample well by rolling it between the palms of your hands, gently inverting the syringe multiple times. Waste the first few drops of blood to remove the volume within the syringe's luer tip. If using a luer lock syringe, avoid dripping blood around the external threads as surface contact will accelerate the clotting time. Adding these steps to the operator's technique may improve precision, especially with a haemodiluted specimen.

- A hospital may have more than one manufacturer's ACT system in its facility and choose to locate the systems by clinical area. Conversely, a hospital may standardise with one manufacturer's instrument, but use a different ACT test dedicated to another clinical area or for specific procedures. However, mixing more than one system in a clinical location, or switching to different ACT test between procedures, or interchanging different ACT tests during the course of a procedure, can have significant untoward consequences due to misinterpretation of results and patient management. Policies and procedures should be developed to guard against cognizant or accidental inappropriate substitution of ACT systems. Some instruments can be set to restrict testing by operators and/or test types. These compliance safety mechanisms can limit the possibility of these events occurring.

- Diatomaceous earth (Celite®) is a naturally occurring, soft, siliceous sedimentary rock. Kaolin is a hydrous aluminium silicate that is abundant in clay. Celite and kaolin are the two most common clot activating reagents used in the manufacture of ACT tests. In the presence of aprotinin (a drug used in some geographic regions to inhibit fibrinolysis during cardiopulmonary bypass procedures), ACT tests that use Celite as its primary activator have been observed to report erroneously higher than expected results. Aprotinin does not appear to have the same interfering effect on ACT tests that use kaolin as a reagent. Selection of an appropriate ACT test should consider the primary activator if aprotinin is likely to be used during patient management.

ACT SYSTEMS AND METHODOLOGIES OF CLOT DETECTION

The **Hemochron® Response Whole Blood Coagulation System** (Accriva Diagnostics, San Diego, CA, USA) is the current generation of the first automated ACT test system. The clot detection module contains two test wells into which disposable, unitised ACT test tubes can be inserted. The test tubes contain the ACT reagent and a precision magnet. Immediately after a 2 mL sample is added, the test tube is vigorously agitated and then placed into a test well by the operator. The instrument automatically rotates the tube at a controlled speed and incubates the sample to 37°C. When a fibrin clot begins to form, it causes the magnet in the test tube to be displaced. Two magnetic detectors located in the test well continuously monitor the precise magnet position. When rotation of the magnet occurs, the elapsed time between the beginning of the test and the clot endpoint is displayed as the ACT time, in seconds.

A variety of ACT test types are available: Celite ACT (indicated for moderate to high heparin concentration), kaolin ACT (indicated for moderate to high heparin concentration) and P214 (glass particle activator, indicated for low heparin concentration). A feature of the Hemochron Response is the option to use special tubes that estimate the dosage of heparin to be given that will achieve a specific procedural target time, and the dosage of protamine to be given at the end of the procedure to neutralise the anticoagulation effect of heparin. In addition, a Protamine Dose Assay test is available to verify that all heparin has been effectively neutralised. These specialty tubes are manufactured in both Celite and kaolin reagent versions.

The **Hemochron® Signature Elite Whole Blood Microcoagulation System** (Accriva Diagnostics, San Diego, CA, USA) is the current generation of the manufacturer's test cuvette based system. The Hemochron Signature Elite system measures whole blood clotting times using disposable single-use cuvettes. Each cuvette contains the reagent necessary for a specified test. The operator inserts a cuvette into the instrument where it is warmed to 37°C and then places one drop of blood into the sample well. When the test procedure starts, a pump draws 15 µL of the specimen into to the test channel where it mixes with the reagent. Next, the pump continuously moves the specimen back and forth through the channel at a set pressure. A series of LED optical detectors, aligned with the test channel, monitor the movement of the oscillating blood. When fibrin strands develop, the viscosity of the blood increases, slowing its rate of movement between the optical sensors. A reduction in flow below a predetermined rate signals the instrument that a clot has formed. An internal timer measures elapsed time between the start of the test and clot formation and displays the ACT time in seconds.

The Hemochron Signature Elite system has two ACT test cuvettes: ACT+ (indicated for heparin concentrations between 1 and 6 IU/mL, silica and kaolin activators) and ACT-LR (indicated for heparin concentrations up to 2.5 IU/mL, primary Celite reagent). PT/INR and APTT tests can also be measured in the Elite system, formulated for both fresh whole blood and citrated samples.

The **i-STAT®** (Abbott Laboratories, Princeton, NJ, USA) analyser is a disposable-test cartridge-based instrument. A 40 µL blood sample is dispensed in the cartridge test well, then inserted into the device. After the cartridge's electrical contacts connect to the analyser, the sample is warmed to 37°C and the blood is mixed with the reagent. Unlike traditional ACT tests, where coagulation is accelerated by mixing a whole blood sample with a particulate activator and clots are detected as thrombin converts fibrinogen to fibrin, the i-STAT ACT endpoint is indicated by conversion of a thrombin substrate other than fibrinogen.

An electroactive compound is sensed amperometrically, and the time of detection is measured in seconds. The i-STAT ACT test is calibrated to match the Hemochron Response Celite ACT test using prewarmed tubes. However, patient results can be customised to report ACT values as calibrated to a non-prewarmed Celite tube.

The i-STAT system has two ACT test cartridges: Celite ACT (intended for procedures that commonly use moderate to high heparin concentrations) and Kaolin ACT (intended for high heparin concentrations). The i-STAT instrument can also test a PT/INR assay using a fresh whole blood sample for monitoring warfarin.

The **ACT Plus Automated Coagulation Timer System** (Medtronic Inc., Minneapolis, MN, USA) uses a disposable dual-channel test cartridge-based system. The cartridge is prewarmed to 37°C for 3 to 5 minutes, followed by a procedure to re-suspend the kaolin reagent. After the sample is collected, two sample channels are filled, each with 0.4 mL of blood. The clot detection process uses a plunger assembly within the cartridge. This assembly is lifted and dropped, mixing blood with the reagent. As the sample clots, fibrin forms at the base of the plunger assembly and impedes the rate of descent. This change in fall rate is detected by a photo-optical sensor located in the instrument. The endpoint of the ACT test is the time at which clot formation is detected and reported in seconds.

Four cartridges are available for use with the ACT Plus system: HR ACT (indicated for moderate and high concentration heparin, kaolin activator), LR ACT (indicated for low concentration heparin, kaolin activator), RACT (Recalcified Activated Clotting Time—For use with citrated whole blood samples at heparin concentrations of 0.0–1.5 I.U./ mL, kaolin activator), and HTC (Heparinase Test Cartridge – indicated to identify the presence of heparin in the patient's blood sample). Medtronic also manufactures the **HMS Plus (Haemostasis Management System)** designed to guide heparin and protamine administration.

The **Cascade Abrazo System** (Helena Laboratories, Beaumont, TX, USA) (not cleared for marketing in the USA) is a disposable card test system. Each test card has a reaction chamber containing paramagnetic iron oxide particles (PIOP) and lyophilised reagents. When the test card is inserted into the device, it is warmed to 37°C and when equilibrated, prompts the operator to dispense a 30–35 µL blood sample onto the test well. The sample is automatically pulled into the reaction chamber where a mixture of particles and reagents is reconstituted. The test begins when a photodetector in the instrument observes a light change from the added sample. While the test is in progress, an electromagnet turns on and off every second. The PIOP particles on the test card stand up when the magnet is on, causing more light to pass to the photodetector. When the magnet is off, the particles fall down, causing less light to be detected. The movement of these particles produces an optical signal that is processed by the analyser. Clotting of the sample causes slowing and eventual cessation of particle movement. The analyser monitors particle movement and records the clotting time in seconds.

The Cascade Abrazo System can analyse two different ACT tests: c-ACT test (indicated for heparin concentrations between 1 and 6 I.U./mL, primary Celite reagent) and c-ACT-LR (indicated for heparin concentrations up to 3.0 I.U./mL, primary Celite reagent). Additional test cards are available to measure Prothrombin Time (PT), International Normalised Ratio (INR) and APTT on either a citrated whole blood specimen or a plasma sample.

Helena Laboratories also manufactures the **Actalyke-XL** system. The methodology of clot detection and ACT test types are modelled after the Hemochron Response Whole Blood Coagulation System.

OTHER POINT-OF-CARE COAGULATION TESTING

The ACT, APTT, and Prothrombin Time (PT) are well characterised methods for assessing the coagulation system in patients. These tests, however, focus only on specific pathways of coagulation and do not necessarily provide information on haemostasis as a whole. For example, the APTT provides clotting time as a measure of the intrinsic coagulation pathway, but provides limited information on fibrinolysis. The endpoint for most coagulation assays is clot formation (the time to clot formation), yet this provides no information on clot strength, rate of clot formation, or fibrinolysis.

Although the APTT and PT assays can be performed at the POC, they are routinely measured in specialised coagulation laboratories, which can lead to delays in providing a result for critical patients.

Viscoelastometrictesting/ thromboelastography

Viscoelastometric testing has emerged as a powerful method for assessing global haemostasis. The general principle of this test involves the addition of whole blood and agonist placed into a cup/cuvette and pin. Depending on the model of instrument, either the cup or pin rotates, and the resistance to this rotation as coagulation occurs is detected over time. A trace of clot formation is obtained that is expressed as time (x-axis) versus an amplitude (y-axis, measured in millimetres). The two main instruments used are **rotational thromboelasometry** (ROTEM®, Tem Innovations GmbH, Germany) or **thromboelasography** (TEG®, Haemonetics, Switzerland).

Each system provides information on a number of parameters of clot formation and lysis (Table 6.1).

The *Rotational Thromboelastometry (ROTEM)* system involves administration of whole blood (300 µL) to a cup in the presence of an agonist. The system is pre-warmed to 37°C. The cup is fixed into place and then elevated into position such that a 1 mm gap is made between the cup and an oscillating pin. This pin oscillates at an axis of ±4.75° throughout the analysis, and light from an LED light source is reflected from a mirror on the oscillating pin to a detector that converts this into a trace (Figure 6.1a). The standard test is run for one hour; however, in critical patients or in patients who require a faster result, the amplitude of the ROTEM trace can be interpreted earlier (after 5 minutes, known as the A5, or after 10 minutes, the A10).

The system has four parallel channels allowing for simultaneous use of four different tests.

Table 6.1 Viscoelasometric parameters using rotational thromboelasometry (ROTEM) and thromboelastography (TEG)

ROTEM	TEG	Measurement	Mechanism
Clotting time (CT)	R-time	Measures the time taken before clot formation commences.	Affected by coagulation factor activity.
Clot Formation Time (CFT)	K-time	Measures the time taken from the commencement of clot formation until the clot firmness is 20 mm.	Affected by platelet function and count, fibrinogen.
Alpha angle	Alpha angle	The angle of the tangent of the curve at the point where the clot firmness is 20 mm.	Affected by platelet function and count, fibrinogen.
Maximum Clot Firmness (MCF)	Maximum Amplitude (MA)	Measures the greatest amplitude of the clot.	Affected by platelets, fibrinogen and Factor XIII.
LI30	LY30	Measures clot lysis at 30 minutes.	Affected by fibrinolytic factors.
A5, A10, A15, A(N)		A measurement of the amplitude at n minutes.	Used as a rapid method of assessing coagulation in critical patients who rely upon quick results.

The ROTEM system uses a number of different agonists in order to measure multiple pathways of coagulation:

EXTEM: A measure of the extrinsic pathway of coagulation. Clotting is stimulated by the addition of human recombinant tissue factor and calcium. Sensitive to coagulation factor deficiencies, hyperfibrinolysis, vitamin K antagonists (such as warfarin), direct thrombin inhibitors, and platelet function.

INTEM: A measure of the intrinsic pathway of coagulation. Clotting is stimulated by ellagic acid and phospholipid. Sensitive to coagulation factor deficiencies, hyperfibrinolysis, heparin, and platelet function.

APTEM: Performed similarly to the EXTEM assay, with addition of aprotinin to the assay to inhibit fibrinolysis. Performed to confirm hyperfibrinolysis when detected in the EXTEM assay.

FIBTEM: Performed similarly to the EXTEM assay, with addition of cytochalasin D to inhibit platelet function. This allows the assay to assess the fibrinogen and platelet contribution to clot formation (an abnormal EXTEM and abnormal FIBTEM suggest a fibrinogen deficiency, while as abnormal EXTEM and normal FIBTEM suggests a platelet deficiency). There is a significant correlation between the FIBTEM MCF and fibrinogen concentration.

NATEM: Performed in the presence of calcium only.

HEPTEM: A measurement of the intrinsic pathway in heparinised patients.

The ROTEM delta system has now been superseded by the ROTEM alpha system. This is a cartridge-based system that eliminates the need for manual pipetting of blood and reagent.

The *Thromboelastography* (TEG) system is performed under similar conditions to the ROTEM system, with a few minor differences. Using the TEG system, blood is administered to the cup/cuvette, and the pin is inserted. Unlike the ROTEM, the pin is fixed into position and the cup rotates. Again the system is pre-warmed to 37°C. The TEG has two parallel channels for testing. The agonists available are:

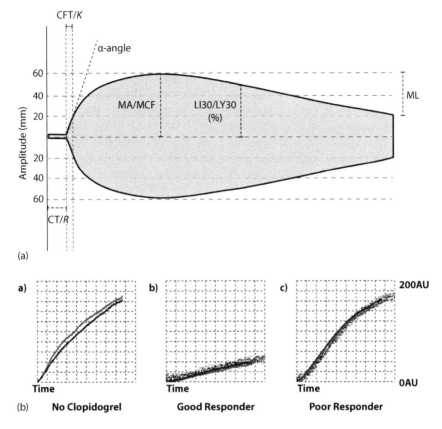

Figure 6.1 **(a)** Typical trace for ROTEM/TEG system with associated measurements. Clotting time (CT/R, sec), Clot Formation Time (CFT/K, sec), Alpha angle (°), Maximum Clot Firmness/Maximum Amplitude (MCF/MA, mm), Lysis Index at 30 minutes (LI30/LY30 Index, %) and Maximum Lysis (ML). **(b)** Plot of ADP test for (a) normal patient; (b) patient on clopidogrel (good responder); (c) patient on clopidogrel (poor responder).

Rapid TEG: A measure of both intrinsic and extrinsic pathways of coagulation.

Kaolin TEG: A measure of the intrinsic pathway of coagulation. Uses kaolin to activate haemostasis. Sensitive to coagulation factor defects, hyperfibrinolysis, heparin, and platelet function.

Kaolin TEG with heparinise: A measure of the intrinsic pathway in heparinised patients.

TEG Functional fibrinogen: A measure of the extrinsic pathway, with addition of a glycoprotein IIb/IIIa inhibitor to inhibit platelet function.

Clinical uses

Both viscoelastometric testing and thromboelastography are valuable in both an intensive care and cardiac surgery setting, with many institutions now adopting transfusion guidelines based on the interpretation of these tests. Introduction of these protocols have been demonstrated to reduce rates of transfusion of blood components.

MULTIPLE ELECTRODE AGGREMOMETRY OF PLATELET FUNCTION

Multiple electrode aggregometry can be used in a point of care setting or in the routine coagulation laboratory for assessment of platelet function. The most commonly available system is the Multiplate® system (Roche Diagnostics). This system uses impedance aggregometry to detect platelet function. Whole blood is added to a test cell containing a magnetic stirrer and two sets of silver-coated probes. As platelets aggregate to the probes in the presence of agonist, the ability of platelets to impede the electrical current between these probes is detected and converted to an aggregation trace (Figure 6.1b) of time (x-axis) and aggregation units (y-axis). The assay is run for 6 minutes, following which an area under the curve is then calculated as a measure of platelet function.

The recommended anticoagulant for blood collection is hirudin, but as this is not always commonly available, the test can be performed in sodium citrate, provided that the sample is recalcified during the initial dilution. The assay is performed in whole blood rather than in platelet-rich plasma, which allows for the assay to be performed with minimal manipulation.

The tests available in the Multiplate system are:

ADPtest. Measures platelet aggregation in the presence of adenosine diphosphate (ADP). Sensitive to ADP receptor defects and P2Y12 inhibitors such as clopiodgrel and prasugrel.

ADPtest HS. A high-sensitivity measure of the ADP P2Y12 pathway through addition of prostaglandin E2.

ASPItest. Measures platelet aggregation in the presence of arachidonic acid. Sensitive to aspirin.

TRAPtest. Measures platelet aggregation in the presence of a thrombin receptor activating peptide (platelet PAR1 thrombin receptor). Antiplatelet agents such as aspirin and clopidogrel have little effect on this assay.

COLtest. Measures platelet aggregation in the presence of collagen. Sensitive to collagen receptor defects.

RISTOtest high and low. Measures platelet aggregation/agglutination in the presence of high and low concentrations of ristocetin. Used to diagnose von Willebrand disease.

Clinical uses

While the utility of Multiplate to diagnose inherited and acquired disorders of platelet function is yet to be determined, and with light transmission aggregometry remaining as the gold standard for this purpose, the utility of the Multiplate system appears to be its ability to provide quantitative results on the effect of antiplatelet agents on platelet function, especially in assessment of clopidogrel inhibition.

SUMMARY

Heparin protocols used in the angiography suite are associated with numerous procedures related to diagnostic imaging and minimally invasive techniques. The heparin dosage administered is dependent on the thromboembolic risk associated with the procedure, combined with the patient's response to the drug. ACT target times are established to set the minimal degree of anticoagulation necessary at various clinical decision-making points throughout the procedure. These target times are developed by each facility and are unique to the test system used for ACT measurement. Evaluation of a new test instrument must assess the sample handling, test operation sequence and how the new system's results correlate to the predicate instrument, thereby evaluating if existing procedural target times are appropriate or need adjustment. In addition, it is essential that during the introductory phase of new system training, staff involved with POC testing become familiar with the limitations and interfering substances that could report an erroneous result. By understanding and addressing these key aspects of POC testing, adoption of new systems can occur in a systematic fashion to foster best practices and safe patient management.

FURTHER READING

A practical guide to laboratory haemostasis. http://www.practical-haemostasis.com

Bates SM, Weitz JI. Coagulation Assays. *Circulation.* 2005;112(4):e53–e60.

Ducrocq G, Jolly S, Mehta SR, Rao SV, Patel T, Moreno R, et al. Activated clotting time and outcomes during percutaneous coronary intervention for non–ST-Segment–elevation myocardial infarction. *Insights From the FUTURA/OASIS-8 Trial.* 2015;8(4):e002044.

Kong R, Trimmings A, Hutchinson N, Gill R, Agarwal S, Davidson S, et al. Consensus recommendations for using the Multiplate® for platelet function monitoring before cardiac surgery. *Int J Lab Hematol.* 2015;37(2):143–147.

Ndrepepa G, Kastrati A. Activated clotting time during percutaneous coronary intervention: A test for all seasons or a mind tranquilizer? *Am Heart Assoc.* 2015;8(4):e002576.

Paniccia R, Fedi S, Carbonetto F, Noferi D, Conti P, Bandinelli B, et al. Evaluation of a new point-of-care Celite-activated clotting time analyzer in different clinical settings: Thei-STAT Celite-activated clotting time test. *Anesthesiology: J Am Society Anesthesiol.* 2003;99(1):54–59.

Shen L, Tabaie S, Ivascu N. Viscoelastic testing inside and beyond the operating room. *J Thorac Dis.* 2017;9(Suppl 4): S299. 6.

Patient care and laboratory safety

7

Radiation safety in the cardiac catheterisation laboratory

CAMERON JEFFRIES

INTRODUCTION

The interventional diagnostic radiology room, and in particular the cardiac catheterisation laboratory (CCL), present a unique environment in which the medical team and patient are exposed to several kinds of hazards. One hazard is radiation exposure to both staff and patients. Staff face the risk of stochastic or late radiation effects, such as cancer, from accumulated radiation dose during their careers. Whereas patients are more likely to experience deterministic radiation effects, such as skin injury, from prolonged radiation exposure during their examination, and can also accumulate risk of late radiation effects. The risk to both groups can be reduced by understanding the physics of radiation production and interaction, and by practising the safety procedures described in this chapter.

PRINCIPLES OF RADIOLOGICAL PROTECTION

Use of penetrating radiation is an essential feature of current medical practice. Diagnostic and interventional imaging most commonly use ionising radiation (i.e. X-rays) that can cause ionisation of molecules in the body. Because of potential damage to living tissue, precautions must be taken when working with ionising radiation. The International Commission on Radiological Protection (ICRP) reviews current knowledge of radiation effects to develop a radiation risk model that is the basis for recommendations and guidance for radiological protection.[1] ICRP publications provide an outline of the best practice approach to radiological protection, which may be adopted into the legislation of individual countries. Australia, for example, adopts such international recommendations in the Radiation Protection Series[2,3] published by the Australia Radiation Protection and Nuclear Safety Agency (ARPANSA).

The radiation risk model makes it impossible to derive a clear distinction between 'safe' and 'dangerous' at typical radiation exposure levels.[1] This uncertainty led to development of the System for Radiological Protection to establish a level of protection that is considered acceptable.[1] This system of protection is based on three fundamental principles of protection:

1. *Justification* of practices and procedures – Any decision that alters radiation exposure should do more good than harm.
2. *Optimisation* of protection – The likelihood of exposure, the number of people exposed and their individual doses should all be kept **as low as reasonably achievable** (ALARA).
3. *Limitation* of individual dose – The total dose to any individual, other than medical exposure of patients, should not exceed recommended limits.

Radiation exposure is classified according to the type of exposure, when applying the principles of radiological protection, as follows:

- *Occupational:* Exposure of workers that is incurred in the course of their work.[2] Relevant workgroups include radiologists, cardiologists, scientists, technologists, and radiographers.
- *Medical:* Exposure of patients as part of their own medical diagnosis or treatment; of carers voluntarily supporting or comforting patients; of volunteers in a biomedical research program.[2]
- *Public:* Exposure incurred by members of the public that is neither occupational nor medical exposure.[3,4]

The potential benefit from radiation will vary according to the type of exposure based on these classifications. Workers who are occupationally exposed to radiation have a greater level of direct benefit (e.g. financial) from that exposure than members of the public, and patients may receive significant benefit in having treatment for their medical conditions. The reason for exposure is thus an important consideration for determining an acceptable level of radiation risk. Accordingly, dose limits have been set related to the exposure situation and the potential benefit from that situation.[1]

MEASUREMENT OF RADIATION DOSE

Assessment of dose from radiation exposure is based on special dosimetric quantities that have been adopted by the system of radiological protection. The dosimetric quantities are designed to provide a system to quantify the relationship between radiation exposure or dose and radiation risk. Radiation dosimetry has a fundamental quantity called **absorbed dose** that is based on measurement of the energy deposited in organs and tissues of the human body.[1] Radiation dose is then related to radiation risk by modifying the absorbed dose to account for the biological impact of different radiations and the sensitivity of organs and tissues to radiation.[1] This modification process gives rise to **equivalent dose** and **effective dose**, which can be assessed from measured operational radiation quantities. These dose quantities are summarised as follows.

Absorbed Dose (D) is the mean energy absorbed by a volume of matter divided by the mass of the irradiated matter.[1] The energy can be averaged over any defined volume of matter. Absorbed dose is the basic physical dose quantity and is applicable to all types of ionising radiation.[1,5] **Kerma**, or a**ir kerma**, is the term used for absorbed dose in air at low energy, i.e. the energy absorbed by a kilogram of irradiated air. The SI unit of absorbed dose is joule per kilogram ($J kg^{-1}$) with the special name **gray (Gy)**.[1] The non-SI unit for absorbed dose is the **rad**, which is predominately used in North America.

Equivalent Dose (H_T) is the mean absorbed dose in a specific organ or tissue multiplied by a radiation weighting factor. The radiation weighting factor is determined by the type and energy of radiation causing the exposure of the organ or tissue.[4] The radiation weighting factor for X-ray radiation used in the CCL, for example, is 1.0, and the weighting factor for the lungs is 0.12, and for the gonads it is 0.20. Equivalent dose to a specified organ or tissue from any type of radiation can be compared directly, and is designed to reflect the amount of damage inflicted.[3] The SI unit for equivalent dose is joule per kilogram ($J kg^{-1}$), the same as for absorbed dose, with the special name **sievert (Sv)**.[1]

Effective Dose (E) takes into account both the type of radiation involved and the radiological sensitivities of individual organs and tissues being irradiated. Effective dose is the sum of the equivalent doses in all irradiated organs and tissues multiplied by a tissue weighting factor for the specific organ or tissue. Effective dose is designed to reflect the radiation harm likely to result from the dose. Effective dose thus allows direct comparison of exposure for any type of radiation and any mode of exposure.[3] The SI unit for effective dose is also joule per kilogram (J kg^{-1}) with the special name **sievert (Sv)**.[1] Table 7.1 provides a list of definitions for radiation terminology.

SOURCES OF RADIATION

Humans are exposed to radiation from a variety of natural and artificial sources. Radioactive materials are in the environment due to the prevalence of naturally occurring radioactive minerals present since the early stages of formation of the universe. The main sources of natural radioactivity are isotopes of uranium, thorium and potassium, which have long half-lives, distributed throughout the earth's crust. Natural radioactivity results in exposure to terrestrial gamma radiation from soil and building materials, release of radon and radon progeny to the atmosphere, and by uptake of radioactive materials in the food and drink that we consume. Natural radioactivity in food results in a natural level of radioactive potassium, uranium, and thorium in our bodies. Radiation exposure also results from cosmic radiation and from man-made radioactivity in the environment in the form of fallout from atmospheric nuclear weapons testing and nuclear accidents.

Worldwide average annual radiation dose due to natural radiation sources has been estimated to

Table 7.1 Definition of radiological terms

Tch	Definition	Units
Exposure	1: In physics, the amount of ionisation per unit mass of air. 2: Generally, being exposed to a radiation source.	Coulomb per kg (C·kg^{-1}), or Roentgen
Absorbed dose	Amount of energy deposited (i.e. absorbed) in 1 kg of matter.	Gray (Gy)
Kerma, Air Kerma	Amount of energy deposited (i.e. absorbed) in 1 kg of air. A specific version of absorbed dose where the matter irradiated is air for X-ray radiation.	Gray (Gy)
Equivalent dose (H$_T$)	Absorbed dose weighted for harmful effects of particular types of radiation.	Sievert (Sv)
Effective dose (E)	Equivalent dose weighted for susceptibility to harm for different tissues.	Sievert (Sv)
Fluoroscopy time (FT)	Duration of fluoroscopy (X-ray on-time).	Minutes
Dose-area Product (DAP), or Kerma-area product (KAP)	Absorbed dose in air multiplied by X-ray beam area as the beam exits the X-ray tube head. Proportional to effective dose to the patient.	Gy·cm^2
Air kerma (AK)	Absorbed dose in air at a fixed point from the isocentre for the X-ray tube. A measure of the amount of energy absorbed by 1 kg of air for the X-ray beam. Useful indicator of skin dose to the patient.	Gray (Gy)
Hp(10)	Measure of personal dose at 10 mm depth of penetration; called Deep Dose Equivalent and is used for monitoring effective dose. Other depths of penetration may be used, e.g. 3 mm or 0.07 mm.	mSv

be 2.4 mSv.[6] The estimated average annual radiation dose due to environmental radioactivity in Australia has been estimated to be approximately 1.5 mSv.[7] Figure 7.1a shows the relative contribution to average annual radiation dose in Australia by natural sources of radiation.

Radiation exposure also results from artificial radiation sources such as medical diagnostic or industrial radiation sources. Exposure to these artificial radiation sources occurs depending on the workplace environment or need to undergo medical diagnosis or treatment. Staff working in the CCL are subject to occupational radiation exposure from artificial radiation sources.

Radiation exposure to workers and the public is subject to internationally recommended dose limits as discussed in Section 'Principles of Radiological Protection'.[1] These have been adopted in Australia within Commonwealth and State government radiation safety legislation.[3] Table 7.2 sets

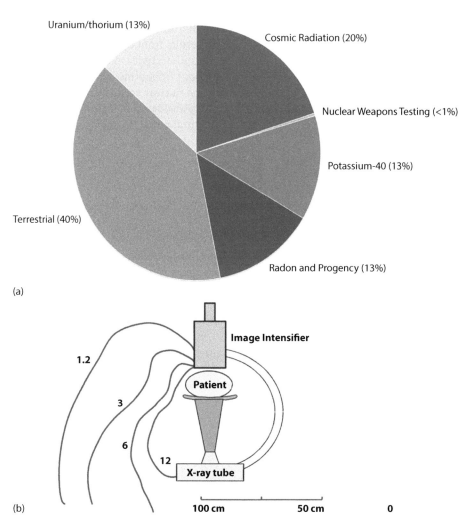

(a)

(b)

Figure 7.1 (a) Average annual dose from background radiation sources in Australia. (b) Example of dose rate contours around a mobile C-arm X-ray machine used for fluoroscopy. ([a] From Australian Radiation Protection and Nuclear Safety Agency, *What is Radiation?* [Internet]. Yallambie, AU, Australian Radiation Protection and Nuclear Safety Agency, [cited 2 May 2018], available from https://www.arpansa.gov.au/understanding-radiation/what-is-radiation; [b] Reproduced courtesy of International Atomic Energy Agency, Training-radiology_all_lectures.zip, RPDIR-L16.2_Fluoroscopy_dose_WEB.ppt [Lecture 16.2 Optimization of Protection in Fluoroscopy] [document on the Internet], Vienna, Austria, International Atomic Energy Agency, [cited 2 May 2018].)

Table 7.2 Recommended annual radiation dose limits

Type of exposure	Occupational exposure	Public exposure
Effective Dose	20 mSv per year, averaged over a period of five consecutive years	1 mSv in a year
Annual equivalent dose to:		
the lens of the eye	20 mSv per year, averaged over a period of five consecutive years	15 mSv
the skin	500 mSv	15 mSv
the hands and feet	500 mSv	

Source: International Commission on Radiological Protection, The 2007 Recommendations of the International Commission on Radiological Protection, ICRP Publication 103, Ann ICRP., 37, 1–332, 2007; Australian Radiation Protection and Nuclear Safety Agency, Code for Radiation Protection in Planned Exposure Situations, Radiation Protection Series C-1, Australian Radiation Protection and Nuclear Safety Agency, Yallambie, AU, 36. 2016.

out the recommended radiation dose limits for occupational and public radiation exposure. The recommended dose limits are intended to represent the maximum suggested level, not the allowable level. Actual radiation dose should always be as low as reasonably achievable (ALARA) and below the recommended dose limits. The average annual dose per capita due to medical radiation in Australia is estimated to be approximately 1.7 mSv.[7] This average is estimated for the entire Australian population, hence individual patients may receive much higher or lower radiation dose.

There is no regulatory limit on the amount of radiation exposure that a patient may receive due to diagnostic, therapeutic, or interventional medical procedures. Radiation exposure to patients is justified by the medical practitioner based on the benefit that may result from the medical treatment. Radiation levels in the CCL may be among the highest encountered during commonly performed radiological studies because of the requirement for extended exposure time. It is important for CCL staff to be aware of radiation dose levels and methods for reduction of exposure consistent with the requirement to obtain images of suitable diagnostic quality.

RADIATION EFFECTS

The effects of radiation exposure are grouped into two general categories:

- Deterministic Effects are radiation-induced injury to a large population of cells or tissue that impairs functioning of organs or tissues. The risk of cataracts is especially important

for cardiologists or radiologists performing interventional procedures using fluoroscopy. Deterministic effects occur above a threshold dose, with the severity increasing as radiation dose increases. Deterministic effects occur shortly after radiation exposure received in a short period of time, i.e. a high dose rate. The most common deterministic effect in the CCL is erythema of a patient's skin exposed within the field of view during the procedure. Higher doses will result in more significant damage to the irradiated skin.

- Stochastic Effects, or Late Effects, are radiation-induced cancer and heritable effects where the probability of an effect occurring increases with radiation dose, but the severity is not related to the radiation dose. Stochastic means 'random', which reflects the probability that such effects occur randomly, irrespective of the radiation dose. Late effects may occur many years after exposure and are believed to occur at any level of radiation dose, i.e. without a threshold. However, for low doses and low dose rates there is conflicting evidence for radiation effects. There is debate about the applicability of the current radiation risk model to low doses, which may be too small to allow detection of excess cancer or hereditary effects within a background of naturally occurring disease.[8,9]

The purpose of radiation protection in the CCL is to prevent immediate effects to the patient, and to minimise the risk of late effects for both staff and patients. The threshold for erythema for a patient is about 2 Gy–3 Gy absorbed dose to the skin,[10,11] although it can be difficult to determine the risk of erythema for complex cases involving multiple views. A medical physicist can provide an accurate estimate of radiation dose to organs and tissues, if required. The theoretical risk of late effects at or below the occupational radiation dose limit is very small compared to the natural incidence of cancer in the general population.

RADIATION SAFETY MEASURES FOR THE OPERATOR AND ASSISTANTS

Radiation dose to staff in the fluoroscopy room is mostly due to radiation scatter from the patient. Radiation scatter occurs from the first few centimetres of the patient, and it is important for staff working with medical fluoroscopy to have a good understanding of the pattern of scattered radiation around a patient. The amount of scattered radiation is related to the complexity of the procedure, size of the patient, modes of operation for the X-ray equipment, and the skill of the operator.[12] The radiation incident on the patient predominately scatters back towards the X-ray tube. Any radiation that is transmitted through the patient is further attenuated by the patient and the image receiver (image intensifier or flat panel detector). The radiation dose rate on the X-ray tube side of the patient is higher than the dose rate on the image receiver side of the patient. The lowest dose rate is typically behind the image receiver itself.

Figure 7.1b shows a typical distribution of scattered radiation around a patient[13] for the preferred positioning, with the x-ray tube underneath the patient. When the tube is positioned below the patient bed, the radiation dose rate to the head, upper body, and hands of the cardiologist and other staff is substantially lower because of the distribution of scattered radiation for this geometry. This is the recommended position for the majority of procedures due to the benefits of reducing radiation dose to staff.[14]

The protection methods used to reduce exposure from scatter radiation are to:

- Minimise TIME
- Maximise DISTANCE
- Maximise SHIELDING

Time

As time spent in a radiation field increases, the radiation dose received also increases. The beam-on time should be kept to an absolute minimum. Exposure time may be controlled at either the control panel or at the table-side by the foot pedal. Keeping fluoroscopic beam-on time and the number of image acquisitions to a minimum will prevent unnecessary radiation dose to the operator, attending personnel and the patient.

Distance

As distance from a radiation source increases, radiation dose decreases very rapidly. Doubling the distance between a person and the source reduces dose by one-fourth (1/4), according to the **inverse square law**. It is good practice for personnel to keep as much distance between themselves and the radiation source as is reasonably possible within the requirements of the procedure.

Shielding

Lead and concrete are the most commonly used materials for shielding against X- rays. The walls of X-ray rooms are usually lined with lead/plywood panels to reduce radiation to areas on the other side of the wall. Viewing areas are additionally protected with transparent lead acrylic windows. The lead equivalent of panels and windows should be assessed for each procedure room through the development of a shielding plan. The shielding thickness is expected to be at least 0.5 mm Pb, which gives about a 90% reduction of the scattered radiation. Portable or hanging transparent lead shields should be available in all modern procedure rooms. Lead shielding should be hanging from the patient bed of the side where most staff are positioned during the procedure. These shields can typically give an 85% dose reduction.

All personnel who are not positioned behind a radiation barrier must wear a protective lead apron and thyroid collar during the procedure. Aprons and collars are usually recommended to have a shielding value of not less than 0.3 mm lead equivalent at a set X-ray energy, but regulatory requirement will vary for each jurisdiction. Lead aprons must be properly stored on a hanger when not in use and handled with care to avoid damage that

Table 7.3 α and β values of the algorithms that best meet the criteria for determining best estimates of effective dose, and an algorithm based on ICRP Publication 103 weighting factors for effective dose

Algorithm	With thyroid shielding		Without thyroid shielding	
	α	β	α	β
Swiss Ordinance (2008)	1	0.05	1	0.1
McEwan (2000)			0.71	0.05
Von Boetticher (2010)	0.79	0.051	0.84	0.100

Source: Jarvinen, H. et al., *Radiat. Prot. Dosimetry.*,129, 333–339, 2008; ICRP, *Ann. ICRP.*, 37, 1–332, 2007; López, P.O. et al., *Ann. ICRP.*, 47, 1–118, 2018.

may compromise their shielding characteristics. Annual inspections should be conducted to detect imperfections in lead aprons. Leaded eyewear, fitted with side panels to reduce penetration of tangential scatter to the cornea, provide an extra measure of protection.

Personal dosimetry

Staff who regularly perform, or who assist in, fluoroscopic procedures are required to wear at least one personal radiation monitoring device. This single monitor is worn underneath the lead apron at the chest or waist position to provide an estimate of whole body radiation dose. There may be limitations to the estimated effective dose from a single monitor due to variability in exposure between protected and unprotected areas of the body. The preferred approach is for staff involved in fluoroscopy to wear two radiation monitors, with the second monitor worn outside the lead and as close to the collar as possible. This second monitor provides an estimate of radiation dose to the lens of the eye. The monitors should be clearly distinguished as to where they are worn to avoid confusion about their readings. Results should be regularly interpreted and reviewed to verify that work practices are adequate.

The best estimate of effective dose (E) for staff using lead aprons can be obtained from the readings of two radiation monitors, using the formula:

$$E = \alpha\, H_u + \beta\, H_o \qquad (7.1)$$

where E is effective dose, H_u and H_o are personal dose equivalents [$H_p(10)$], with H_u measured underneath the lead apron (either on the chest or the waist), and H_o is measured on the collar over the apron, and where α and β are pairs of weighting

factors. The limitation of this method for estimating effective dose is that there is no single α and β pair that can adequately represent occupational exposure for all geometries and all types of procedure. A comparison of α and β values[15] proposed by other authors has identified a set of values that best meet the criteria of no underestimation and minimum overestimation for typical geometries.[1] These values are presented in Table 7.3, along with α and β values based on the weighting factors for effective dose in ICRP Publication 103.[5]

RADIATION SAFETY MEASURES FOR THE PATIENT

The medical value of fluoroscopic X-rays is well recognised, but the potential risk is not, the usual assumption being that the benefit to the patient outweighs any radiation risk. It is important that measures are introduced to reduce the likelihood and severity of deterministic effects from fluoroscopically guided interventional procedures.

Skin injuries attributable to X-rays from fluoroscopy has been reported over recent decades[10] and the number of fluoroscopically guided interventions have increased dramatically over the last 30 years, and procedures have become more complex, more frequent and longer-lasting. More patients are obese, with patient size being a significant contributing factor to a high radiation dose. Radiation-induced skin injuries and epilation are the most commonly reported side effects of high-dose procedures,[10] and the severity of effects is related to the skin radiation dose. The most common effect is early, transient erythema that can occur within a few hours or up to 24 hours following an exposure of more than 2 Gy.[10] More serious effects, such as acute radiation injury and chronic radiation injury, following higher radiation exposure to the skin may occur weeks, months or years after exposure. As radiation-induced ulcers may occur with a long time delay and without obvious relationship to radiation exposure, it is important to provide information to the patient and to the referring doctor about a high radiation dose to assist in the correct diagnosis of skin injury, should it occur in the future.

Typically, the regulatory authority in each country sets output dose rate limits for fluoroscopy units. For example, in Australia, for continuous or pulsed fluoroscopy, the maximum allowable dose rate in air at the surface of the patient is 50 mGy/min without automatic exposure control, and 100 mGy/min with exposure control. However, for fluoroscopy with cine or digital image acquisition, there is no regulation or standard specifying a limit for the dose rate, either at the input to the image receiver or to the patient surface. In the past, evaluation of radiation doses received by patients required that radiation dose rates be known for the specific fluoroscopy system and for each mode of operation used during the various procedure types. These dose rates would ideally be derived from measurements performed by a medical physicist at the particular facility. Those measurements would then allow calculation of the screening time and number of cine runs that would lead to a given skin dose. Calculations such as these had to be documented for all the protocols used in the CCL.

Regulatory requirements have been updated such that fluoroscopic X-ray equipment is required to have a transmission ionisation chamber fitted into the X-ray tube head, post-collimation, to measure the **dose area product (DAP)**. This detector is often called a DAP meter. DAP is the absorbed dose in air multiplied by the area of the beam at the ionisation chamber, and may also be called **kerma area product (KAP)**; therefore, the unit for DAP is $Gy{\cdot}cm^2$, but the magnitude of the dose may be displayed as mGy, cGy, or μGy, depending of the preference of the equipment manufacturer. Common variations of displayed DAP units are $cGy{\cdot}cm^2$, $mGy{\cdot}cm^2$, or $μGy{\cdot}cm^2$. It is important to carefully note the units when comparing DAP between procedures undertaken on different X-ray equipment. DAP provides the most reliable dose measurement technique for dynamic radiological examinations involving varying projection directions and technique factors.

Because of the risk of immediate radiation effects, the focus of concern regarding harm from to patient radiation exposure is usually the absorbed dose to irradiated skin area in the primary beam. Radiation exposure to internal organs not in the path of the direct beam and possible late radiation effects are also a concern. Prior to the widespread use of DAP meters, estimation of dose to irradiated skin required records of the tube voltage, tube current, and total screening time; and for cine, the tube voltage and current, pulse width, frame rate, number of cine runs, and a list of projections used during a procedure. Measurement of DAP for a procedure simplifies the process of estimating radiation dose both to skin and to the patient. DAP, independent of field size and focal distance, is proportional to the effective dose, and hence radiation risk, to a patient. DAP is also proportional to the effective dose to staff working in a procedure room, so minimising patient dose also reduces radiation dose to staff.

The maximum skin entrance dose can be deduced from DAP if field size and X-ray focal spot to skin distance are known, but DAP alone does not allow determination of skin entrance dose. Fluoroscopy equipment fitted with a DAP meter will also measure absorbed dose in air, air kerma, at a fixed reference point from the X-ray tube (usually absorbed dose at a point 15 cm from the isocentre towards the focal spot). Air kerma at this point in space provides a good initial estimate of radiation dose to skin and should be used to determine the risk of immediate radiation effects for a patient. CCL staff may want to set an air kerma action level to determine the potential for skin injury and hence further follow up with the patient or the referring doctor (e.g. if >3 Gy, follow up for possible skin damage).

Modern fluoroscopy equipment provides a dose report at the end of a procedure that should be recorded and archived. The dose report will typically include total DAP and air kerma, as well as DAP and air kerma for each projection used during a procedure. Dose information may include DAP, air kerma, skin dose distribution, projection details, and peak skin dose.[14] Fluoroscopy time is not a useful indicator of patient radiation dose as it does not include the effect of fluoroscopy dose rate, nor the additional dose from cine-acquisition.

RECOMMENDATIONS FOR SAFE FLUOROSCOPY PRACTICE

Factors that determine radiation dose and dose rate to the patient (and to personnel) during fluoroscopy/fluorography are as follows:

Size of the patient

As the beam is positioned over more dense areas of a patient, the penetration of X-rays decreases. To maintain image quality, the tube voltage and/or tube current are adjusted automatically and/or manually. How this is done will determine the degree of increase in dose rate with increasing patient size.

Dose rates will be greater and dose will accumulate faster in larger patients

Tube current (mA)

Tube current determines the number of electrons involved in the production of radiation in the X-ray tube. X-ray production increases as tube current is increased. Tube current controls the number of X-rays that are available to be detected by the image receiver for a fixed tube voltage. Entrance dose rates are in direct proportion to tube current.

Keep the tube current as low as practicable

Tube voltage (kVp or kV)

Tube voltage determines the energy of the radiation produced by an X-ray tube. Higher voltage is generally required with the larger patient for increased beam penetration (image brightness) but this is accompanied by a lowering of image contrast and increase in X-ray energy, the latter being proportional to voltage. From the patient viewpoint, a higher energy beam is advantageous since it contains less of the softer or low energy X-rays that contribute to a higher skin dose, but it is not beneficial to image resolution to have a high-energy beam. Reducing tube current will lower X-ray production but will not affect penetration. Thus, it is preferable to operate with a higher voltage and low current than with a low voltage and a high current.

Keep the tube voltage as high as possible to achieve a compromise between image quality and low patient dose

Proximity of X-ray tube to the patient

It is important in all procedures to maintain the X-ray source at maximum distance from the patient's surface due to the protection offered by the inverse square law. This distance may be limited by the design of the unit, and arising from this it should be remembered that in the lateral and oblique projections, entrance dose rates at the patient's skin can be much higher than those measured in the anteroposterior (or postero-anterior) view, therefore avoid unnecessary oblique orientation.

Keep the X-ray tube at maximum distance from the patient

Proximity of image receiver to the patient

When the image intensifier or flat panel detector is close to the patient, image quality can improve, because of distortion of anatomy and image blurring resulting from geometric factors. Also, the intensity of X-rays required to produce a sufficiently bright image also decreases, resulting in a better image with lower patient dose.

Keep the image receiver as close to the patient as possible

Image magnification (most important for image intensifiers)

Entrance dose rate at the patient's skin is related to the magnification selected. A good approximation is that dose rates scale inversely with the area of the image intensifier's field size. Thus, compared to a 23 cm (9″) diameter field, a 15 cm (6″) field will require double the dose, and 31 cm (12″) will require half the dose. Image resolution on an image intensifier will improve with the use of magnification, but there is a greater relative increase in dose to the patient.

In modern fluoroscopy, flat panel detectors will increase dose when magnification is increased, but the relative dose increase is less than with image intensifiers. However, there may be very little or no improvement in image resolution at higher magnification.

Do not over-use the magnification (small field) mode of operation

X-ray field collimation

Collimators can be manually adjusted to reduce or enlarge the area of the X-ray field. Collimating to the area of interest reduces scattered radiation to the detector and so improves image quality. Reducing field size also reduces the volume of patient tissue being irradiated and consequently reduces the dose to personnel, since less scatter is generated. Counter-intuitively, because collimation will reduce the amount of scattered radiation reaching the image receiver, the automatic exposure control can increase the dose rate to compensate for very tight collimation,[16] and the dose rate to the patient's skin can increase significantly. Care should be taken to avoid collimation that is too tight. Modern units give a real-time reading of Gy·sec, which can inform the user if this scenario is happening.

Always use appropriate collimation where possible

Beam-on time

Minimising fluoroscopic beam-on time and the number of image acquisitions for a procedure will prevent unnecessary radiation dose to the patient, operator and other personnel. Do not screen when the live image on the TV monitor is not being used. Use the last-image hold after the beam is turned off for continued visualisation.

Keep beam-on time to an absolute minimum

SUMMARY

In brief, it is most important ALARA principles be adhered to. The potential for approaching or exceeding the threshold for skin injury must be recognised and that steps for avoidance be implemented. Safety procedures that minimise dose to patients and staff must always be adopted. Accurate and complete records of radiation dose used during procedures should be kept. Periodic review of dose metrics for each type of procedure should be encouraged to ensure patient dose remains **as low as reasonably achievable**. Further radiation safety information can be obtained from the radiation safety officer or a medical physicist at the hospital or institution.

ACKNOWLEDGEMENT

The author acknowledges the work of Dr Peter Cross, who contributed to the development of this chapter.

REFERENCES

1. International Commission on Radiological Protection (ICRP). The 2007 Recommendations of the International Commission on Radiological Protection. ICRP Publication 103. *Ann ICRP.* 2007;37(2–4):1–332.
2. Australian Radiation Protection and Nuclear Safety Agency. *Fundamentals for Protection Againstilonising Radiation.* Yallambie(AU): Australian Radiation Protection and Nuclear Safety Agency; 2014:32. Radiation Protection Series F-1.
3. Australian Radiation Protection and Nuclear Safety Agency. *Code for Radiation Protection in Planned Exposure Situations.* Yallambie, AU: Australian Radiation Protection and Nuclear Safety Agency; 2016:36. Radiation Protection Series C-1.
4. Australian Radiation Protection and Nuclear Safety Agency. *Code of Practice for Radiation Protection in the MedicalaApplicationsOfilonzingRadiation.* Barton, MI: Australian Radiation Protection and Nuclear Safety Agency; 2008:36. Radiation Protection Series No. 14.
5. López PO, Dauer LT, Loose R, Martin CJ, Miller DL, Vañó E, et al. ICRP Publication 139: Occupational radiological protection in interventional procedures. *Ann ICRP.* 2018;47(2):1–118.
6. United Nations Scientific Committee on the Effects of Atomic Radiation. *Sources and Effects of Ionizing Radiation: Volume 1 Sources.* New York: United Nations Publications; 2000:654.
7. Australian Radiation Protection and Nuclear Safety Agency. *What Is Radiation?* [Internet]. Yallambie, AU: Australian Radiation Protection and Nuclear Safety Agency; no date [cited 2 May 2018]. Available from: https://www.arpansa.gov.au/understanding-radiation/what-is-radiation.

8. Dauer LT, Brooks AL, Hoel DG, Morgan WF, Stram D, Tran P. Review and evaluation of updated research on the health effects associated with low-dose ionising radiation. *RadiatProt Dosimetry*. 2010;140(2):103–136.

9. Calabrese EJ, O'Connor MK. Estimating risk of low radiation doses: A critical review of the BEIR VII report and its use of the linear no-threshold (LNT) hypothesis. *Radiat Res*. 2014;182(5):463–474.

10. Jaschke W, Schmuth M, Trianni A, Bartal G. Radiation-Induced skin injuries to patients: What the interventional radiologist needs to know. *Cardiovasc IntervRadiol*. 2017;40(8):1131–1140.

11. Stewart F, Akleyev A, Hauer-Jensen M, Hendry J, Kleiman N, Macvittie T, et al. ICRP publication 118: ICRP statement on tissue reactions and early and late effects of radiation in normal tissues and organs–threshold doses for tissue reactions in a radiation protection context. *Ann ICRP*. 2012;41(1):1–322.

12. Vano E, Sanchez RM, Fernandez JM, Bartal G, Canevaro L, Lykawka R, et al. A set of patient and staff dose data for validation of Monte Carlo calculations in interventional cardiology. *RadiatProt Dosimetry*. 2015;165(1–4):235–239.

13. International Atomic Energy Agency. Training-radiology_all_lectures. zip: RPDIR-L16.2_Fluoroscopy_dose_WEB.ppt [Lecture 16.2 Optimization of Protection in Fluoroscopy]. Vienna, Austria: International Atomic Energy Agency; no date [cited 2 May 2018]. Available from: https://www.iaea.org/file/2017/training-radiologyalllectureszip.

14. Cousins C, Miller DL, Bernardi G, Rehani MM, Schofield P, Vañó E, et al. ICRP Publication 120: Radiological protection in cardiology. *Ann ICRP*. 2013;42(1):1–125.

15. Jarvinen H, Buls N, Clerinx P, Jansen J, Miljanic S, Nikodemova D, et al. Overview of double dosimetry procedures for the determination of the effective dose to the interventional radiology staff. *Radiat Prot Dosimetry*. 2008;129(1–3):333–339.

16. Koenig TR, Mettler FA, Wagner LK. Skin injuries from fluoroscopically guided procedures: Part 2, review of 73 cases and recommendations for minimizing dose delivered to patient. *Am J Roentgenol*. 2001;177(1):13–20.

8

Infection control procedures

DAVID ANDRESEN AND GIULIETTA PONTEVIVO

INTRODUCTION

In infection control, as in other areas of risk management, interventions may be prioritised according to two factors: the likelihood of the adverse event (infection), and the consequences if it does occur. While infection is uncommon in both coronary and electrophysiological procedures, the consequences can be severe–from ruptured mycotic aneurysms from infected femoral closure devices, to complete implanted device removal and prolonged antibiotic therapy for infected endocardiac leads. Happily, the scientific basis of infection prevention has evolved in the last two decades from the flimsy foundations of expert opinion and biological plausibility, to high quality observational–and in some cases randomised–data. While infection prevention is a responsibility of every healthcare worker, units with sound management, training, equipment, environment, and infection prevention protocols will be the best place to manage these important clinical and reputational risks.

DEFINITIONS

Accepted definitions in infection control ensure that we are speaking a common language and that our infection prevention data have external validity. Table 8.1 includes a list of the important and more frequently used terms applicable to any clinical or laboratory area.

RISKS AND CONSEQUENCES

Infectious risks of interventional cardiology procedures may be classified in several ways. We find it useful to consider separately the risk of blood-borne viruses, infections associated with vascular access or incision sites, and infections related to permanently retained devices. Blood-borne virus infections are uncommon so long as single-use devices are not reprocessed or reused. Such transmission events are generally either patient-to-healthcare-worker, or rarely, healthcare-worker-to-patient. Vascular access infections are uncommon in electrophysiology, due to predominantly venous

Table 8.1 Definitions in infection control

Aseptic technique/Aseptic non-touch technique (ANTT)	Aseptic technique consists of a set of specific practices and procedures performed under carefully controlled conditions. Aseptic technique protects patients during clinical procedures by applying infection prevention measures that minimise the presence of microorganisms on key parts of the equipment.
Clinical waste	Waste with potential to cause sharps injury, infection, or offence. When packaged and disposed of appropriately, there is virtually no public health significance. Clinical waste includes human tissues, bulk body fluids and blood, visibly blood-stained body fluids, and visibly blood-stained disposable material and equipment.
Colonisation	Detection of an organism from a site (usually skin, throat, nose, or perineum, and/or chronic ulcers or medical devices) that shows no sign of invasive infection.
Decolonisation (see load reduction)	Treatment of colonised persons with antimicrobials or antiseptics to eradicate a colonising microorganism with pathogenic potential.
Disinfection	Reduction of the number of viable microorganisms on a product or item to a level previously specified as appropriate for its intended further handling or use.
Hand hygiene	A general term referring to any action of hand cleansing. Includes washing hands with use of water, soap or a soap solution, either non-antimicrobial or antimicrobial, or applying a waterless alcohol-based hand rub (ABHR) to the surface of the hands (e.g. alcohol-based hand rub). When performed correctly, hand hygiene results in a reduction of microorganisms on hands.
MSSA	Methicillin-susceptible *Staphylococcus aureus.*
MRSA	Methicillin-resistant *Staphylococcus aureus*. A strain of S. aureus that is resistant to beta-lactam antibiotics including penicillins (such as flucloxacillin and nafcillin) and cephalosporins (such as cephalexin and cefazolin).
PPE	Personal protective equipment. Refers to a variety of infection prevention and control barriers and respirators used alone, or in combination, to protect mucous membranes, skin and clothing from contact with recognised and unrecognised sources of microorganisms in healthcare settings.
Pre-operative load reduction	Use of topical and/or systemic antibiotics to reduce *Staphylococcus aureus* or MRSA colonisation prior to surgical procedures, to reduce the infection risk associated with that procedure.
Screening	Microbiological testing for the purpose of detection of multi-resistant organisms carriage within a patient or population. By intent, screening is different to clinical diagnostic testing that is used in the setting of suspected infection.
Standard precautions	Standard precautions represent the minimum infection prevention measures that apply to all patient care, regardless of suspected or confirmed infection status of the patient in any setting where healthcare is delivered. These encompass precautions including healthcare worker vaccination, use of PPE, hand hygiene, sharps safety, and environment/equipment cleaning.

catheterisation sites and short device dwell-times. Arterial vascular access sites are more prone to infection, particularly if arteriotomy closure devices are used. Infection of coronary stents is remarkably rare.

Two large observational studies have suggested that infectious complications of coronary catheterisation occur at a rate of 0.1%–0.65%.[1,2] Electrophysiological device infections may be of the leads, the generator device, or both simultaneously. The rate of such device infections is typically 0.5%–2%,[3,4] or around 2 per 1,000 device-years, and may be rising. About half of these occur within a year of implantation and are thus presumed to be related to periprocedural device contamination. Risk factors for electrophysiological device infections include diabetes mellitus, heart failure, renal impairment, revision procedures, anticoagulation, and operator inexperience.[5] Infection prevention issues are briefly discussed in the American College of Cardiology Foundation angiography consensus statement.[6] The following sections address generic infection prevention issues and those specifically related to angiography, followed by a discussion of issues unique to electrophysiology procedures when they exist.

THE PATIENT

Many risks for cardiac disease such as smoking, obesity, and diabetes are also recognised risks for periprocedural infection, so patient selection and pre-procedure smoking cessation is important. Periprocedural blood sugar control is also important, with recent Centers for Disease Control guidelines[7] advocating a target of <11.1 mmol/L. Patients with active infections at the time of a procedure is planned should have these optimally treated, when possible, prior to the cardiological procedure.

PERSONNEL

Healthcare workers should be trained in general principles of infection prevention, hand hygiene,[8] and aseptic non touch-technique (ANTT) in addition to procedure-specific training. Use of standard precautions is the primary strategy for minimising transmission of healthcare-associated infections. Healthcare service organisations should ensure that standard precautions are implemented and consistent with current national/international guidelines. Additional ('transmission-based') precautions may need to be implemented to support standard precautions if the patient is known or suspected to have a communicable infection/disease and the procedure cannot safely be deferred. Borrowing from safety principles in other high-reliability industries, all staff should be empowered to speak up and stop procedures if they believe that infection control procedures have been breached.

Clinical healthcare workers and other staff who have patient contact should be vaccinated against hepatitis B, and be aware of their post-vaccination immunity status (vaccine response). Access to a suitable staff health service for counselling, management, and follow-up after occupational exposures such as sharps injuries or splash from body fluid exposure is mandatory. All healthcare workers in the perioperative environment have high risk of sustaining percutaneous injuries related to use of sharp devices. It is the responsibility of all involved to maintain a safe working environment while handling sharp instruments and needles.

Use of personal protective equipment, such as eye wear and/or face protection, impervious gowns, and sterile gloves by all members of the multidisciplinary team can minimise the risk of wound infection and protect staff from occupational exposure to microorganisms. Masks and eye protection should be removed after hand hygiene to minimise mucous membrane exposure to body fluids. All healthcare workers should have short-clipped nails, and artificial nails are not suitable. Nail polish should not be worn, and this includes shellac-type polish. Healthcare workers with dermatitis or other skin conditions should seek expert advice and not participate in procedures when their hands are affected. Watches, jewellery, and bracelets can harbour microorganisms and reduce the efficiency of hand hygiene, particularly of the skin under a ring.

The operator and assistants should wear an impervious surgical gown, fluid-resistant surgical mask (changed between each procedure) and eye protection. A clean hair cover (preferably disposable caps) covering all hair including sideburns, facial hair, and the nape of the neck should be worn. Sterile gloves should be used, and alternative products should be available for any staff with latex allergies. 'Double-gloving' has been advocated when patients have known blood-borne virus infections, but this may limit manual dexterity and is contrary to the principle of standard precautions. Use of surgical masks is of uncertain benefit but may assist in preventing contamination of the sterile field.[9]

ENVIRONMENT

The environment of the interventional cardiology laboratory should be fit for purpose, uncluttered, and have adequate storage facilities such that equipment and supplies are protected from dust and body fluid contamination. Recent evidence shows that a contaminated healthcare environment plays a significant role in the transmission of microorganisms.[10] Reference to local design and construction standards is essential. Contemporary British standards stipulate 15 air changes per hour, but 25 changes (as for an operating theatre) would seem desirable. Designated staff should be given maintenance and cleaning duties, and regular audits of the physical environment should occur.

Physical cleaning with a neutral detergent is an essential first step to remove dirt, debris, and other organic material. The floor should be wet-mopped between cases if soiling is evident. Two-in-one products with a detergent action and disinfectant properties are available, but their compatibility with equipment and surfaces should be checked. If disinfectants are used, they must be prepared and diluted to manufacturer's instructions. Noncritical items (such as procedure trolleys, sphygmomanometer cuffs, transducers, and monitors) should be adequately cleaned between patients. Clean mop heads and clean water/detergent should be used between each case. In addition to this between-case and as-required cleaning, comprehensive environmental cleaning at the end of each procedure list should include floors, bench tops, and other horizontal surfaces, furniture, and reusable equipment.

EQUIPMENT

Infection prevention and control experts should be consulted regarding purchasing and procurement decisions, allowing appropriate risk-assessment. The manufacturer's guidance should be followed unless there are strong reasons to the contrary. If there are such departures from product or device manufacturers' directions, these should be documented and approved through appropriate governance channels. Single-use devices should be traceable, and inventory management must ensure appropriate storage and adherence to shelf-life advice and use-by dates. For all invasive procedures, particularly those involving permanent device implantation, sterile technique is essential. Sterile drapes (preferably disposable) should be sufficiently large to cover the entire patient. Equipment immediately adjacent to the sterile field (e.g. image intensifier) should also be fully covered with suitable sterile drapes.

Femoral artery closure techniques are addressed in an American Heart Association Scientific Statement.[11] Arteriotomy closure devices have been associated with local infections and vascular complications such as arterial occlusion and false aneurysm formation, usually with staphylococci.[12,13] The role of antibiotic prophylaxis in this setting is unproven, but a single dose of 2 grams IV cefazolin may be considered when such closure devices are deployed. Routine use of prophylactic antibiotics in diabetic patients having arteriotomy closure devices has been advocated.[14]

Sharps must be disposed of directly into suitable puncture-proof containers, and disposal of contaminated equipment (bloodstained drapes, non-reusable items, etc.) must follow appropriate clinical waste streams according to local institutional policies.

THE PROCEDURE

Aseptic technique protects patients and healthcare workers during invasive clinical procedures by employing infection control measures that minimise the potential presence of pathogenic organisms on key parts of the equipment or invasive devices. ANTT is a framework for aseptic practice and its effective implementation has reduced rates of healthcare-associated infection. The principles of asepsis remain the same for all procedures, as each health service organisation has a duty to monitor and assess perioperative healthcare worker compliance with aseptic technique.

Hand hygiene is a general term referring to any action of hand cleansing. To prevent surgical site infections, the application of 'surgical hand antisepsis scrub' where hands are cleansed to the elbows for 2–5 minutes is required before the first procedure of a session,[9,15] with all wrist and finger bands, nail polish or artificial nails, and any other jewellery removed. Between cases, visible hand soiling should be removed with soap and water, and then hand hygiene performed with an approved antiseptic product prior to donning fresh sterile gloves for the next case. Surgical scrub using alcohol-based hand rub has recently been introduced for cases after the initial 5 minute scrub with water and an antimicrobial product.

If hair removal is required, use of electric clippers immediately before the procedure is preferred to shaving with a razorblade, which may create skin abrasions. Skin preparation in the sterile field should be with an alcoholic agent, as these have superior rapid bacterial killing to aqueous products.[16] There is no good evidence regarding choice of residual antiseptic agent (chlorhexidine or providone iodine), so this may be determined by local preferences and availability. Prophylactic antibiotics are not required for coronary procedures.

ISSUES SPECIFIC TO ELECTROPHYSIOLOGICAL PROCEDURES

Screening of preoperative general surgery patients for *Staphylococcus aureus* nasal carriage, followed by 5 days of preoperative staphylococcal decolonisation of carriers with nasal mupirocin and chlorhexidine body washes reduced all postoperative staphylococcal surgical site infection by 60% and deep infections by 80%.[17] While this has not been demonstrated specifically in electrophysiological procedures, the topical agents used are safe and not expensive. However, standardising the screening and prescribing may be difficult in some settings, in which case universal rather than targeted preoperative decolonisation may be considered. For instance, a Pittsburgh unit employs 5 days of pre-procedure Chlorhexidine washes for outpatients, and from the day of admission for inpatient (emergency) procedures.[18] British guidelines[4] advocate periprocedural load reduction in known methicillin sensitive *Staphlococcus aureus* (MSSA) or Methicillin-resistant *Staphylococcus aureus* (MRSA) carriers.

Haematoma in the pectoral pocket is a risk factor for device infection. The American Heart Association/Heart Rhythm Society guideline[5] recommends careful technique to avoid local haematoma formation, and avoidance of postoperative heparin administration.

Preoperative intravenous antibiotic therapy reduces the risk of device infection by 60%–95%.[19] Both the American Heart Association/Heart Rhythm Society guidelines[5] and the British Heart Rhythm Society/British Cardiovascular Society guidelines[4] endorse the use of single dose intravenous anti-staphylococcal antibiotic prophylaxis for insertion of electrophysiological devices. This is usually cefazolin, or sometimes vancomycin in centres where resistance rates among staphylococci are high (or for known MRSA carriers).

More recent data have shown that vancomycin is an inferior prophylactic agent against MSSA, so if a glycopeptide antibiotic is required it should probably be added to cefazolin rather than replacing it. Preoperative nose and throat swab screening for *Staphylococcus aureus* with susceptibility determination would allow more precise targeting of procedural prophylaxis. The glycopeptide teicoplanin has considerable advantages over vancomycin, being administered as a slow push rather than an infusion over several hours, but is usually more expensive. An optimised procedural prophylaxis regimen might therefore be:

- *MRSA carriers:* 2 grams cefazolin (3 g > 120 kg body weight) statim **plus** 800 mg teicoplanin statim
- *MSSA carriers:* 2 grams cefazolin (3 g > 120 kg body weight)
- *Non-carriers:* 2 grams cefazolin (3 g > 120 kg body weight)

There are no data supporting the ongoing administration of either intravenous or oral antimicrobials beyond completion of the procedure. Such use will increase side-effects, promote antimicrobial resistance, and possibly defer recognition of early device infections.[5] A large Canadian randomised clinical trial (RCT)[20] has just reported its results verbally: In almost 20,000 electrophysiological device recipients, an intensified antibiotic prophylaxis strategy of pocket antibiotic lavage and two days of postoperative oral antibiotics was no better than standard single dose prophylaxis. Allergic reactions were significantly increased in the intensified strategy group, and resistance outcomes were not assessed. If these findings are confirmed after peer review and full publication, this trial will confirm single dose systemic antibiotic prophylaxis as the contemporary standard of care. Use of topical antibiotic agents (e.g. pocket irrigation) should be regarded as having unproven safety and efficacy and should be avoided.

An 'antibacterial envelope' has recently been marketed for electrocardiac device insertion that contains rifampin and minocycline, antibacterials with a good track record as impregnated agents in central lines. Preliminary safety data for this device are encouraging,[21] but efficacy assessment awaits the results of a current RCT. The high acquisition cost may be a barrier to use in some settings. Wound dressing with sterile gauze and/or a sterile transparent semipermeable dressing is recommended.[18]

OUTCOMES

Rare infectious outcomes (such as arteriotomy site infections, blood-borne virus transmission) should be investigated individually by Root Cause Analysis methodologies by a multidisciplinary team. Other infections (such as electrophysiological device infections within 12 months of insertion) should be monitored systematically using process control techniques, to detect increases above baseline or benchmark infection rates. Adverse infectious outcomes should be reported via existing institutional processes, such as incident management systems. If 'clusters' occur, then deeper investigation such as a RCA process or quality improvement intervention may be required, with external input from people with appropriate skill sets.

SUMMARY

It is ultimately up to the individual operator to implement all appropriate infection control guidelines, and to unit leadership to provide the policies, resources, and training to ensure that this occurs. In team-oriented environments such as the electrophysiology and cardiac catheterisation laboratories, suitable staff training, equipment, supervision, and clear protocols are essential to maintain satisfactory standards and ensure the lowest possible infection rate. Ongoing monitoring of procedure-associated infections and prompt investigation of adverse incidents or increasing infection rates will provide a second line of defence against these high-consequence infection events.

REFERENCES

1. Muñoz P, Blanco JR, Rodríguez-Creixéms M, García E, Delcan JL, Bouza E. Bloodstream infections after invasive nonsurgical cardiologic procedures. *Arch Inter Med.* 2001:161: 2110–2115.

2. Samore MH, Wessolossky MA, Lewis SM, Shubrooks S, Karchmer AW. Frequency, risk factors, and outcome for bacteremia after percutaneous transluminal coronary angioplasty. *Am J Cardiol.* 1997:79(7): 873–877.

3. Bongiorni MG, Marinskis G, Lip GYH, Svendsen JH, Dobreanu D, Blomström-Lundqvist C. How European centres diagnose, treat, and prevent CIED infections: Results of a European heart rhythm association survey. *EP Europace.* 2012:14(11): 1666–1669.

4. Sandoe JAT, Barlow G, Chambers JB, Gammage M, Guleri A, Howard P, et al. Guidelines for the diagnosis, prevention and management of implantable cardiac electronic device infection. Report of a joint working party project on behalf of the British Society for antimicrobial chemotherapy (BSAC, host organization), British Heart Rhythm Society (BHRS), British Cardiovascular Society (BCS), British Heart Valve Society (BHVS) and British Society for Echocardiography (BSE). *J Antimicrob Chemother.* 2015:70(2): 325–359.

5. Baddour LM, Epstein AE, Erickson CC, Knight BP, Levison ME, Lockhart PB, et al. Update on Cardiovascular Implantable Electronic Device Infections and Their Management: A Scientific Statement From the American Heart Association, endorsed by the Heart Rhythm Society. *Circulation.* 2010: 121:458–477.

6. Bashore TM, Balter S, Barac A, Byrne JG, Cavendish JJ, Chambers CE, et al. American College of Cardiology Foundation/Society for Cardiovascular Angiography and Interventions Expert Consensus Document on Cardiac Catheterization Laboratory Standards Update: A report of the American College of cardiology foundation task force on expert consensus documents. *J Am Coll Cardiol.* 2012:59(24): 2221–2305.

7. Berríos-Torres SI, Umscheid CA, Bratzler DW, Leas B, Stone EC, et al. Centers for disease control and prevention guideline for the prevention of surgical site Infection. *JAMA Surgery.* 2017:152(8): 784–791.

8. Centers for Disease Control and Prevention. Guideline for hand hygiene in health-care settings: Recommendations of the health-care infection control practices Advisory Committee and the HICPAC/SHEA/APIC/IDSA hand hygiene task force. *Morbidity and Mortality Weekly Review* 2012:51(No. RR-16).

9. World Health Organization. *Global Guidelines for the Prevention of Surgical Site Infection.* Geneva, Switzerland: WHO. 2016. Accessed 3 January 2018 at http://apps.who.int/iris/bits tream/10665/250680/1/9789241549882-eng. pdf.

10. Dancer SJ. Controlling hospital acquired infection: Focus on the role of the environ-ment and new technologies for decon-tamination. *Clin Microbiol Rev.* 2014:27(4): 665–690.

11. Patel MR, Jneid H, Derdeyn CP, Klein LW, Levine GN, Lookstein RA, et al. Arteriotomy closure devices for cardiovascular pro-cedures: A scientific statement from the American Heart Association. *Circulation.* 2010:122: 1882–1893.

12. Johanning JM, Franklin DP, MD, Elmore JR, MD, Han DC. Femoral artery infections associated with percutaneous arterial clo-sure devices. *J Vasc Surg.* 2010:34: 983–985.

13. Carey D, Martin JR, Moore CA, Valentine MC, Nygaard TW. Complications of femoral artery closure devices. *Catheter Cardiovasc Interv.* 2001:52: 3–7.

14. Baddour LM, Bettmann MA, Bolger AF, Epstein AE, Ferrieri P, Gerber MA, et al. Nonvalvular cardiovascular device-related infections. *AHA Scientific Statement. Circulation.* 2003:108: 2015–2031.

15. Australian College of Operating Room Nurses. *Standards for Perioperative Nursing in Australia.* 14th ed. Adelaide, Australia:ACORN. 2016.

16. Darouiche RO, Wall MJ, Itani KMF, Otterson MF, Webb AL, Carrick MM, et al. Chlorhexidine-Alcohol versus povidone: Iodine for surgical site antisepsis. *N Engl J Med.* 2010:362 (1): 18–26.

17. Bode LGM, Kluytmans JAJW, Wertheim HFL, Bogaers D, Vandenbroucke-Grauls CMJE, Roosendaal R, et al. Preventing surgical site infections in nasal carriers of *Staphylococcus aureus. New England J Med.* 2010:362(1):9–17.

18. Sastry S, Rahman R, Yassin MH. Cardiac implantable electronic device infection: From an infection prevention perspec-tive. *Advances in Preventative Medicine* 2010:Article ID 357087: 8 pages. doi:10.1155/2015/357087.

19. Darouiche R, Mosier M, Voigt J. Antibiotics and antiseptics to prevent infection in car-diac rhythm management device implanta-tion surgery. *PACE.* 2012:35: 1348–1360.

20. Krahn AD, Philippon F, Exner DV, Birnie DH, Saginur R, Mangat I, et al. Prevention of arrhythmia device infection trial (PADIT): Pilot study results. *Can J Cardiol.* 2012: 28: S394.

21. Henrikson CA, Sohail R, Acosta H, Johnson EE, Rosenthal L, Pachulski D, et al. Antibacterial envelope is associated with low infection rates after implantable cardioverter-defibrillator and cardiac resyn-chronization therapy device replacement. Results of the Citadel and Centurion stud-ies. *JACC: Clin Electrophysiol.* 2017:3(10): 1158–1167.

9

Nursing care of the cardiac catheterisation patient

JULIE PARKINSON, JO-ANNE M. VIDAL AND EVA KLINE-ROGERS

INTRODUCTION

Contemporary nursing practice in the cardiac catheterisation laboratory (CCL) has changed significantly over the past decade with the introduction of percutaneous procedures for a variety of indications, including structural heart disease. Most of the new structural heart treatments are now performed using a percutaneous approach, resulting in fewer adverse events, shorter recovery times and hospital lengths of stay, and lower healthcare costs. In general, patients undergoing cardiac catheterisations are better informed, demand more access to their medical care records, and expect shorter waiting and procedural times with quick hospital discharge, better outcomes, and improved communication from the cardiac team.

Cardiac catheterisation nurses are now, more than ever, challenged to diversify and broaden their skills. Procedures are more complicated and patients have comorbidities requiring involvement from anaesthetic, cardiothoracic, vascular and surgical teams. Patients requiring cardiac catheterisation arrive via the emergency department, hospital ward, the coronary care unit, from other hospitals and from the general community. Hence, CCL nurses are required to facilitate coordination of multiple team members, and to be more knowledgeable in their ability to assess and anticipate potential adverse events in addition to rapidly detecting and treating such events. Furthermore, as members of the multidisciplinary team, nurses are in a unique position to clarify the benefits and risks associated with different procedures, ensure adherence to safety protocols, and to anticipate and manage unexpected complications. Provision of nursing care should be culturally sensitive, and a non-English speaking patient must have access to professional interpreter services, in addition to pre/during/post care periods, especially for consent. This ensures accuracy and impartiality in communicating information.

PRE-CARDIAC CATHETERISATION PROCESS

Prior to admission, patients are reviewed by the relevant medical specialist. Upon determining the need for a coronary angiogram, supportive services and referrals are established, encompassing geriatrics, vascular, social and other services. Cardiac catheterisation procedures are commonly performed on an elective basis. This allows time to obtain the following information:

- Demographic information including full name, date of birth, contact details, next of kin.
- Symptoms, past medical history.
- Current medications including supplements (dose and frequency), allergies.
- Previous cardiac procedures and diagnostic testing, e.g. an electrocardiogram (ECG), computed tomography cardiac catheterisation (CTCA), stress test or stress echocardiogram, myocardial perfusion scan, previous cardiac catheterisation performed and results, previous percutaneous coronary intervention (PCI), previous cardiac surgery (including coronary artery bypass graft [CABG] operation report or post-CABG angiography delineating number, location and territory of vessels).
- Relevant input from other specialties such as renal and respiratory physician, endocrinologist, vascular surgeon and others.
- Full physical workup, assessment of potential arterial access sites.
- Pre-procedure airway assessment and pre-notification of high-risk patients e.g. body mass index >35, prior difficulty with sedation analgesia, substance abuse, expected length of procedure >6 hours, sleep apnea, significant pulmonary disease (peripheral capillary oxygen saturation [SpO_2] <94% on room air), significant renal/hepatic impairment or low ejection fraction.[1]
- Pathology results such as electrolytes, renal function (urea, creatinine, estimated glomerular filtration rate [eGFR] or creatinine clearance [CrCl]), full blood count (FBC) and coagulation studies, obtained as close to the procedure date as possible. Expert consensus, however, recommends 2–4 weeks prior to the planned procedure.[2] These should be repeated prior to the planned procedure if there has been a clinical or medication change within that period, or recent contrast media administration.[2] Similarly, coagulations studies or international normalised ratio (INR) may need to be assessed just prior to the procedure date to ensure procedural safety.
- Baseline 12-lead electrocardiogram (ECG) is useful for comparison, particularly during the immediate post-procedural phase.

PATIENT PREPARATION

Patient education

Patient education is initially commenced by the cardiologist once the decision for the procedure has been made and continues through the patient's hospital stay. Importantly, information should be provided in small amounts and appropriate to each stage of the admission, so as not to overwhelm the patient. Upon admission, the education focus should include preparation for the procedure, with only a brief mention of discharge considerations such as activity/work/driving restrictions. A brief overview of the day can occur during the initial patient interview and assessment. It is important to discuss the procedure in terms the patient can understand, without technical jargon and aimed at a level appropriate for the patient. Ideally, family members should be included in the conversation and any written materials should be prepared at a 5th grade reading level.

Education should then focus on likely access routes, expected sensations, the steps of the procedure, approximate timeline and what happens at the end of the procedure. Patients should also know when to expect the procedural results and future recommendations. For a patient undergoing cardiac catheterisation, results may be communicated as (1) normal heart arteries; (2) minor disease or narrowing of the heart arteries best treated with medications (medical management); (3) stents and/or balloons to the heart arteries (PCI); (4) heart bypass surgery; or (5) for further discussion with the heart team involving the patient and family.

Post-procedural patient education should progress to haemostasis techniques and expected sensations, frequency of observations and assessments, mobilisation protocols and when the patient can resume drinking and eating. Discharge considerations such as recommencement of medications (or changes to medications), vascular access site care, referral to cardiac rehabilitation, and more detailed explanations regarding activity, work and driving restrictions should be given.

At each stage of the patient's journey, good communication and patient education by a confident, reassuring, professional and friendly team is the patient's ultimate confidence builder.[3(p7)]

Consent

Written, informed consent is a legal and ethical prerequisite for all CCL procedures and is obtained by the performing clinician. An informed consent should contain information about the planned procedure and cover all possible scenarios (e.g. emergency CABG or unplanned procedures such as PCI), reasons for recommendations, risks and benefits, alternatives (e.g. medical management in the very elderly if so indicated), contain no abbreviations (e.g. CABG for coronary artery bypass graft) and have adequate opportunity for questions. Patients with cognitive impairment and unable to provide informed consent must have a responsible person present (e.g. legal guardian), including during the Time-Out process immediately before commencement of the procedure. Informed consent for emergency procedures while difficult, must demonstrate an attempt to provide information to the patient and family about risk, and benefit, and balance this with rapid intervention.[4]

Documentation

Documentation in the CCL is commenced with a referral that is thorough, complete, and provides enough information for staff preparation to commence before the patient is seen by the cardiologist (or delegated medical officer). Documentation encompasses both electronic and paper records, and each hospital has its own policies related to recording and documentation of CCL procedures, including the archiving of cineangiography images. Documentation includes patient history, medications and allergies, risk factors, physical assessments including vital signs, vascular access site and baseline neurovascular observations, dentures, prostheses, belongings, fasting, voiding, falls and pressure area risk, intravenous (IV) fluids, blood tests, blood glucose level (BGL) and specifics regarding the procedure being performed. Patients should bring in their current medications so they can be documented, dosage checked and administered if required. Outpatients who are admitted can then use their own supply as long as charted by the medical officer.

Patient identification requires at least three unique patient identifiers—full name, date of birth and hospital medical record number. Patient identification must include double-checking the patient's name, date of birth and allergies against hospital identification bands. As per local hospital policy, colour-coded identification bands can be applied to separate limbs to identify allergies. It is suggested that allergies should be ascertained with every admission, so only the patient's aforementioned details can be found on the band. Patient identification should occur at each transfer of care, e.g. from admission area to recovery, entry to procedure room, during Team Time-Out, on return to recovery or discharge area, and in other areas as appropriate for each unique hospital setting.

Fasting

There is a paucity of evidence guiding the optimal period of fasting required for the range of procedures that involve local anaesthesia, procedural sedation or general anaesthesia in the CCL. Historically, nil by mouth was strictly imposed, primarily due to first-generation contrast agents (ionic and high-osmolar contrast media) that induced nausea and vomiting (4.58% and 1.84%, respectively)[5,6] with increased risk of aspiration. However, low osmolar, non-ionic contrast media rarely induce vomiting (0.3%).[7] The historical nil by mouth culture in CCLs may be based on anaesthesiologist guidelines in the past. Routine fasting of patients prior to cardiac catheterisation and PCI is not justifiable, with no increase in intra-procedural endotracheal intubation and/or aspiration pneumonia[8] and is not recommended by Australian,[9] North American[4] or European guidelines.[10] This is particularly relevant with emergent procedures where fasting status is of lower priority than the emergency itself. Pre-procedural fasting is still strongly recommended by some[9] as sedative agents may impair airway reflexes and place the patient at increased risk of aspiration of gastric contents.[3(p14)] In procedures requiring general anaesthesia, fasting may be indicated, and local policy should be followed.

Cannulation

IV cannulation allows immediate IV access during routine or emergency procedures for the administration of IV fluids (for routine prehydration and IV bolus in the emergency setting), sedation, analgesia, antibiotics, blood transfusion and vasoactive medications, if required. Positioning of the IV cannula must be appropriate to the procedure and has recently evolved with the increase in radial access procedures. Considerations include avoiding the wrist and back of the hand on the planned radial access limb, use of a proximal large-bore IV cannula for administration of IV adenosine for fractional flow reserve study, and IV cannula insertion on the same arm as the access site for non-invasive blood pressure (NiBP) measurements and non-obstruction of IV fluids on the ipsilateral arm. An IV port should be available close to the IV entry site for emergency medications, but also an additional port should be accessible once the patient is draped (e.g. halfway up the IV line for administration of sedation, but avoiding unnecessary radiation to the circulating nurse).

Special patient preparation

PATIENTS WITH DIABETES

Patients with diabetes requiring procedures within the CCL are at an increased risk of poor glycaemic control due to fasting, interruptions to usual medication regimens and predispose the patient to an increased risk of adverse outcomes.[11] Furthermore, preparation of the diabetic patient is often managed on an ad-hoc basis by those with limited expertise in this area, and evidence to support practice is lacking. Medical guidelines generally provide limited direction for CCL nurses in the management of diabetic patients including fasting, monitoring of BGLs oral hypoglycaemic agents (other than metformin) and insulin regimens.[2,12–14] Nursing guidelines are also similarly limited in recommendations for the nursing care of diabetic patients.[9]

The Australian Diabetes Society,[11] for example, provides guidelines for management of diabetic patients in the peri-operative period. While not specifically designed for CCLs, radiological procedures are covered and peri-operative diabetic management principles can be applied to the CCL setting. Pre-procedural evaluation to determine the type of diabetes and optimal management aims to ensure the patient with diabetes is well prepared, that the diabetes is well controlled, and to ensure the patient is capable of pre- and post-procedure instructions. Distinction between Type 1 and Type 2 diabetes can be difficult with both Type 1 and long-standing Type 2 diabetics at an increased risk of diabetic ketosis or ketoacidosis within hours if insulin is withdrawn or omitted, especially at times of physiological stress when counter-regulatory hormone production is increased.[11]

To minimise disruption to glycaemic control, diabetic patients should undergo elective procedures early on morning procedural lists, where fasting is as short as possible (if required at all). For non-elective, complex procedures or procedures required later in the day, medications should be reduced or withheld. Specific guidelines are problematic due to the variety of diabetes classifications, medications and types of procedures offered in the CCL; however, the Australian Diabetes Society[11] provides the following guide:

Insulin-treated patients on a morning list:

- Patients scheduled first on a morning list may be able to delay their insulin and breakfast until after their procedure, provided the procedure is short and they are capable of eating by 10:00 am.
- Patients scheduled for later procedures (morning list) may have a half-dose in the form of intermediate or long-acting insulin, although short-acting insulin should be avoided. Following procedures, a half dose of short-acting insulin can be administered prior to lunch.
- Patients should resume their usual insulin and diet in the evening.

Insulin-treated patients on an afternoon list:

- Patients may have a small dose of short-acting insulin together with a half-dose of usual intermediate- or long-acting insulin together with breakfast.
- Patients should resume their usual insulin and diet in the evening.
- If glycaemic control becomes erratic during or following the procedure, the patient should be admitted overnight for observation and/or stabilisation.

Patients on oral anti-hyperglycaemic (AHG) medications:

- AHGs should be withheld on the day of procedure and resumed at normal mealtime at night.
- Metformin should be omitted 24 hours prior to the procedure and resumed 48 hours after the procedure (as long as renal function has not changed significantly). This recommendation is related to the risk of severe and persistent lactic acidosis associated with metformin and contrast media, especially in the setting of chronic kidney disease (CKD). However, metformin should not be used in patients with severe CKD[2] and the dose reduced in patients with moderate CKD.[15] However, evidence is lacking regarding patients with normal renal function and some guidelines recommend taking metformin normally.[15]

- Sodium glucose co-transporter 2 inhibitors (SGLT2i), a newer class of AHG agents used in Type 2 diabetes (e.g. dapaglifozin [Forxiga®, Bristol-Myers Squibb], empagliflozin [Jardiance, Boehringer Ingelheim] or a combination with metformin [Xigduo, Astra Zeneca; Jardiamet, Boehringer Ingelheim]) should be withheld 2 days prior to procedures due to the risk of severe euglycaemic diabetic ketoacidosis with near normal or only mildly elevated BGLs.[16]

Blood Glucose Level (BGL) monitoring frequency:

- All diabetic patients must have a BGL on admission pre-procedure.
- Insulin-treated patients must have regular BGLs (e.g. 2 hourly).
- AHG-treated patients must have regular BGLs (e.g. 4 hourly).
- Diabetic patients on diet alone should have increased frequency of BGLs (e.g. 4 hourly). Hyperglycaemia may require supplemental insulin and/or initiation of AHG.
- Any patient with a BGL falling outside 5–10 mmol/L should have increased monitoring frequency of BGLs.
- If BGL is less than 4.0 mmol/L, glucose should be given.
- An insulin-glucose infusion is the best way to maintain normoglycaemia.

PATIENTS WITH CHRONIC KIDNEY DISEASE (CKD) AND POST-CONTRAST ACUTE KIDNEY INJURY (PC-AKI)

Contrast media is predominantly excreted by the kidneys[17] with patients suffering CKD at an increased risk of developing post-contrast acute kidney injury (PC-AKI) (also known as contrast induced nephropathy [CIN]). PC-AKI is defined as an acute reduction in kidney function, a relative increase in serum creatinine (≥25%, or 44 µmol/L [0.5 mg/dL]) or a decrease in glomerular filtration rate (GFR) or creatinine clearance (CrCl) 48–72 hours post-contrast exposure.[18(p275)] The overall incidence of PC-AKI in the general population is <3% but can rise to 50% or more in patients with multiple risk factors.[19(p245),20] The risk of needing dialysis as a result of PC-AKI remains small.[18(p275)] The true incidence of PC-AKI may be overestimated, as there are many causes of AKI following cardiac catheterisation and PCI, e.g. haemodynamic instability resulting in cholesterol or thrombotic embolisation to the renal arteries caused by catheter manipulations.[21]

Major risk factors for PC-AKI include fixed risk factors (CKD, diabetes mellitus, congestive heart failure, advanced age, female gender) and modifiable risk factors (hypotension, anaemia, nephrotoxic drugs, hypercholesterolemia, peri-procedural dehydration/hypovolemic states, pre-procedural hyperglycaemia, contrast type and contrast volume).[22]

The mechanism of CIN is not completely understood, and is thought to be attributed to direct renal toxicity and acute tubular necrosis.[18(p275)] The only proven major strategies to reduce CIN include IV pre-hydration and minimising the amount of contrast media, which are supported by Australian,[9] North American[2,13] and European[14] guidelines. Intravascular volume expansion through the use of 0.9% sodium chloride maintains renal blood flow, preserves nitric oxide production, prevents medullary hypoxemia, and enhances contrast elimination.[23] There is no clear evidence of benefit for IV sodium bicarbonate, or adjunctive pharmaceuticals including N-acetylcysteine, mannitol, ascorbic acid, dopamine, haemofiltration/dialysis among others.[22,24-28] Additional advantages of IV sodium chloride 0.9% are low cost, ease of use and no risk of compounding errors. Iso-osmolar non-ionic contrast (iodixanol e.g. Visipaque™) may be superior to low-osmolar ionic contrast (iohexol e.g. Ultravist®, Omnipaque™), especially in octogenarian diabetic patients.[23]

Pre-procedure assessment and counselling are important to determine patient risk and to employ preventative measures to mitigate the adverse consequence of PC-AKI post administration of contrast.[24] Nurses are therefore in an ideal position to improve at-risk patient outcomes by:

- Encouraging IV pre-, peri- and post-hydration regimens.
- Identifying potential nephrotoxic medications (e.g. non-steroidal anti-inflammatory drugs).
- Suggesting left ventricular end diastolic pressure (LVEDP) guided hydration management.[24]
- Discussing an agreed contrast volume limit with the proceduralist at Time-Out.[2]
- Avoiding 'test' or 'puff' injections, reminders of CKD if ventriculography/aortography suggested, and limiting number of angiographic views.[2]
- Monitoring contrast volume during procedures (using volumes that are as low as reasonably achievable [ALARA] and notifying the proceduralist once agreed contrast volume has been reached e.g. contrast volume should not exceed twice the baseline eGFR,[23] noting there is no absolutely safe limit of contrast dose).
- Discussing patient risk if ad hoc procedure is considered. A preferred strategy may involve staging procedures 72 hours apart.
- Encouraging oral intake of fluids (in addition to IV hydration) to maintain volume expansion.
- Maintaining strict fluid balance charting.
- Ensure patient education and encourage general practitioner follow-up including electrolytes, urea and creatinine (EUCs) at 72–84 hours post contrast administration.
- In dialysis patients, the coordination of an extra haemodialysis session or exact timing of dialysis to remove contrast medium post-procedure is unnecessary unless avoiding volume overload.[15]

Several pre-, peri- and post-procedural hydration regimens have been proposed, including sodium chloride 0.9% 1–1.5 mL/kg/h 3–12 hours before and 12–24 hours after the procedure;[22,23] however, this does not suit the outpatient day procedure population, where total time in hospital may be 6 hours or less. In these patients it has been proposed a 3 mL/kg infusion of sodium chloride 0.9% over 1 hour pre-procedure and 1–1.5 mL/kg/hour for 4–6 hours post-procedure be administered.[29] For an LVEDP guided approach, the alternative has been suggested:

- LVEDP < 13 mmHg–5 mL/kg/h × 4 hours
- LVEDP 13–18 mmHg –3 mL/kg/h × 4 hours
- LVEDP > 18 mmHg –1.5 mL/kg/h × 4 hours[24,30]

Forced diuresis to maintain euvolemia using LVEDP, while novel, requires further research.[15] Patients with severe heart failure (NYHA grade 3–4) hydration protocols should be individualised for type, volume and duration.[15]

ANTICOAGULATED PATIENTS

Pre- and peri-procedural management of patients taking anticoagulant medications is a common clinical conundrum frequently involving multidisciplinary teams and specialties, and practices vary greatly between institutions.[31] Procedures performed in the CCL range from low, intermediate to high risk of bleeding with the American College of Cardiology Interventional, Electrophysiological and Surgeons section leadership councils providing consensus guidelines on various procedures and bleeding risk level[31] (online appendix):

- Low-risk – cardiac catheterisation/PCI via transradial route, right heart catheterisation, most atrial fibrillation (AF)/flutter ablations, permanent pacemaker, implantable cardioverter defibrillator
- Low to intermediate risk – cardiac catheterisation via transfemoral route
- Intermediate risk – PCI via transfemoral route, intra-aortic balloon pump, pericardiocentesis, percutaneous mitral valve repair, left atrial appendage occlusion, endovascular grafting
- High risk – transaortic valve replacement (TAVR, also known as transaortic valve implantation, TAVI), aortic valvuloplasty, mechanical circulatory support

However, procedural complexity may impact procedural risk of bleeding and even procedures with low risk of bleeding may have significant bleeding sequelae in the event of complications. In addition, individual patient factors such as pre-procedure anaemia or coagulation disorder may also impact on the bleeding risk.

Vitamin K antagonist (VKA) therapy (most commonly, warfarin) remains the most common anticoagulant worldwide although non-vitamin K antagonist oral anticoagulants (NOACs) (also known as direct oral anticoagulants [DOACs]) are now a mainstream therapy for non-valvular AF and the treatment and prevention of thromboembolism. Warfarin has a half-life of approximately 36–42 hours whereas for NOACs the half-life is dependent on renal function, ranging from 6–27 hours (normal renal function [CrCl ≥ 80 mL/min] to CrCl 15–29 mL/min).[31]

For patients on warfarin therapy, the traditional approach has been to interrupt warfarin 3–5 days prior to cardiac catheterisation to ensure that the international normalised ratio (INR) is <1.8,[2] and some still recommend this approach especially in the setting of femoral access or higher bleeding-risk procedures.[18(p96)] However, transradial access procedures with lower bleeding risks have resulted in more relaxed recommendations including non-interruption of warfarin therapy (in absence of patient-related factors that increase the risk of bleeding),[18(p96),31] and non-interruption, ensuring the INR is <2.2.[2] However some institutions may be more conservative in their approach and nurses should refer to local policy.

For all patients on warfarin therapy, advanced planning is required to ensure therapeutic goals are maintained, increased risks are not inadvertently caused and procedural safety is maintained. The patient should have an INR 5–7 days before the procedure so that a high INR (e.g. >3.0) may be identified and there is adequate time to rectify. Where a normal INR is desired for a procedure, the following guidance statement is useful. For patients with; (a) an INR 1.5–1.9, warfarin should be discontinued 3–4 days before; (b) an INR 2.0–3.0, warfarin should be discontinued 5 days before; and (c) an INR > 3.0, warfarin should be discontinued for at least 5 days before.[31] An INR should be repeated 24 hours before in high-risk patients or on the procedural day for low-risk patients. In high-risk patients (e.g. metallic heart valves) unable to have radial procedures, a bridging protocol with unfractionated heparin (UFH) or low molecular weight heparin (LMWH) is indicated.

The shorter half-life associated with NOACs theoretically should result in reduced duration of therapy interruption compared to warfarin, although this is dependent on procedural risk, specific agent and estimated creatinine clearance. Table 9.1 outlines current recommendations for therapy interruption for low-bleeding risk procedures that are dependent on renal function (and specifically CrCl using the Cockcroft-Gault formula).

Australian, North American and European guidelines recommend patients with acute coronary syndrome receive anticoagulation in addition to antiplatelet therapy, until definitive invasive

Table 9.1 Current renal-function guided recommendations for the interruption of NOAC medications for patients undergoing low-risk bleeding procedures

NOAC agent	Creatinine clearance mL/min			
	≥80 (normal renal function)	50–79 (mildly impaired renal function)	30–49 (moderately impaired renal function)	15–29 (severely impaired renal function)
Dabigatran	≥24 hr	≥36 hr	≥48 hr	≥72 hr (contraindicated for use in Australia)
Apixaban, Rivaroxaban	≥24	≥24	≥24	≥36

Source: Doherty, J.U. et al., *J. Am. Coll. Cardiol.*, 69, 871–898, 2017; Clinical Excellence Commission. Non-vitamin K antagonist oral anticoagulant (NOAC) guidelines. In: Commission CE, Ed., Sydney, Australia, NSW Health 1–40, 2017.

therapy is achieved (e.g. PCI).[12,14,33] LMWH (e.g. enoxaparin) may be preferred over IV UFH as it does not require activated partial thromboplastin time (aPTT) monitoring and is simpler to administer.[33] The standard recommended dose for enoxaparin is 1 mg/kg subcutaneous (SC) twice daily, and reduced to 1 mg/kg SC daily in patients with CKD.[33] In patients receiving enoxaparin together with thrombolysis during STEMI, additional dosing is not required during PCI if the last dose was <8 hours before (although additional boluses are required if >8 hours).[33] UFH should be ceased ≥4 hours, and LMWH should be ceased at least 24 hours prior to cardiac catheterisation or PCI.[31]

Most procedures performed in the CCL involve administration of intravenous or intra-arterial anticoagulation. In diagnostic cardiac catheterisation where arterial time is >20 minutes, UFH 2000–5000 IU is commonly administered.[3(p113)] Additional UFH dosing during PCI is recommended as 70–100 IU/kg (or 50–70 IU/kg if concomitant glycoprotein IIb/IIIa inhibition) is administered.[33] Target-activated clotting time (ACT) during PCI should be 250–350 seconds (or 200–250 seconds if GPIIb/IIIa inhibitors have been used).[18(p88),34(p830),]

Alternatively, direct IV thrombin inhibition with bivalirudin is the most widely used anticoagulant in the United States for PCI,[3(p431)] with reduced bleeding events and short half-life (25 minutes) enabling prompt sheath removal.[18(p95)]

UFH and enoxaparin should be stopped immediately after PCI, except in specific situations (e.g. thrombotic complication, AF).[34(p830)] The duration of triple antithrombotic therapy (aspirin, P2Y12 and vitamin K antagonist) should be minimised to limit the risk of bleeding, and a lower INR (e.g. 2.0 to 2.5) may be reasonable in appropriate patients.[12]

PATIENTS WITH ALLERGIES

Allergies must be identified, documented and communicated at each transfer of care during the patient's hospital admission to prevent topical antiseptic, medication, adhesive, or contrast media allergic reaction. Alternatives should be discussed with the patient and arranged as appropriate.

Allergic reactions to contrast media are rare and range from mild hypersensitivity (<3%), to moderate to severe reactions (0.04%), with mortality occurring in less than 1 in 100,000 patients.[35] Delayed reactions are usually cutaneous and begin one hour or longer (usually 6–12 hours, but up to one week) following administration, likely associated with T lymphocyte-mediated hypersensitivity.[35,36] Immediate-type reactions occur up to one hour after contrast administration and are virtually always non-immunoglobulin (Ig)-E mediated (previously termed 'anaphylactoid reactions').[37,38] The immediate moderate-to-severe reactions include bronchospasm and wheezing, angio-oedema, coronary artery spasm, hypotension, cardiac arrhythmia, cardiac failure (including hypovolemic shock and pulmonary oedema), convulsions and loss of consciousness.[35,38]

A previous reaction to contrast represents a 20%–60% absolute risk during subsequent exposure and is the most important risk factor, with asthma also increasing the risk, particularly of bronchospasm.[35] A history of multiple food and drug allergies, advanced age and women also represent a higher risk.[2,3(p364)]

Premedication is recommended for patients with a known prior allergy to contrast. Common protocols include:

- Corticosteroids, e.g. prednisone 50 mg administered at 13 hours, 7 hours and 1 hour prior to procedure
- Antihistamine, for example diphenhydramine 50 mg (e.g. benadryl) or promethazine (e.g. phenergan) 1 hour prior to procedure
- For emergent procedures, IV hydrocortisone 100–200 mg and IV promethazine 12.5–25 mg[2,3(p364),4]

The need for conscious sedation should be assessed and may not be required in patients receiving antihistamines due to the possible side effect of drowsiness.[38]

Management strategies for patients at high risk of developing an immediate moderate to severe reaction include close observation and team preparedness to treat a reaction. Treatment depends on the type of reaction, but usually requires epinephrine 0.3–0.5 mg intramuscular every 5–15 minutes or adrenaline 50 micrograms IV dose-titrated to effect, oxygen, large volume fluids, corticosteroids, anti-emetic and inotropic support.[2,3(p365),38] Most patients recover from reactions without long-term morbidity.[35]

The common misconception that seafood allergies are related to the iodine content in seafood and that this confers an increased risk to contrast media persists.[3(p364),37,39] The allergen is actually in the tropomycin protein in shellfish and parvalbumin in fish, and appears unrelated to iodine.[2,39] Anaphylactoid prophylaxis for patients with a history of allergic reactions to shellfish or seafood is not beneficial,[4] and some suggest stopping the outdated practice of enquiring about seafood allergy before administration of contrast media and that this would likely help end propagation of the misconception.[37]

PATIENTS WITH CHRONIC OBSTRUCTIVE PULMONARY DISEASE

Chronic obstructive pulmonary disease (COPD) is a common condition with an estimated global prevalence of almost 12% in adults over the age of 30.[40] Symptoms include dyspnea, cough, sputum production, wheeze, chest tightness, exercise limitation and at the severe spectrum, complicated by fatigue, weight loss, sleep disturbance and anorexia.[40] COPD often co-exists with cardiovascular disease,[3(p366)] and to rule out concomitant disease processes that contribute to dyspnea and exercise intolerance, cardiac catheterisation and echocardiography may reveal additional therapeutic options such as PCI or TAVR.

COPD is characterised by a chronically high level of carbon dioxide and a low level of oxygen in the blood, with the physiological mechanisms involving a ventilation-perfusion (Va/Q) mismatch and the haldane effect.[41] Patients most susceptible to oxygen-induced hypercapnia are those with severe hypoxemia, and cautious administration of oxygen using titrated administration to achieve an oxygen saturation of 88%–92% is the best approach.[41] Routine use of oxygen therapy in any patient with a blood oxygen saturation (SaO2) >93% is not recommended, and in COPD patients, the target of 88%–92% is also supported in current guidelines.[33]

For COPD patients presenting for procedures in the CCL, it is important that patients who are experiencing acute exacerbations of COPD have their procedure postponed if possible.[3(p366)]

Chronic obstructive sleep apnea (OSA) is an underdiagnosed problem[3(p366)] and associated with an increased risk of coronary artery disease, hypertension, left ventricular dysfunction, arrhythmias and sudden cardiac death.[42] Patients may be unaware they have OSA, and it is often reported first by bed-partners[43] or may become apparent during procedures such as in the CCL. OSA is characterised by disruptive snoring, witnessed apnea or gasping, hypersomnolence and morning headache, among other signs and risk factors (e.g. obesity).[44]

Nurses in the CCL are well placed to identify patients with snoring, apneic periods, labile oxygen saturations, and hypoxia often associated with sedation and should communicate this so that patients can be referred appropriately for follow-up. Patients who use non-invasive ventilation devices (continuous positive airway pressure [CPAP] or bi-level positive airway pressure [BiPap]) should bring these to the hospital.[3(p366)]

Access site and circulation assessment

A comprehensive assessment and documentation of all potential arterial access sites and circulation prior to the procedure is important as a baseline to compare with post procedure. Frequently different staff may be involved in patient care; therefore, a consistency of assessment ensures that circulation changes are noticed. Circulation assessment includes colour, sensation, warmth, movement, capillary refill, and quality of access site pulse in addition to presence of distal pulses.

If the femoral approach is used, the femoral artery, dorsalis pedis and posterior tibial arteries should be assessed, graded and recorded on a scale of 0 to 4+ (absent to bounding).[3(p91)] Pulses that are unable to be palpated should be assessed using Doppler and documented using a similar scale. Distal pulses are marked with a single-use marker pen.

If the radial approach is anticipated, similar circulation assessment is required; however, further assessment is recommended using the Allen's and/or Barbeau tests. With the Allen's test, the radial and ulnar arteries are occluded simultaneously while the patient opens and closes his or her hand until colour changes. If the patient then relaxes the hand, subsequent release of the ulnar artery should result in a return to normal colour within 8–10 seconds.[3(p57)]

The Barbeau test uses oximetry and plethysmography and is a more objective assessment of circulation, ensuring adequate ulnar artery supply to the hand. With the pulse oximeter placed on the patient's index finger, compress the radial artery. The following three types may proceed with radial access if return to a normal waveform occurs within 2 minutes: (Type A), return to normal waveform; (Type B), initial damping but eventual recovery to normal waveform, (Type C), initial damping that does not completely recover or normalise. Type D, where there is no return of waveform after 2 minutes, should not proceed to arterial access via the radial route. A reverse Barbeau test similarly tests the calibre of the radial (rather than ulnar) artery. By compressing the ulnar artery with the oximetry probe on the little finger, the same assessment can be used. Both right and left hands should be assessed.

All potential access sites should have hair removed so that drapes and dressings can be applied securely and removed without causing patient discomfort.

PERI-PROCEDURAL NURSING CARE

Time-Out

After transfer to the procedure room, clinical handover is performed and the patient positioned supine on the X-ray table according to the procedure being performed. The patient should be made comfortable and warm. Time-Out is a mandatory pre-procedure safety review to prevent wrong-site surgery and is also used to collectively discuss the case.[13] Components of Time-Out include (but are not limited to) the following: (1) correct patient name; (2) correct procedure; (3) consent form completed and signed; (4) confirmation of any allergies; (5) any antibiotic, anticoagulant, diabetic or other medication requiring team discussion prior to proceeding; (6) correct site and side is being used; (7) confirmation of pre-wash if required; and (8) availability of any special equipment and/or imaging that will be required during the procedure.[2] Involving the patient in this process with all team members allays patients' anxiety, ensures patients are fully informed and should be completed prior to administration of procedural sedation.

Haemodynamic monitoring

The patient is connected to haemodynamic monitoring equipment and appropriate additional equipment if required. Patients at higher risk of discomfort or anxiety should be offered sedation and analgesia[9] and should be administered prior to arterial puncture as this is frequently the most painful part of the procedure. Sedation should only be given once baseline observations are recorded. Observations should include continuous ECG, respiratory rate, SpO_2 monitoring, and blood pressure.[9] Ongoing haemodynamic monitoring and documentation is performed regularly throughout the procedure.

If procedural sedation is used, nurses should continuously monitor pulmonary ventilation and oxygen using pulse oximetry, combined with clinical observation of respiration to detect hypopneic hypoventilation, bradypnea, apnea or partial airway obstruction.[1] Furthermore, adequacy of ventilation and oxygenation should be recorded at least every 10 minutes, with any indication of respiratory compromise promptly reported to the proceduralist and corrective interventions implemented immediately. End-tidal carbon dioxide monitoring (capnography) and respiratory rate monitoring are better indicators of respiration than SpO_2 monitoring, especially in the CCL environment where the patient is almost completely covered in sterile drapes and direct visual assessment of ventilation is difficult. Capnography should be used for all patients at higher risk of impaired respiratory function, including patients with COPD, STEMI, haemodynamically unstable patients, and patients requiring higher doses of procedural sedation or any anaesthesia-supported procedure.

The most appropriate ECG leads to use for detection of ischaemia during a PCI procedure are V_2–V_4, III and aVF, depending on the artery being treated.[9,45] Many haemodynamic systems have certain default leads; however, this should not prevent the changing of lead choices, dependent on the clinical scenario.

Additional equipment for pacing or defibrillation may also be required, depending on the clinical scenario.

The role of the haemodynamic monitoring nurse, technician or technologist is to monitor and communicate changes in cardiac pressures and rhythms; therefore, staff must be competent in interpreting the full range of pressure and ECG waveforms.[3(p24)] Responsibility extends to the recording and documentation of all procedural elements in the catheterisation report (depending on individual hospital systems), and all staff must practice within their legal scope of practice.

Arterial access

To ensure an ideal arterial puncture and limit the risk of vascular complications, fluoroscopy and ultrasound have both been shown to have a positive effect. This is particularly important in femoral arterial punctures, although it is also helpful for radial punctures, especially for high risk patients (borderline Allen's or Barbeau test during pre-procedure assessments) or when resistance is felt during sheath insertion or during wire and catheter advancements.

An ideal femoral puncture is located within the common femoral artery (CFA), rather than a high puncture (above the inguinal ligament) or below the bifurcation, and hence in the superficial or profunda branches of the femoral artery. Use of fluoroscopy to locate angiographic markers and ensure the arteriotomy is found in the common femoral artery has reduced the risk of pseudoaneurysm, haematoma, arteriovenous fistula, retroperitoneal bleeding or any arterial access site complication requiring intervention.[46]

The use of ultrasound in guiding femoral punctures has further improved success rates for common femoral artery (CFA) punctures and also reduced vascular complications such as haematoma (>5 cm), pseudoaneurysm, retroperitoneal bleeding, arterial dissection or thrombosis, or major bleeding.[47] The benefit of ultrasound guidance in reducing vascular complications has not been realised with radial artery access.[48] Ultrasound guidance does not significantly increase costs associated with the single-use sterile sleeve or procedure time once processes are embedded within the team.

Catheterisation laboratories have gradually adopted fluoroscopy and ultrasound-guided access protocols, especially in training centres where uptake has increased. There is a significant learning curve associated with ultrasound guidance, from 82.4% (fewer than 6 ultrasound guided procedures) to 87.6% (≥15 ultrasound guided procedures).[47] The increased adoption of ultrasound may be related to the overall decrease in femoral access experience associated with the increase in radial procedures and possible concerns regarding the 'radial paradox'.[49] Vascular access site complications have been shown to be lower in radial artery access compared to femoral access; however, in predominantly radial-access operators, vascular complications may increase when required to use femoral access.

An alternative arterial route may be required in certain situations and these are ideally discussed during Time-Out. Patients with borderline Allen's or Barbeau tests during pre-procedure assessments may need cross-over to the contralateral side, or femoral access in case of puncture failure. STEMI patients with anticipated radial access should have femoral access also prepped up-front to reduce delays, in case larger equipment is needed, or for haemodynamic support if required (e.g. intra-aortic balloon pump).

Procedural documentation

The minimum components of a procedural report are variable among institutions but should include a structured report of indications for procedure, patient demographic information, relevant patient history and risk factors, all staff involved (including technical, visiting or relieving staff), procedure performed, access route, all stock used for the procedure, all procedural times (including time in/out of lab, sheath in/out), haemodynamic values/rhythm/calculations and pressure waveforms, medications including dosages, PCI information (e.g. balloon/stents/inflation times and atmospheres, final diameters), contrast used, radiation dose, pre/post sedation scores (e.g. Aldrete scoring system), complications and adverse events, pre/post Thrombolysis In Myocardial Infarction (TIMI) score, and a full summary of events/actions/effects during the case.[2]

POST-PROCEDURE NURSING CARE

Following cardiac catheterisation, patients are transferred to the recovery area where vital signs, neurovascular status and access site(s) are closely monitored. Nurses should be vigilant for possible complications and should be able to manage them accordingly. The patient, family members or next of kin are all notified of the results of the procedure.

Vital signs and neurovascular observations, arterial access site monitoring

All patients must have regular vital signs, neurovascular observations and assessment of the arterial access site in the post procedure period to detect for the development of complications.

Vital signs should include regular assessment of NiBP, pulse, respiratory rate and SpO_2. Frequency of assessments are recommended as follows: every 15 minutes for 1 hour, then every 30 minutes for 2 hours, and hourly for 4 hours (or until discharge if same-day), then every 4 hours. However there are no specific nursing guidelines for this recommendation.

Once the arterial sheath is removed (e.g. when activated clotting time ([ACT] < 160 seconds[9]), frequency of observations should increase for sheath removal and in the post-sheath removal period. Moreover, vital signs should be performed more frequently if the patient develops chest pain, arrhythmias, access site complication or other complications. There are no recommendations for cardiac monitoring post routine diagnostic cardiac catheterisation, although automatic vital sign monitoring at intervals set according to individual CCL policy is commonly followed.

All PCI patients should have continuous ECG monitoring post PCI in order to detect signs of ischemia and arrhythmias,[9,50] although duration of monitoring is dependent on patient risk. An elective and stable PCI patient for same-day discharge may only require ECG monitoring for 4 hours post PCI. High-risk patients (e.g. patients with STEMI/NSTEMI) should be monitored for a minimum of 24 hours,[50] and some patients require extended monitoring durations (e.g. patients with severe left main disease waiting for CABG). The most appropriate leads to monitor for ischemic changes are leads III, aVL and V_2.[45] All patients should have a 12-lead ECG post PCI to assess for changes compared to the pre-procedural ECG and in the event of post-procedure complications (e.g. acute stent thrombosis). Monitor alarms should be tailored to individual patient requirements and ST-segment monitoring commenced especially in leads best reflecting the territory treated. However, it should be noted ST-segment monitoring remains widely underused, with reasons being a 'lack of physician support,' high number of false ST alarms, lack of education about the technology, and what to do in response to ST alarms.[50]

Neurovascular observations include the same circulation assessments as for pre-procedure: colour, sensation, warmth, movement, capillary refill, and presence of distal pulses. These should be compared to the contralateral limb. Frequency of neurovascular and access site assessments should be the same as vital signs, i.e. every 15 minutes for 1 hour, then every 30 minutes for 2 hours and so on. Abnormal neurovascular observations should warrant further evaluation to investigate causes and rule out development of complications.

The arterial access site should be assessed at the same time as other observations and documented on each occasion. Assessment includes a visual inspection and palpation of the access site and surrounding tissue. Femoral access sites may require deep palpation over the site, proximally, medially, laterally and distally for signs of haematoma, retroperitoneal bleed, pseudoaneurysm or other complications. For radial punctures, palpation of the whole arm is important to rule out haematomas that may have resulted from wire perforation rather than related to haemostasis at the wrist area. If more than one arterial access site, careful attention is required for documentation of both sites to avoid confusion. In the early period post procedure, the access site should remain visible (while maintaining patient dignity) to easily observe for complications such as bleeding. The patient should be instructed to watch and report without delay if bleeding, pain, swelling, or other sensations such as feeling faint, dizzy, nausea or chest pain.

Haemostasis

Haemostasis, or the cessation of bleeding post sheath removal, is achieved by various methods, with manual compression the gold standard to which all subsequent methods and devices have been compared.

FEMORAL HAEMOSTASIS

For femoral haemostasis using manual compression, firm compression is applied 1 cm superior to the skin puncture site for a minimum of 10 minutes, with gradual easing of pressure over 5 minutes. Longer compression may be required and should be individualised according to risks such as hypertension, larger sheath size, anticoagulation and antiplatelet medications, etc. Other methods of manual compression have also been described, including 5 minutes of compression is applied per French size of sheath,[3(p77)] with 4 minutes of occlusive pressure, then a gradual release until distal pulses return[51] and compression ranging from 15 to 30 minutes.[9,52] Each institution will have variations to these protocols.

Mechanical compression was developed as an alternative to manual compression to reduce the amount of nursing time and effort required to ensure haemostasis. Mechanical compression may also be preferred when longer haemostasis time is required, as with: (1) larger sheaths; (2) excessively anticoagulated patients; (3) treatment of complications such as haematoma, bleeding or retroperitoneal bleeding; (4) ongoing femoral support (e.g. after removal of IABP using manual compression, or post ultrasound guided compression (USGC) for treatment of pseudoaneurysm); or (5) after failure of other methods. The FemoStop™ remains the most common mechanical compression system, allowing visual inspection and the ability to palpate the groin to assess for complications. The FemoStop™ system consists of an air-filled dome locked into a plastic arch, with a strap passed under the patient hips to secure firmly. The amount of pressure is controlled by a sphygmomanometer. Protocols vary among institutions, but generally there is a short period of occlusive pressure at 10–20 mmHg higher than the patient's systolic blood pressure (SBP), followed by gradual reductions until zero pressure is reached then the FemoStop™ is removed. Generally, the time taken for haemostasis is longer with the FemoStop™ compared to manual compression. Another mechanical compression device, the C-clamp system is rarely used in contemporary practice.

Vascular closure devices (VCDs) provide immediate haemostasis, eliminate the need for prolonged arterial compression, reduce the period of bedrest, and facilitate early mobilisation and potentially earlier discharge. They have not, however, reduced complication rates,[3(p78)] are costly, and may be associated with an increase in complications such as haematoma, pseudoaneurysm, infection and VCD embolisation.[53] VCDs may be helpful in patients who are unable to lay flat for long periods, for example patients with COPD, patients with back pain, or patients with memory problems unable to remember post procedure instructions. Types of VCDs include haemostatic plugs (e.g. Angio-Seal, Exoseal, Mynx), clips (e.g. StarClose) and suture mediated closure devices (e.g. Perclose). In structural heart procedures where very large-sized sheaths are used (e.g. 20 French or larger), pre-closure of arterial and venous sites using suture-mediated VCDs are common.

RADIAL HAEMOSTASIS

Radial haemostasis is most commonly achieved by removal of the arterial sheath at the end of the procedure (while the patient is still in the laboratory) with application of a radial compression device (e.g. TR Band™, Radistop, TRAcelet). Once radial haemostasis is achieved, patent haemostasis should be promptly achieved to reduce the risk of radial artery occlusion. Patent haemostasis is the cessation of bleeding while ensuring continued blood flow through the radial or ulnar artery to the hand.

With the TR Band™, patent haemostasis may be achieved by several methods: (1) slow deflation of compression until bleeding occurs, then reinsert 1–2 mL of air; or (2) with the oximetry probe on the index finger, remove air in 1 mL increments while compressing the ulnar artery until the oximetry waveform returns. If unable to achieve patent haemostasis due to bleeding, leave compression device in place for 15 minutes then reattempt deflations.[3(p65)]

There is no consensus in optimal duration for device application to achieve haemostasis, prevent complications and preserve radial patency. Ultrashort compression duration (20 minutes) has not been shown to improve radial patency or reduce complications.[54] Kern et al.[3(p65)] advocate the commencement of weaning compression after 90 minutes, although they more recently suggest 1–2 hours for diagnostic procedures and 2–4 hours for interventional procedures.[18(p74)] If bleeding recurs the compression band can be reapplied.

Bleeding post sheath removal reflects a loss of haemostasis and nurses are often required to manage bleeding (and other complications) in the post procedural period. It is imperative that nurses caring for patients who have undergone diagnostic and interventional procedures are competent in the full range of haemostasis techniques and act promptly if additional treatment is needed.

Arterial access sites must be covered with a transparent occlusive dressing to allow for visual assessment and palpation for detection of complications.

Post-procedure documentation

Contemporaneous documentation in the post procedural period is required in case of sudden changes in condition, escalation of symptoms or transfer of care. Once the patient arrives to recovery (or the ward in case of direct transfer) a full clinical handover must be undertaken with staff receiving the patient. Clinical handover elements include:

- Patient identification, demographics, allergies
- Arterial or other access sites (and any attempts or crossovers), sheath size, multiple punctures

- Medications and fluids administered, further medications to be given or infusions ordered, medication changes
- Procedure performed, prosthetics used such as stents (e.g. number, size, position, results)
- Arterial pressures, complications such as arrhythmias, chest pain, access site complications, actions and effects of treatment, sedation scores, respiratory and neurological status
- Results, further orders (e.g. EUCs to monitor for PC-AKI), referrals (e.g. cardiac rehabilitation, cardiac surgeon, social worker) or future plans of care
- A review of all documentation of procedural elements including haemodynamics, waveforms, vital signs and procedural results, to ensure completeness and chase up outstanding components

Documentation post-procedure depends on local institution protocols, and many electronic medical records provide a synthesised summary of the patient admission, including details of interventions performed. Neurovascular observations, vital signs and access site assessments are mandatory for post procedure documentation. Other elements may include but are not limited to fluid balance chart (oral and IV fluids, urine output), resumption of diet, IV cannulation scores and IV cannula removal if patient for discharge, general nursing assessments if patient is to be admitted (including falls risk, pressure area risk, infection risk, belongings, smoking, drug and other medication history, bowel chart, etc.), plan of care, patient education and so on.

Post-procedure mobilisation

Mobilisation following haemostasis is dependent on the type of procedure performed, the arterial access site, development of complications, ongoing need for monitoring, other comorbidities, as well as other factors. There is no consensus regarding the optimal period of bedrest following cardiac catheterisation or PCI. Rolley et al.[9] point to the heterogeneous methodology in studies investigating cardiac catheterisation and PCI in relation to haemostasis, complications and optimal mobilisation periods. Patients should be managed on bedrest for at least 2 hours but not exceeding 4 hours unless clinical condition indicates otherwise.[9]

For delayed sheath removal post PCI, this may result in bedrest periods of 6 hours and often longer. Patients on prolonged bedrest should be offered position changes such as elevating the head of the bed no more than 15–30 degrees, a pillow under the knees to relieve back pain, or rolling the patient and supporting with pillows on the side the sheath is located.

For patients with femoral access procedures, bedrest is determined by time of haemostasis and varies widely from institution to institution. Resumption of diet and fluids can occur once the patient can sit up and support the arterial access site in case of coughing. For patients having radial access procedures, the need for bedrest is almost negated, apart from that needed to perform vital signs and assessments. Recovery from procedural sedation may require the patient to remain in bed until it is safe to transfer to a chair. For any patients in whom access site or other complications develop, bedrest periods are longer until the patient is stable.

PREVENTING AND MANAGING COMPLICATIONS

Vascular complications

Invasive procedures such as cardiac catheterisation and PCI were originally performed via cut-down technique, and then progressed to the percutaneous femoral artery approach in the 1980s. Once new device angioplasty procedures became commonplace in the 1990s, there was a concurrent increased in vascular complications rates with access via the femoral artery. Brachial access was also used but was not advantageous compared to femoral access[55,56] and is rarely used today. Femoral access became mainstream until the last decade when radial arterial access gained popularity and surpassed femoral artery access in many countries.[19(p56)] The advantages of radial artery access include patient comfort with immediate sheath removal and reduced need for prolonged bedrest; and by nature an easily compressible site allowing for decreased nursing care post procedure and early hospital discharge.[57–59]

Procedures performed in the CCL are usually well tolerated by most patients; however, accessing the arterial blood system is not without risk. While the risk of major complications such as death, myocardial infarction and stroke are low, vascular access site complications are more common but less frequently explained to patients in the pre-procedure period. Vascular access site complications range from small to severe, from unsightly such as bruising, to limb- or life-threatening such as compartment syndrome or retroperitoneal bleed. The abundance of studies over the past 30 years have reported an incidence of vascular access site complications that ranges considerably from less than 0.5%[60] to 76%.[61]

BLEEDING

Bleeding is the most visible of vascular access site complications and has a reported incidence from 0.07%[62] to 23.9%.[63] The wide variability in reported incidence is related to the definition of bleeding with (1) descriptive definitions involving some form of visible bleeding (ooze, trickling, brisk or spurting blood)[61,64,65]; (2) quantitative definitions including a drop in blood count[66–69]; and (3) treatment-based definitions requiring a response to the bleeding such as administration of blood products.[70,71] Nursing studies most frequently use descriptive definitions of bleeding and report a higher incidence of bleeding compared to medical studies.

Risk factors for bleeding include advanced age, female gender, severe renal impairment, multiple punctures, larger sheath size, glycoprotein IIb/IIIa inhibitor, longer sheath dwell time, vascular closure device.[72–77] Radial access has consistently shown a lower incidence of bleeding than femoral access.[75,78,79] Lower bleeding rates may be related to the closer proximity of the radial artery to the skin surface, with a potential easier arterial puncture and haemostasis, and easier visual inspection and control of the site compared to femoral sites.

Nursing management of bleeding depends on the nature of the bleeding. A minor 'tracking' ooze, while annoying, may require 5 minutes manual compression and application of a new transparent dressing. Minor ooze that continues may require application of a mechanical compression device, or wad of gauze under a transparent dressing and, as a last resort, a haemostatic alginate wound dressing (e.g. surgicel, kaltostat). Due to the increased risk of infection as a result of blood and gauze providing a culture media,[18(p83)] these dressings must be removed at the earliest opportunity.

Sudden bleeding that is large or spurting indicates arterial bleeding and loss of haemostasis. Immediate manual compression is required to re-establish haemostasis and all nurses caring for post cardiac catheterisation or PCI should be competent in the management of bleeding. Additional compression may be required using a mechanical compression device as per local hospital preference.

HAEMATOMA

Haematoma is defined as a palpable mass at the puncture site caused from bleeding via the arteriotomy site, and ranges in size from small (<5 cm), moderate (5–10 cm) to large (>10 cm). Haematomas may occur at any stage of the procedure from initial arterial puncture, during or after the procedure when haemostasis occurs, or in the hours or days following the procedure. Initially, there is a soft spongy feeling on palpation (especially femoral haematomas), but as further blood collects results in a hard, painful lump.[80(p255)] As the haematoma progresses it can become very serious resulting in diminished distal pulses, lower extremity oedema, loss of sensory or motor function, impaired skin viability, tachycardia or shock, and it sometimes requires surgical decompression. Risk factors for the development of haematoma include female gender,[75,77,81,82] pre-procedure UFH or LMWH,[81] multiple punctures,[81,83] and VCD use.[69]

Femoral haematoma

There is heterogeneity in the definition of haematoma among studies with a reported range in incidence from 0.1%[84] to 35.1%,[85] and in Australia, 15.5%.[75] Nursing studies tend to capture all haematomas whereas medical studies limit the definition to large haematomas or those resulting in serious sequelae. Haematomas may occur during sheath insertion, incomplete or failed vascular closure device deployment, during haemostasis using manual or mechanical compression, or related to patient restlessness or non-compliance to instructions. Treatment involves re-establishing haemostasis and compression of the remaining haematoma, as this may result in an increased risk of further complications such as pseudoaneurysm.

Radial haematoma (including compartment syndrome)

Radial access has resulted in a lower incidence of haematoma (and other vascular complications combined) compared to femoral[48,58,62,84] and is one of the driving forces behind the increased uptake of radial access procedures. Most haematomas develop during transradial sheath removal, although can develop during the procedure, which is difficult to identify and treat while the arm is draped.[18(p74)] Patients complaining of pain or paresthesia (numbness) warrant close evaluation during the procedure. Haematomas can be managed by manual compression in the first instance, followed by careful wrapping using a compression bandage, elevation and application of ice. Haematomas at the level of the elbow or upper arm (including subclavian) are likely related to wire dissection or perforation related to retrograde dissection and can usually be managed conservatively with compression.[48] Prevention includes avoidance of straight hydrophilic guidewires and use of small J-tipped wires (e.g. 1.5 mm J-tip rather than standard 3 mm J-tip wires routinely used with femoral access), with particular attention to wire resistance or pain at any stage.[18(p268)] Angiography of the arm is used to identify causes of wire or catheter resistance and the development of complications such as dissection or perforation.[48]

Compartment syndrome is a rare (<0.01%)[86] but serious extension of an uncontrolled haematoma and is a medical emergency. Open fasciotomy can be usually avoided if preventative measures are employed, such as: (1) stopping IV anticoagulation, (2) controlling pain and blood pressure, and (3) using transient external compression with a blood pressure cuff.[48] Any suspected expanding haematoma should be closely monitored using frequent arm circumference measurements, and if uncontrolled, urgent medical review is indicated. Tizón-Marcos & Barbeau[86] recommend the immediate application of a blood pressure cuff at 10-15 mmHg less than systolic blood pressure to allow distal pulsatile flow to the hand (monitored with oximetry/plethysmography) so bleeding stops and diffuses into the arm. Usually 2 periods of 15 minutes are required to control bleeding.[86]

RETROPERITONEAL BLEEDING

Retroperitoneal bleeding is a serious complication related to femoral arterial access procedures but occurs rarely, with a contemporary incidence of between 0.2%[75] to 0.7%.[87,88] Risk factors for retroperitoneal bleeding include a high arterial puncture, posterior-wall puncture, female gender, small body surface area, vascular closure devices, large sheath size or long sheath dwell time, intensity and duration of anticoagulation and IV glycoprotein IIb/IIIa inhibitor use.[88–92]

A retroperitoneal bleed should be suspected in patients with hypotension, tachycardia, pallor, lower abdominal or back pain, fall in Hb/HCT, or signs and symptoms similar to a vagal reaction but not responsive to medications.[18(p85)] Nursing management includes immediate femoral puncture compression, frequent monitoring of observations, using a large bore cannula to draw urgent blood for a full blood count, blood type crossmatching, rapid infusion of IV fluids, IV analgesia for pain, reversal of anticoagulation, and preparation for urgent transfer to CT for diagnosis. Management is often conservative and supportive in patients with a sealed site of bleeding, but may require urgent transfer back to the CCL for contralateral artery access and treatment, or transfer to theatre for vascular surgery.

With the increase in radial access procedures, both proceduralists and nursing staff have a lower exposure to femoral access procedures than in previous years. This is especially relevant with training medical, nursing and technical staff in the contemporary era and may lead to an increased risk associated with lack of experience with femoral procedures. It is important that all staff receive ongoing training in the prevention, recognition, diagnosis and prompt treatment required for retroperitoneal bleeding.

RADIAL ARTERY SPASM (RAS)

If a patient complains of significant pain in the region of the radial artery during the passage of a sheath, guidewire, or catheter radial artery spasm should be suspected.[93] RAS is a common complication, occurring in around 10%–20% of patients and is often due to significant alpha$_1$ adenoreceptors within the medial layer of the vessel.[18(p268),94] RAS prevents the completion of the procedure via transradial route in 2%–5% of patients and can result in endothelial injury and dysfunction.[94] The radial artery is small in size compared to the femoral artery, commonly 1.8–2.99 mm,[95,96] with men usually having a larger diameter than women (2.7 vs. 2.4 mm).[97]

Risk factors for RAS include younger age, female gender, diabetes mellitus, smaller wrist circumference, low body mass index (BMI) and the use of non-hydrophilic coated sheaths.[98] RAS is also associated with excessive catheter manipulations, multiple catheter exchanges and with less operator experience.[3(p64)]

Prevention and management of RAS (Grade I–II) frequently involves administration of intra-arterial vasodilators such as verapamil and/or nitroglycerin, hydrophilic sheaths, sedation and analgesia. If spasm continues despite these repeated measures (Grade III), crossover to a femoral approach may be required to complete the procedure. Very rarely, severe spasm (Grade IV) may require a short general anaesthetic to remove an entrapped catheter or sheath.[93] An entrapped device with even a gentle pull can be agonising for the patient.

RADIAL ARTERY OCCLUSION

Radial artery occlusion (RAO) is known as the Achilles' heel of transradial catheterisation,[99] and is reported to occur in <1%–10% of procedures.[3(p67)] Three possible mechanisms include: (1) arterial wall injury, endothelial denudation and local vascular reactions induced by sheath insertion, (2) interruption of antegrade flow during the procedure, and (3) both of these factors may facilitate local thrombus, and/or chronic inflammatory process, leading to intimal hyperplasia and thickening of intima media which may result in delayed luminal obliteration or reduction.[99] Predictors of RAO are either patient related (e.g. diabetes, female gender, low BMI) or procedure related (e.g. inadequate anticoagulation, large diameter of sheath and catheters, successive transradial procedures and occlusive haemostasis).[18(p268),99]

While most RAOs are asymptomatic and benign due to the dual circulation to the hand, there are rare reported cases of hand ischemia, with symptoms including pain, numbness and pallor. The clinical consequences of RAO are not only related to repeat catheterisations but also as a conduit for coronary artery bypass surgery or in patients who need an arteriovenous fistula for haemodialysis.[94]

Reducing the incidence of RAO therefore remains a challenge, with some treatments already accepted as best practice (e.g. patent haemostasis)[100] and others showing potential for improving practice. A promising large study (PROPHET II) of 3000 randomised patients involving the ipsilateral ulnar compression combined with patent haemostasis (compared to patent haemostasis alone) of the radial artery showed a significant reduction in the incidence of RAO.[101] Other non-pharmacologic treatments include mechanical recanalisation of the occluded artery, medicated sheaths and sheathless guides.[99] Potential pharmacologic treatments include LMWH,[102] thrombolysis or subcutaneous nitroglycerin[103] although these need further randomised studies. A recent meta-analysis of 66 studies involving more than 31,000 participants reported a 5.5% RAO incidence at >1 week follow-up and recommend high-dose heparin, shorter compression times and patent haemostasis as measures to reduce RAO.[104]

THROMBOEMBOLISM

Thrombus formation within the arterial system is a rare but serious complication that results from thrombus dislodgement and embolisation into the cerebral, pulmonary, coronary, or peripheral circulation. Peripheral thromboembolism (or atheroembolism) is a limb and potentially life-threatening complication which has been reported in 0.2%–0.4% of cases.[19(p62),105] Thromboembolism has several causes that may be identified and include arterial thrombosis secondary to intimal dissection, the scraping of guidewires and catheters against the aortic wall, inadequate anticoagulation, or aggressive haemostasis technique in the setting of peripheral vascular disease (PVD).[18(p270),80(p256)] VCDs have been associated with peripheral thromboembolism with some studies reporting femoral artery thrombosis or limb ischaemia due to embolisation of foreign material or in-situ device components.[19(p62)]

Patients with the following signs and symptoms should be evaluated promptly for possible flow-obstructing thrombus or dissection; lower extremity pain or paresthesia, reduced or absent distal pulses, pallor or cold limb compared to the contralateral side.[52]

Risk factors for thromboembolism include female gender, advanced age, PVD and CKD, patients undergoing high-risk procedures, morbid obesity and conversely, patients with a small BMI, placement of a large diameter catheter or sheath (e.g. intra-aortic balloon pump), prolonged occlusive pressure during haemostasis, femoral artery dissection, and non-aspiration of arterial sheath prior to removal (especially after prolonged sheath-dwell duration).[3(p89),52,18(p270),80(p256)] Techniques to prevent or minimise thromboembolism involve consistent aspiration of blood from catheters to clear any debris that might have been noticed during catheter advancement, clearing Y-connector valves and other devices (e.g. aspiration catheters), and careful haemostasis techniques to prevent total obliteration of distal peripheral pulses.[18(p270),80(p256)]

PSEUDOANEURYSM

Pseudoaneurysm is an uncommon complication that forms when an arterial puncture site fails to heal, thus allowing arterial blood to ooze or jet into the extravascular space forming a pulsatile, aneurysm-like haematoma.[106,107] Pseudoaneurysms usually occur several days after the procedure and often in the setting of a large haematoma and bruising, mostly associated with localised pain and swelling (a firm palpable lump) and diagnosed with femoral ultrasound. The incidence of pseudoaneurysm has gradually fallen from the highest reported incidence of 5.6% in the femoral era[108] to 0.4% in the combined femoral and radial era[58,75,105] to less than 0.1% in dedicated radial studies.[62,84]

Risk factors for pseudoaneurysm include low femoral puncture (e.g. in the superficial femoral artery), larger diameter sheaths, inadequate compression technique post sheath removal and abnormal haemostasis including that induced by prolonged use of anticoagulation, especially in the post-procedure period.[108-111] Small pseudoaneurysms (<2 cm) often close spontaneously within 1 month; however, if larger or treatment is required, thrombin injection or ultrasound-guided compression are the two most common treatments.[18(p261-262)] Thrombin injection has several advantages over USGC: greater success, effective on patients with anticoagulation, can be used on pseudoaneurysms above the inguinal ligament, less pain to the patient and technician, and there is a risk of stress-related wrist injury to the ultrasound technician with USGC.[18(p264)]

ARTERIOVENOUS (AV) FISTULA

AV fistula is a very rare complication (<0.1%)[58,84] which results from puncture of the artery as well as the vein, resulting in a fistulous communication between the two vessels. The majority of AV fistulae are small in size and immediate treatment is not necessary due to the high likelihood of spontaneous closure or remain asymptomatic.[18,112,113]

Risk factors are difficult to determine due to the rarity and studies usually combine rare complications, but may include female gender, arterial hypertension, high or low femoral puncture, multiple puncture attempts, left groin puncture, high procedural anticoagulation and warfarin therapy.[112,114] Surgery or stent grafting may be required if symptomatic (moderate pain) in 10% of patients with AV fistulae or high output heart failure occurs.[3(p89),18(p264)]

INFECTION

Infection at the arterial access site is a rare but serious complication occurring in 0.64% of interventional cases with septic complications occurring in only 0.24% of patients.[18(p264)] Types of infections include infected pseudoaneurysms and haematomas, groin abscesses and endarteritis.[115–118] Signs and symptoms may involve pain, swelling, erythema, fever or chills, purulent discharge, raised white cell count and symptom onset frequently occurs after the patient is discharged.

Risk factors for the development of infection include diabetes, repeated vascular access at the same site, long indwelling sheath time and VCDs.[19(p62),119] The literature is equivocal regarding the risk of infection with VCD use; while many studies report the safety of various VCDs, no significant increase in infection rates has been associated with their use,[120–123] case report series consistently identify VCDs have an association with groin infections.[115–118] While routine antibiotic prophylaxis is not recommended before procedures, contamination of the sheath (delayed sheath exchanges or patient touching site) or as recommended as per VCD product recommendations, it is standard to give 1 g cephalexin as a prophylactic measure.[18] Vancomycin 1 g may be given alternatively in case of allergy.

BRUISING

Bruising or ecchymosis at the vascular site is one of the least frequently reported but most commonly experienced complications, occurring in 36%–68% of patients.[73–75,124–127] Vascular access site bruising is sometimes considered a minor complication and indeed an acceptable outcome following angiography or PCI; it is not a life threatening complication, usually does not prolong the hospital stay and there is no reliable method of measuring bruising.[124] Patients, however, often see bruising as unsightly and associated with pain if bruising was the result of a haematoma.

Bruising is defined as a bluish purple discolouring of the skin surrounding the arteriotomy site resulting from bleeding or haematoma formation, classified as small (<5 cm), moderate (5–10 cm) or large (>10 cm). Risk factors include older age, female gender, hypertension (SBP ≥ 140 mmHg), primary PCI (rather than elective procedures), left sided access and multiple punctures.[73,75,124,128] Radial access, diabetes and a history of previous angiography or PCI is associated with lower risk of bruising.[75]

Non-access site complications

CORONARY DISSECTION

Coronary dissection is frequently associated with PCI and is angiographically visible in 30%–50% of angioplasty procedures, and in the pre-stent era, was a significant risk factor for abrupt vessel closure.[18(p273)] In modern PCI, implanted stents seal the dissected tissue flaps that result from 'controlled injury' induced by balloon dilatation, and are generally considered benign.[52] Minor dissections (Type A–B) are probably best treated conservatively[34(p723)] and PCI delayed if elective. Major dissections (dissection Type C–F), however, carry significant morbidity and mortality if left untreated, and require stabilisation with stenting.[34(p723)]

Guide catheter related dissections occur more commonly with the right coronary artery (RCA) than left main (LM) due to the relative size differences of the ostia, selection of guiding catheter shape, or non-coaxial guiding catheter alignment combined with forceful contrast injections.[34(p723–724)] Guide catheter dissections extending into the aorta are very rare (0.02% for diagnostic angiography and 0.07% for PCI) and almost all resulting from retrograde dissection from the RCA, and less frequently from the left main.[18(p723),34(p273)] Dissections involving the aortic cusp +/− extending <40 mm up the aorta, generally have a good prognosis, and the evolving dissection can be followed by computed tomography (CT) or transesopageal echocardiogram.[18(p274)] Systolic blood pressure must be controlled to prevent extension of the dissection. Dissections involving the aortic cusp and extending >40 mm up the aorta are treated surgically and are associated with a high mortality rate.[18(p274)]

CORONARY PERFORATION, PERICARDIAL EFFUSION, TAMPONADE AND PERICARDIOCENTESIS

Coronary perforation is a rare and life-threatening complication and occurs in 0.5%–0.84% of patients during PCI.[129–131] Perforation is a breach of the integrity of the artery wall, caused by oversized balloons or stents, balloon rupture, aggressive post stent dilatation, excessive rotablation or guidewire exit, resulting in extravasation of blood into the myocardium, pericardium or a cardiac chamber.[34(p731)] As little as 80–200 mL additional fluid in the pericardial sac (i.e. pericardial effusion) can cause pressure to rise and exert force on the myocardium sufficient to reduce cardiac output and result in tamponade.[34(p734)]

Risk factors for coronary perforation, pericardial effusion and tamponade include female gender and ablative (debulking) techniques;[131] however, the decreased use of these mean a greater proportion are caused by guidewires, particularly in the setting of primary PCI and chronic total occlusion (CTO) intervention.[34(p731)] Other risk factors include advanced age, previous CABG, intravascular ultrasound (IVUS) use, and tortuous, calcified and small arteries; predictors are likely interrelated.[34(p731),130,132(p168)]

Symptoms of perforation include pain (chest, neck or throat), vagal symptoms, hypotension (with or without tachycardia), ventricular ectopy, although the patient may be asymptomatic. Signs include extravasation of contrast, an errant wire positioning, and in massive tamponade, the 'dead heart' sign.[34(p733)]

Initial management includes: (1) prolonged balloon tamponade at the perforation site with low pressure for at least 10 minutes if tolerated by the patient (further repeat or longer inflations as required and tolerated); (2) conventional stents; (3) covered stents for larger perforations; and (4) check angiograms to ensure no progression of perforation. A distal perforation with failure to seal may require thrombin, microcoil, fat embolism, clotted autologous blood or microparticles. Urgent portable transthoracic echocardiography is very useful but not mandatory in time critical tamponade (an obtunded and hypotensive patient with a respiratory variation in aortic pressure is adequate to diagnose tamponade). For unstable patients with haemodynamic compromise due to tamponade, urgent pericardiocentesis is required with autologous transfusion (or blood products) as appropriate. Anticoagulation should not be immediately reversed with the wire and balloon in the vessel during attempted perforation occlusion; this could result in thrombosis of the whole vessel and leads to a higher mortality rate than the perforation itself.[18(p279)] Further echocardiography at 4 and 24 hours is important to monitor progression or confirm cessation of bleeding.

Nursing actions include calling for help (urgent echocardiography, anaesthetist, surgeon or interventional radiologist as appropriate) including summonsing additional nursing or technical staff, preparing for pericardiocentesis and ensuring all equipment is available and ready, organising equipment for autologous blood transfusion, managing the patient with unstable haemodynamics, reversing heparin if required, urgent group and hold for administration of blood products, frequent vital signs and haemodynamic monitoring, attaching patient to defibrillation/pacing pads, communication and reassurance to the patient.

NO-REFLOW

The no-reflow phenomenon describes the abrupt cessation of coronary flow without evidence of mechanical coronary obstruction, typically during primary PCI (PPCI) and complex PCI (particularly vein graft intervention or when rotational atherectomy devices are used).[34(p728)] No re-flow occurs infrequently (0.6%–3%)[132(p168),133] and common to all procedures is the liberation and distal embolisation of significant amounts of plaque coupled with vasoconstriction of the distal arterial bed.[132(p168)] No re-flow is associated with significant morbidity including reduced myocardial salvage, larger infarct size, reduced left ventricular ejection fraction at 6 months and increased risk of 1-year mortality.[133,134]

Prevention and treatment strategies for no re-flow are either pharmacological or mechanical but evidence is generally weak and anecdotal, hence the proposed treatments depend on differential diagnosis. If no re-flow is due to thrombus or new plaque rupture, then manual catheter aspiration is appropriate, along with anticoagulation with IIb/IIIa inhibitors.[18(p278)] If no-reflow is due to dissection, additional stenting is indicated. No re-flow due to severe spasm may be treated with intracoronary nitrogylcerin. No re-flow as a result of distal microembolisation, the following may be effective and is recommended; (1) adenosine 100 mcg/mL 1–2 mL bolus; (2) nitroprusside 100 mcg/mL 1–2 mL bolus; (3) verapamil 100 mcg/mL 1–2 mL bolus, with several grams required in total to treat this phenomenon.[13,18(p279)]

AIR EMBOLISM

Air embolisation is an iatrogenic complication of cardiac catheterisation and PCI and while half are asymptomatic (0.2%), others are significant air embolism events (0.19%), the most serious resulting in prolonged cardiac arrest.[135] The patient may complain of chest pain with accompanied ST elevation and rhythm disturbance leading to asystole or ventricular fibrillation.

The primary cause of air embolism is personnel, particularly with junior staff (both medical and nursing), in the first few months of training, with events being more common during PCI than diagnostic angiography.[34(p727)] Common causes for inadvertent introduction of air into the coronary system are manifolds, syringes, pressure tubing connections, Tuohey-Borst (Y-connection adaptor), three-way taps, inadequate flushing or aspiration of catheters, automatic contrast injector syringes, poor monitoring of contrast levels and balloon rupture.[34(p727)]

Several treatment options exist, including anecdotal reports of alternative approaches for successful management of air embolism. Treatment consists of administration of 100% oxygen by facemask to help minimise ischemia and produce a diffusion gradient favouring reabsorption of the air.[18(p277)] Large volume, forceful saline flushes may attempt to disperse smaller bubbles.[135] If a large bubble exists, this has been reported to be successfully aspirated using a thombectomy catheter.[136,137] Guidewire bougie to disperse a bubble occluding a coronary artery has also been reported.[34(p728)] Advanced life support is required for prolonged cardiac arrest with an eventual spontaneous return of circulation.

Prevention involves ensuring all equipment is flushed and air-free, connections are firm, syringes kept bubble-free and contrast injections or flushes into the patient are always performed methodically (syringe plunger always held upwards and tapped prior to injecting to ensure any air rises to the top of the plunger rather than into the patient). Faulty stock or equipment must be reported to management.

ACUTE AND SUB-ACUTE STENT THROMBOSIS

Acute and sub-acute stent thrombosis occurs rarely (<1%)[13] but is a potentially catastrophic complication that often presents as ST-segment elevation myocardial infarction (STEMI) within 30 days post procedure. This is associated with high mortality rates of 20%–45%[138] and is regarded as a medical emergency.[139] Mechanisms of acute ST include: (1) stent-related (hypersensitivity, incomplete endothelialisation, stent design); (2) procedure-related (inadequate stent expansion/sizing, incomplete stent apposition, residual edge dissection), (3) lesion-related (lesion/stent length, vessel/stent diameter, complex lesions, saphenous graft, stasis); or (4) patient-related factors (PCI for acute coronary syndrome/STEMI, diabetes mellitus, acute renal failure, impaired left ventricular function, premature cessation of dual antiplatelet therapy, aspirin or clopidogrel non responsiveness, prior brachytherapy).[138] It is important to consider the aetiology of stent thrombosis as it guides further therapy and is useful for avoidance of recurrence, with non-adherence or resistance to dual antiplatelet therapy (DAPT) the most common causes.[138] Patient education to ensure compliance to DAPT is paramount in preventing this serious complication.

Treatment is almost always emergent PCI with options for restoring perfusion, including thrombectomy (routine thombectomy in PCI is no longer recommended in the 2017 European Society of Cardiology guidelines, however is reasonable practice in cases of large residual thrombus)[140] and or balloon angioplasty. Treatment may also include administration of more potent pharmacologic agents such as IV glycoprotein IIb/IIIa inhibitors.[18(p197)] Understanding the underlying aetiology by using IVUS or OCT to determine presence of stent underexpansion/malapposition or residual dissection is reasonable before further PCI is performed with balloon inflations or stenting. Finally, evaluation for a hypercoagulable state, thrombocytosis or aspirin/clopidogrel resistance with escalation of antiplatelet therapy to prasugrel or ticagrelor is standard.[18(p197)]

ARRHYTHMIAS

Serious arrhythmias are rare during diagnostic cardiac catheterisation (less than 0.5%),[3(p3)] more common during PCI (1.5%)[34(p710)] and PPCI (5.7%),[141] and increase with procedures such as TAVR.[142,143] The origins of arrhythmias in cardiac catheterisation are related to ischemia or reperfusion (either spontaneous or iatrogenic) or vagally mediated reflexes.

Arrhythmias may occur during the passage of catheters through heart chambers, and in particular, with manipulation of catheters or pacing wires, resulting in atrial stretching that may cause atrial arrhythmias such as atrial fibrillation and supraventricular tachycardia. Stimulation of the right ventricular outflow tract or papillary muscles by catheter contact may cause ventricular arrhythmias.[3(p370)] Moreover ventricular arrhythmias occur commonly when associated with crossing the aortic valve during left ventriculography or associated with crossing a narrowed aortic valve in TAVI, and with the stiff pre-shaped wire positioned in the left ventricle.[3(p152),18(p393)]

Occlusive catheter engagement of coronary arteries may lead to dampened or ventricularised pressures, and injecting contrast in this setting may lead to ventricular fibrillation.[144] Damped or ventricularised pressures occur when the outer diameter of a catheter is larger than the ostial diameter or when the tip of a catheter is pressed against a vessel wall. Damping results in falsely low systolic and falsely high diastolic pressure readings with a narrow pulse pressure and delayed upstroke and downstroke, and is a sign of severe partial obstruction.[144] Ventricularisation is a less severe form of damping, where the diastolic pressure drops to a greater extent than the systolic. The incidence of coronary pressure damping has been reported by Her et al.[145] in a series of 2,926 patients as occurring in 2.3%, with true atherosclerotic lesions occurring in 40.8% of patients with damped pressures. Coronary spasm can also result in damped pressure waveforms and is reversible.[145] Damped pressures occur more frequently in the right coronary artery, whereas ventricularisation occurs more commonly in the left main coronary artery (LMCA).[144] In a series of 46 patients with significant LMCA stenosis, ventricularisation occurred in 9% of patients.[146] The conus branch of the right coronary artery is a common source of ventricular fibrillation, related to catheter induced ischemia and as a result of injection of contrast into a small coronary vessel.[34(p740)]

Arrhythmias during PCI are related to either ischemia or reperfusion, with vagally mediated reflexes responsible for the majority of events.[34(p739)] Coronary occlusion alters myocardial cell refractory periods, prolongs QT intervals and slows conduction, with catecholamine surges associated with intervention and ischemia.[34(p739)] Tachyarrhythmias and bradyarrhythmias occur during the coronary occlusion and reperfusion as action potentials and conduction normalise in a haphazard manner. Ventricular tachycardia (VT) and ventricular fibrillation (VF) occurring during PPCI for STEMI are not benign events and are associated with increased morbidity and mortality.[141] Risk factors for VT/VF during PPCI include patients with comorbid conditions, early presentation from symptom onset to the emergency department (ED) arrival (<180 minutes), baseline heart rate >70 bpm, lack of β-blockers in ED, initial TIMI flow grade 0 and right coronary as infarct-related artery.[141,147–149] Bradyarrhythmias due to vagal responses emanating from afferents in the inferoposterior wall of the left ventricle, or efferents to the AV node are more common in fearful or anxious patients, dehydrated patients or patients in pain.[34(p741)] Prolonged bradycardia is more likely associated with ischemia or reperfusion of the right coronary artery and in particular the dominant artery supplying the sinus or AV nodal arteries.[34(p741)] Reperfusion arrhythmias immediately following PPCI, in order of frequency, involve increased ventricular ectopics (52%), acute idioventricular rhythm (33%), bradycardia (17%), atrial fibrillation (10%), non-sustained VT (5%) and VF (2%).[150]

Arrhythmias associated with TAVI commonly occur peri-procedurally and extend beyond the procedure itself. Conduction disturbances include bradyarrhythmias such as heart block and bundle branch blocks and are related to the close anatomical relationship between the aortic valve and fundamental structures of the heart conduction system.[151] New onset LBBB (10.2%–52%)[151] RBBB, advanced AV blocks (8.3%–36%)[151] and result in permanent pacemaker implantation (PPI) post TAVI in 6.5%–36.0% of patients;[151–153] however, many conduction abnormalities resolve prior to discharge and over time, rates of PPI are decreasing.[151] The wide range in incidence of conduction disturbances is related to patient and procedure factors including premorbid conditions, size of valve, depth of implantation, overexpansion of native aortic annulus and in particular balloon-expandable valves resulting in lower rates of LBBB than self-expandable valves and to a greater extent mechanically expandable valves.[152–154]

VASOVAGAL REACTION

Vasovagal reaction is a complication resulting from parasympathetic nervous system stimulation and subsequent vagus nerve activation. Vagal activation results in bradycardia, hypotension, and cerebral hypoxia and ischaemia, causing syncope.[155] The most severe responses result in asystole and require cardiopulmonary resuscitation (CPR).[2] A vasovagal reaction from hypotension can occur with no change in heart rate, occurring most commonly in the elderly.[3(p77)] Peri-procedurally, vasovagal reactions may be associated with the initial administration of lidocaine, arterial needle insertion or sheath advancement.[3(p76)] Vasovagal reaction may also be caused by IV contrast saturation in the coronary tree, creating competitive flow and localised ischaemia. Patients are asked to cough to increase vagal tone, increase intrathoracic pressure and dispel contrast from coronary tree. Post-procedure risk is higher in femoral than radial access procedures, especially during sheath removal and is associated with pain.[3(p138)]

Treatment of vasovagal reaction includes removal of the noxious stimuli causing the vagal response (e.g. releasing pressure application on the arterial access site while maintaining haemostasis), bolus administration of IV fluids, administration of atropine and metaraminol (if not easily reversed or prolonged), metoclopramide (or similar) for nausea and vomiting if required, and closely monitoring vital signs and neurovascular observations.

NURSE'S ROLE IN THE CCL TEAM IN PREVENTION AND IDENTIFICATION OF COMPLICATIONS

The role of the nurse during cardiac catheterisation and PCI is critical in the identification of serious complications and they are an integral part of the team approach in managing them. Nurses are in an ideal position to improve patient outcomes by:

- Observing for complications, i.e. 'another set of eyes'
- Reporting suddenly changing or trending haemodynamics, e.g. pressure damping

- Reporting cardiac rhythm changes
- Assessing patients, pain, level of consciousness
- Suggesting alternative equipment available
- Awareness of, familiarisation with (and how to use or prepare), location of all stock held in the laboratory
- Reporting distal wire migration, dislodgement or retraction
- Reporting contrast hang-up or extravasation
- Anticipating of worst-case scenarios and responsibilities. Connecting external defibrillator/pacing pads in high risk patients
- Confirming standard medications have been administered and reporting deviations from protocols, double-checking discrepancies with relevant staff
- Suggesting pharmacotherapy options or alternatives
- Reporting agreed key performance indices, e.g. verbalising time since last dose of heparin, checking activated clotting times at agreed intervals
- Clear, closed-loop communication to ensure understanding between team members
- Using graded assertiveness if required to ensure patient safety and standards are adhered to ensuring deteriorating patients receive higher level care if required (e.g. rapid response team)
- Being aware of 'fixation error',[156] recognising all physiological cues in deteriorating patients and escalating as appropriate

PATIENT DISCHARGE

Patient education

Patient education is integral to preparation for discharge and occurs throughout the patient's entire admission. In preparation for discharge there is a shift in focus to ensure the patient understands:

- Care of the arterial access site – for example, supporting the groin firmly when getting in and out of the car on the way home, coughing, laughing, crying, defecating, etc.
- What to do if bleeding or haematoma occurs – instruct the patient to apply firm pressure for a specified period of time (each institution will have their own guidelines) and if uncontrolled, they should call an ambulance or seek urgent

medical help. Some CCLs provide their contact details so patients have a point of contact if they have questions or to report complications.

- Activity restrictions – for same-day procedures patients should be advised to have a quiet evening resting at home with no lifting, sport, housework, or work. This may be recommended for a few days after the procedure, and activity gradually increased thereafter. Refrain from swimming, bathing or use of a spa until puncture site wound has healed.
- Driving restrictions – after invasive arterial procedures and procedures involving procedural sedation, driving restrictions can occur depending on country and state regulations. Driving following cardiac catheterisation and elective PCI can usually recommence in a few days; after a STEMI, NSTEMI, or permanent pacemaker it may be a few weeks[9]; commercial driving restrictions are usually longer and this includes patients having had a cardiac arrest.
- Removal of the dressing – ensure the patient understands the importance of removing the dressing as instructed. Patients may be instructed to remove dressing in the shower the following morning, wash the site gently and pat dry with a towel. If the patient remains in hospital, the dressing should be removed by staff and the site documented appropriately in the patient file. A moist site with a dressing that has not been removed for many days (even reportedly, weeks)[75] has a higher risk of infection. Instruct the patient to observe for signs and symptoms of infection, especially patients most at risk of infection such as diabetic patients.
- The normal course of recovery – the patient may be tired for a day or so, often related to anxiety in the lead-up to the procedure and subsequent lack of sleep, etc. Bruising at the arterial site is normal and will fade in a week or so; however, if bruising is ongoing or other symptoms develop (e.g. alterations in sensation, temperature, movement or strength) the patient should seek help.
- Chest pain or other acute symptoms (appropriate to their diagnosis) – do they have a management plan (if chronic condition) or know who to contact and how?
- Medications – ensure the patient understands when to recommence medications such as metformin and other diabetic medications, NOACs or warfarin, especially if instructions are complex or patient comprehension is an issue.
- Encourage the patient to continue to drink fluids on the same day as the procedure to help clear contrast. Care is required with patients with an impaired LVEF so not to overload.
- Patients with memory problems – education should be directed to a responsible person in addition to the patient.
- The result of the procedure – to reassure (if a normal result) or to provide a course of action if symptoms develop (especially if at risk of STEMI/NSTEMI or acute coronary syndrome, present to hospital if symptoms do not resolve with an agreed timeframe).
- Follow-up with patient's general practitioner, cardiologist or other specialist as directed (e.g. cardiac surgeon). Are the appointments made or do they have to make them? Ensure the patient has the contact details for other health professionals they are required to see.
- Has the patient been referred to cardiac rehabilitation as appropriate?
- Activity and diet guidelines.
- If patient smokes, provide smoking cessation resources.

Finally, the patient should be provided with written instructions covering most of the topics listed above.

Day-only PCI (or same-day discharge)

Patients who undergo elective PCI via the radial approach are increasingly being considered for day-only PCI procedures. Day-only PCI programs offer several advantages including increased patient satisfaction, reduced nursing workload and optimising an efficient care delivery system.[157(p285)] Day-only PCI is not only limited to radial procedures and may be used in femoral procedures where patients are stable and meet discharge-lead criteria. In order to facilitate day-only PCI the following criteria should be considered:

- Proceduralist agrees the patient is appropriate for same-day discharge.
- No procedural or arterial access site complications that would prevent discharge.

- Patient lives within a pre-specified distance deemed acceptable to proceduralist, has private transport to return to hospital in case of complications, agrees to return if complications develop.
- No self-care issues, compliant with instructions including activity and driving restrictions, does not live alone.
- Written instructions are provided and understood.
- Discharge occurs at a time acceptable to patient, significant other and staff.
- Other criteria as developed by individual program.
- Patient should be contacted the next day to ensure wellbeing and discuss any concerns.

Follow-up

Patients should be contacted within 7 days following discharge for the purpose of checking on the arterial access site (removal of dressing; development of any haematoma, bleeding, bruising, limb sensation, movement or strength variances), advocating for cardiac rehabilitation program involvement, questions regarding medications or follow-up appointments, and referral to services where needed.[9,75] This information should be entered into the patient record in case of representation to hospital.

SUMMARY

Nursing in the CCL is a highly specialised and constantly changing discipline where nurses are required to adapt to contemporary evidence constantly evolving interventional techniques. Nurses also work across and are required to be competent in all areas of the CCL, including the preadmission process with the patient, admission and patient-preparation, performing a variety of roles during the procedure (haemodynamic monitoring, medication administration, providing advanced life support measures), and post procedure follow-up (haemostasis techniques), monitoring and managing complications (both vascular and non-access site related), mobilisation instructions, and patient and family education. These highly motivated teams of nurses work very closely with medical, technical, radiography, administrative and other support personnel to provide the highest quality of care to all patients presenting for procedures within the CCL.

REFERENCES

1. Conway A, Rolley J, Page K, Fulbrook P. Clinical practice guidelines for nurse-administered procedural sedation and analgesia in the cardiac catheterization laboratory: A modified Delphi study. *J Adv Nurs.* 2013;70(5):1040–1053.
2. Bashore TM, Balter S, Barac A, Byrne JG, Cavendish JJ, Chambers CE, et al. 2012 American College of Cardiology Foundation/Society for Cardiovascular Angiography and Interventions Expert Consensus Document on Cardiac Catheterization Laboratory Standards Update: A report of the American College of Cardiology Foundation Task Force on Expert Consensus Documents. *J Am Coll Cardiol.* 2012;59(24):2221–2305.
3. Kern MJ, Sorajja P, Lim MJ. *The Cardiac Catheterization Handbook.* 6th ed. Philadelphia, PA: Elsevier; 2016.
4. Levine G, Bates E, Blankenship J, Bailey S, Bittl J, Cercek B, et al. ACCF/AHA/SCAI guidelines for percutaneous coronary intervention: Executive summary: A report of the American College of Cardiology Foundation/American Heart Association Task Force on Practice Guidelines and the Society for Cardiovascular Angiography and Interventions. *J Am Coll Cardiol.* 2011;58(24):e44–e122. Plus Data Supplements 3–4.
5. Katayama H, Yamaguchi K, Kozuka T, Takashima T, Seez P, Matsuura K. Adverse reactions to ionic and nonionic contrast media: A report from the Japanese Committee on the Safety of Contrast Media. *Radiology.* 1990;175(3):621–628.
6. Bush WH, Swanson DP. Acute reactions to intravascular contrast media: Types, risk factors, recognition, and specific treatment. *Am J Roent.* 1991;157(6):1153–1161.
7. Gomi T, Nagamoto M, Hasegawa M, Katoh A, Sugiyami M, Murata N, et al. Are there any differences in acute adverse

reactions among five low-osmolar non-ionic iodinated contrast media? *Eur Radiol.* 2010;20(7):1631–1635.

8. Hamid T, Aleem Q, Lau Y, Singh R, McDonald J, McDonald J, et al. Pre-procedural fasting for coronary interventions: Is it time to change practice? *Heart.* 2014;100:658–661.

9. Rolley J, Salamonson Y, Wensley C, Dennison C, Davidson P. Nursing clinical practice guidelines to improve care for people undergoing percutaneous coronary interventions. *Aust Crit Care.* 2011;24:18–38.

10. Wijns W, Kolh P, Danchin N, Di Mario C, Falk V, Folliguet T, et al. Guidelines on myocardial revascularization: The Task Force on Myocardial Revascularization of the European Society of Cardiology (ESC) and the European Association for Cardio-Thoracic Surgery (EACTS). *Eur Heart J.* 2010;31:2501–2555.

11. Australian Diabetes Society. Peri-operative diabetes management guidelines – Australian Diabetes Society 2012[05/07/2018]. Available from: https://diabetessociety.com.au/documents/perioperativediabetesmanage-mentguidelinesfinalcleanjuly2012.pdf.

12. Amsterdam EA, Wenger NK, Brindis RG, Casey DE, Jaffe AS, Jneid H, et al. 2014 AHA/ACC Guideline for the management of patients with Non-ST-Elevation Acute Coronary Syndromes: Executive Summary. *J Am Coll Cardiol.* 2014;64(24):2645–2687.

13. Levine GN, Bates ER, Blankenship JC, Bailey SR, Bittl JA, Cercek B, et al. 2011 ACCF/AHA/SCAI guideline for percutaneous coronary intervention. *Catheter Cardiovasc Interv.* 2013;82(4):E266–E355.

14. Windecker S, Kolh P, Alfonso F, Collet J-P, Cremer J, Falk V, et al. 2014 ESC/EACTS Guidelines on myocardial revascularization 2014 2014-08-28 00:00:00.

15. van der Molen AJ, Reimer P, Dekkers IA, Bongartz G, Bellin M-F, Bertolotto M, et al. Post-contrast acute kidney injury. Part 2: Risk stratification, role of hydration and other prophylactic measures, patients taking metformin and chronic dialysis. *Eur Radiol.* 2018;28:2856–2869.

16. Australian Diabetes Society. Alert – Severe euglycaemic ketoacidosis with sglt2 inhibitor use in the perioperative period 2018[05/07/2018]. Available from: https://diabetessociety.com.au/documents/2018_ALERT-ADS_SGLT2i_PerioperativeKetoacidosis_v3__final2018_02_14.pdf.

17. Wymer DC. CHAPTER 5 – Imaging. In: Floege J, Johnson RJ, Feehally J, editors. *Comprehensive Clinical Nephrology*, 4th ed. Philadelphia, PA: Mosby; 2010. pp. 56–74.

18. Kern MJ, Sorajja P, Lim MJ. *The Interventional Cardiac Catheterization Handbook.* 4th ed. Philadelphia, PA: Elsevier; 2018.

19. Eeckhout E, Serruys PW, Wijns W, Vahanian A, van Sambeek M, de Palma R, editors. *Percutaneous Interventional Cardiovascular Medicine: The PCR-EAPCI Textbook.* Vol 1. Toulouse, France: PCR Publishing; 2012.

20. Mehran R, Aymong ED, Nikolsky E, Lasic Z, Iakovou I, Fahy M, et al. A simple risk score for prediction of contrast-induced nephropathy after percutaneous coronary intervention: Development and initial validation. *J Am Coll Cardiol.* 2004;44(7):1393–1399.

21. van der Molen AJ, Reimer P, Dekkers IA, Bongartz G, Bellin M-F, Bertolotto M, et al. Post contrast acute kidney injury – Part 1: Definition, clinical features, incidence, role of contrast medium and risk factors. *Eur Radiol.* 2018;28:2845–2855.

22. Faggioni M, Mehran R. Preventing Contrast-induced Renal Failure: A Guide. *Interv Cardiol Review.* 2016;11(2):98–104.

23. Merschen R. An overview of chronic kidney disease and useful strategies for clinical management. *Cath Lab Digest.* 2012;20(3).

24. McCullough PA, Choi JP, Feghali GA, Schussler JM, Stoler RM, Vallabhan RC, et al. Contrast-induced acute kidney injury. *J Am Coll Cardiol.* 2016;68(13):1465–1473.

25. Weisbord SD, Gallagher M, Jneid H, Garcia S, Cass A, Thwin S-S, et al. Outcomes after angiography with sodium bicarbonate and acetylcysteine. *N Engl J Med.* 2018;378:603–614.

26. Majumdar SR, Kjellstrand CM, Tymchak WJ, Hervas-Malo M, Taylor DA, Teo KK. Forced euvolemic diuresis with mannitol and furosemide for prevention of contrast-induced nephropathy in patients with ckd undergoing coronary angiography: A randomized controlled trial. *Am J Kid Dis.* 2009;54(4):602–609.

27. Solomon R, Gordon P, Manoukian SV, Abbott JD, Kereiakes DJ, Jeremias A, et al. Randomized trial of bicarbonate or saline study for the prevention of contrast-induced nephropathy in patients with CKD. *CJASN.* 2015;10(9):1519–1524.

28. ACT Investigators. Acetylcysteine for prevention of renal outcomes in patients undergoing coronary and peripheral vascular angiography – main results from the Randomized Acetylcysteine for Contrast-Induced Nephropathy Trial (ACT). *Circulation.* 2011;124(11):1250–1259.

29. Rudnick MR. Prevention of contrast induced nephropathy associated with angiography – UpToDate 2018[cited 2018 02/07/2018]. Available from: https://www.uptodate.com.acs.hcn.com.au/contents/prevention-of-contrast-nephropathy-associated-with-angiography?search=prevention%20of%20contrast%20induced%20nephropathy&source=search_result&selectedTitle=1 ~ 97&usage_type=default&display_rank=1.

30. Brar SS, Aharonian V, Mansukhani P, Moore N, Shen AYJ, Jorgensen M, et al. Haemodynamic-guided fluid administration for the prevention of contrast-induced acute kidney injury: The POSEIDON randomised controlled trial. *Lancet.* 2014;383(9931):1814–1823.

31. Doherty JU, Gluckman TJ, Hucker WJ, Januzzi JL, Ortel TL, Saxonhouse SJ, et al. 2017 ACC expert consensus decision pathway for periprocedural management of anticoagulation in patients with nonvalvular atrial fibrillation: A report of the American College of Cardiology Clinical Expert Consensus Document Task Force. *J Am Coll Cardiol.* 2017;69(7):871–898.

32. Clinical Excellence Commission. Non-vitamin K antagonist oral anticoagulant (NOAC) guidelines. In: Commission CE, Ed. Sydney, Australia: NSW Health; 2017. pp. 1–40.

33. Chew DP, Scott IA, Cullen L, French JK, Briffa TG, Tideman PA, et al. National Heart Foundation of Australia & Cardiac Society of Australia and New Zealand: Australian clinical guidelines for the management of acute coronary syndromes 2016. *Heart, Lung Circ.* 2016;25:895–951.

34. Eeckhout E, Serruys PW, Wijns W, Vahanian A, van Sambeek M, de Palma R, editors. *Percutaneous Interventional Cardiovascular Medicine: The PCR-EAPCI Textbook.* Vol 2. Toulouse, France: PCR Publishing; 2012.

35. Thomson KR, Varma DK. Safe use of radiographic contrast media. *Aust Prescr.* 2010;33(1):35–37.

36. Gharekhanloo F, Torabian S. Comparison of allergc adverse effects and contrast enhancement between iodixanol and iopro-mide. *Ir J Radiol.* 2012;9(2):63–66.

37. Beaty AD, Lieberman PL, Slavin RG. Seafood allergy and radiocontrast media: Are physicians propagating a myth? *Am J Med.* 2008;121(2):158.e1–e4.

38. Nyakale N, Lockhat Z, Sathekge M. Nuclear medicine-induced allergic reactions. *Curr Allergy Clin Im.* 2015;28(1):10–17.

39. Huang S-W. Seafood and iodine: An analysis of a medical myth. *Allergy Asthma Proc.* 2005;26(6):468–469.

40. Ferguson GT, Make B. *Management of Refractory Chronic Obstructive Pulmonary Disease.* Philadelphia, PA: Wolters Kluwer; 2018.

41. Abdo WF, Heunks LMA. Oxygen-induced hypercapnia in COPD: myths and facts. *Crit Care.* 2012;16(5):323–326.

42. Gami AS, Olson EJ, Shen WK, Wright RS, Ballman KV, Hodge DO, et al. Obstructive sleep apnea and the risk of sudden cardiac death: A longitudinal study of 10,701 adults. *J Am Coll Cardiol.* 2013;62(7):610–616.

43. Gami AS, Olson EJ, Shen WK, Wright RS, Ballman KV, Hodge DO, et al. Sleep apnea increases risk of sudden cardiac death. *Cath Lab Digest.* 2013;62(7):610–616.

44. Somers VK, White DP, Amin R, Abraham WT, Costa F, Culebras A, et al. Sleep apnea and cardiovascular disease: An American Heart Association/American College of Cardiology Foundation scientific statement From the American Heart Association Council for High Blood Pressure Research Professional Education Committee, Council on Clinical Cardiology, Stroke Council, and Council on Cardiovascular Nursing in Collaboration With the National Heart, Lung, and Blood Institute National Center on Sleep Disorders Research (National Institutes of Health). *J Am Coll Cardiol.* 2008;52(8):686–717.

45. Green M, Ohlsson M, Forberg J, Bjork J, Edenbrandt L, Ekelund U. Best leads in the standard electrocardiogram for the emergency detection of acute coronary syndrome. *J Electrocardiol.* 2007;40(3):251–256.

46. Fitts J, Lee P, Hofmaster P, Malenka D. Fluoroscopy-guided femoral artery puncture reduces the risk of PCI-related complications. *J Interv Cardiol.* 2008;21(3):273–278.

47. Seto AH, Abu-Fadel MS, Sparling JM, Zacharias SJ, Daly TS, Harrison AT, et al. Real-time ultrasound guidance facilitates femoral arterial access and reduces vascular complications: FAUST (Femoral Arterial Access With Ultrasound Trial). *JACC: Cardiovasc Interv.* 2010;3(7):751–758.

48. Bertrand OF, Rao SV. Complications of transradial catheterization. In: Bertrand OF, Barbeau G, Kiemeneij F, editors. *Best Practices for Transradial Approach in Diagnostic Angiography and Intervention.* Philadelphia, PA: Wolters Kluwer; 2015. pp. 139–148.

49. Azzalini L, Jolicoeur EM. The use of radial access decreases the risk of vascular access-site-related complications at a patient level but is associated with an increased risk at a population level: The radial paradox. *EuroIntervention.* 2014;10(4):531–532.

50. Drew BJ, Califf RM, Funk M, Kaufman ES, Krucoff MW, Laks MM, et al. Practice standards for electrocardiographic monitoring in hospital settings: An American Heart Association Scientific Statement From the Councils on Cardiovascular Nursing, Clinical Cardiology, and Cardiovascular Disease in the Young: Endorsed by the International Society of Computerized Electrocardiology and the American Association of Critical-Care Nurses. *Circulation.* 2004;110(17):2721–2746.

51. Gupta PN, Salam Basheer A, Sukumaran GG, Padmajan S, Praveen S, Velappan P, et al. Femoral artery pseudoaneurysm as a complication of angioplasty. How can it be prevented? *Heart Asia.* 2013;5(1):144–147.

52. Carrozza JP, Cutlip D, Saperia GM. Complications of diagnostic cardiac catheterization 2018[cited 2018 13/07/2018]. Available from: www.uptodate.com.

53. Koreny M, Riedmuller E, Nikfardjam M, Siostrzonek P, Mullner M. Arterial puncture closing devices compared with standard manual compression after cardiac catheterization: systematic review and meta-analysis. *JAMA* 2004;291(3):350–357.

54. Lavi S, Cheema A, Yadegari A, Israeli Z, Levi Y, Wall S, et al. Randomized trial of compression duration after transradial cardiac catheterization and intervention. *J Am Heart Assoc: Cardiovasc Cerebrovasc Dis.* 2017 02/03./09/received/28/ accepted;6(2):e005029.

55. Benit E, Missault L, Eeman T, Carlier M, Muyldermanns L, Materne P, et al. Brachial, radial, or femoral approach for elective Palmaz-Schatz stent implantation: A randomized comparison. *Catheter Cardiovasc Diag.* 1997;41:124–130.

56. Johnson L, Esente P, Giambartolomei A, Grant W, Loin M, Reger M, et al. Peripheral vascular complications of coronary angioplasty by the femoral and brachial techniques. *Catheter Cardiovasc Diag* 1994;31(3):165–172.

57. Cohen M, Alfonzo C. Starting a transradial vascular access program in the cardiac catheterization laboratory. *J Inv Cardiol.* 2009;21(Supplement A):11A–7A.

58. Jolly SS, Yusuf S, Cairns J, Niemela K, Xavier D, Widimsky P, et al. Radial versus femoral access for coronary angiography and intervention in patients with acute coronary syndromes (RIVAL): A randomised, parallel group, multicentre trial. *Lancet.* 2011;377(23 April):1409–1420.

59. Tremmel J. Launching a successful transradial program. *J Inv Cardiol.* 2009;21(Supplement A):3A–8A.

60. Eggebrecht H, Von Birgelen C, Naber CK, Kroeger K, Schmermund A, Wieneke H, et al. Impact of gender of femoral access complications secondary to application of a collagen-based vascular closure device. *J Inv Cardiol.* 2004;16(5):247–250.

61. Chlan L, Sabo J, Savik K. Effects of three groin compression methods on patient discomfort, distress, and vascular complications following a percutaneous coronary intervention procedure. *Nurs Res.* 2005;54(6):391–398.

62. Tewari S, Sharma N, Kapoor A, Syal SK, Kumar S, Garg N, et al. Comparison of transradial and transfemoral artery approach for percutaneous coronary angiography and angioplasty: A retrospective seven-year experience from a north Indian center. *Indian Heart J.* 2013;65(4):378–387.

63. Warren BS, Warren SG, Miller SD. Predictors of complications and learning curve using the Angio-Seal closure device following interventional and diagnostic catheterization. *Catheter Cardiovasc Interv.* 1999;48(2):162–166.

64. Kussmaul 3rd W, Buchbinder M, Whitlow P, Aker U, Heuser R, King S, et al. Femoral artery hemostasis using an implantable device (Angio-Seal) after coronary angioplasty. *Catheter Cardiovasc Diag.* 1996;37:362–365.

65. McCabe PJ, McPherson LA, Lohse CM, Weaver AL. Evaluation of nursing care after diagnostic coronary angiography. *Am J Crit Care.* 2001;10(5):330–340.

66. Applegate RJ, Grabarczyk MA, Little WC, Craven T, Walkup M, Kahl FR, et al. Vascular closure devices in patients treated with anticoagulation and IIb/IIIa receptor inhibitors during percutaneous revascularization. *J Am Coll Cardiol.* 2002;40(1):78–83.

67. Chandrasekar B, Doucet S, Bilodeau L, Crepeau J, deGuise P, Gregoire J, et al. Complications of cardiac catheterization in the current era: A single-center experience. *Catheter Cardiovasc Interv.* 2001;52:289–295.

68. Sanborn TA, Ebrahimi R, Manoukian SV, McLaurin BT, Cox DA, Feit F, et al. Impact of femoral vascular closure devices and anti-thrombotic therapy on access site bleeding in acute coronary syndromes: The acute catheterization and urgent intervention triage strategy (ACUITY) trial. *Circulation: Cardiovasc Interv.* 2010;3(1):57–62.

69. Dangas G, Mehran R, Kokolis S, Feldman D, Satelr L, Pichard A, et al. Vascular complications after percutaneous coronary interventions following hemostasis with manual compression versus arteriotomy closure devices. *J Am Coll Cardiol.* 2001;38(3):638–641.

70. Amin F, Yousufuddin M, Stables R, Shamin W, Al-Nasser F, Coats A, et al. Femoral haemostasis after transcatheter therapeutic intervention: A prospective randomised study of the angio-seal device vs. the femostop device. *Int J Cardiol.* 2000;76:235–240.

71. Ramana RK, Singh A, Dieter RS, Moran JF, Steen L, Lewis BE, et al. Femoral angiogram prior to arteriotomy closure device does not reduce vascular complications in patients undergoing cardiac catheterization. *J Interv Cardiol.* 2008;21(2):204–208.

72. Doyle BJ, Ting HH, Bell MR, Lennon RJ, Mathew V, Singh M, et al. Major femoral bleeding complications after percutaneous coronary intervention – incidence, predictors and impact on long-term survival among 17,901 patients treated at the Mayo Clinic from 1994 to 2005. *J Am Coll Cardiol: Cardiovasc Interv.* 2008;1(2):202–209.

73. Cheng KY, Chair SY, Choi KC. Access site complications and puncture site pain following transradial coronary procedures: A correlational study. *Int J Nurs Stud.* 2013;50(10):1304–1313.

74. Lansky AJ, Pietras C, Costa RA, Tsuchiya Y, Brodie BR, Cox DA, et al. Gender differences in outcomes after primary angioplasty versus primary stenting with and without abciximab for acute myocardial infarction: Results of the Controlled Abciximab and Device Investigation to Lower Late Angioplasty Complications (CADILLAC) trial. *Circulation.* 2005;111(13):1611–1618.

75. Parkinson J. An evaluation of peripheral vascular access site complications following coronary angiography and percutaneous coronary intervention (PCI). University of Sydney, NSW; 2015.

76. Tavris DR, Gallauresi BA, Lin B, Rich SE, Shaw RE, Weintraub WS, et al. Risk of local adverse events following cardiac catheterization by hemostasis device use and gender. J Inv Cardiol. 2004;16(9):459–464.

77. Tavris DR, Gallauresi BA, Dey S, Brindis R, Mitchel K. Risk of local adverse events by gender following cardiac catheterization. Pharmacoepidemiol Drug Saf. 2007;16(2):125–131.

78. Kiemeneij F, Laarman GJ, Odekerken D, Slagboom T, van der Wieken R. A randomized comparison of percutaneous transluminal coronary angioplasty by the radial, brachial and femoral approaches: The access study. J Am Coll Cardiol. 1997;29(6):1269–1275.

79. Mamas M, Ratib K, Routledge H, Neyses L, Fraser D, de Belder M, et al. Influence of arterial access site selection on outcomes in Primary Percutaneous Coronary Intervention. J Am Coll Cardiol: Cardiovasc Interv. 2013;6(7):698–706.

80. Watson S, Gorski KA. Invasive Cardiology – A Manual for Cath Lab Personnel. 2nd ed. Royal Oak, MI: Physicians' Press; 2005.

81. Andersen K, Bregendahl M, Kaestel H, Skriver M, Ravkilde J. Haematoma after coronary angiography and percutaneous coronary intervention via the femoral artery frequency and risk factors. Eur J Cardiovasc Nurs. 2005;4(2):123–127.

82. Tizón-Marcos H, Bertrand OF, Rodés-Cabau J, Larose É, Gaudreault V, Bagur R, et al. Impact of female gender and transradial coronary stenting with maximal antiplatelet therapy on bleeding and ischemic outcomes. Am Heart J. 2009;157(4):740–745.

83. Berry C, Kelly J, Cobbe S, Eteiba H. Comparison of femoral bleeding complications after coronary angiography versus percutaneous coronary intervention. Am J Cardiol. 2004;94(3):361–363.

84. Burzotta F, Trani C, Mazzari MA, Tommasino A, Niccoli G, Porto I, et al. Vascular complications and access crossover in 10,676 transradial percutaneous coronary procedures. Am Heart J. 2012;163:230–238.

85. Walker S, Cleary S, Higgins M. Comparison of the FemoStop device and manual pressure in reducing groin puncture site complications following coronary angioplasty and coronary stent placement. Int J Nurs Prac. 2001;7(6):366–375.

86. Tizón-Marcos H, Barbeau G. Incidence of compartment syndrome of the arm in a large series of transradial appoach for coronary procedures. J Intervl Cardiol. 2008;21(5):380–384.

87. Maluenda G, Delhaye C, Gonzalez MA, Ben-Dor I, Gaglia MA, Collins SD, et al. Conservative versus invasive management strategy for retroperitoneal hemorrhage after percutaneous coronary intervention. J Am Coll Cardiol. 2010;55(10 Supplement):A215.E2039.

88. Farouque HMO, Tremmel JA, Raissi Shabari F, Aggarwal M, Fearon WF, Ng MKC, et al. Risk factors for the development of retroperitoneal hematoma after percutaneous coronary intervention in the era of glycoprotein IIb/IIIa inhibitors and vascular closure devices. J Am Coll Cardiol. 2005;45(3):363–368.

89. Ellis SG, Bhatt D, Kapadia S, Lee D, Yen M, Whitlow PL. Correlates and outcomes of retroperitoneal hemorrhage complicating percutaneous coronary intervention. Catheter Cardio Inte. 2006;67(4):541–545.

90. Kent KC, Moscucci M, Mansour KA, DiMattia S, Gallagher S, Kuntz R, et al. Retroperitoneal hematoma after cardiac catheterization: Prevalence, risk factors, and optimal management. J Vasc Surg. 1994;20(6):905–913.

91. Tiroch KA, Arora N, Matheny ME, Liu C, Lee TC, Resnic FS. Risk predictors of retroperitoneal hemorrhage following percutaneous coronary intervention. Am J Cardiol. 2008;102(11):1473–1476.

92. Young K, Earl T, Selzer F, Marroquin OC, Mulukutla SR, Cohen HA, et al. Trends in major entry site complications from

percutaneous coronary intervention (from the Dynamic Registry). *Am J Cardiol.* 2014;113(4):626–630.

93. Patel T, Shah S, Pancholy SB, editors. *Anantomy, Tortuosities and Access Difficulties.* Philadelphia, PA: Wolters Kluwer; 2015.

94. Rathore S, editor. *Radial Artery Spasm and Abnormal Flow Reserve.* Philadelphia, PA: Wolters Kluwer; 2015.

95. Amoroso G, Laarman G-J, Kiemeneij F. Overview of the transradial approach in percutaneous coronary intervention. *J Cardiovasc Med.* 2007;8(4):230–237.

96. Loh YJ, Nakao M, Tan WD, Lim CH, Tan YS, Chua YL. Factors influencing radial artery size. *Asian Cardiovas Thorac Ann.* 2007;15(4):324–326.

97. Caputo RP, Tremmel JA, Rao S, Gilchrist IC, Pyne C, Pancholy S, et al. Transradial arterial access for coronary and peripheral procedures: Executive summary by the transradial committee of the SCAI. *Catheter Cardiovasc Interv.* 2011;78:829–839.

98. Rathore S, Stables RH, Pauriah M, Hakeem A, Mills JD, Palmer ND, et al. Impact of length and hydrophilic coating of the introducer sheath on radial artery spasm during transradial coronary intervention: A randomized study. *JACC: Cardiovasc Interv.* 2010;3(5):475–483.

99. Abdelaal E, Bernat I, Pancholy SB, editors. *Hemostasis and Radial Artery Occlusion.* Philadelphia, PA: Wolters Kluwer; 2015.

100. Rao SV, Tremmel JA, Gilchrist IC, Shah PB, Gulati R, Shrof AR, et al. Best practices for transradial angiography and intervention: A consensus statement from the society for cardiovascular angiography and intervention's transradial working group. *Catheter Cardiovasc Interv.* 2014;83(2):228–236.

101. Pancholy SB, Bernat I, Bertrand OF, Patel TM. Prevention of Radial artery occlusion after transradial catheterization: The PROPHET-II Randomized Trial. *JACC: Cardiovasc Interv.* 2016;9(19):1992–1999.

102. Zankl AR, Andrassy M, Volz C, Ivandic B, Krumsdorf U, Katus HA, et al. Radial artery thrombosis following transradial coronary angiography: Incidence and rationale for treatment of symptomatic patients with low-molecular-weight heparins. *Clin Res Cardiol.* 2010;99(12):841–847.

103. Chen Y, Ke Z, Xiao J, Lin M, Huang X, Yan C, et al. Subcutaneous injection of nitroglycerin at the radial artery puncture site reduces the risk of early radial artery occlusion after transradial coronary catheterization: A randomized, placebo-controlled clinical trial. *Circulation: Cardiovasc Interv.* 2018;11(7):e006571.

104. Rashid M, Kwok CS, Pancholy S, Chugh S, Kedev SA, Bernat I, et al. Radial artery occlusion after transradial interventions: A systematic review and meta-analysis. *J Am Heart Assoc.* 2016;5(1):e002686.

105. Dencker D, Pedersen F, Engström T, Køber L, Højberg S, Nielsen MB, et al. Major femoral vascular access complications after coronary diagnostic and interventional procedures: A Danish register study. *Int J Cardiol.* 2016;202:604–608.

106. Ates M, Sahin S, Konuralp C, Gullu U, Cimen S, Kizilay M, et al. Evaluation of risk factors associated with femoral pseudoaneurysms after cardiac catheterization. *J Vasc Surg.* 2006;43(3):520–524.

107. Lenartova M, Tak T. Iatrogenic pseudoaneurysm of femoral artery: Case report and literature review. *Clin Med Res.* 2003;1(1):243–247.

108. Moscucci M, Mansour KA, Kent C, Kuntz RE, Senerchia C, Baim DS, et al. Peripheral vascular complications of directional coronary atherectomy and stenting: Predictors, management, and outcome. *Am J Cardiol.* 1994;74:448–453.

109. Knight CG, Healy DA, Thomas RL. Femoral artery pseudoaneurysms: Risk factors, prevalence, and treatment options. *Ann Vasc Surg.* 2003;17(5):503–508.

110. Kresowik TF, Khoury MD, Miller BV, Winniford MD, Shamma AR, Sharp WJ, et al. A prospective study of the incidence and natural history of femoral vascular complications after percutaneous transluminal coronary angioplasty. *J Vasc Surg.* 1991;13(2):328–333; discussion 33–35.

111. Quarmby JW, Engelke C, Chitolie A, Morgan RA, Belli AM. Autologous thrombin for treatment of pseudoaneurysms. *Lancet.* 200216;359(9310):946–947.

112. Kelm M, Perings SM, Jax T, Lauer T, Schoebel FC, Heintzen MP, et al. Incidence and clinical outcome of iatrogenic femoral arteriovenous fistulas: Implications for risk stratification and treatment. *J Am Coll Cardiol.* 2002;40(2):291–297.

113. Samal AK, White CJ. Percutaneous management of access site complications. *Catheter Cardio Interv.* 2002;57(1):12–23.

114. Waksman R, King SB, 3rd, Douglas JS, Shen Y, Ewing H, Mueller L, et al. Predictors of groin complications after balloon and new-device coronary intervention. *Am J Cardiol.* 1995;75(14):886–889.

115. Cherr GS, Travis JA, Ligush J, Jr., Plonk G, Hansen KJ, Braden G, et al. Infection is an unusual but serious complication of a femoral artery catheterization site closure device. *Ann Vasc Surg.* 2001;15(5):567–570.

116. Cooper C, Miller A. Infectious complications related to the use of the Angio-Seal hemostatic puncture closure device. *Catheter Cardiovasc Interv.* 1999;48:301–303.

117. Pipkin W, Brophy C, Nesbit R, Mondy JS. Early experience with infectious complications of percutaneous femoral artery closure devices. *J Vasc Surg.* 2000;32(1):205–208.

118. Smith TP, Cruz CP, Moursi MM, Eidt JF. Infectious complications resulting from use of hemostatic puncture closure devices. *Am J Surg.* 2001;182(6):658–662.

119. Samore MH, Wessolossky MA, Lewis SM, Shubrooks Jr SJ, Karchmer AW. Frequency, risk factors, and outcome for bacteremia after percutaneous transluminal coronary angioplasty. *Am J Cardiol.* 1997;79(7):873–877.

120. Chevalier B, Lancelin B, Koning R, Henry M, Gommeaux A, Pilliere R, et al. Effect of a closure device on complications rates in high-local-risk patients: Results of a randomized multicenter trial. *Catheter Cardiovasc Interv.* 2003;58:285–291.

121. Kahn Z, Kumar M, Hollander G, Frankel R. Safety and efficacy of the perclose suture-mediated closure device after diagnostic and interventional catheterizations in a large consecutive population. *Catheter Cardiovasc Interv.* 2002;55:8–13.

122. Kapadia S, Raymond R, Knopf W, Jenkin S, Chapekis A, Ansel G, et al. The 6F angio-seal arterial closure device: Results from a multimember prospective registry. *Am J Cardiol.* 2001;87(6):789–791.

123. Kussmaul 3rd W, Buchbinder M, Whitlow P, Aker U, Heuser R, King S, et al. Rapid arterial hemostasis and decreased access site complications after cardiac catheterization and angioplasty: Results of a randomized trial of a novel hemostatic device. *J Am Coll Cardiol.* 1995;25(7):1685–1692.

124. Cosman TL, Arthur HM, Natarajan MK. Prevalence of bruising at the vascular access site one week after elective cardiac catheterisation or percutaneous coronary intervention. *J Clin Nurs.* 2011;20(9–10):1349–1356.

125. Jaspers L, Benit E. Immediate sheath removal after PCI using a Femostop is feasible and safe: Results of a registry. *Acta Radiologica.* 2003;58(6):535–537.

126. Jones T, McCutcheon H. A randomised controlled trial comparing the use of manual versus mechanical compression to obtain haemostasis following coronary angiography. *Intensive Crit Care Nurs.* 2003;19(1):11–20.

127. Robb C, McLean S. Using pressure dressings after femoral artery sheath removal. *Professional Nurse.* 2000;15(6):371–374.

128. Sabo J, Chlan LL, Savik K. Relationships among patient characteristics, comorbidities, and vascular complications post-percutaneous coronary intervention. *Heart & Lung.* 2008;37(3):190–195.

129. Stankovic G, Orlic D, Corvaja N, Airoldi F, Chieffo A, Spanos V, et al. Incidence, predictors, in-hospital, and late outcomes of coronary artery perforations. *Am J Cardiol.* 2004;93(2):213–216.

130. Ellis SG, Ajluni S, Arnold AZ, Popma JJ, Bittl JA, Eigler NL, et al. Increased coronary perforation in the new device era: Incidence, classification, management, and outcome. *Circulation.* 1994;90(6):2725–2730.

131. Fasseas P, Orford JL, Panetta CJ, Bell MR, Denktas AE, Lennon RJ, et al. Incidence, correlates, management, and clinical

outcome of coronary perforation: Analysis of 16,298 procedures. *Am Heart J.* 2004;147(1):140–145.

132. Kern MJ, Berger PB, Block P, Klein L, Laskey W, Uretsky BF, editors. *SCAI Interventional Cardiology Board Review Book.* Philadelphia, PA: Lippincott, Williams & Wilkins; 2007.

133. Resnic FS, Wainstein M, Lee MKY, Behrendt D, Wainstein RV, Ohno-Machado L, et al. No-reflow is an independent predictor of death and myocardial infarction after percutaneous coronary intervention. *Am Heart J.* 2003;145(1):42–46.

134. Ndrepepa G, Tiroch K, Keta D, Fusaro M, Seyfarth M, Pache J, et al. Predictive factors and impact of no reflow after primary percutaneous coronary intervention in patients with acute myocardial infarction. *Circulation: Cardiovasc Interv.* 2010;3(1):27–33.

135. Khan M, Schmidt DH, Bajwa T, Shalev Y. Coronary air embolism: Incidence, severity, and suggested approaches to treatment. *Catheter Cardiovasc Diag.* 1995;36(4):313–318.

136. Prasad A, Banerjee S, Brilakis ES. Hemodynamic consequences of massive coronary air embolism. *Circulation.* 2007;115(4):e51–e3.

137. Patterson MS, Kiemeneij F. Coronary air embolism treated with aspiration catheter. *Heart.* 2005;91(5):e36.

138. Holmes DR, Kereiakes DJ, Garg S, Serruys PW, Dehmer GJ, Ellis SG, et al. Stent thrombosis. *J Am Coll Cardiol.* 2010;56(17):1357–1365.

139. Carrozza JP. Periprocedural complications of percutaneous coronray intervention. Wolters Kluwer; 2018[updated 08/02/2018; cited 2018 13/07/2018].

140. Ibanez B, James S, Agewall S, Antunes MJ, Bucciarelli-Ducci C, Bueno H, et al. 2017 ESC Guidelines for the management of acute myocardial infarction in patients presenting with ST-segment elevationThe Task Force for the management of acute myocardial infarction in patients presenting with ST-segment elevation of the European Society of Cardiology (ESC). *Eur Heart J.* 2018;39(2):119–177.

141. Mehta MH, Starr AZ, Lopes RD, Hochman JS, Widimsky P, Pieper KS, et al. For the APEX AMI Investigators. Incidence of and outcomes associated with ventricular tachycardia or fibrillation in patients undergoing primary percutaneous coronary intervention. *JAMA.* 2009;3001(17):1779–1789.

142. Eeckhout E, Serruys PW, Wijns W, Vahanian A, van Sambeek M, de Palma R, editors. *Percutaneous Interventional Cardiovascular Medicine: The PCR-EAPCI Textbook.* Vol 3. Toulouse, France: PCR Publishing; 2012.

143. Montone RA, Testa L, Fraccaro C, Montorfano M, Castriota F, Nerla R, et al. Procedural and 30-Day clinical outcoes following transcatheteter aortic replacement with Lotus Valve: Results of the RELEVANT Study. *Catheter Cardiovac Interv.* 2017;90:1206–1211.

144. Klein LW,Korpu D. Damped and ventricularized coronary pressure waveforms. *J Invasive Cardiol.* 2017;29(11):387–389.

145. Her AY, Ann SH, Singh GB, Kim YH, Koo BK, Shin ES. Prediction of coronary atherosclerotic ostial lesion with a damping of the pressure tracing during diagnostic coronary angiography. *Yonsei Med J.* 2016;57(1):58–63.

146. Mahajan N, Hollander G, Malik B, Temple B, Thekkoott D, Abrol S, et al. Isolated and significant left main coronary artery disease: Demographics, hemodynamics and angiographic features. *Angiology.* 2006;57(4):464–477.

147. Mehta RH, Harjai KJ, Grines L, Stone GW, Boura J, Cox D, et al. Primary Angioplasty in Myocardial Infarction (PAMI) Investigators. Sustained ventricular tachycardia or fibrillation in the cardiac catheterization laboratory among patients receiving primary percutaneous coronary intervention: Incidence, predictors and outcomes. *J Am Coll Cardiol.* 2004;43(10):1765–1772.

148. Piccini JP, Berger JS, Brown DL. Early sustained ventricular arrhythmias complicating acute myocardial infarction. *Am J Med.* 2008;121(9):797–804.

149. Ohlow MA, Geller C, Richter S, Farah A, Müller S, Fuhrmann JT, Lauer B. Incidence and predictors of ventricular arrhythmias

after ST-segment elevation myocardial infarction. *Am J Emergency Med.* 2012;30(4):580–586.

150. Wehrens XHT, Doevendans PA, Ophuis TJO, Wellens HJJ. A comparison of electrocardiographic changes during reperfusion of acute myocardial infarction by thrombolysis or percutaneous transluminal coronary angioplasty. *Am Heart J.* 2000;139:430–436.

151. Mangieri A, Montalto C, Pagnesi M, Lanzillo G, Demir O, Testa L, et al. TAVI and post procedural cardiac abnormailities. *Frontiers Cardiovasc Med.* 2018;5(85):1–12.

152. Fadahunsi OO, Olowoyeye A, Ukaigwe A, Li Z, Vora AN, Vemulapalli S, et al. Incidence, predictors and outcomes of permanent pacemaker implantation following transcatheter aortic valve replacement. Analysis of the U.S Society of Thoracic Surgeons/American College of Cardiology TVT Registry. *JAMA: Cardiovasc Interv.* 2016;9(21):2189–2199.

153. Sathananthan J, Ding L, Yu M, Catlin B, Chan A, Charania J, et al. Implications of transcatheter heart valve selection on early and late pacemaker rate and on length of stay. *Canadian J Cardiol.* 2018;34:1165–1173.

154. Auffret V, Puri R, Urena M, Chamandi C, Rodriguez-Gabella T, et al. Conduction disturbances after transcatheter aortic valve replacement – current status and futureperspectives. *Circulation.* 2017;136:1049–1069.

155. Kern M. Hypotension in the Cath Lab? Think Vagal Reaction Early. *Cath Lab Digest.* 2012;20(2).

156. Fioratou E, Flin R, Glavin R. No simple fix for fixation errors: Cognitive processes and their clinical applications. *Anaesthesia.* 2010;65(1):61–69.

157. Speiser BS, Amoroso G, editors. *Nursing Workload.* Philadelphia, PA: Wolters Kluwer; 2015. p. 285.

10

Vascular access site management and arterial closure

PETER HADJIPETROU

INTRODUCTION

Percutaneous catheterisation access and vascular access site care have remained at the forefront of innovation in order to optimise procedural success, reduce complications and maintain patient satisfaction and comfort. The transradial route has gained popularity and is now the preferred access site in many centres around the world, due to patient convenience and safety by reducing vascular access site complications such as retroperitoneal bleeding and allowing early ambulation. The traditional transfemoral approach, however, remains an important skill to master particularly in patients requiring large-bore sheath access such as in complex high-risk interventions, structural procedures and procedures requiring mechanical circulatory support. It is recognised, irrespective of the access site choice, that there is an association between bleeding at the vascular access site and mortality and this has fostered various techniques to optimise vascular access site preparation and management. When the procedure is completed, the sheath(s) are removed

and pressure must be applied to the artery until haemostasis is achieved. Meticulous management of the vascular access site is an integral part of patient care in order to avoid puncture-related complications. The number and complexity of catheterisations performed worldwide continues to increase, with vascular complications estimated to occur in 0.2%–1.9% of patients undergoing elective diagnostic angiography depending on the access site used, and up to 10% in patients undergoing certain interventional procedures.[1–5]

There has been considerable expansion in the indications for diagnostic and percutaneous coronary, cardiac and non-cardiac vascular interventions. More high-risk patients and chronic, complex coronary lesions are being included, necessitating a variety of new devices to improve success rates. In addition, there is now an entire subspecialty of percutaneous cardiac structural intervention that requires large-bore sheath access, performed predominantly via the transfemoral route but also increasingly using axillary, subclavian and transapical approaches. The incidence of complications varies widely because of the diversity of procedures in an increasingly ageing population. Predictors associated with an increased incidence of vascular hazards include older age, presence of peripheral vascular disease, puncture of the superficial femoral artery, smaller body surface area, use of larger-calibre introducing sheaths, the brachial approach, duration and intensity of periprocedural anticoagulants and use of glycoprotein IIb/IIIa receptor inhibitors.[6,7]

PUNCTURE TECHNIQUE AND COMPLICATIONS

Femoral arterial access

Historically, vascular access to the femoral artery and vein has been obtained by palpation and use of the Seldinger technique. The aim is to puncture the common femoral artery at the level of the femoral head in order to facilitate manual compressibility when the sheath is removed and optimise haemostasis. Knowledge of anatomical and bony landmarks as well as a careful puncture technique is important to avoid risks associated with superficial femoral artery puncture or puncture of the retroperitoneal segment and simultaneous artery and vein puncture. As a general guide, it is safer to puncture the artery directly above the inferior border of the femoral head. This may be facilitated by fluoroscopic guidance if necessary. The inguinal skin crease should be avoided as an anatomical landmark because of its variable location in relation to the common femoral artery.

Contemporary vascular access procedures should ideally use the most optimal vessel site, fluoroscopy, ultrasound and meticulous vascular puncture technique including micro-puncture access. The advent of complex procedures requiring large-bore sheaths, longer procedural time and anticoagulation has led to renewed interest in ultrasound-guided vascular access in order to reduce the relatively higher complication rate associated with those procedures. Routine use of ultrasound-guided access has been shown to reduce the likelihood of inadvertent posterior wall arterial puncture, simultaneous arterial/venous puncture, and avoiding puncture of the superficial femoral artery and the retroperitoneal arterial segment. This in turn can potentially reduce the likelihood of failed access and clinical complications such as haematomas, false aneurysms, arterio-venous fistulae, vascular trauma and retroperitoneal haemorrhage.

Complications of femoral access

Femoral vascular access complications range from simple haematomas to more serious injuries that may require surgical repair, false aneurysms, arterio-venous fistulae, infection, arterial thrombosis leading to critical limb ischaemia, femoral neurological deficits and significant bleeding requiring transfusion, with its attendant risks of disease transmission. Unintentional puncture of the femoral artery above the inguinal ligament should be avoided because of the increased risk of retroperitoneal haematoma. Retroperitoneal bleeding is one of the most serious and feared femoral access complications because it can lead to haemodynamic collapse and increased mortality. Bleeding in the retroperitoneal space does not tamponade; it is hidden with no sign of external bleeding and is difficult to diagnose early, with the first sign often being hypotension and haemodynamic collapse.

Every attempt should be made to optimise vascular access and minimise the risk of complications that can lead to potentially avoidable prolonged hospital stays, increased patient discomfort, inconvenience, periprocedural morbidity and added cost, regardless of how successful or elegant the procedure may have otherwise been. It is important to recognise peripheral vascular complications early, which can often be made at the bedside. External haemorrhage is easily recognised and should be managed by immediate compression. Retroperitoneal bleeding is often more difficult to diagnose. It should be suspected in any patient with unexplained hypotension or falling haemoglobin levels following femoral instrumentation. Common presenting symptoms include significant back or flank pain and suprainguinal tenderness and fullness.[8] It is more commonly seen following intensive anticoagulation in conjunction with glycoprotein IIb/IIIa receptor antagonists and prolonged sheath dwelling times. The diagnosis is often made clinically but can be confirmed, if necessary, by computed tomographic scanning. Femoral artery thrombosis is associated with loss of peripheral pulses and clinical signs of limb ischaemia. The diagnosis is usually confirmed by duplex sonography or angiography. Vascular duplex scanning is useful to distinguish a large haematoma from an expanding pseudoaneurysm or arterio-venous fistula. Duplex scanning is also an effective tool for non-surgical repair of pseudoaneurysms. This is achieved by Doppler-guided compression until flow into the pseudoaneurysm is obliterated, or by ultrasound guided thrombin injection into the false aneurysm sac.

Radial artery access site

The femoral approach has historically been used for access in the majority of patients. The radial artery as an alternative and default to femoral access is appealing because it is superficial, easily accessible and compressible and avoids the many vascular complications described with femoral access. As the techniques and catheter equipment have evolved, the transradial artery approach is becoming increasingly popular as the primary access site. In contemporary practice, radial access is preferred by many operators for routine diagnostic and interventional coronary procedures as well as a spectrum of acute clinical syndromes such as ST segment elevation myocardial infarction where the risk of bleeding may be increased from the femoral approach because of the need for potent anticoagulants. Despite the smaller calibre of the radial artery compared to the femoral artery there is no disadvantage to procedural success. With current techniques it has become routine to use 5-French and 6-French procedural sheaths as a result of the steady improvement in accessibility to the lesion site in standard and complex angioplasty. The radial approach has the advantage of minimising access site complications and is relatively easy to use, allowing immediate sheath removal even in anticoagulated patients. It is very comfortable for patients and operator time is shorter, with earlier ambulation also a distinct advantage.

Radial artery complications occur less frequently and tend to be less severe compared to femoral access. These include difficulties related to access and tortuosity necessitating crossover to the contralateral radial or femoral conversion, radial artery spasm and radial artery occlusion rates varying between 1% and 10%. Because of the extensive collateralisation of the hand, clinical ischaemic events are rare.

ACHIEVING HAEMOSTASIS AND CLOSURE OF PUNCTURE SITE

Vascular access complications, as well as the discomfort associated with manual compression and prolonged bed rest have led to several new haemostatic devices for closure of the arterial puncture. These have been studied in several trials evaluating their safety, effectiveness and ease of handling compared with the conventional method of manual compression. There is also potential for improved cost-effectiveness from earlier ambulation and decreased hospital stays.

Direct closure by open suturing of the brachial artery was the first technique described by Sones for achieving haemostasis at the access site. Alternatively, with the introduction of Judkin's percutaneous femoral method for cardiac catheterisation, haemostasis is achieved with direct compression either manually or with a C-clamp device for 10–40 minutes. A pneumatic vascular compression device (Femostop, C.R. Bard, Billerica, MA) has also been developed to apply external femoral artery compression after sheath removal with comparable success and complication rates.

Radial access haemostasis

The ease of achieving haemostasis after radial artery access and early ambulation are the main drivers for the uptake of this technique in contemporary practice. The radial artery is superficial, easily compressible and easy to perform with the assistance of various simple compression bands. It is comfortable for the patient and haemostasis is easily achieved even in fully anticoagulated states.

Femoral access haemoastasis

The main issues with regard to management of the vascular access site are safe removal of the catheter or sheath and accomplishing haemostasis without bleeding or arterial injury. This is most commonly achieved by digital or mechanical compression of the artery to control bleeding and to allow coagulation to occur. In manual compression, arterial sheath removal is usually delayed 4–6 h after interventional procedures or heparin discontinuation. Application of pressure is necessary for periods up to 20 minutes or longer and both hands are usually required for digital compression.

MECHANICAL DEVICES

Mechanical devices such as the C-Clamp consist of a disk-shaped pressure pad attached to an inverted U-shaped structure that is in turn attached to a vertical shaft so that it can slide up and down.

The device is supported by a broad base, which is slipped beneath the patient's hip. When the sheath is removed, downward pressure is applied on the arm, which lowers the disk-pad over the puncture site to compress the artery. The arm automatically locks in this position and is released when coagulation is estimated to have occurred. The height of the arm and the pressure applied can be easily adjusted. The main advantage of this device is that of convenience, allowing the operator to perform other duties while coagulation is taking place. In a randomised trial comparing the effectiveness of manual or C-clamp mechanical compression it was found that patients receiving mechanical compression had a lower incidence of haematoma formation and shorter time to haemostasis.[9,10]

The Femostop pneumatic compression device consists of an inflatable transparent bubble attached to an arch made of hard plastic (Figure 10.1). The plastic guard is secured with an adjustable belt around the patient's hips. Pressure is applied by gradually inflating the bubble as the sheath is removed to temporarily occlude the vessel until haemostasis occurs. Advantages include the ability to accurately control compression pressure using the manometer and the low risk of device malposition with patient movement. This device is safe and effective and seems to cause less discomfort than the C-clamp. It also allows application of gentle compression for prolonged periods, which

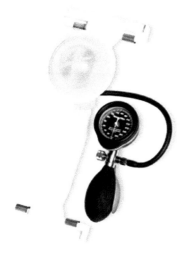

Figure 10.1 FemoStop pneumatic compression device. (Femostop® Vascular Closure Device image provided courtesy of Abbott. ©2018 Abbott. All Rights Reserved.)

may lead to a lower incidence of false aneurysm formation. This should be able to be performed with minimum patient discomfort allowing early recovery, ambulation and discharge.

In general, several hours of bed rest with the patient immobilised are necessary following the haemostasis procedure.

DIRECT ARTERIAL CLOSURE DEVICES

The major disadvantages of compression techniques are that they are time-consuming and anticoagulation has to be reduced before it can be performed safely. This prolongs bed rest, causes patient discomfort and delays convalescence. This has led to the development of several devices to facilitate direct closure of the femoral arteriotomy site, including collagen plug devices (VasoSeal, AngioSeal), and percutaneous suture closure (Perclose, Proglide). These devices can achieve satisfactory haemostasis with equivalent success rates to manual and mechanical compression. If used successfully they provide the advantage of allowing immediate sheath removal and early patient ambulation, shortening the convalescence period.

COLLAGEN PLUGS

Several commercially available devices have been developed to allow delivery of collagen at the exterior of the vessel to achieve haemostasis after arterial puncture. These include the Vascular Haemostatic Device (VHD VasoSeal, Datascope Corp., Montvale, NJ) and Angioseal (Sherwood Davis & Geck, St Louis Missouri), which is a collagen plug with an anchor mechanism.

VasoSeal

The VasoSeal haemostatic device is the prototype bovine collagen device. It consists of purified collagen plugs that induce the formation of a haemostatic cap directly over the arterial puncture site. The biodegradable collagen plug induces local platelet activation and aggregation, releasing coagulation factors and resulting in the formation of fibrin and thrombus. Collagen is ultimately degraded by granulocytes and macrophages. The delivery system uses two 90 mg collagen cartridges advanced through an 11.5 F sheath directly over the arterial surface guided by pre-procedure needle depth measurements and use of a blunt-tipped dilator. After the application of the collagen plug, light pressure is sustained for 3–5 minutes to obtain haemostasis.

Collagen plugs are relatively safe and effective, allowing for earlier patient mobilisation compared to manual compression after diagnostic angiography and are particularly helpful when haemostasis has to be achieved and uninterrupted anticoagulation is desirable. The time needed to attain haemostasis is decreased by about 14 minutes after diagnostic catheterisation (using 6F–8F) and by about 25–30 minutes after angioplasty using the collagen plug compared to conventional manual compression.[2,8] Shorter time to haemostasis is achieved if sealing is performed at a comparable prothrombin time, with similar sheath dwell times as for manual compression.[11] Whereas VasoSeal does not influence the rate of minor local complications, there appears to be an increase in the incidence of major complications. In a retrospective review of the vasoseal haemostasis device in predominantly anticoagulated patients, complications included vascular surgery in 5%, failure to achieve haemostasis (2%), late external bleeding (2%), purulent discharge (1.5%) and large (>6 cm) haematomas (6%). Smaller (<6 cm) haematomas occurred in 7% and minor blood oozing in 7%. One or more complications were noted in 30.5% of cases.[12] These complication rates are similar to other reports and appear to be higher than with manual compression.[13] There is no difference regarding local complications compared to manual compression, when sheath dwell times are identical at similar levels of anticoagulation. There are some other disadvantages for using this device. Delayed application carries a potential risk of infection and is not recommended. Re-puncture of the same artery within 1 month should be avoided because of the risk of intraluminal dislocation of the collagen, which can cause local thrombosis or distal embolisation. Also, the late proliferative reaction induced by the collagen can lead to subcutaneous scar formation and make future arterial access more difficult.

Because of the relatively higher incidence of access site complications associated with this device, its use has been mainly limited to those situations where immediate haemostasis is desirable in patients with high levels of anticoagulation. It has not been recommended for routine use after angioplasty.

Implantable collagen devices

The Haemostatic Puncture Closure Device (AngioSeal) produces direct femoral arterial haemostasis by deploying a bio-absorbable anchor through a carrier sheath to the anterior vascular wall. The anchor is drawn up tightly against the arteriotomy, by means of an absorbable suture while drawing down a small collagen plug. This combination of the anchor with the collagen plug retained by the suture forms a mechanical 'sandwich' around the arteriotomy (Figure 10.2).

The success rate of device deployment is high and the time to haemostasis is considerably shorter even in patients with higher levels of anticoagulation. In most patients this is almost immediate (within 1 minute). Compared with manual compression, complication rates appear to be lower for bleeding

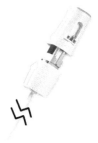

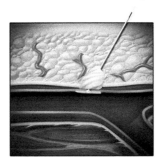

Figure 10.2 The AngioSeal device has 3 absorbable components: An anchor deployed intra-arterially, a collagen sponge positioned on the outer wall of the artery, and a suture. The procedure involves locating the artery, setting the anchor, and sealing the puncture by applying tension on the suture to draw the collagen sponge and anchor together, 'sandwiching' the arteriotomy. (AngioSeal® Vascular Closure Device image provided courtesy of Terumo Medical Corporation.)

and haematoma but there is no difference in the incidence of pseudo-aneurysm, arterio-venous fistulae, limb ischaemia, or infection.[14-16]

This device allows earlier haemostasis and ambulation without associated decrease in safety compared to traditional methods such as manual compression. This device is therefore particularly useful in patients who receive heparin and in those undergoing interventional procedures, allowing shorter sheath dwell times and earlier ambulation and discharge. Its major disadvantage is that re-puncture of the artery is not recommended for at least three months after use of the device.

Percutaneous suturing devices

Devices have been designed for percutaneous deployment of surgical sutures to the common femoral arterial puncture site during diagnostic or interventional procedures (Proglide, Perclose, Techstar/Prostar). The needles with attached sutures are housed in a sheath delivery system, which is advanced through the arteriotomy over a wire. A dedicated marker lumen is incorporated to indicate that the needles and sutures are within the vessel lumen by pulsatile blood return. The needles carrying the sutures are then deployed through the edges of the arteriotomy and tied with a sliding knot and knot pusher to ensure apposition of the knot to the vessel wall (Figure 10.3). These devices are a safe and effective method of achieving haemostasis to allow early or immediate ambulation. They significantly shorten time to haemostasis even when used in fully anticoagulated patients without significant increase in the incidence of major access

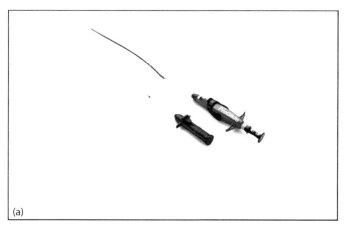

(a)

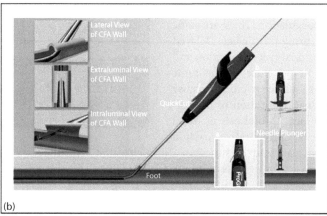

(b)

Figure 10.3 (a) Illustration of the percutaneous suture closure device (Proglide) and (b) insertion into its correct position, indicated by pulsatile blood return from the dedicated marker lumen. The needles are unlocked and pulled through the arterial wall during deployment. The knot pusher is used to oppose the knot to the arterial wall. (Courtesy of Abbott. ©2018 Abbott. All Rights Reserved.)

site related complications.[17,18] For larger sheath access that can range from 8F to 24F, haemostasis can also be achieved by deployed two proglide devices. There is a relatively prolonged learning curve with high volume users of the device generally achieving a higher success rate.

CONCLUSIONS

Where possible, radial artery access is preferred as it is associated with greater patient comfort, earlier ambulation and increased safety and time to haemostasis. In femoral arterial and venous access, a strategy of manual compression or closure devices can be used but suboptimal haemostasis can result in prolonged hospital stay, patient discomfort, and vascular complications. Various strategies to achieve more complete haemostasis and earlier patient ambulation have included use of smaller sheath sizes, C-clamps or pneumatic compression devices, as well as a variety of arterial and venous closure devices. Their effectiveness has been enhanced by the current practice in percutaneous interventions of reducing peri- and post-procedural anticoagulation. However, these various methods of securing haemostasis must be compared with the 'gold standard' of manual compression, which is also safe and effective for smaller sheath sizes. Recently there has been a shift towards the use of ancillary devices to achieve haemostasis, as these permit immediate sheath removal and haemostasis and are successful in achieving haemostasis in larger sheath size access.

Various factors influence the choice of haemostasis technique. Patient factors include the risk of complications and patient tolerance for the technique, taking into consideration body size, discomfort, and the expected duration of compression. Operator factors include individual preference for a device based on previous experience and the learning curve associated with the technique, ease of use and patient safety. Institutional factors include cost, availability of equipment and length of hospital stays. Regardless of the haemostatic device used, it is important for the groin access management scheme to be performed safely and with minimal discomfort to the patient.

REFERENCES

1. Johnson LW, Lozner EC, Johnson S, Krone R, Pichard AD, Vetrovec GW, et al. Coronary arteriography 1984–1987: A report of the registry of the society for cardiac angiography and interventions. I. Results and complications. *Cathet Cardiovasc Diagn.* 1989; 17:5–10.

2. Messina LM, Brothers TE, Wakefield TW, Zelenock GB, Lindenauer SM, Greenfield LJ, et al. Clinical characteristics and surgical management of vascular complications in patients undergoing cardiac catheterization: Interventional versus diagnostic procedures. *J Vasc Surg.* 1991; 13:593–600.

3. Spokojny AM, Sanborn TA. Management of arterial puncture site. *J Interv Cardiol.* 1994; 7:187–193.

4. Johnson LW, Esente P, Giambartolomei A, Grant WD, Loin M, Reger MJ, et al. Peripheral vascular complications of coronary angioplasty by the femoral and brachial techniques. *Cathet Cardiovasc Diagn.* 1994; 31:165–172.

5. Kaufman J, Moglia R, Lacy C, Dinerstein C, Moreyra A. Peripheral vascular complications from percutaneous transluminal coronary angioplasty. A comparison with transfemoral cardiac catheterisation. *Am J Med Sci.* 1989; 297(1):22–25.

6. EPIC investigators. Use of a monoclonal antibody directed against the platelet glycoprotein IIb/IIIa receptor in high-risk coronary angioplasty. *N Engl J Med.* 1994; 330:956–961.

7. EPILOG investigators. Platelet glycoprotein IIb/IIIa blockade with abciximab with low-dose heparin during percutaneous coronary revascularization. *N Engl J Med.* 1997; 336:1689–1696.

8. Kent KC, Moscucci M, Mansour KA, DiMattia S, Gallagher S, Kuntz R, et al. Retroperitoneal haematoma after cardiac catheterisation: Prevalence, risk factors, and optimal management. *J Vasc Surg.* 1994; 20:905–913.

9. Semler HJ. Transfemoral catheterization: Mechanical versus manual control of bleeding. *Radiology*. 1985; 154:234–235.
10. Semler HJ, Experience with an external clamp to control bleeding following transfemoral catheterization. *Radiology*. 1974; 110:225–226.
11. Silber S, Bjorvik A, Rosch A. Usefulness of collagen plugging with VasoSeal after PTCA as compared to manual compression with identical sheath dwell times. *Cathet Cardiovasc Diagn*. 1998; 43:421–427.
12. Carere RG, Webb JG, Miyagishima R, Djurdev O, Ahmed T, Dodek A. Groin Complications associated with collagen plug closure of femoral arterial puncture sites in anticoagulated patients. *Cathet Cardiovasc Diagn*. 1998; 43:124–129.
13. Camenzind E, Grossholz M, Urban P, Dorsaz PA, Didier D, Meier B. Collagen application versus manual compression: A prospective randomized trial for arterial puncture site closure after coronary angioplasty. *J Am Coll Cardiol*. 1994; 24:655–662.
14. Cremonesi A, Castriota F, Tarantino F, Troiani E, Ricci E, El BJ, et al. Femoral arterial haemostasis using the angio-seal system after coronary and vascular percutaneous angioplasty and stenting. *J Invas Cardiol*. 1998; 10:464–469.
15. Fry SM. Review of the Angio-Seal hemostatic puncture closure device. *J Invas Cardiol*. 1998; 10(2):111–120.
16. Kussmaul WG, Buchbinder M, Whitlow PL, Aker UT, Heuser RR, King SB, et al. Rapid arterial haemostasis and decreased access site complications after cardiac catheterization and angioplasty: Results of a randomized trial of a novel haemostatic device. *J Am Coll Cardiol*. 1995; 25:1685–1692.
17. Chamberlin JR, Lardi AB, McKeever LS, Wang MH, Ramadurai G, Grunenwald P, et al. Use of vascular sealing device (VasoSeal and Perclose) versus assisted manual compression (Femostop) in transcatheter coronary interventions requiring Abciximab (Reopro). *Cathet Cardiovasc Interv*. 1999; 47:143–147.
18. Gerckens U, Cattelaens N, Lampe E-G, Grube E. Management of arterial puncture site after catheterization procedures: Evaluating a suture mediated closure device. *Am J Cardiol*. 1999; 83(12):1658–1663.

11

Medical management of the cardiac patient undergoing coronary angiography

SARA HUNGERFORD, PETER RUCHIN AND GERARD CARROLL

INTRODUCTION

Increased access to cardiac catheterisation units and the ongoing evolution of interventional cardiology techniques have revolutionised the treatment of acute coronary syndromes in the last few decades. Emergency percutaneous coronary intervention (PCI), including angioplasty and coronary artery stenting, together with the ongoing development of newer anti-platelet agents, have dramatically altered the management of acute myocardial infarction (AMI) and unstable angina pectoris (UAP).

Beyond interventional cardiology techniques for the coronary circulation, the field has also expanded to include interventions for structural heart disease. The term structural heart disease is used frequently to discuss a broad group of non-coronary heart disease, including congenital and acquired valvular heart disease. Structural heart disease interventions, such as transcatheter aortic valve implantation (TAVI) and transcatheter mitral valve implantation (TMVI), represent a rapidly evolving branch of percutaneous treatments to correct lesions that were previously treated surgically, or simply not addressed.[1]

This chapter examines the indications for cardiac catheterisation, preparation of the coronary care patient prior to angiography or structural heart disease intervention, potential complications of cardiac catheter procedures, and the management of patients on return to the coronary care unit after intervention for coronary or structural heart disease.

INDICATIONS FOR CARDIAC CATHETERISATION

A prominent role of the coronary care unit is to determine which presentations of chest pain are due to acute coronary syndromes (i.e. UAP or AMI). Other frequent indications for admission and cardiac catheterisation include acute dyspnoea of cardiac origin or acute haemodynamic compromise due to arrhythmias, pump failure or valvular disease. These may be classified under the following five major categories:

Diagnostic clarification of chest pain and acute ischaemic syndromes

The decision and timing of cardiac catheterisation in individuals with chest pain and acute ischaemic

syndromes is variable worldwide. Patients presenting with ST-elevation myocardial infarction (see section 'Primary management in acute ST-elevation myocardial infarction') should have, where possible, immediate cardiac catheterisation. Randomised trials have shown benefit and support the principle of an early invasive approach in other 'high-risk' patients (i.e. non ST-elevation myocardial infarction, fluctuating ST segments, prolonged rest pain, pulmonary oedema with ischaemia, recurrent or sustained ventricular arrythmias, new mitral regurgitation, and elevated troponins in the first eight hours after onset of pain). While the optimal timing is uncertain, the majority of patients undergo coronary revascularisation early (i.e. within 24 hours where feasible). This early timing was shown to be of clear benefit in high-risk patients in the TIMACS trial, and subgroup analyses of major trials support this approach in elderly patients as well as younger patients.[2]

Patients with 'completed' myocardial infarction may develop in-hospital complications, the most common of which is ongoing ischemia. Hence, usual practice is the recommendation for coronary angiography during admission. Ongoing ischemia may be evident as rest angina or an abnormal stress test.

Primary management in acute ST-elevation myocardial infarction

With the advent of improved antiplatelet therapies and the more widespread use of drug-eluting stents, immediate intervention for acute coronary occlusion presenting as ST-elevation myocardial infarction has now become a feasible and efficacious first-line treatment option.[3] Many large metropolitan and some well-resourced regional centres offer a 24-hour primary angioplasty and stenting service for the unequivocal acute coronary occlusion presenting as ST-elevation myocardial infarction. The argument for this approach is strongest when the patient is haemodynamically compromised, particularly with cardiogenic shock, which has a very poor prognosis when treated conservatively.

Indeed, since the early pioneering days of coronary angioplasty, multiple randomised trials have now shown that PCI enhances survival and results in a lower rate of intracranial haemorrhage and recurrent myocardial infarction (MI) compared to fibrinolysis.[4] As such, the American College of Cardiology Foundation/American Heart Association guideline for the management of ST-elevation myocardial infarction recommends use of primary percutaneous coronary intervention (PCI) for any patient with an acute ST-elevation myocardial infarction who can undergo the procedure in a timely manner by persons skilled in the procedure.[5] Timely is defined as an ideal first medical contact to PCI time of 90 minutes or less for patients transported to PCI-capable hospital, or 120 minutes or less for patients who initially arrive at or are transported to a non-PCI capable hospital and are then taken to a PCI-capable hospital. For patients presenting with ST-elevation myocardial infarction 12–14 hours after symptom onset, randomised trials of routine late PCI have shown an improvement in left ventricular function, but not in hard clinical outcomes. If primary PCI cannot be achieved in a timely manner (i.e. <90 minutes from patient arrival to balloon angioplasty), then systemic lysis is preferred to ensure timely reperfusion. Lysis remains the reperfusion strategy of choice in the setting of excessive distance or anticipated prolonged 'door-to-balloon' time.

The recommendation for primary PCI in ST-elevation is based on the results of multiple randomised trials comparing PCI to fibrinolytic therapy. In a quantitative meta-analysis of 23 randomised trials, Keeley et al. found that primary PCI was better than thrombolytic therapy at reducing overall short-term death (7% n = 270 vs. 9% n = 360; p = 0.002), death (5% n = 199 vs. 7% n = 276; p = 0.0003), non-fatal re-infarction (3% n = 80 vs. 7% n = 222; p < 0.001), stroke (1% n = 30 vs. 2% n = 64; p = 0.0004), and the combined endpoint of death, non-fatal re-infarction, and stroke (8% n = 253 vs. 14% n = 442; p < 0.0001).[6] The positive outcome from this meta-analysis is driven almost completely by reinfarction in the lysis arm and serves to highlight the importance of early catheterisation when systemic lysis is used as the reperfusion strategy in ST-elevation myocardial infarction. In situations where it is unclear which reperfusion strategy to choose, prolonged duration of presumed coronary occlusion (greater than 3 hours) favours primary PCI over lysis, with respect to outcome.

Rescue PCI for failed thrombolysis, especially in the setting of ongoing ST-segment and haemodynamic compromise

Fibrinolysis immediately before primary PCI, previously called facilitated PCI, is no longer recommended. However, rescue PCI for persistent occlusion of the infarct-related artery in the case of failed thrombolytic therapy, especially when there are signs of haemodynamic compromise, is ideal. This is most relevant to patients in smaller metropolitan and regional coronary care units that may not have access to 24-hour interventional cardiology services and is the reason for a 'drip-and-ship' policy (i.e. systemic lysis followed by immediate transfer to a PCI-capable centre). In a meta-analysis by Topol et al., there was a trend towards a reduction in both the 6-week and 1-year mortality in patients treated with rescue angioplasty compared to those treated with thrombolysis alone.[7]

The elective patient with other indications for undergoing cardiac catheterisation

Aside from chest pain and acute coronary syndromes, there are several other potential indications for the elective patient to undergo cardiac catheterisation (see Table 11.1).

Dyspnoea at rest or on exertion is a common indication for elective cardiac catheterisation. This may be elicited on history or during an exercise stress test. An equivocal or positive functional and/or anatomical cardiovascular screening examination may also prompt referral for elective cardiac catheterisation. These include a positive stress echocardiogram (i.e. ST-segment depression/elevation, dyspnoea or chest pain, ventricular arrhythmias, or evidence of reversible myocardial ischemia on stress echocardiography), and/or a computed tomography (CT) coronary angiogram with evidence of a stenosis >70% lumen diameter.

Table 11.1 Indications for elective cardiac catheterisation

- Dyspnoea
- Positive stress echocardiogram
- CT coronary angiogram with >70% stenosis
- Left ventricular dysfunction
- Pre-operative assessment prior to other cardiac surgery
- Pulmonary hypertension
- Intra-cardiac shunt
- Primary arrhythmias

Cardiac catheterisation also plays an important diagnostic role in determining the aetiology of left ventricular dysfunction (i.e. secondary to either coronary artery disease or cardiomyopathy); the exclusion of coronary artery disease and invasively quantifying pressure-volume relationships in the presence of valvular heart disease; quantification of, and pharmacological challenge in, the setting of pulmonary hypertension, and; the diagnosis and quantification of an intra-cardiac shunt. Patients with primary arrhythmias, such as ventricular tachycardia, atrial fibrillation and even existing left bundle branch block may also benefit from early definition of their coronary anatomy.

Management of valvular and congenital heart disease

AORTIC STENOSIS AND TRANSCATHETER AORTIC VALVE IMPLANTATION (TAVI)

Balloon valvuloplasty for degenerative calcific aortic stenosis (AS) in adults has no long-term haemodynamic or symptomatic benefit, and has been surpassed by rapid advances in transcatheter aortic valve implantation (TAVI) technologies.[8,9] There is a high restenosis rate with balloon valvuloplasty (50% by 6 months) as well as a risk of aortic regurgitation, aortic rupture, leaflet avulsion, ventricular perforation, systemic embolisation or stroke and local vascular injury. It is therefore reserved for patients with critical AS who are extremely unwell and are awaiting surgical or transcatheter aortic valve replacement, or who require urgent non-cardiac surgery.

TAVI is now recognised as a viable therapeutic option for patients with severe, symptomatic AS who are high-risk for conventional surgery. TAVI can be accomplished in selected high-risk patients with outcomes that compare favourably with the outcomes of standard valve replacement as predicted by validated operative risk assessment tools.[10–13] In intermediate-risk patients the rate of death from any cause is similar in the TAVI group when compared to surgical patients. TAVI in intermediate-risk patients has also been shown to result in lower rates of acute kidney injury, severe bleeding, and new onset atrial fibrillation; however, surgery results in fewer major vascular complications and less paravalvular aortic regurgitation.[14]

The procedure is performed with the patient under general anaesthesia and requires use of fluoroscopy and transoesophageal guidance. The ideal transcatheter aortic prosthesis position is to restrain the native leaflets and relieve the stenosis without unnecessary contact with the surrounding structures. A valve extending excessively into the ventricle or the aorta might be associated with adverse events such as mitral insufficiency, arrhythmias or aortic injury.

MITRAL REGURGITATION AND TRANSCATHETER MITRAL VALVE IMPLANTATION (TMVI)

Mitral valve surgery is still the gold standard treatment of mitral regurgitation (MR), and yet, up to 40% of patients with severe MR may not receive conventional surgery because they are deemed too high-risk.[15] Several percutaneous TMVI technologies have been developed over the past few years for patients who are unable to undergo surgical correction of MR, and are at varying stages of investigation and clinical implementation. The existing and upcoming TMVI technologies are best categorised by functional mechanisms, including edge-to-edge repair, chordal repair, indirect or direct annuloplasty, enhanced coaptation, or valve replacement.

The greatest experience exists with MitraClip™, which was first implanted in humans in 2003. The landmark Endovascular Valve Edge-to-Edge Repair Study (EVEREST) demonstrated that percutaneous repair with the MitraClip™ system could be accomplished with low rates of morbidity and mortality and with acute MR reduction to <2+ in the majority of patients.[16,17] There is also an expanding portfolio of transcatheter annuloplasty options (e.g. Cardioband, Mitralign, Carillion and Millipede). These devices either make use of the coronary sinus to achieve indirect annuloplasty, or achieve direct annuloplasty or ventriculoplasty.[18] A number of transcatheter replacement systems are also in the early stages of clinical implementation (e.g. Tendyne, Neovasc, CardaQ and Twelve) and have been shown to be effective and safe therapies for selected patients with symptomatic native MR.[19–23] All TMVI procedures are performed with the patient under general anaesthesia and require the use of fluoroscopy and transoesophageal guidance.

MITRAL AND PULMONARY STENOSIS AND BALLOON VALVULOPLASTY

Long-term success rates of percutaneous mitral balloon valvotomy (see Chapter 38) for mitral stenosis in selected patients are comparable to surgical commissurotomy.[24] Echocardiography is a useful investigative tool in identifying patients who will have favourable outcomes (i.e. those with little or no valve calcification, good valve mobility, minimal valve thickening, minimal mitral regurgitation, no involvement of subvalvular structures and no intercurrent left atrial thrombus).[25] Complications of mitral valvuloplasty include death (0.5%), atrial septal defect (10%) (most are small and close spontaneously), severe mitral regurgitation (2%), ventricular perforation (1%), stroke (1%) and restenosis (10%).[26] Percutaneous balloon valvuloplasty for congenital pulmonary stenosis has been highly successful and is now the procedure of choice provided the valve is not heavily calcified. Long-term 'curative' outcomes have been achieved with very low procedural mortality (0.2%).[27]

PERCUTANEOUS ATRIAL SEPTAL DEFECT (ASD) AND PATENT FORAMEN OVALE (PFO) CLOSURE DEVICES

The first congenital heart lesion to be treated with non-surgical transcatheter devices over 50 years ago was a patent ductus arteriosus (PDA). Since then, a number of other innovative devices have been developed for closure of ASD and PFO. The greatest experience exists with the Amplatzer Septal Occluder Device, which consists of a self-expanding double-disc Nitinol wire mesh with polyester layers. The Amplatzer device may be deployed via a 6–12 French sheath under guidance of simultaneous transoesophageal echocardiography. Complete shunt obliteration is achieved in approximately 94% of patients by 3 months.[28] Complication rates are low and include:[29]

Right ventricular embolism	0.9%
Transient ischaemic attack	0.4%
Endocarditis	0.4%

Patients undergoing transcatheter closure of an ASD, PFO or PDA are admitted on the same day of the procedure and are usually discharged the following morning. In addition to aspirin for 48 hours prior to the procedure, perioperative heparin (5000–15000 international units) and antibiotic prophylaxis are given in the cardiac catheter suite. Post-procedure, a regimen of aspirin 100 mg daily for six months and clopidogrel 75 mg daily for one month is commenced. To determine whether successful closure has occurred, transthoracic echocardiograms are performed at 1, 3 and then 12 months post deployment. Despite shorter 'length-of-stays', high efficacy rates and comparable costs with surgery, non-surgical techniques for ASD and PDA closures still require further large multicentre trial outcomes.

PREPARATION FOR CARDIAC CATHETERISATION

An important function of the coronary care unit is the preparation of the patient prior to coronary angiography.

Consent

Even before admission to the cardiac catheterisation laboratory, patient education should be performed, and informed consent obtained. The risks associated with cardiac catheterisation are described in the following section. The importance of obtaining consent prior to transfer to the laboratory is crucial due to the fact that many patients will receive a premedication comprising of an oral benzodiazepine and/or a sedating antihistamine in the catheterisation laboratory.

Patients at risk of contrast nephropathy

Patients with pre-existing renal disease and reduced eGFR are at increased risk of contrast nephropathy from the iodinated contrast used at cardiac catheterisation. Although there is some debate in the literature, the risk of contrast nephropathy may be minimised by intravenous (IV) hydration immediately prior to, during and after the procedure, as well as strict limitation of contrast volume (i.e. omission of ventriculography or aortography) and use of iso- or low-osmolar contrast (e.g. Visipaque). Pre-procedure N-acetylecysteine (NAC) is used by some operators; however, the benefit of NAC in preventing contrast-induced nephropathy is not well established.[30] It is critical that all patients have recently measured serum urea and creatinine prior to cardiac catheterisation, as contrast nephropathy is dependent on contrast dose, and knowledge of renal risk may alter the approach in individual patients, to limit contrast load.

Patients with diabetes mellitus

Patients with diabetes mellitus make up a large proportion of patients undergoing coronary angiography and have a markedly increased risk of coronary artery disease. Patients with diabetes in the PROCAM study had at least twice the risk of myocardial infarction compared to those without diabetes.[31] The presence of other cardiovascular risk factors was found to increase this risk even further. Patients in the PROCAM population with both diabetes and hyperlipidaemia had a 15-fold increased risk of myocardial infarction. As reported by Haffner, patients with diabetes without a history of ischaemic heart disease have as high a risk of infarction as non-diabetic patients with previous myocardial infarction.[32]

Patients with diabetes require several special precautions prior to cardiac catheterisation, including prehydration to minimise the risk of contrast nephropathy in those with diabetics with even mild renal impairment. The attending physician needs to modify oral hypoglycaemic agents and insulin therapy before and after angiography. As should occur perioperatively, patients with diabetes should omit their sulphonylurea while fasting. If the patient is taking metformin or a sodium-glucose co-transporter 2 inhibitor (e.g. empagliflozin or dapaglifozin), this should be ceased 48 hours prior to angiography if possible, to minimise the potential risk of drug accumulation and lactic acidosis in the setting of contrast-related renal impairment.

Patients with a contrast allergy

Patients with a history of contrast allergy should be considered for pre-treatment with corticosteroid therapy. Those with a history of anaphylaxis to contrast media should receive at least 25 mg prednisone orally or 100 mg hydrocortisone IV at least six hours prior to the procedure. Some physicians recommend oral prednisolone (1 mg/kg/day to a maximum of 50 mg/day) for 72 hours prior to cardiac catheterisation. The 2007 focused update of the American College of Cardiology/American Heart Association/Society for Cardiovascular Angiography and Intervention 2005 percutaneous coronary intervention guidelines recommended the use of iso-osmolar in preference to low osmolar agents in patients with chronic kidney disease.[33]

Antiplatelet therapy

For the majority of patients who are referred for elective coronary angiography, aspirin 100 mg per oral (PO) daily will be commenced prior, with the exception of those who may have an aspirin allergy, have had recent gastro-intestinal ulceration, or who are planned for near-future procedures where antiplatelet therapy may be contraindicated. In patients who are presenting acutely with a ST-elevation myocardial infarction or other high risk acute coronary syndromes, in addition to aspirin loading (300 mg per PO stat evidence suggests an advantage for ticagrelor loading [180 mg per PO stat] over clopidogrel [600 mg per PO stat] in these patients undergoing primary PCI, but at a cost of increased bleeding, particularly if the patient proceeds to subsequent surgical coronary artery bypass grafting.[34-37] Importantly, ticagrelor is not recommended in the context of lysis. Ticagrelor and prasugrel both have the advantage of rapid onset of action compared to clopidogrel, when front loading before PCI. However, clopidogrel is inexpensive, easily available, is a once daily dose, and hence is still widely used in Australia as the second antiplatelet agent to go with aspirin in patients being considered for PCI.

Anticoagulation

In the setting of lysis, either IV/subcutaneous enoxaparin or IV heparin will be administered. In the setting of patients presenting acutely with ST-elevation myocardial infarction or other 'high-risk' acute coronary syndromes for immediate PCI, either enoxaparin or heparin is administered IV simultaneously with the initial anti-platelet loading doses. Heparin is generally preferred over enoxaparin by many operators worldwide due to its easy measurability (i.e. activated clotting time), quick offset, and in limited circumstances, its potential to be reversed with protamine sulphate. For patients undergoing elective cardiac catheterisation, a small dose of IV heparin is frequently administered at the time of sheath insertion at the beginning of the procedure.

COMPLICATIONS OF CARDIAC CATHETERISATION

Coronary angiography and PCI

A variety of adverse events, ranging from minor problems without long-term sequelae to major complications requiring immediate corrective action, may arise from diagnostic cardiac catheterisation and percutaneous coronary intervention. Newer structural interventional procedures may be associated with different, and in some cases, more frequent complications. The most common complications associated with cardiac catheterisation with PCI and TAVI are discussed below.

The Second Registry of the Society for Cardiac Angiography and Interventions reported on over 220,000 patients who underwent cardiac catheterisation over a 3-year period. They found the following complication rates.[38]

Death	0.10%
Myocardial infarction	0.06%
Stroke	0.07%
Local vascular complications (sheath haematomas, false aneurysms, arteriovenous fistulae and infection)	0.46%
Contrast reactions	0.23%

Other well-recognised complications include:[39]

Nephropathy	<0.5%
Serious arrhythmia	0.3%–0.5%
Vasovagal reactions	1.5%–2.5%

The rates of local vascular complications have dramatically decreased with the uptake of the radial rather than brachial approach. Patients identified at highest risk of death were those with left main coronary artery disease (0.55%), left ventricular ejection fractions <30% (0.3%), NYHA functional class IV (0.29%)[38] and severe comorbidities (e.g. diabetes mellitus, renal impairment, chronic lung disease and peripheral vascular disease).

Structural heart disease interventions

Despite being less invasive than open-chest surgery, structural heart disease interventions remain associated with the potential for serious complications. Access and delivery complications pertain mostly to the sheath size and delivery system. Dissection or perforation of the iliofemoral arteries can occur in the setting of traumatic sheath insertion or vessel tortuosity. Further up the arterial tree, vascular perforation leading to retroperitoneal haemorrhage should be suspected when unexplained hypotension occurs. Stroke is also thought to be most likely due to atheroembolism from the ascending aorta or arch as the delivery system is advanced. The incidence of stroke varies but with current devices and experiences, the stroke rate ranges from 0% to 10% in TAVI patients.[40,41]

While device embolisation after deployment is rare, more common complications related to positioning and deployment include paravalvular regurgitation, native valve injury and coronary artery obstruction. With the newer-generation devices, moderate to severe paravalvular regurgitation is infrequent.[10,42,43] Obstruction of a coronary artery may occur during TAVI when an obstructive portion of the frame overlies the ostium, or more concerningly, when a bulky and calcified native leaflet is pinned over the coronary ostium.

Atrioventricular block is known to occur in up to 8.2% of patients undergoing surgical aortic valve replacement.[44] Atrioventricular block also occurs in TAVI patients, presumably as a consequence of the pressure applied on the conducting tissues located subendocardially in the left ventricular outflow tract and interventricular septum. Early experience suggests that prostheses extending farther in the ventricle are associated with a higher incidence of conduction abnormalities, most commonly left bundle branch block.[45] TAVI-induced heart block requiring permanent pacemaker insertion ranges from 7%–18%.[46,47] Serious but extremely rare complications include annular and root rupture, cardiac perforation, cardiogenic shock, acute renal failure and structural valve failure.

POST-ANGIOGRAPHIC MANAGEMENT IN THE CORONARY CARE UNIT

Haemostasis following sheath removal

Following routine cardiac catheterisation via the femoral approach, the femoral sheath is removed and femoral haemostasis is achieved with digital pressure for approximately 10–20 minutes. Several femoral artery closure devices that achieve haemostasis via a suture system or a patch on the wall of the affected femoral artery (e.g. Perclose and Angioseal respectively) have been developed to minimise bleeding and are frequently deployed at the time of sheath removal (see Chapter 10), especially in those patients on dual antiplatelet therapy and anticoagulants. Regardless of the means to achieve haemostasis in patients undergoing a femoral approach, all patients should observe a minimum 4-hours of bed rest post procedure, and be closely monitored for re-bleeding or bruising.

The overall aim of effective haemostasis following femoral sheath removal is to prevent major blood loss, groin haematomas and false aneurysm formation. The physician should auscultate for a femoral bruit; if a false aneurysm is suspected, an ultrasound should be arranged, and manual compression with analgesia is recommended. Doppler ultrasound can be both diagnostic and therapeutic by compressing and closing the neck of the false aneurysm using the ultrasound probe. For more complex femoral arterial complications, CT-angiography, thrombin injection, or interventional or vascular surgical repair can occasionally be required.

Following cardiac catheterisation via the radial approach, the radial sheath is removed and radial haemostasis is routinely achieved using a radial artery compression device rather than digital pressure haemostasis. A mechanical device such as a TR band allows selective compression of the radial artery to allow blood return to the distal hand and preserve patency of the radial artery. The device is transparent so that visual inspection of the puncture site can be maintained. The patient should observe a minimum of 1–2 hours of bed rest, and be closely monitored for re-bleeding or bruising.

Radial artery access is associated with lower rates of post-procedural bleeding than the femoral approach. Nevertheless if re-bleeding at the radial puncture site occurs, the radial band should be reapplied and the local hospital deflation protocol resumed. If swelling or bruising develops in the forearm or upper arm proximal to the initial puncture site, arterial perforation should be suspected and manual pressure applied at the area of maximal swelling for at least 20 minutes until swelling abates. In the event of loss of the distal radial pulse and/ or neurovascular compromise, radial artery dissection should be suspected.

Haemodynamic compromise following cardiac catheterisation

There may be several reasons as to why a patient may develop haemodynamic compromise following cardiac catheterisation. These include, but are not limited to: allergic or anaphylactic reactions; a profound vagal episode following femoral sheath removal or femoral artery compression; blood loss at the puncture site or occult bleeding into the retroperitoneal space; cardiac tamponade; device embolisation; cardiac arrhythmia and/or; re-infarction due to acute stent thrombosis.

Choice of antiplatelet therapy post-procedurally

As soon as possible after the diagnosis of acute coronary syndrome is made, 300 mg of uncoated aspirin should be administered. Once the reperfusion strategy of PCI is confirmed, a P2Y12 receptor blocker, such as ticagrelor, clopidogrel or prasugrel, should be administered in a loading dose.[34-37] For most ST-elevation myocardial infarction patients, a glycoprotein IIb/ IIIa inhibitor is no longer routinely administered, but may be used in the cardiac catheterisation laboratory for evidence of no or slow reperfusion or thrombus or for clinical instability related to worsening ischemia.[48-53] The following day the patient is commenced on aspirin 100 mg daily indefinitely, as well as ticagrelor, clopidogrel or prasugrel for 12 months. This corresponds to the time at which the risk of thrombosis of the coronary artery stent is increased. Careful consideration to individual product information should be followed if switching from one P2Y12 receptor blocker to another in the post-procedure period.

Choice of anticoagulant therapy peri-procedurally

As mentioned above, all patients with ST-elevation myocardial infarction are treated with anticoagulant therapy, which should be given as soon as possible after the diagnosis. For patients undergoing primary PCI, unfractionated heparin is generally preferred in preference to bivalirudin (Grade 2c), on the assumption that the patient will also receive a potent oral antiplatelet agent.[54,55] Anticoagulant therapy is sometimes continued post-procedurally if the thrombus burden is high; however, this is operator-dependent. Otherwise, routine deep venous thrombosis prophylaxis with subcutaneous enoxaparin or heparin is recommended while the patient is cardiac-monitored.

REFERENCES

1. Palacios I, Arzamendi D. Structural heart intervention: Beyond transcatheter valve therapy. *Rev Esp Cardiol.* 2012; 65:405–413.
2. Alexander KP, Newby LK, Cannon CP, Armstrong PW, Gibler WB, Rich MW, et al. Acute coronary care in the elderly, part I: Non-ST-segment-elevation acute coronary syndromes: A scientific statement for healthcare professionals from the American heart association council on clinical cardiology: In collaboration with the society of geriatric cardiology. *Circulation.* 2007; 115(19):2549: https://www.clevelandclinicmeded.com/medicalpubs/diseasemanagement/hematology-oncology/hypercoagulable-states/ Accessed: 7 May 2018.
3. Stone GW, Brodie BR, Griffin JJ, Morice MC, Costantini C, Goar FGS, et al. Prospective, multicentre study of the safety and feasibility of primary stenting in acute myocardial infarction: In-hospital and 30-day results of the PAMI stent pilot trial. *J Am Coll Cardiol.* 1998; 31:23–30.
4. Keeley EC, Boura JA, Grines CL. Primary angioplasty versus IV thrombolytic therapy for acute myocardial infarction: A quantitative review of 23 randomised trials. *Lancet.* 2003; 361(9351):13.
5. O'Gara PT, Kushner FG, Ascheim DD, Casey DE Jr, Chung MK, de Lemos JA, et al. CW2013 ACCF/AHA guideline for the management of ST-elevation myocardial infarction: A report of the American College of Cardiology Foundation/American Heart Association task force on practice guidelines. *Circulation.* 2013; 127(4):e362.
6. Topol EJ, Califf RM, George BS, Kereiakes DJ, Abbottsmith CW, Candela RJ, et al. A randomised trial of immediate versus delayed elective angioplasty after IV tissue plasminogen activator in acute myocardial infarction. *N Engl J Med.* 1987; 317:581–588.
7. Lieberman EB, Bashore TM, Hermiller JB, Wilson JS, Pieper KS, Keeler GP, et al. Balloon aortic valvuloplasty in adults: Failure of procedure to improve long-term survival. *J Am Coll Cardiol.* 1995; 26:1522–1528.
8. Otto CM, Mickel MC, Kennedy JW, et al. Three year outcome after balloon aortic valvuloplasty: Insights into prognosis of valvular aortic stenosis. *Circulation.* 1994; 89:642–650.
9. Grube E, Schuler G, Buellesfeld L, Gerckens U, Linke A, Wenaweser P, et al. Percutaneous aortic valve replacement for severe aortic stenosis in high-risk patients using the second- and current third-generation self-expanding CoreValve prosthesis: Device success and 30-day clinical outcome. *J Am Coll Cardiol.* 2007; 50:69–76.
10. Webb JG, Pasupati S, Humphries K, Thompson C, Altwegg L, Moss R, et al. Percutaneous transarterial aortic valve replacement in selected high-risk patients with aortic stenosis. *Circulation.* 2007; 116:755–763.
11. Smith C, Leon M, Mack M, Miller C, Moses J, Svensson L, et al. PARTNER 1 trial investigators. Transcatheters versus surgical aortic valve replacement in high-risk patients. *New Engl J Med.* 2011: 364:2187–2198.

12. Mack M, Leon M, Smith C, Moses J, Tuzcu E, Webb J, et al. PARTNER 1 trial investigators. 5-year outcomes of transcatheter aortic valve replacement or surgical aortic valve replacement for high surgical risk patients with aortic stenosis (PARTNER 1): A randomized controlled trial. *Lancet*. 2015; 385(9986):2477–2484.

13. Leon M, Smith C, Mack M, Makkar R, Svensson L, Kodali S, et al. the PARTNER 2 trial investigators: Transcatheter or surgical aortic valve replacement in intermediate-risk patients. *N Engl J Med*. 2016; 374:1609–1620.

14. Iung B, Baron G, Butchart EG, Delahaye F, Gohlke-Bärwolf C, Levang OW, et al. A prospective survey of patients with valvular heart disease in Europe: The Euro heart survey on valvular heart disease. *Eur Heart J*. 2003; 24:1231–1243.

15. Feldman T, Kar S, Rinaldi M, Fail P, Hermiller J, Smalling R, et al. Percutaneous mitral repair with the MitraClip system: Safety and mid-term durability in the initial EVEREST cohort. *J Am Coll Cardiol*. 2009; 54:8:686–694.

16. Feldman T, Foster E, Glower D, et al. Percutaneous repair or surgery for mitral regurgitation. *N Engl J Med*. 2011; 364:1395–1406.

17. Nickenig G, Hammerstingl C, Schueler R, Topilsky Y, Grayburn PA, Vahanian A, et al. Transcatheter mitral annuloplasty in chronic functional mitral regurgitation: 6-month results with the CardioBand percutaneous mitral repair system. *JACC Cardiovasc Interv*. 2016; 9(19):2039–2047.

18. Muller D, Jansz P, Shaw M, Conellan M, Spina R, Pedersen W, et al. Transcatheter mitral valve replacement for patients with symptomatic mitral regurgitation: A global feasibility trial. *J Am Coll Cardiol*. 2017; (69/94):381–391.

19. Cheung A, Webb J, Verheye S, Moss R, Boone R, Leipsic J, et al. Short-term results of transapical transcatheter mitral valve implantation for mitral regurgitation. *J Am Coll Cardiol*. 2014; 64:1814–1819.

20. Bapat V, Buellesfeld L, Peterson MD, Hancock J, Reineke D, Buller C, et al. Transcatheter mitral valve implantation (TMVI) using the Edwards FORTIS device. *EuroIntervention*. 2014; 10(suppl U):U120–U128.

21. Quarto C, Davies S, Duncan A, Lindsay A, Lutter G, Lozonschi L, Moat N. Transcatheter mitral valve implantation. 30-day outcome of first-in-man experience with an apically tethered device. *Innovations*. 2016; 11:174–176.

22. Dahle G, Rein K, Fiane A. Single centre experience with transapical transcatheter mitral valve implantation. *Interact Cardiovasc Thorac Surg*. 2017; 1(25):177–184.

23. Reyes VP, Raju BS, Wynne J, Stephenson LW, Raju R, Fromm BS, et al. Percutaneous balloon valvuloplasty compared with open surgical commissurotomy for mitral stenosis. *N Engl J Med*. 1994; 331:961–967.

24. Wilkins G, Weyman AE, Abascal V, Block P, Palacios I. Percutaneous mitral valvotomy: An analysis of echocardiographic variables related to outcome and the mechanism of dilatation. *Br Heart J*. 1988; 60:299–308.

25. Braunwald E. *Heart Disease A Textbook of Cardiovascular Medicine* 5th ed. Philadelphia, PA: W. B. Saunders. 1997:1016–1017.

26. Stanger P, Cassidy SC, Girod DA, Kan JS, Lababidi Z, Shapiro SR. Balloon pulmonary valvuloplasty: Results of the valvuloplasty and angioplasty of congenital anomalies registry. *Am J Cardiol*. 1990; 65(11):775–783.

27. Thanopoulos BVD, Laskari CV, Tsaousis GS, Zarayelyan A, Vekiou A, Papadopoulos GS. Closure of atrial septal defects with the Amplatzer occlusion device: Preliminary results. *J Am Coll Cardiol*. 1998; 31(5)1110–1116.

28. Masura J, Lange P, Wilkinson J, Kramer H, Alwi M, Goussous Y, et al. US/International multicenter trial of atrial septal catheter closure using the Amplatzer septal occluder: Initial results (Abstract 804-1). *J Am Coll Cardiol*. 1998; 31(2):57A.

29. Li J, Jin E, Yu L, Li Y, Liu N, Dong Y, et al. Oral N-acetylcysteine for prophylaxis of contrast-induced nephropathy in patients following coronary angioplasty: A meta-analysis. *Exp Ther Med*. 2017; 14(2):1568–1576.

30. Assmann G, Schulte H. Diabetes and hypertension in the elderly: Concomitant hyperlipidaemia and coronary heart disease risk. *Am J Cardiol.* 1989; 63:33H–37H.

31. Haffner SM, Lehto S, Rönnemaa T, Pyörälä K, Laakso M, et al. Mortality from coronary heart disease in subjects with type 2 diabetes and in non diabetic subjects with and without prior myocardial infarction. *N Engl J Med.* 1998; 339:229–234.

32. King SB, 3rd, Smith, SC Jr, Hirshfeld, JW Jr, Jacobs AK, Morrison DA, Williams DO, et al. 2007 Focused update of the ACC/AHA/SCAI 2005 guideline update for percutaneous coronary intervention: A report of the American College of Cardiology/American Heart Association task force on practice guidelines: 2007 writing group to review new evidence and update the ACC/AHA/SCAI 2005 guideline update for percutaneous coronary intervention, writing on behalf of the 2005 writing committee. *Circulation.* 2008; 117:261. Available at: www.circ.ahajournals.org (Accessed 29 January 2008).

33. Xian Y, Wang TY, McCoy LA, Effron MB, Henry TD, Bach RG, et al. Association of discharge aspirin dose with outcomes after acute myocardial infarction: Insights from the treatment with ADP receptor inhibitors: Longitudinal assessment of treatment patterns and events after acute coronary syndrome (TRANSLATE-ACS) Study. *Circulation.* 2015; 132(3):174–181.

34. Wiviott SD, Braunwald E, McCabe CH, Montalescot G, Ruzyllo W, Gottlieb S, et al. TRITON-TIMI 38 Investigators. Prasugrel versus clopidogrel in patients with acute coronary syndromes. *N Engl J Med.* 2007; 357(20):2001.

35. Steg PG, James S, Harrington RA, Ardissino D, Becker RC, Cannon CP, et al. PLATO study group. Ticagrelor versus clopidogrel in patients with ST-elevation acute coronary syndromes intended for reperfusion with primary percutaneous coronary intervention: A Platelet Inhibition and Patient Outcomes (PLATO) trial subgroup analysis. *Circulation.* 2010; 122(21):2131.

36. Motovska Z, Hlinomaz O, Miklik R, Hromadka M, Varvarovsky I, Dusek J, et al. PRAGUE-18 study group circulation. Prasugrel versus ticagrelor in patients with acute myocardial infarction treated with primary percutaneous coronary intervention: Multicenter randomized PRAGUE-18 Study. *Circulation.* 2016; 134(21):1603.

37. Johnson LW, Lozner EC, Johnson S, Krone R, Pichard AD, Vetrovec GW, Noto TJ. Coronary arteriography 1984–1987: A report of the registry of the Society for Cardiac Angiography and Interventions. I. Results and complications. *Cathet Cardiovasc Diagn.* 1989; 17:5.

38. Adair OV, Havranek EP. *Cardiology Secrets.* Philadelphia, PA: Hanley & Belfus; 1995. 50.

39. Webb JG, Altwegg L, Boone RH, Cheung A, Ye J, Lichtenstein S, et al. Transcatheter aortic valve replacement: Impact on clinical and valve-related outcomes. *Circulation.* 2009; 119:3009–3016.

40. Cribier A, Eltchaninoff H, Tron C, et al. Treatment of calcific aortic stenosis with the percutaneous heart valve: Mid-term follow-up from the initial feasibility studies: The French experience. *J Am Coll Cardiol.* 2006; 47:1214–1223.

41. Walther T, Simon P, Dewey T, Wimmer-Greinecker G, Falk V, Kasimir MT, et al. Transapical minimally invasive aortic valve implantation: Multicenter experience. *Circulation.* 2007; 116:I240–I245.

42. Dawkins S, Hobson AR, Kalra PR, Tang ATM, Monro JL, Dawkins KD. Permanent pacemaker implantation after isolated aortic valve replacement: Incidence, indications, and predictors. *Ann Thorac Surg.* 2008; 85:108–112.

43. Piazza N, Onuma Y, Jesserun E, Kint PP, Maugenest AM, Anderson RH, et al. Early and persistent intraventricular conduction abnormalities and requirements for pacemaking after percutaneous replacement of the aortic valve. *J Am Coll Cardiol Intv.* 2008; 1:310–316.

44. Sinhal A, Altwegg L, Pasupati S, Humphries KH, Allard M, Martin P, et al. Atrioventricular block after transcatheter balloon expandable aortic valve implantation. *J Am Coll Cardiol Intv.* 2008; 1:305–306.

45. Sinhal A, Altwegg L, Pasupati S, Humphries KH, Allard M, Martin P, et al. Early and persistent intraventricular conduction abnormalities and requirements for pacemaking after percutaneous replacement of the aortic valve. *J Am Coll Cardiol Intv.* 2008; 1:310–316.

46. Goodman SG, Menon V, Cannon CP, Steg G, Ohman EM, Harrington RA. Acute ST-segment elevation myocardial infarction: American College of Chest Physicians evidence-based clinical practice guidelines. 8th ed. *Chest.* 2008; 133(6 Suppl):708S.

47. Valgimigli M, Campo G, Percoco G, Bolognese L, Vassanelli C, Colangelo S, et al. Multicentre evaluation of single high-dose bolus tirofiban vs abciximab with sirolimus-eluting stent or bare metal stent in acute myocardial infarction study (MULTISTRATEGY) Investigators. Comparison of angioplasty with infusion of tirofiban or abciximab and with implantation of sirolimus-eluting or uncoated stents for acute myocardial infarction: The MULTISTRATEGY randomized trial. *JAMA.* 2008; 299(15):1788.

48. Gurm HS, Smith DE, Collins JS, Share D, Riba A, Carter AJ, et al. The relative safety and efficacy of abciximab and eptifibatide in patients undergoing primary percutaneous coronary intervention: Insights from a large regional registry of contemporary percutaneous coronary intervention. (BMC2). *J Am Coll Cardiol.* 2008; 51(5):529.

49. De Luca G, Ucci G, Cassetti E, Marino P J. Benefits from small molecule administration as compared with abciximab among patients with ST-segment elevation myocardial infarction treated with primary angioplasty: A meta-analysis. *J Am Coll Cardiol.* 2009; 53(18):1668.

50. Zeymer U, Margenet A, Haude M, Bode C, Lablanche JM, Heuer H, et al. Randomized comparison of eptifibatide versus abciximab in primary percutaneous coronary intervention in patients with acute ST-segment elevation myocardial infarction: Results of the EVA-AMI Trial. *J Am Coll Cardiol.* 2010; 56(6):463.

51. Akerblom A, James SK, Koutouzis M, Lagerqvist B, Stenestrand U, Svennblad B, Oldgren JJ. Eptifibatide is noninferior to abciximab in primary percutaneous coronary intervention: Results from the SCAAR (Swedish Coronary Angiography and Angioplasty Registry). *J Am Coll Cardiol.* 2010; 56(6):470.

52. Raveendran G, Ting HH, Best PJ, Holmes DR Jr, Lennon RJ, Singh M, et al. Eptifibatide vs abciximab as adjunctive therapy during primary percutaneous coronarys intervention for acute myocardial infarction. *Mayo Clin Proc.* 2007; 82(2):196.

53. Valgimigli M, Frigoli E, Leonardi S, et al. Bivalirudin or unfractionated heparin in acute coronary syndromes. *N Engl J Med.* 2015; 373:997.

12

Patient risk assessment: Use of risk calculators

EDWINA WING-LUN AND DAVID SMYTHE

INTRODUCTION

Risk calculators within the cardiovascular community have increased exponentially over recent decades, aided by the technology to create and maintain large databases, and hand-held devices to compute them. Users include healthcare workers ranging from medical students to allied health professionals, to physicians standardising their assessment criteria, and to specialists conducting clinical trials.

There are now well over a hundred risk calculators for coronary heart disease (CHD) or cardiovascular disease (CVD) alone, and many hundreds of calculators to assess the many facets of cardiology practice. It is impossible to assess all of these risk scores or calculators in one chapter, but this treatise provides an introduction to some of the more commonly used calculators, and serves as a guide to their application. In using any of these calculators, it is imperative that the setting and the goal (pre-test and post-test probability) are matched to the calculator or assessment program chosen.

These calculators are essentially predictive statistical models. They are often derived from databases with many hundreds of thousands of subjects. Individual risk factors are identified and then multivariate analysis is used to develop a predictive model. Often the model is derived from one half of the cohort and then tested on the other half to determine its predictive accuracy. One helpful indicator of the predictive accuracy of the model is the C-statistic. A C-statistic of 1.0 indicates a perfect model where no false positives are identified at the same time as no false negatives are missed. A model with a C-statistic of 0.5 is as useful as a coin toss. For the models discussed below, the C-statistic are of the order of 0.7.

CARDIOVASCULAR RISK ASSESSMENT

Cardiovascular risk assessment is performed in a multitude of settings, including primary care, the physician's office and emergency departments. The outcome determines further testing and management choices. It is worth noting that some studies have found significant inconsistencies between risk calculator estimates: They only concur two-thirds of the time, and this is somewhat equivalent to a trained physician's assessment of risk.[1] Yet, despite this limitation, risk assessment has proven to be a useful and effective tool in guiding medical therapy, and is widely accepted as an essential prognostic adjunct.

Framingham score

The original cardiovascular risk assessment is the Framingham Coronary Heart Disease Risk Score, which estimates the likelihood of acute coronary syndrome (ACS) or cardiac death within a 10-year period. The Framingham Study is the original epidemiological enquiry into heart disease, founded in 1948 in Framingham, a small town just west of Boston, Massachusetts, with the ideal statistical and geographical climate to study the natural history of disease.[2,3] From the early results published in 1957, where hypertension, serum cholesterol and relative weight were first identified as correlates for atherosclerotic heart disease, over 4,000 publications now refer to this database, and more information continues to accrue.

OTHER VARIATIONS

There are a number of other coronary heart disease and cardiovascular disease 'risk functions' created from the Framingham heart study, and different online risk calculators use different factors as guidelines for treatment recommendations.

For example, the 1998 Framingham Coronary Heart Disease (10-year risk) Score was intended for use in individuals age 30–74 years without any evidence of coronary heart disease at baseline, to estimate the 10-year risk of developing coronary heart disease. It uses age, diabetes, smoking status, JNC-V blood pressure categories (JNC-V: The Fifth Report of the Joint National Committee of Detection, Evaluation, and Treatment of High Blood Pressure)[4] NCEP total cholesterol categories (NCEP: National Cholesterol Education Program), and low-density lipoprotein (LDL) cholesterol categories.

THE HARD CORONARY HEART DISEASE ASSESSMENT

In 2001 the Framingham cohort was used to develop the Hard Coronary Heart Disease (10-year-risk) assessment.[5] It uses age, total cholesterol, high density lipoprotein (HDL), systolic blood pressure (SBP), treatment for hypertension and smoking status in a complex plus-and-minus points system to establish a 10-year estimate of coronary artery disease (myocardial infarction or coronary death) for men and women who do not have coronary disease, peripheral vascular disease or diabetes from the ages of 30–79 years. Total points range from <0 to ≥17 for men, and <9 to ≥25 for women. Ten-year risk ranges from <1 to ≥30.

ARIC score

The Framingham heart study, while critical in developing our understanding of cardiovascular disease and establishing risk, was derived from a fairly homogenous cohort, which has been criticised for lack of diversity of the population included (e.g. no races other than white). Many guidelines have therefore looked to other scores derived from other cohorts.[6] This includes the Atherosclerosis Risk in Communities (ARIC) study, which was a prospective study, held in four communities across an ethnic mix from 1897.[7] The population included, and therefore assessable by this score, is the age group 45–65 with no history of cardiovascular disease. The ARIC score is a 10-year risk predictor, using gender, race (black or white), smoking status, age, total cholesterol, HDL cholesterol, SBP, hypertension medication and diabetes to calculate cardiovascular risk.

Other models

Other cardiovascular risk assessment models include the American Heart Association cardiovascular risk score, the Australian Absolute CVD Risk, the New Zealand CVD Risk Charts and the Global risk assessment tools. These have been used to provide 10-year risk for atherosclerotic cardiovascular disease (ASCVD) in sex- and race-specific estimates. Each of these has different implications in terms of medical investigations, follow up and medical management, which may include lifestyle modifications or commencement of medications. For example, using the Australian Absolute cardiovascular disease risk calculator results in a 5-year risk of CVD of <10% (low risk), 10%–15% (moderate risk) and >15% (high risk). These risks translate to lifestyle modification and consideration of blood pressure lowering therapy if hypertensive, lifestyle modification and consideration of pharmacotherapy for blood pressure and lipid control, more regular medical reviews and, last, lifestyle modification with simultaneous pharmacotherapy for blood pressure, lipids and more regular reviews respectively.[8]

FURTHER CARDIOVASCULAR RISK STRATIFICATION SCORES

Duke treadmill score

In 1987, a group from Duke University examined almost 2,000 patients to establish a simple score to predict a patient's cardiovascular mortality using the Bruce Protocol. It added prognostic value to other clinical data available for the patient, including known coronary disease and ejection fraction.[9]

The calculation of what has been termed the 'Duke Treadmill Score' is extremely simple:

$$\text{Exercise Time} = (5 \times \text{ST Segment Deviation})$$
$$= (4 \times \text{Treadmill Angina Index})$$

where exercise time is in minutes on the Bruce protocol; the ST deviation was taken from the largest deviation from the baseline electrocardiogram (ECG) ST segment in any of the 12 leads on three consecutive beats and occurred during exercise or in recovery; and angina index was 0 if no angina was experienced, 1 if typical angina occurred but did not require cessation of exercise and 2 if angina was the reason exercise was terminated. The exercise time could be limited by symptoms such as angina, dyspnoea or fatigue, rhythm abnormalities, marked hyper- or hypotension, or ST displacement of >0.2 mV with angina symptoms.

Scores can range from +15, indicative of the lowest risk, to −25 indicating the highest risk. For example, patients who achieved stage 5 on the Bruce protocol with no ST changes or angina symptoms would score +15. This compares to a patient who did not progress to stage 2 of the Bruce protocol, ceased the test due to angina symptoms and had 4 mm of ST depression and who would score −25.

Table 12.1 Duke treadmill risk score, risk classification and four-year survival risk

		Four-year survival (inpatients)	Four-year survival (outpatients)
Low risk	≥ + 5	98%	99%
Moderate risk	−10– + 4	92%	95%
High risk	<−10	71%	79%

Two-thirds of outpatients were classified as low-risk according to the Duke Treadmill Score, which gives them a 99% 4-year survival (see Table 12.1). This has compared favourably with the 1% risk of an adverse outcome associated with skilled angiography. Further evaluation of this score has been performed in subsequent years and has been argued to establish a group of patients who are of such low risk that revascularisation would not change their survival, and hence coronary angiography to assess vasculature is unnecessary and would pose an unnecessary risk to the patient.

REVASCULARISATION SCORES

SYNTAX score

The Syntax score is a lesion-based assessment tool designed to grade the complexity of disease in the entire coronary anatomy of a patient via angiographic assessment. This score aims first to predict revascularisation outcomes and second to predict the risk of occlusion as a result of the procedure. As such, it incorporates the American Heart Association (AHA) definition of the coronary tree segments,[10] the Leaman Score that allocates relative weights to those segments, based on the percentage of blood supply to the left ventricle, the American College of Cardiology (ACC) and AHA lesion classification system (which essentially assesses the difficulty in treating a lesion), the Total Occlusion Classification system, and the Duke and Institut Cardiovasculaire Paris Sud (ICPS) bifurcation lesion classification system. The Syntax score can range from Low: 0–22, Intermediate: 23–32, to High: ≥33[11] (see Table 12.2). Accurate calculation of the Syntax score is quite complex and is most easily performed via a handheld device or other electronic calculator.

The Syntax trial was a prospective randomised controlled trial across the United States and Europe,

Table 12.2 Results of the SYNTAX trial at five years for de novo three-vessel disease

	PCI	CABG
Overall MACE 5 years	37.5%	24.3%
Composite of death/stroke/MI	22.0%	14.0%
All cause death	14.6%	9.2%
MI	9.2%	4.0%
Repeat revascularisation	25.4%	12.6%
Stroke	3.0%	3.5%

Source: Head, S.J. et al., Eur. Heart J., 35, 2821–2830, 2014.
Abbreviations: PCI, percutaneous coronary intervention; CABG, coronary artery bypass surgery; MACE, major adverse cardiac events; MI, myocardial infarction.

Table 12.3 Five-year estimates of adverse events as per SYNTAX terciles

	MACE			Repeat revascularisation		
Syntax Score	PCI	CABG		PCI	CABG	
Low (0–22)	33.3%	26.8%	Similar	23.1%	14.9%	Similar
Intermediate (23–32)	37.9%	22.6%	Significantly higher in PCI	25.1%	11.0%	Significantly higher in PCI
High (≥33)	41.9%	24.1%	Significantly higher in PCI	28.2%	12.6%	Significantly higher in PCI

Source: Head, S.J. et al., Eur. Heart J., 35, 2821–2830, 2014.
Abbreviations: MACE, major adverse cardiac events; PCI, percutaneous coronary intervention; CABG, coronary artery bypass surgery.

which enrolled 1,800 all-comers with de novo left main or three-vessel disease, and sought to compare revascularisation strategies of coronary artery bypass grafting (CABG) or stenting with Taxus drug eluting stents. Of these, 1,095 had triple vessel disease, with almost 550 of these randomly assigned to either CABG or percutaneous coronary intervention (PCI). Patients were assessed at 30 days and then followed yearly. The 5-year outcomes for triple vessel disease indicated that, overall, PCI was an independent risk factor for major adverse cardiac events (MACE); however, at the lowest syntax tercile (score 0–22) MACE was similar, and therefore could be considered as an alternative to CABG (see Tables 12.3 and 12.4). A sub-analysis for medically treated diabetes mellitus showed that this cohort had higher MACE in the PCI group, suggesting that three-vessel disease in the presence of diabetes should be treated with CABG.[12]

Seven hundred and fifty patients were randomised with left main disease and, unlike the triple vessel cohort, no significant difference was found in total MACE, composite safety end point of death/stroke/myocardial infarction (MI), all-cause death, cardiac death and MI. The incidence of stroke was

Table 12.4 Thrombolysis in myocardial infarction (TIMI) risk score components

Criteria	Value
Age ≥65	+1
≥3 CAD risk factors	+1
Known CAD (stenosis ≥50%)	+1
Aspirin use in the past 7 days	+1
Severe angina (≥2 episodes in 24 hr)	+1
ECG changes ≥0.5 mm at presentation	+1
Elevated serum cardiac markers	+1

Abbreviations: CAD, coronary artery disease; ECG, electrocardiogram.

significantly higher in the CABG group and repeat revascularisation was increased in the PCI group. In the lowest two syntax terciles (scores 0–32), MACE was similar between CABG and PCI, but mortality was higher in the CABG group. In patients with a high syntax score (≥33) MACE was higher in the PCI group. The result of this analysis suggests that PCI may be equivalent to CABG for treatment of left main stem disease if the syntax score is <33.[13]

CHEST PAIN IN THE ACUTE CARE SETTING

Chest pain presentations in Australian Emergency Departments are the second most common complaint. Pain in the throat and chest account for 3.4% of presentations and 14.2% of admissions from emergency; 6.5% are diagnosed with angina pectoris.[14]

The ideal algorithm in the acute care setting is one that can quickly and accurately identify those patients that can be safely discharged, those that need further assessment and those that need more aggressive or urgent attention. There have been debates as to the exact statistics that are required, but in our current clinical climate, it seems to be a negative predictive value <1% with sensitivity and specificity close to 100%, within a time line of <2 hours.[15] Needless to say, this has been nearly impossible to achieve, and has led to the development, redevelopment, and either incomplete or inconclusive validation of many risk-scoring systems.

TIMI score

The grandfather of chest pain scoring systems could be said to be the TIMI (Thrombolysis in myocardial infarction) risk score.[16] It was created in the 1990s from the Thrombolysis in Myocardial Infarction 11B trial and Efficacy and Safety of Subcutaneous Enoxaparin in Unstable Angina and Non-Q-Wave Coronary Event Trial.[17] The TIMI risk score provides a simple estimate of the 30-day mortality in patients with a confirmed diagnosis of acute coronary syndrome (ACS) and has been used to base more aggressive therapy. It must be noted that this is not a score to stratify indeterminate chest pain as to likelihood of ischemia.

It is a simple scoring system in which each factor is allocated a value of one (see Table 12.4), the addition of which provides the total score, which indicates 14-day all-cause mortality, new or recurrent MI, and severe or recurrent ischaemia requiring urgent revascularisation. The higher the score, the higher the likelihood of this combined end-point. Originally, this score was hoped to enable decisions regarding treatment including antithrombotic therapy choices and conservative vs. invasive strategies.[16]

GRACE score

The GRACE score is similar to the TIMI score in that it predicts outcomes in patients with ACS.[18] There were two scores derived from the GRACE Project,[19] the first predicting in-hospital mortality with nine variables (age, heart rate, SBP, creatinine or history of renal dysfunction, cardiac arrest on admission, ST segment changes, abnormal cardiac enzymes and Killip Class), and has a complex scale of scoring, making it difficult to remember or operate without an electronic device. Age, for example, is divided into <30 years, then in 10-year increments until ≥90 years of age, and each of these divisions is allocated an uneven number of points: <30 is 0°points, 30°–39°is 8°points, 40°–49°is 25 points and so on. A second GRACE score predicting 6-month outcomes also involves nine variables: Older age, history of MI, history of heart failure, increased pulse rate, lower SBP, elevated initial serum creatinine level, elevated serum cardiac biomarkers, ST segment depression on presenting ECG, and not having PCI in hospital. It is again not easy to calculate without a device. The GRACE score, similar to the TIMI score, hoped to provide guidelines for management.[20] (See Tables 12.5 and 12.6 for NSTEMI and STEMI risk categories, GRACE score and mortality risk.)[21]

Again, similarly to the TIMI score, the GRACE score has been trialled for use in undifferentiated chest pain; however, it failed to be sensitive enough to be of clinical use.[15]

HEART score

One of the more commonly used scoring systems for undifferentiated chest pain is the HEART score. It was specifically designed for use in the acute care setting for patients ≥21 years of age to establish requirement for admission. The HEART score was developed to be simple, using six factors or fewer, based on clinical acumen and medical literature to establish factors that prompted admission and further assessment by physicians. Five factors were chosen: presenting history, ECG changes, age, risk factors, and troponin. Each of the five factors could have a possible score of 0, 1 or 2 (see Table 12.7) that when totalled would result in a low score (0–3), a moderate score (4–6) or a high score (7–10), which dictates management (see Table 12.8). With a HEART

Table 12.5 GRACE score and mortality risk for NSTEMI

Risk category	NSTEMI in-hospital mortality		NSTEMI 6 month post-discharge mortality	
	GRACE score	Probability of death (%)	GRACE score	Probability of death (%)
Low	1–108	1	1–88	<3
Intermediate	109–140	1–3	89–118	3–8
High	141–372	>3	119–263	>8

Table 12.6 GRACE SCORE and mortality risk for STEMI

Risk category	STEMI in-hospital mortality		STEMI 6 Month post-discharge mortality	
	GRACE score	Probability of death (%)	GRACE score	Probability of death (%)
Low	49–125	<2	27–99	<4.4
Intermediate	126–154	2–5	100–127	4.5–11
High	155–319	>5	128–263	>11

Table 12.7 The HEART score

Parameter	Categories	Points
History	Slightly suspicious	0
	Moderately suspicious	+1
	Highly suspicious	+2
ECG	Normal	0
	Non-specific repolarisation changes /LBBB/PM	+1
	Significant ST depression	+2
Age	<45 years	0
	45–65 years	+1
	≥65	+2
Risk factors • Hypercholesterolaemia • Hypertension • Cigarette smoking • Positive family history • Diabetes Mellitus • Obesity (BMI > 30) • Atherosclerotic disease	None	0
	1 or 2 risk factors	+1
	≥3 risk factors	+2
Troponin	≤ Normal limit	0
	1–3 × Normal limit	+1
	>3 × Normal limit	+2

Abbreviations: ECG, electrocardiogram; DM, diabetes mellitus; BMI, body mass index; MI, myocardial infarction; PCI, percutaneous coronary intervention; CABG, coronary bypass grafting; CVA, cerebral vascular aneurysm; TIA, transient ischaemic attack.

Table 12.8 The HEART score, showing total score, major adverse cardiac events (MACE) and suggested management

Points	Risk of MACE	Management
0–3: Low score	0.9%–1.7%	Discharge may be considered
4–6: Moderate score	12%–16.6%	Admission
7–10: High score	50%–65%	Admission and early invasive management

score of 0–3, MACE rates were <2%, which may indicate minimal risk for discharge, but in the current clinical climate, a MACE rate of <1% is the accepted standard.[15]

HEART Pathway

The HEART Pathway was an add-on development to the HEART score to clarify which patients could be discharged in the low HEART score group that would achieve a discharged MACE rate of <1%. It uses serial troponins, measured at 0 and 3 hours, in addition to the Heart score to achieve a discharged patient MACE of 0% at 30 days.[15]

There are a number of other scores that have been applied in acute care settings to determine the likelihood of MACE and, in particular, to identify a cohort of patients that can be safely discharged.

THORACIC SURGERY RISK SCORES

There are a number of Thoracic Surgery Risk Scores, some of which apply to specific surgeries, such as CABG only, while some are more generalised.

The National Database for Cardiac Surgery was established in 1989 by The Society of Thoracic Surgeons (STS),[22] and rapidly grew to include hundreds of participating sites and millions of procedures. Using logistic regression analysis, risk models were established for various procedures and operations and these were updated each calendar year. This includes CABG only, aortic valve replacement only, mitral valve replacement only and mitral valve repair only, and a combination of these. It is applicable to adult patients aged 18 to 110 years and includes a long list of variables including demographics such as age, sex and weight, but also many clinical considerations, such as type of operation and comorbidities such as previous operations and immunocompromise.

The outcomes of the STS Risk model are operative in-hospital mortality (regardless of time), and post-discharge but within 30 days, permanent stroke (not resolving within 24 hours), renal failure, prolonged ventilation (>24 hours) or re-intubation, deep sternal wound infection, reoperation, major morbidity or operative mortality, and length of stay (short <6 days) and long (>14 days).[23]

The STS score is often used in identifying patients as high risk for surgical aortic valve replacement, particularly in this era of an alternative to surgery—transcatheter aortic valve replacement (TAVR) and has recently been shown to be a valid predictor of TAVR risk as well.[24]

EuroSCORE

The EuroSCORE is the European System for Cardiac Operative Risk Evaluation, which again was deduced from a large (almost 20,000 patient) database.[25] This database was contributed to by many European countries, the largest of which were Germany, UK, Spain, Finland, France and Italy. The EuroSCORE II risk factors and information can be seen in Table 12.9, and is possible to apply using mental arithmetic. There is a more detailed version, the Logistic EuroSCORE that can be more accurate in predicting risk for high-risk patients. This is shown in Table 12.9, and requires computed calculations. It is advised that using the online risk calculator is the most accurate and easiest way of calculating risk with the EuroScore II.

ATRIAL FIBRILLATION STROKE RISK SCORES

CHADS$_2$ score

The CHADS$_2$ score is the original risk calculator for stroke in patients with non-valvular atrial fibrillation. First published in 2001, the CHADS$_2$

Table 12.9 EuroSCORE II risk factors

EuroSCORE II		Notes
Age	Years (1 score for each 5 years or part thereof over 60 years)	Questionable validity >90 years
Gender	Male or female (1 for F)	
Renal impairment	Normal, moderate, severe, dialysis (serum creatinine >200 micromol/L)	Creatinine clearance. Normal >85 mL/min, moderate 50–85 mL/min, severe <50 mL/min, dialysis disregards serum creatinine
Extracardiac arteriopathy	Yes or no (2 for yes)	Claudication, carotid occlusion or >50% stenosis, amputation for arterial disease, previous/planned intervention on the abdominal aorta, limb arteries or carotids
Poor mobility	Yes or no (2 for yes)	Due to musculoskeletal or neurological dysfunction
Previous cardiac surgery	Yes or no (3 for re-do)	
Chronic lung disease	Yes or no (1 for yes)	Bronchodilators or steroid use long-term
Active endocarditis	Yes or no (3 for yes)	Active antimicrobial treatment
Critical preoperative state	Yes or no (3 for yes)	VT, VF, CPR or aborted SCD, perioperative ventilation, inotropes, intraaortic balloon pump, acute renal failure
Diabetes on insulin	Yes or no	
New York heart association class	I–IV	
CCS class 4 angina	Yes or no (2 for yes)	
Left ventricular function	Good, moderate (1), poor (3), very poor	Good: >50%, moderate: 31%–50%, poor: >20%–30%, very poor: ≤20%
Recent myocardial infarction	Yes or no (2 for yes)	<90 days prior to surgery
Pulmonary hypertension	No, moderate, severe (2 for >60 mmHg)	
Urgency of operation	elective, urgent, emergency (2), salvage	Routine; required this admission; procedure required prior to the start of the next working day; CPR en route to hospital
Weight of intervention	Isolated CABG (0) and single non-CABG (2), 2 procedures (2), 3 procedures (2), post infarct septal rupture (3)	CABG, valve repair or replacement, part of the aorta replacement, structural defect repair, maze procedure, cardiac tumour resection
Surgery on thoracic aorta	Yes or no (3)	

Abbreviations: VT, ventricular tachycardia; VF, ventricular fibrillation; SDC, sudden cardiac death; CCS, Canadian Cardiovascular Score; CPR, cardiopulmonary resuscitation; CABG, coronary bypass grafting.

Table 12.10 CHADS$_2$ score risk factors for atrial fibrillation

Component	Score
Congestive heart failure	1
Hypertension	1
Age ≥75 years	1
Diabetes mellitus	1
Stroke/TIA	2

Abbreviation: TIA, transient ischaemic attack.

Table 12.11 CHADS$_2$ score and adjusted stroke risk for non-valvular atrial fibrillation

CHADS$_2$ score	Adjusted stroke risk (%) per annum	Risk classification
0	1.9	Low risk
1	2.8	
2	4	Moderate risk
3	5.9	
4	8.5	High risk
5	12.5	
6	18.2	

Table 12.12 CHA$_2$DS$_2$-VASc scoring

Component	Score
Congestive heart failure	1
Hypertension	1
Age ≥75 years	2
Diabetes mellitus	1
Stroke/TIA/Thromboembolic event	2
Vascular disease (previous MI, PAD, aortic plaque)	1
Age 65 to 74 years	1
Female sex	1

Abbreviations: TIA, Transient ischaemic attack; MI, myocardial infarction; PAD, pulmonary artery disease.

index identified independent risk factors that were included in pre-existing stroke risk prediction schemes (Atrial Fibrillation Investigators [AFI] or Stroke Prevention and Atrial Fibrillation [SPAF] Investigators), and included factors such as history of previous cerebral ischemia (previous stroke or transient ischaemic attack [TIA]), hypertension, diabetes mellitus, congestive heart failure, and age 75 years or greater.[26] The scoring and adjusted stroke risk (%) is shown in Table 12.10, remembering that the stroke rate in this cohort was based on hospitalisation for stroke, which may differ in current practice. While appealingly simple, the CHADS$_2$ score failed to differentiate the truly low-risk population, with the low-risk group having 1.9%–2.8% per year and thus did not aid in differentiating those that did not require anticoagulation well enough.

Over the next decade or so the CHADS$_2$ was updated to the CHA$_2$DS$_2$-VASc score, which included **three** new risk factors of vascular disease, age 65–74 years and female sex.[27] This updated score better determined stroke risk among those in the low-risk (CHADS$_2$ score of 0 or 1) and therefore allows differentiation of management recommendations. A score of 0, for oral anticoagulation (OAC) is not recommended, a score of 1 indicates recommendation for OAC and ≥2 represents a 'definite recommendation' for OAC (see Tables 12.11 through 12.13).

BLEEDING RISK SCORES

Many of the above risk scores, be they for treatment for ACS or for management of atrial fibrillation, provide some weight or suggestion of management that invariably involves one version or another of anticoagulation. Therefore, bleeding risk scores have been established in an attempt to balance our calculations and consider both the pros and cons of treatment.

CRUSADE score

In acute coronary syndromes, the most commonly used bleeding risk score is the CRUSADE calculator score that stratifies the risk of major bleeding.[28] It is meant to be used after diagnosis of non ST-elevation MI (NSTEMI) or ST-elevation MI (STEMI), but before treatment initiation. This bleeding risk score can contribute to decision making regarding anti-thrombotic and invasive therapy. Major bleeding was defined as intracranial

Table 12.13 CHA$_2$DS$_2$-VASc score, stroke risk per annum and anticoagulation recommendations

CHA$_2$DS$_2$-VASc score	Adjusted stroke risk (%) per annum	Recommendations
0	0	No OAC
1	1.3	Possible OAC
2	2.2	Recommend OAC
3	3.2	
4	4.0	
5	6.7	
6	9.8	
7	9.6	
8	6.7	
9	15.2	

Abbreviation: OAC, oral anticoagulation.

haemorrhage, retroperitoneal bleed, haematocrit drop ≥12%, or red blood cell transfusion. Components used are heart rate, SBP, hematocrit, creatinine clearance, sex, signs of congestive heart failure at presentation, history of vascular disease, history of diabetes mellitus with variable weightings to establish an individual's score. The most predictive components in this risk calculator are renal function and haematocrit. The importance of this score has been underpinned by findings that mortality risk is strongly correlated with bleeding risk. However, high risk is also associated with

Table 12.14 CRUSADE score and risk of major bleeding

Bleeding score	Risk of major bleeding
Very low risk: ≤20	3.1%
Low risk: 21–30	5.5%
Moderate risk: 31–40	8.5%
High risk: 41–50	11.9%
Very high risk: >50	19.5%

high reward with treatment, therefore this risk calculator can help guide awareness and appropriate dosing. The CRUSADE score is a complex one that is best performed with a device; however, the scoring outcome and risk of major bleeding is listed in Table 12.14.

HAS-BLED score

The HAS-BLED score is a commonly used estimate of major bleeding risk in 1-year in patients with atrial fibrillation, which aids in the risk-benefit assessment of anticoagulation prescription.[29] It is usually balanced with the CHA$_2$DS$_2$-VASc Score (see above). The HAS-BLED pnemonic stands for hypertension, abnormal renal and liver function, stroke, bleeding, labile international normalised ratio (INR), elderly, and drugs or alcohol (see Table 12.15). Many of the online calculators space this out or change the order, but they pertain to the same parameters, which have weighted values between 0 and 2. The total score can

Table 12.15 HAS-BLED score

		Points
H	Hypertension: uncontrolled, >160 mmHg systolic	1
A	Abnormal renal function: dialysis, transplant, creatinine >200 umol/L,	1
	Abnormal liver function: Cirrhosis, bilirubin >2 × ULN, AST/ALT, AP >3 × ULN	1
S	Stroke: prior history of stroke	1
B	Bleeding: previous major bleed or bleeding diathesis	1
L	Labile INR: unstable or high, time in therapeutic range <60%	1
E	Elderly: >65 years of age	1
D	Drug use: history of drug or alcohol use (≥8 drinks/week);	1
	medications increasing bleeding risk such as NSAIDs or antiplatelet agents	1

Abbreviations: AST/ALT, aspartate transaminase/alanine transaminase; AP, alkaline phosphatas; ULN, upper limit of normal; INR, international normalised ratio; NSAIDS, non-steroidal inflammatory drugs.

Table 12.16 HAS-BLED total score, predicted bleeding risk and management recommendations

Score	Major bleeding risk in one year	Bleeds per 100 patient years	Risk for major bleeding/overall management
0	0.9%	1.13	Consider anticoagulation
1	3.4%	1.01	Consider anticoagulation
2	4.1%	1.88	Moderate risk, consider anticoagulation
3	5.8%	3.72	High risk, consider alternatives to
4	8.9%	8.7	anticoagulation
5	9.1%	12.5	
6–9	Likely over 10%, rare to score >5 in validation trial		

range from 0–9, where a score of ≥ 3 denotes high risk of major bleeding, requiring regular review and some caution in prescription (see Table 12.16). It should be noted that there is some cross-over between the components of the CHA_2DS_2-VASc score and the HAS-BLED score, resulting often in a reflection of risk in both, and therefore a physician's discretion and a patient's preference contribute to decision making.

SUMMARY

The calculators and scores discussed in this chapter are but the tip of the iceberg in terms of medical calculators available. With the advent of hand held devices the number and range of calculators available continue to increase not only within the field of cardiology, but in all areas of medicine. It can be difficult to tease out which of these are validated, that is, whether their suggested score or risk assessment is reliable. It can also be difficult to establish whether a particular score is applicable to a population or patient of interest. The simple fact that a calculator is familiar, popular or available on many of the hand held apps does not guarantee either.

Knowledge of the origins and intention of a scoring system is imperative to appropriate application, interpretation and treatment decision making. This chapter has not only introduced some of the founding and most common risk assessment tools, but also provides a framework by which such assessment tools should themselves be assessed.

REFERENCES

1. Allan GM, Nouri F, Korownyk C, Kolber MR, Vandermeer B, McCormack J. Agreement among cardiovascular disease risk calculators. *Circulation*. 2013; 127:1948–1956.
2. Dawber TR, Meadors GF, Moore FR Jr. Epidemiological approaches to heart disease: The Framingham Study. *Am J Public Health*. 1951; 41:279–286.
3. Dawber TR, Kannel WB. The Framingham Study an epidemiological approach to coronary heart disease. *Circulation*. 1966; 34(4):553–555.
4. The Fifth Report of the Joint National Committee on Detection, Evaluation, and Treatment of High Blood Pressure (JNC V) *Arch Intern Med*. 1993;153(2):154–183.
5. Pogue VA, Ellis C, Michel J, Francis CK. New staging system of the Fifth Joint National Committee Report on the Detection, Evaluation and Treatment of High Blood Pressure (JNC-V) alters assessment of the severity and treatment of hypertension. *Hypertension* 1996; 28:713–718.
6. Goff DC, Jr., Lloyd-Jones DM, Bennett G, Coady S, D'Agostino RB, Gibbons R, et al. 2013 ACC/AHA guideline on the assessment of cardiovascular risk: A report of the American College of Cardiology/ American Heart Association Task Force on practice guidelines. *Circulation*. 2014; 129(25 Suppl 2):S49–S73.

7. The ARIC investigators. The atherosclerosis risk in communities (ARIC) study: Design and objectives. *Am J Epidemiol.* 1989; 129(4):687–702.

8. Lalor E. National Vascular Disease Prevention Alliance. Guidelines for the management of absolute cardiovascular disease risk. 2012. ISBN 978–0–9872830–1–6. https://strokefoundation.com.au/~/media/strokewebsite/resources/treatment/absolutecvd_gl_webready.ashx.

9. Mark DB, Shaw L, Harrell FE Jr, Hlatky MA, Lee KL, Bengtson Jr., et al. Prognostic value of a treadmill exercise score in outpatients with suspected coronary artery disease. *N Engl J Med.* 1991; 325:849–853.

10. Austen WG, Edwards JE, Frye RL, Gensini GG, Gott VL, Griffith LS, et al. A reporting system on patients evaluated for coronary artery disease. Report of the Ad Hoc Committee for Grading of Coronary Artery Disease, Council on Cardiovascular Surgery, American Heart Association. *Circulation.* 1975; 51(4):5–40.

11. Sianos G, Morel MA, Kappetein AP, Morice MC, Colombo A, Dawkins K, et al. The Syntax Score: An angiographic tool grading the complexity of coronary artery disease. *Euro Intervention.* 2005; 1:219–227.

12. Head SJ, Davierwala PM, Serruys PW, Redwood SR, Colombo A, Mack MJ, et al. Coronary artery bypass grafting vs. percutaneous coronary intervention for patients with three-vessel disease: Final five-year follow-up of the SYNTAX trial. *Eur Heart J.* 2014; 35(40):2821–2830.

13. Morice MC, Serruys PW, Kappetein AP, Feldman TE, Stahle E, Colombo A, et al. Five-year outcomes in patients with left main disease treated with either percutaneous coronary intervention or coronary artery bypass grafting in the Synergy between Percutaneous Intervention with Taxus and Cardiac Surgery Trial. *Circulation.* 2014; 129:2388–2394.

14. Australian Institute of Health and Welfare 2016. Emergency department care 2015–2016: Australian hospital statistics. Health services series no. 72. Cat. No. HSE 182. Canberra, Australia: AIHW.

15. Alley W, Mahler S. Clinical decision aids for chest pain in the emergency department: Identifying low-risk patients. *Open Access Emergency Medicine.* 2015; 7:85–92.

16. Antman EM, Cohen M, Bernink PJ, McCabe CH, Horacek T, Papuchis G, et al. The TIMI risk score for unstable angina/non-ST elevation MI: A method for prognostication and therapeutic decision making. *JAMA* 2000; 284:835–842.

17. Antman EM, McCabe CH, Gurfinke, EP, Turpie AG, Bernink PJ, Salein D, et al. Enoxaparin prevents death and cardiac ischaemic events in unstable angina/non-q-wave myocardial infarction. Results of the Thrombolysis in Myocardial Infarction (TIMI) 11B trial. *Circulation.* 1999; 100:1593–1601.

18. Yan AT, Yan RT, Tan M, Eagle KA, Granger CB, Dabbous OH, et al. In-hospital revascularization and one-year outcome of acute coronary syndrome patients stratified by the GRACE risk score. *Am J Cardiol.* 2005; 96(7):913–916.

19. The GRACE investigators. Rationale and design of the GRACE (Global Registry of Acute Coronary Events) project: A multinational registry of pateints hospitalized with acute coronary syndromes. *Am Heart J.* 2001; 141:190–199.

20. Devlin G, Anderson FA, Heald S, Lopez-Sendon J, Avezum A, Ellio J, et al. Management and outcomes of lower risk patients presenting with acute coronary syndromes in a multinational observational registry. *Heart* 2005; 91(11):1394–1399.

21. GRACE ACS risk model calculator website: www.outcomes-umassmed.org/grace/acs_risk/acs_risk_content.html.

22. Ferguson TB, Dziuban SW, Edwards FH, Eiken MC, Shroyer LW, Pairolero PC, et al. The STS national database: Current changes and challenges for the new millennium. *Ann Thorac Surg.* 2000; 69:680–691.

23. The Society of Thoracic Surgeons website: www.sts.org.

24. Balan P, Zhao Y, Johnson S, Arain S, Dhoble A, Estrera A, et al. The Society of Thoracic Surgery Risk Score as a predictor of 30-day mortality in transcatheter vs surgical aortic valve replacement: A single-centre experience and its implications for the development of a TAVR risk-prediction model. *J Invasive Cardiol.* 2017; 29(3):109–114.

25. European System for Cardiac Operative Risk Evaluation website: www.euroSCORE.org.

26. Gage BF, Waterman AD, Shannon W, Boechler M, Rich M, Radford MJ. Validation of clinical classification schemes for predicting stroke: Results from the National Registry of Atrial Fibrillation. *JAMA.* 2001; 285(22):2864–2870.

27. Lip GY, Nieluwlaat R, Pister, R, Lane DA, Crijins HJ. Redefining clinical risk stratification for predicting stroke and thromboembolism in atrial fribrillation using a novel risk factor-based approach: The Euro Heart Survey on Atrial Fibrillation. *Chest* 2010; 137:263–272.

28. CRUSADE bleeding score calculator website: www.Crusadebleedingscore.org.

29. Pisters R, Lane DA, Nieuwlaat R, De Vos CB, Crijns HJ, Lip GY. A novel user-friendly score (HAS-BLED) to assess 1-year risk of major bleeding in patients with atrial fibrillation: The Euro Heart Survey. *Chest.* 2010; 138(5):1093–1100.

13

An evidence-based guide to cardiac catheterisation

STEVEN FADDY AND GARY J. GAZIBARICH

INTRODUCTION

Evidence-based medicine (EBM) uses the scientific literature to guide the management of individual patients and has become the standard in clinical practice in recent years. It relies on a thorough literature search, appraisal of relevant papers, analysis of study results, and application of these results to a population or clinical condition. The *JAMA* series titled 'Users' Guide to the Medical Literature'[1-19] provides complete guidelines for appraising all types of studies and clinical questions, and is strongly recommended for those wishing to further their expertise in this area. This chapter summarises the EBM protocol for randomised controlled trials, observational studies and diagnostic tests. EBM uses the quality of scientific evidence and grading of recommendations to guide clinicians with individual patient management.

THE LITERATURE SEARCH

The literature search is the first and possibly most important step in the process. The emphasis is on finding results of **all** studies performed in the area of interest. This will include searching several electronic databases such as Medline, EMBASE and the Cochrane Database of Systematic Reviews. Reference lists of papers uncovered by the literature search should also be examined for references that have not previously been identified.

A complete literature search also involves searching clinical trials registries[20-21] to find trials that are still underway; and may involve contact with experts in the field to find results of unpublished trials. This step, which may seem somewhat extreme, avoids publication bias: Trials that show positive results are more likely to be submitted and accepted for publication than trials which fail to demonstrate a significant effect.

SOURCES OF EVIDENCE

A literature search will commonly uncover many types of studies and publications. It is important to identify which studies may give satisfactory results and which studies have results that are subject to bias. A summary of the most common sources of evidence is presented below.

Systematic review

A systemic review (also referred to as an 'overview') summarises all the scientific evidence pertinent to a clinical question, including a thorough literature search, critical appraisal of the studies identified, analysis of pooled results (meta-analysis), and identification of the population to which these results apply. Clinicians need only assess the systematic review to evaluate the quality of the literature search, adequacy of the methods of appraisal, and the applicability of the results to their individual patient(s). If these criteria are satisfactorily met, the results of the systematic review can be easily applied to the patient or clinical condition in question.

Randomised controlled trial (RCT)

The RCT is considered the best study design to show evidence of association between an exposure and outcome (Figure 13.1a). The strength of RCTs lies largely in the random assignment of patients to the exposure under examination (a drug, intervention or therapy) or a control (current therapy or placebo). Completely random allocation of patients to the study groups should ensure that baseline characteristics of the groups are almost identical provided enough patients are included in the study. Confounders are variables that alter the strength of association between an exposure and an outcome. Study results can be adjusted for confounders if they are known to occur. However, unidentified confounders have the potential to alter the observed strength of association. By randomly assigning patients to either study group, unidentified confounders should be evenly distributed between the groups and should not bias the strength of association. In this way, the only difference between study groups should be exposure to the study factor. The study groups are followed prospectively to the end of the trial and assessed for the outcome.

Cohort study

A cohort study follows patients prospectively from an exposure to an outcome but the assignment of exposure is non-random and based on patients' individual characteristics (such as cigarette smoking or cholesterol level) (Figure 13.1b). Non-random assignment introduces bias from confounding factors. For example, consider a study investigating the relationship between smoking and coronary artery disease. The exposure factor is cigarette smoking and it is neither ethical nor sensible to randomise patients to be smokers or non-smokers. Instead, allocation to a study group is guided by the patients' own habits. Cigarette smoking may be associated with higher coffee consumption, higher stress levels, less exercise, or a tendency towards other negative lifestyle habits. These confounding factors may thus have an independent association with coronary artery disease. The absence of randomisation may result in these factors being unevenly distributed between the smoking and non-smoking groups and bias the observed strength of association between smoking and coronary artery disease.

Case-control study

A case-control study identifies positive outcomes first and works backwards to identify the levels of exposure (Figure 13.1c). A control population can be chosen from a number of sources. A poorly defined control group (hospital-based controls) is chosen from a narrow section of the community and is often not representative of the whole population. A well-defined control group (population-based controls) is drawn from the same geographical areas at the same time as the cases being evaluated and is often well representative of the section of the community from which it is drawn.

In an attempt to obtain some equality in baseline characteristics of the study groups, controls are often age- and sex-matched to cases. However, matching has been shown to have little effect on the estimate of association and extreme care must be taken to ensure that results are not biased by other unidentified confounding variables.

The advantages of a case-control study are the ability to study exposures for which it is unethical to randomise patients and the ability to study outcomes that are rare. For example, consider a study

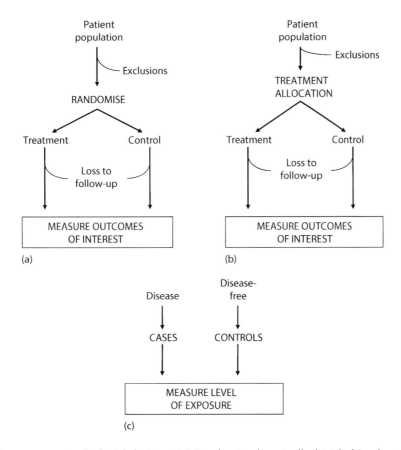

Figure 13.1 Common controlled trial designs. **(a)** Randomised controlled trial, **(b)** cohort study, **(c)** case-control study.

examining the relationship between a hypothetical industrial solvent (HIS) and atrial myxoma. Obviously it would be unwise to expose patients to this chemical simply to see if atrial myxoma develops. Further, atrial myxoma is a rare disease and it may be necessary to expose many thousands of subjects to the chemical in order to detect two or three cases. In these situations it would be far better to identify as many cases as possible, obtain a suitable control group, and study both groups for the relative rates of exposure to HIS.

Case descriptions

Case series and case reports are simply a description of the course of treatment for small groups of patients or individual patients, respectively. The benefits of randomisation are lost since only those patients treated are reported and there is generally no control group to compare with the group receiving the new treatment or medication. As such, it is not possible to draw any conclusions about cause and effect from these reports.

CRITICAL APPRAISAL

Having identified all sources of evidence addressing the clinical question, it is necessary to analyse the quality and content of these papers. The exact method of appraisal will vary with different study types, publication types and clinical questions. The 'Users' Guide to the Medical Literature' series[1–19] divides most appraisals into two basic units: 'Are the results of the study valid?' and 'What are the results and how will they help me in caring for my patients?'

Critical appraisal of a systematic review starts with validation of the criteria used to select articles for inclusion, including the literature search. The review is assessed to ensure that the validity of each primary study has been appraised. The results are reviewed to ensure consistency and reproducibility between trials. When these criteria have been met it is possible to adopt the results, assuming there is adequate precision (results lie within a statistically suitable range). The study population is assessed for relevance to the physician's own patient population.[8]

Papers concerning therapies or interventions are checked for random allocation of patients to treatment groups, adequate retention of subjects, sufficient follow-up, similarity of baseline characteristics, adequate blinding and analysis by intention-to-treat. Assessment can then be made of the significance of the treatment effect, the precision of the results and the relevance of the patient population to the clinician's own patients.[2,3]

Trials assessing harms of an exposure require a clearly defined comparison group with similar baseline characteristics, outcomes measured the same way for both groups, sufficient follow-up and investigation for a dose-response gradient. Appraisal of the strength of association between exposure and outcome (and the precision of this estimate) is made along with the relevance to the clinician's practice.[6] The relative harms of a therapy can then be weighed against benefits for individual patients.[22]

Articles concerning diagnostic tests require an independent, blind comparison of all patients with a reference standard. All patients should have the reference test to be compared with the new test. The patient population should be representative of those patients on whom the test would normally be performed. Likelihood ratios, sensitivity, specificity, positive predictive value and negative predictive value can be assessed to determine whether the new test provides any additional benefit in diagnosis of the target disease.[4,5]

ASPECTS OF STUDY DESIGN

Randomisation

The benefits of randomisation have already been discussed. They primarily revolve around equality of baseline characteristics. If the study groups are similar for all measurable variables it can be assumed that the distribution of any unidentified confounding variables will also be evenly distributed. In this way, study groups should be similar in every aspect except for the treatment or intervention being applied. The results will reflect the true effect of the new treatment without bias from uneven distribution of covariates.

Power and sample size

In any analysis of cause and effect, chance plays a part in the interpretation of test results. A study may correctly detect an effect of treatment when such an effect truly exists or correctly not detect an effect when no effect exists. In either case, no error has been made. However, a study may detect a treatment effect when no effect exists. This is referred to as Type I (or α) error and is equal to the P value. If the significance level is set at $P = 0.05$ then there is a 5% chance that the difference observed between the study groups has occurred entirely by chance. Type II (or β) error occurs when a study fails to detect a treatment effect where one actually exists. The power of a study ($=1 - \beta$) is defined as the probability that the study will correctly detect a treatment effect when one actually exists. Hence, if $\beta = 20\% = 0.20$, the power of the study is $1 - \beta = 1 - 0.20 = 0.80 = 80\%$. This means that there is an 80% chance of correctly detecting a treatment effect for the specified sample size.

Sample size is calculated taking into account the expected magnitude of the treatment effect (from previous research or pilot studies), the Type I error and required power of the study. If a large treatment effect is expected, a relatively small number of patients may be required to demonstrate the effect. Conversely, if a small treatment effect is expected, a larger number of patients may be required to establish that the small difference among study groups is due to treatment and not to chance. A trial loses power when the sample size is not large enough to detect the difference expected. That is, the probability that the trial will demonstrate a statistically significant effect of the specified magnitude is diminished.

In the planning stage of a study, sample size calculations should be performed to determine how many patients are required to have a reasonable chance of demonstrating the specified treatment effect. In the appraisal of a study that does not show a significant treatment effect, sample size calculations will determine whether there are sufficient patients to adequately detect the observed effect. Conversely, the sample size calculation can be used to evaluate the power of the study according to the number of patients actually enrolled.

Ideally, a study should have a power of at least 80% to detect the specified treatment effect.

Blinding

An important aspect of any study is the blinding of study participants and investigators to the patient's treatment group. Surveillance bias occurs when an investigator is aware of the patient's treatment group and preferentially investigates more thoroughly for an outcome or side effect. Any investigator involved in collecting data should not be aware of the patient's treatment group, particularly in the case of subjective measurements such as pain that are open to interpretation. A physician may treat a patient differently if he or she is aware of the study group to which the patient has been randomised. This is referred to as treatment bias. A patient's response to a disease is also affected by his or her perception of the adequacy of the treatment being applied. Patients who know they are receiving a placebo or the currently accepted treatment may not respond as well as patients who know they are receiving the new 'wonder drug', simply by virtue of the former group's perception of sub-optimal treatment. The 'placebo effect' is a response to a placebo treatment simply because patients think they are being treated and has been reported to be higher than 30%.[23,24] Others have disputed that this phenomenon exists[25] and suggest other mechanisms for the apparent cure of untreated patients. The placebo effect will bias results towards 'no effect of treatment' and should always be considered when interpreting results. This principle has been applied recently to interventional procedures such as renal denervation, in which a 'sham' procedure is performed in the control group to minimise risk of treatment bias.

Control group

Choice of an appropriate control group is vital to ensure applicability of the results of a study to the patient population. If a current treatment or practice exists, this should be the intervention applied to the control group in the study. Patients are often unaware of this and incorrectly assume that a control group receives no treatment, whereas a control group in fact receives the best known alternative treatment to that of the experimental group. A placebo control is only appropriate if no current treatment exists for the disease.

Analysis by intention-to-treat

Study participants in a RCT should be analysed in the group to which they were randomised, regardless of the treatment they received. This is referred to as analysis by intention-to-treat. There are many reasons why a patient may not comply with a medication regimen including adverse effects of the drug, cost of the treatment, clerical errors or misinterpretation of the dosing instructions. All of these factors are likely to occur if the drug is made widely available. The overall efficacy of the drug will be altered by the level of compliance in the general community. Hence, analysis of the effect of a drug should include those patients who were intended to take the drug but for one reason or another failed to do so.

Loss to follow-up

A clinical trial should strive to account for most, if not all, patients enrolled. Loss of contact with some patients is inevitable, particularly in trials with a long follow-up period. With careful planning and data collection, however, it is often possible to collect data on almost all patients enrolled in the trial. Omission of data from missing patients can alter the observed strength of association between an exposure and outcome. In trials where loss to follow-up is excessive (more than about 20%) a best case/worst case analysis should be performed. The best case assumes that all missing patients from the active treatment group have survived (or been cured) and all missing controls have died (or still have the disease). Conversely, the worst case assumes that all missing patients receiving the active treatment have died and all missing controls have survived. The true level of effect will lie somewhere between these two values.

Generalisability

Results of a study cannot always be applied to every patient or population. If a patient is different in some way to those involved in the study there may be a characteristic that alters the strength of effect in this patient. A classic example is the aborted Cardiac Arrhythmia Suppression Trial (CAST) clinical trial,[26] in which patients who had suffered myocardial infarction were given flecainide with the intention of suppressing ventricular ectopy and improving survival. It had been demonstrated previously that suppressing ventricular ectopic beats improved survival, and studies had shown that flecainide was effective in suppressing ventricular ectopics. The CAST trial investigators found a death rate 3.5 times higher in the flecainide group than the control group. The previous studies with flecainide had been performed on patients with long QT syndromes and were not applicable to post-MI patients with ischaemic myocardial disease.

DEVELOPING GUIDELINES USING THE GRADE SYSTEM

When making healthcare management decisions, patients, clinicians, and policy makers must consider the benefits and risks of alternative strategies. Authors of clinical practice guidelines ideally prefer to base their recommendations on high quality evidence that shows consistent treatment results and minimal risk of serious side effects to patients. There may be very few well-conducted randomised controlled trials that offer high quality evidence in some areas of medicine (e.g. cardiac arrest).

In 2004, the Grading of Assessment, Development and Evaluation (GRADE) system was developed to rate the quality of evidence (as high, moderate, low, or very low) and grade the strength of recommendations (as strong or weak).[27] The GRADE system outlines the requirements for study design, consistency of findings and directness of findings. GRADE emphasises that high-quality evidence alone does not necessarily imply strong recommendations, and strong recommendations can arise from low quality evidence.[28] For example, a well-conducted randomised controlled trial that demonstrates a clear treatment benefit but has significant methodological shortcomings may be downgraded from a strong to a weak recommendation. RCTs can also have their evidence downgraded based on study limitations, inconsistent results, indirect evidence, imprecision, and reporting bias. Although observational studies (e.g. cohort, case-control) are always given a low quality evidence rating, they may be upgraded from a weak to strong recommendation, if there is a large treatment effect, dose-response relationship, or consistent findings across several studies. The strength of recommendations also depends on patient values and preferences, and on whether the treatment is cost-effective. The GRADE system

is gaining popularity and has been used by the American College of Chest Physicians in the latest clinical guidelines for antithrombotic therapy in venous thromboembolic disease.[29]

Evidence from well-conducted randomised controlled trials may result in 'recommendations' for or against a course of action. For example, 'It is **recommended** that a patient with acute chest pain or other symptoms suggestive of an acute coronary syndrome receives a 12-lead eletrocardiogram and this is assessed for signs of myocardial ischaemia by an experienced clinician within 10 minutes of first acute clinical contact.[30]

Evidence from observational studies or randomised trials that have been downgraded result in 'suggestions' for or against an intervention. For example, 'We **suggest** that communities may train bystanders in compression-only CPR for adult out-of-hospital cardiac arrest as an alternative to training in conventional CPR.[31]

There are other systems used in cardiology for translating scientific evidence into clinical practice guidelines. For example, the American College of Cardiology and American Heart Association recommendations provide a widely used set of treatment guidelines based on a classification system rating the strength of the recommendation (Class I to III) and the quality of evidence (Level A to C).[32]

EVALUATING DIAGNOSTIC TESTS

Clinicians use a threshold (or cut-off) value in a diagnostic test to establish the presence or absence of disease. There is generally an overlap in the distribution of values for diseased and non-diseased populations, and the selected threshold value must consider the need to correctly identify patients with disease against the need to correctly identify patients without disease. Consequently, diagnostic tests cannot be 100% accurate. This concept is illustrated in Figure 13.2, where most of the test values for the Diseased population exceed the non-diseased population and there are three different threshold values (a, b or c). For threshold value 'a', many patients with disease will be correctly identified (Test values ≥ 'a' for the Diseased population) but some will be missed (Test values < 'a' for the Diseased population). Many patients who are non-diseased will be correctly identified (Test value < 'a' for the Non-diseased population) but some will be misclassified as having disease

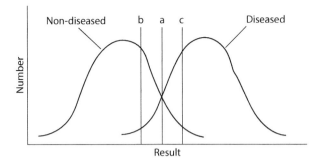

Figure 13.2 Distribution of continuous results of a test in diseased and non-diseased patients, with three possible threshold values for distinguishing positive from negative results.

(Test value ≥ 'a' for the Non-diseased population). For threshold value 'b', nearly all patients with disease will be correctly identified, but more of the non-diseased patients will be misclassified as having disease. For threshold value 'c', very few non-diseased patients will be misclassified as having disease, but more diseased patients will be missed.

A diagnostic test is positive when the test value is greater than or equal to the threshold value, and negative when the test value is less than the threshold value. When a diagnostic test is applied to a population of diseased and non-diseased patients, there are four possible test outcomes as summarised in Table 13.1. The properties of a diagnostic test are defined in Table 13.1 and discussed in the following.

The validity of a diagnostic test is determined by comparing the test results to the 'gold standard' (assumed to be 100% accurate) method of detecting disease. Sensitivity measures the ability of a test to correctly detect patients with disease. It is also called the 'True Positive Rate' and can be remembered as 'Positive in Disease'. Specificity measures the ability of a test to correctly exclude non-diseased patients. It is called the 'True Negative Rate' and can be remembered as 'Negative in Health'. Sensitivity and specificity summarise the performance of a diagnostic test for a population but cannot be used to interpret test results for an individual patient.[33]

Receiver-Operator curves show the sensitivity and specificity for all threshold values, and can be used to determine the optimal sensitivity and specificity of a diagnostic test.[34]

The positive predictive value is the proportion of patients with a positive test who actually have the disease, and the negative predictive value is the proportion of patients with a negative test who do not have disease. Predictive values depend on disease prevalence and are therefore not transferable between patients or clinical settings.[33]

The likelihood ratio indicates how many times more (or less) likely a patient with disease is to have a specific test result compared to a patient without disease. The positive likelihood ratio examines the positive test results and compares them in patients with disease to those without disease. The best diagnostic test to 'rule in' disease has a large positive likelihood ratio (>10). The negative likelihood ratio examines the negative results and compares them in patients without disease to those with disease. The best diagnostic test to 'rule out' disease has a very small negative likelihood ratio (<0.1).[35] The likelihood ratio is independent of disease prevalence and allows the clinician to calculate the probability of disease for an individual patient.[33]

EBM emphasises that diagnostic tests are only of value if they result in improved patient outcomes.[35] Improved patient outcomes from diagnostic tests may result from the availability of an effective treatment, reductions in test related adverse events or anxiety, or if disease confirmation provides prognostic information for patients with an untreatable condition. The GRADE system has been applied to diagnostic tests to grade the quality of scientific evidence and rate the strength of recommendations. For example, there was only a weak recommendation for coronary computed tomography scanning to replace invasive coronary angiography to diagnose coronary artery disease in a population with low (20%) pre-test probability. Understandably, patients are willing to accept invasive coronary angiography given the risks associated with 21% false positives (unnecessary

Table 13.1 Test outcomes and properties of a diagnostic test

Test Outcomes

	GOLD STANDARD (100% Accurate)		
	Disease present	Disease absent	TOTALS
Positive Test Result	True positive TP	False positive FP	TP + FP
Negative Test Result	False negative FN	True negative TN	FN + TN
TOTALS	TP + FN	FP + TN	

Definition of Properties

Sensitivity	= Proportion of patients with disease who have a positive test = TP/(TP + FN)
Specificity	= Proportion of patients without disease who have a negative test = TN/(FP + TN)
Positive Predictive Value	= Proportion of patients with a positive test that truly have disease = TP/(TP + FP)
Negative Predictive Value	= Proportion of patients with a negative test that truly do not have disease = TN/(TN + FN)
Positive Likelihood Ratio	= Probability of positive test in those with disease/probability of positive test in those without disease = TP rate/FP rate = (TP/(TP + FN))/(FP/(FP + TN)) = Sensitivity/(1 – Specificity)
Negative Likelihood Ratio	= Probability of negative test in those with disease/probability of negative test in those without disease = FN rate/TN rate = (FN/(TP + FN))/(TN/(FP + TN)) = (1 – Sensitivity)/Specificity
Pre-Test Probability	= p1 = Probability of disease before diagnostic testing = prevalence
Pre-Test Odds	= p1/(1 – p1)
Post-Test Odds	= Pre-Test Odds x Likelihood Ratio
Post-Test Probability	= Post-Test Odds/(1 + Post-Test Odds) = probability of disease after diagnostic testing
Accuracy	= (TP + FN)/(TP + FN + FP + TN)

patient anxiety and further testing) and approximately 1% false negatives (missing out on effective treatment).[36]

CONCLUSIONS

EBM provides clinicians with the best scientific evidence to guide treatment of individual patients. EBM emphasises critical appraisal of the scientific literature in search of the best source(s) of evidence to address a clinical or research question. It encourages the clinician to seek out high quality studies and avoid those that may provide biased or misleading results.

These concepts can also be applied to the design stage of a clinical trial to ensure that the best quality results are obtained. Knowledge of the techniques for producing high-quality results allows careful design and implementation of the study and ensures that future researchers need not repeat a poorly designed or poorly conducted trial, but can direct their funds and efforts towards improving further the advances already made.

REFERENCES

1. Oxman AD, Sackett DL, Guyatt GH, Browman G, Cook D, Gerstein H, et al. Users' guides to the medical literature: I. How to get started. JAMA. 1993;270(17):2093–2095.
2. Guyatt GH, Sackett DL, Cook DJ, Guyatt G, Bass E, Brill-Edwards P, et al. Users' guides to the medical literature: II. How to use an article about therapy or prevention A. Are the results of the study valid? JAMA. 1993;270(21):2598–2601.
3. Guyatt GH, Sackett DL, Cook DJ, Guyatt G, Bass E, Brill-Edwards P, et al. Users' guides to the medical literature: II. How to use an article about therapy or prevention B. What were the results and will they help me in caring for my patients? JAMA. 1994;271(1):59–63.
4. Jaeschke R, Guyatt G, Sackett D. Users' guides to the medical literature. III. How to use an article about a diagnostic test. A. Are the results of the study valid? Evidence-based medicine working group. JAMA. 1994;271(5):389–391.
5. Jaeschke R, Guyatt GH, Sackett DL, Guyatt G, Bass E, Brill-Edwards P, et al. Users' guides to the medical Literature: III. How to use an article about a diagnostic test B. What are the results and will they help me in caring for my patients? JAMA. 1994;271(9):703–707.
6. Levine M, Walter S, Lee H, Haines T, Holbrook A, Moyer V. Users' guides to the medical literature. JAMA. 1994;271(20):1615–1619.
7. Laupacis A, Wells G, Richardson S, Tugwell P for the evidence-based medicine working group. User's guides to the medical literature: IV. How to use an article about prognosis. JAMA 1994;272(3):234–237.
8. Oxman AD, Cook DJ, Guyatt GH, Bass E, Brill-Edwards P, Browman G, et al. Users' guides to the medical literature: VI. How to use an overview. JAMA. 1994;272(17):1367–1371.
9. Richardson WS, Detsky AS. Users' guides to the medical literature: VII. How to use a clinical decision analysis A. Are the results of the study valid? JAMA. 1995;273(16):1292–1295.
10. Richardson WS, Detsky AS, Guyatt G, Cook D, Gerstein H, Hayward R, et al. Users' guides to the medical literature: VII. How to use a clinical decision analysis B. What are the results and will they help me in caring for my patients? JAMA. 1995;273(20):1610–1613.
11. Hayward RS, Wilson MC, Tunis SR, Bass EB, Guyatt G. Users' guides to the medical literature: VIII. How to use practical guidelines. A. Are the recommendations valid? JAMA. 1995;274(7):570–574.
12. Wilson MC, Hayward RS, Tunis SR, Bass EB, Guyatt G, Cook D, et al. Users' guides to the medical literature: VIII. how to use clinical practice guidelines B. what are the recommendations and will they help you in caring for your patients? JAMA. 1995;274(20):1630–1632.
13. Guyatt G, Sackett D, Sinclair J, Hayward R, Cook D, Cook R. For the evidence-based medicine working group: Users' guides to the medical literature: IX. A method for grading health care recommendations. JAMA. 1995;274(22):1800–1804.
14. Naylor CD, Guyatt GH, Bass E, Gerstein H, Heyland D, Holbrook A, et al. Users' guides to the medical literature: X. How to use an article reporting variations in the outcomes of health services. JAMA. 1996;275(7):554–558.
15. Naylor CD, Guyatt GH, Dans AL, Dans LF, Glasziou P, Green L, et al. Users' guides to the medical literature: XI. How to use an article about a clinical utilization review. JAMA 1996;275(18):1435–1439.
16. Guyatt GH, Naylor CD, Juniper E, Heyland DK, Jaeschke R, Cook DJ. Users' guides to the medical literature: XII. How to use articles about health-related quality of life. JAMA. 1997;277(15):1232–1237.
17. Drummond MF, Richardson WS, O'brien BJ, Levine M, Heyland D. Users' guides to the medical literature: XIII. How to use an article on economic analysis of clinical practice. A. Are the results of the study valid? JAMA. 1997;277(19):1552–1557.

18. O'Brien B, Heyland D, Richardson W, Levine M, Drummond M. Users' Guides to the medical literature XIII: How to use an article on economic analysis of clinical practice. B. What are the results and will they help me in caring for my patients? *JAMA.* 1997;277(22):1802–1806.

19. Dans AL, Dans LF, Guyatt GH, Richardson S, Group E-BMW. Users' guides to the medical literature: XIV. How to decide on the applicability of clinical trial results to your patient. *JAMA.* 1998;279(7):545–549.

20. Anonymous. World Health Organization. International Clinical Trials Registry Platform Search Portal. http://apps.who.int/trial-search/ Accessed 13 February 2018.

21. Anonymous. US National Library of Medicine. ClinicalTrials.gov. https://clinical-trials.gov/ Accessed 13 February 2018.

22. Glasziou PP, Irwig LM. An evidence based approach to individualising treatment. *BMJ.* 1995;311(7016):1356–1359.

23. Finniss DG, Kaptchuk TJ, Miller F, Benedetti F. Biological, clinical, and ethical advances of placebo effects. *Lancet.* 2010;375(9715):686–695.

24. Benedetti F, Mayberg HS, Wager TD, Stohler CS, Zubieta JK. Neurobiological mechanisms of the placebo effect. *J Neurosci.* 2005;25(45):10390–10402.

25. Hróbjartsson A, Gøtzsche PC. Is the placebo powerless? Update of a systematic review with 52 new randomized trials comparing placebo with no treatment. *J Int Med.* 2004;256(2):91–100.

26. Price DD, Finniss DG, Benedetti F. A comprehensive review of the placebo effect: Recent advances and current thought. *Ann Rev Psychol.* 2008;59:565–590.

27. Guyatt G, Oxman AD, Akl EA, Kunz R, Vist G, Brozek J, et al. GRADE guidelines: 1. Introduction—GRADE evidence profiles and summary of findings tables. *J Clin Epidemiol.* 2011;64(4):383–394.

28. Guyatt GH, Oxman AD, Vist GE, Kunz R, Falck-Ytter Y, Alonso-Coello P, et al. GRADE: An emerging consensus on rating quality of evidence and strength of recommendations. *BMJ* (Clin Res ed). 2008;336(7650):924–926.

29. Kearon C, Akl EA, Ornelas J, Blaivas A, Jimenez D, Bounameaux H, et al. Antithrombotic therapy for VTE disease: CHEST guideline and expert panel report. *Chest.* 2016;149(2):315–352.

30. Chew DP, Scott IA, Cullen L, French JK, Briffa TG, Tideman PA, et al. National Heart Foundation of Australia & Cardiac Society of Australia and New Zealand: Australian clinical guidelines for the management of acute coronary syndromes. 2016. *Heart Lung Circ.* 2016;25:895–951.

31. Finn J, Bhanji F, Lockey A, Monsieurs K, Frengley R, Iwami T, et al. Part 8: Education, implementation, and teams. 2015 International consensus on cardiopulmonary resuscitation and emergency cardiovascular care science with treatment recommendations. *Resus.* 2015;95:e203–e224.

32. Yancy CW, Jessup M, Bozkurt B, Butler J, Casey Jr DE, Colvin MM, et al. 2017 ACC/AHA/HFSA focused update of the 2013 ACCF/AHA guideline for the management of heart failure. *J Am Coll Cardiol.* 2017;70:776–803.

33. Attia J. Moving beyond sensitivity and specificity: Using likelihood ratios to help interpret diagnostic tests. *Aust Prescr.* 2003;26(5):111–113.

34. Anonymous. Medical Biostatistics and Research. ROC Curve. MedicalBiostatistics. com www.medicalbiostatistics.com/roc-curve.pdf. Accessed 5 March 2018.

35. Deeks JJ, Altman DG. Diagnostic tests 4: Likelihood ratios. *BMJ.* 2004;329(7458):168–169.

36. Schünemann HJ, Oxman AD, Brozek J, Glasziou P, Jaeschke R, Vist GE, et al. Rating quality of evidence and strength of recommendations: GRADE: Grading quality of evidence and strength of recommendations for diagnostic tests and strategies. *BMJ.* 2008;336: 1106–1110.

PART 3

Physiology and pharmacology

14

Pressure waveforms in the cardiac cycle

JOHN EDWARD BOLAND AND DAVID W. BARON

INTRODUCTION

Dynamic blood pressure is the propulsive force generated in the cardiovascular system by rhythmic ventricular contractions that generate pulsatile blood flow in arteries. This dynamic arterial pressure dissipates into constant low-pressure flow in the capillary circulation. Right or left heart cardiac catheterisation records pressures as continuous rhythmic waveforms from the intracardiac chambers and great vessels by means of catheters inserted directly into arteries or veins, each chamber or vessel having its own distinctive pulsatile pattern with characteristics that reflect underlying pathologies. This chapter describes how the mechanical and physiological responses to pressure variations during the cardiac cycle assist investigations of valve disease and other cardiac abnormalities.

PRESSURE MEASUREMENT

The human or mammalian heart is a four-chambered pump with dual circuits to the pulmonary and systemic circulations. Pressures in left and right sides of the heart need to be measured separately. Recordings of right heart or pulmonary circulation consist of right atrium, right ventricle, pulmonary artery and pulmonary artery wedge (PAW) pressures. The PAW pressure is a measure of left atrial pressure transmitted retrogradely via pulmonary veins to a right heart catheter 'wedged' in a distal pulmonary artery and is accepted as a representative value of left atrial pressure, noting that there is a time lag (or phase shift) of some 50–80 msec between recordings of left atrium and PAW pressures. This is the time it takes for left atrial pressures to travel across pulmonary veins to the pulmonary arteries.

The left heart or systemic circulation consists of measurements of aortic, left ventricular and occasionally left atrial pressures measured by crossing the mitral valve retrogradely from the left ventricle, which is sometimes possible. Left atrial pressure is usually recorded via the PAW position, or by transseptal puncture from the right atrium, or by crossing a patent foramen ovale.

In sinus rhythm, right atrium, left atrium and pulmonary arterial wedge pressures are biphasic in contour (i.e. have two distinct waves per heartbeat, Figure 14.1a) reflecting the rise and fall in atrial pressures caused by sequential filling and drainage of blood in the atria. Venous pulse recordings such as superior and inferior venae cavae that supply the right atrium, and the pulmonary veins, that fill the left atrium, are also biphasic because there are no valves separating the atria from their filling source. Ventricles, which are separated from inflow and outflow ports by valves, reflect mainly monophasic pressure traces (i.e. one wave per heartbeat, Figure 14.1b) as do arterial pressures.

Left and right heart catheterisation was once routinely performed for all patients undergoing cardiac catheterisation, whether for investigation of ischaemic heart disease or other reasons. In time it was

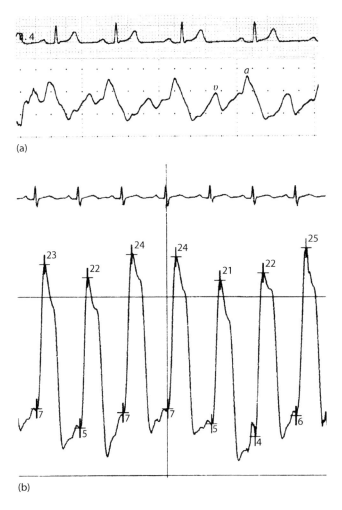

(a)

(b)

Figure 14.1 (a) Right atrial pressure waveform showing distinct biphasic trace consisting of repeated a and v waves. The a wave of the atrial pressure trace follows the P wave of the electrocardiogram, the v wave follows the T wave. The downslope of the a wave is the x descent, the downslope of the v wave is the y descent. (b) Right ventricular pressure showing one deflection per heartbeat. Ventricular end-diastole aligns with the R wave of the electrocardiogram and reflects activity of the a wave of the right atrium. The right heart is a low-pressure system and pressures are usually monitored on a scale 0–40 mmHg.

realised that right heart catheterisation was unnecessary for patients presenting only with angina. Right heart catheterisation, either by itself or in conjunction with left heart catheterisation, is now performed selectively for patients presenting with certain conditions such as valvular heart disease, congenital heart disease, constrictive pericarditis, cardiomyopathy, pulmonary hypertension or heart transplant assessment for calculation of pulmonary vascular resistance. Information obtained by these investigations is essential for further clinical management.

THE CARDIAC CYCLE

The cardiac cycle may be defined as the sequence of events occurring between two consecutive cardiac contractions. Each cycle begins with the right atrium and may be separated into atrial and ventricular components, or according to events in the left or right heart. With each heartbeat, blood returning from the peripheral circulation is channelled by the right ventricle to the lungs for oxygenation and recirculated to the periphery via the left ventricle. A complete description of the cardiac cycle describes changes in electrocardiogram (ECG), blood pressure, volume, blood flow and flow velocity in all cardiac chambers and follows events occurring in both right and left heart systems. The ECG serves as a baseline on which to synchronise different cardiac events.

The cardiac cycle is a continuous cycle that begins with electrical activation of the sinoatrial node. This induces depolarisation and causes contraction of both atria (P wave of the ECG), followed by stimulation of the atrioventricular node and contraction of both ventricles (QRS complex of the ECG). Before atria or ventricles can contract, however, the chambers must first fill with blood. This description of the cardiac cycle therefore begins with the atrial filling that occurs immediately prior to atrial contraction and follows the direction of blood flow through the heart.

Right atrium

The key to understanding the haemodynamics of the cardiac cycle lies in understanding the biphasic nature of the atrial pressure waveforms. Blood returns to the right atrium via superior and inferior venae cavae that permit continuous filling of the right atrium during atrial diastole. The right atrioventricular valve (tricuspid) is closed during early atrial diastole, causing atrial pressure and volume to increase as the atrium fills. This pressure increase is evident as an upward deflection of the atrial waveform and is recorded as a v wave (Figure 14.2a). The tricuspid valve then opens in mid-atrial diastole, when the atrium is only partly filled, and blood drains passively from the atrium into the ventricle. Following this decrease in volume load, atrial pressure drops accordingly (seen as the descent of the v wave, Figure 14.2b). Blood continues to drain freely from the venae cavae into the atrium and flows directly across the open tricuspid valve into the right ventricle. With the valve open there is virtually no resistance to flow between atrium and ventricle, therefore pressures in these two chambers will equalise temporarily.

Atrial diastole lasts until the atrium contracts in response to atrial depolarisation at the time of the P wave of the ECG. This causes another small but forceful increase in atrial pressure (the a wave), which empties additional atrial blood into the ventricle (Figure 14.2c). Note that the a wave aligns with the P wave on the ECG and the v wave aligns with the T wave.

Up to 80% of ventricular filling occurs by passive venous drainage across the open tricuspid valve before the atrial contraction or 'atrial kick' occurs. The right ventricle then begins to contract, increasing its pressure relative to the right atrium; the tricuspid valve closes, the atrium relaxes (Figure 14.2d) and atrial pressure drops (seen as the descent of the a wave). Passive venous return across the tricuspid valve continues with a new v wave (Figure 14.2a) during ventricular systole and the atrial cycle begins anew with the next a wave.

As each cycle begins with atrial contraction, the a wave is the first upward deflection of the atrial pressure waveform and the v wave follows the a wave in the same cycle. Each a wave is haemodynamically paired with the preceding v wave, not the one following. This pairing is considered to be part of the same cycle of movement of valve leaflets, atrioventricular valve motion and possible regurgitant flow across the valve. Atrial pressure waveforms are reported as an a wave, v wave and mean value (e.g. the right atrial waveform in Figure 14.1a is reported as $a = 5$, $v = 4$, m = 3, or 5/4/3), where the value for the v wave is taken from the waveform preceding the a wave. In practice there is usually little difference between two consecutive a and v waves.

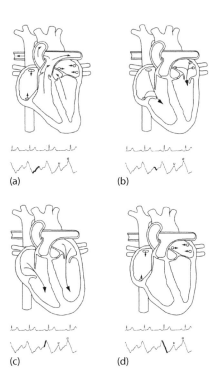

Figure 14.2 Sequence of events depicting valve opening and closure with corresponding changes in the electrocardiogram and atrial pressure waveform. Passive venous return to the atria causes the upstroke of the v wave during atrial diastole/ventricular systole (a). Opening of the atrioventricular valves allows passive ventricular filling, resulting in a fall in atrial pressure and the downstroke of the atrial v wave (b). Atrial contraction increases atrial pressure, causing the upstroke of the a wave and completing ventricular filling (c). As blood empties from the atria, atrial pressure drops, causing the descent of the a wave as ventricular contraction begins with isovolumetric contraction (d) with closure of all four cardiac valves. The atria refill and the cycle continues anew with (a).

In sinus rhythm, each atrial depolarisation is paired with a single subsequent ventricular contraction. In atrial fibrillation, however, atrial depolarisation is continuous and exceeds the rate of ventricular contraction. On the ECG the QRS is irregular, and atrial activity is evident as a series of weak and irregular waves (called F waves) preceding each QRS complex. As there is loss of direct atrial contraction, the corresponding atrial pressure waveform shows an absence of a waves, appearing only as a sequence of single irregular v waves, although a biphasic wave pattern can still be evident.

The c wave

A third wave, the c wave may also be evident as a slight upward deflection during the descent of the a wave. Just after the tricuspid valve closes, ventricular pressure continues to increase from its systolic contraction, causing the valve leaflets to bulge

backwards into the atrium. This results in a small pressure increase in the atrial waveform, seen as the c wave. In practice, this third waveform is not clearly apparent and can generally be dismissed. A perfect atrial waveform therefore consists of three upward deflections (the a, c and v waves respectively). The downslope of the a wave is called the x descent, and the downslope of the v wave is called the y descent. The same factors identified in atrial pressure waveforms can be identified in the jugular venous trace, which is transmitted retrogradely from the right atrium.

Left atrium

The preceding description of the right heart cycle applies equally to both right and left heart systems. In the same way that venae cavae fill the right atrium, the left atrium acts as a reservoir for venous blood return during ventricular systole as pulmonary veins fill the left atrium. Passive left atrial filling against a closed mitral valve during ventricular systole forms the left atrial *v* wave. This is followed by mitral valve opening, then atrial contraction and an *a* wave. Both left and right atria empty their loads near-simultaneously into each ventricle. Atrial pressure then parallels ventricular pressure until ventricular contraction begins and the mitral valve closes along with the tricuspid valve. The *a* and *v* waves thus reflect atrial systole and diastole respectively.

Combined atrial cycle

Right and left atria contract and relax (almost) simultaneously, as do right and left ventricles. The electrical stimulus from the sinoatrial node reaches the right atrium a fraction of a second before the left atrium, creating a slight time lag in left atrial response. Similarly, although the AV node conducts its electrical signal simultaneously along the Bundle of His, for various reasons the left ventricle starts to contract before the right, but right ventricular ejection begins first, lasts longer and ends later than that of the left ventricle. It follows that the mitral valve closes slightly ahead of the tricuspid valve and the aortic valve closes slightly earlier than the pulmonary valve. Such detail can only be appreciated with an echogram (for exact details of timing see subsequent text). Generally, changes in left atrial pressure parallel those of the right atrium, changes in the left ventricle parallel those of the right and changes in aorta parallel those of the pulmonary artery.

Ventricular cycle

Valves are almost entirely passive structures that open and close according to the pressure difference in chambers on either side of the valve. When the atria begin to fill at the very beginning of atrial diastole, the ventricles are still contracting from the previous systole. The ventricles then relax and ventricular pressure starts to fall. When ventricular pressure falls below that of atrial pressure, the tricuspid and mitral valves are forced open and permit ventricular filling. At first, ventricular pressure increases only slightly with its initial passive atrial inflow. Atrial systole causes a sudden late rise in pressure coincident with a late inflow of blood, seen as a small sharp rise in ventricular pressure at end-diastole. This value is identical to the atrial *a* wave and is referred to as ventricular end-diastolic pressure or EDP (Figure 14.3). Following atrial

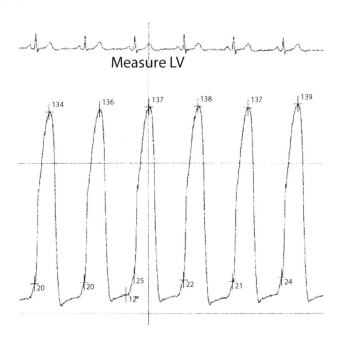

Figure 14.3 Left ventricular pressure waveform showing systole and end-diastole (the a wave). The lower value (12*) indicates the plateau preceding the a wave (see later text for explanation). Note this patient has diastolic values higher than normal, indicating some ventricular impairment. Left ventricular pressures are usually monitored on a scale of 0–200 mmHg.

systole, ventricular muscles begin to constrict, causing ventricular pressure to rise above atrial pressure and forcing closure of the atrioventricular valves.

End-diastolic pressure (EDP)

Left ventricular EDP is the pressure in the ventricle immediately preceding ventricular contraction and is called preload. According to the Frank-Starling principle, preload is a measure of presystolic muscle fibre stretch, is proportional to ventricular end-diastolic volume, and directly determines the force of cardiac contraction. Aortic end-diastole, the pressure against which the ventricle has to work to open the aortic valve, is called afterload (as a surrogate for systemic vascular resistance). The higher these respective values, the greater the load imposed on ventricular pumping activity.

Ventricular filling

It should be noted that there are three distinct phases of ventricular filling. The first, early ventricular filling, or rapid filling phase, is an active energy-consuming process resulting from relaxation of ventricular forces as the ventricle recovers from systole and involves uncoiling of the ventricular muscle fibres. Hence, myocardial contraction is not the only energy-consuming period of ventricular activity. The second phase is the period of diastasis consisting of ventricular filling after the preceding uncoiling activity. Diastasis is the passive filling stage that dominates the ventricular filling period. The third phase is the atrial contribution to ventricular filling, or a wave, which boosts passive ventricular filling by forceful atrial contraction and at rest delivers an additional 20%–40% volume load to the ventricle.

During diastole, pressure in the ventricle drops to a very low value, not quite reaching zero. The lowest value reached is usually an artefactual downward spike (see Figures 14.1b and 14.3) and is ignored. True ventricular diastole is therefore taken as the pressure reached immediately prior to systole. The question arises as to what constitutes true ventricular end-diastole. Some operators consider the a wave as their preferred value for end-diastole. The a wave, however, although occurring

immediately prior to ventricular contraction and thus a true measure of EDP, is a mixture of atrial and ventricular function and cannot be accepted as a true value of ventricular forces. A more accurate measure of passive stiffness of ventricular forces is the plateau before the a wave (see Figure 14.3). The second phase of ventricular filling, diastasis, is consequently the preferred value for EDP. Optimum information can be conveyed by reporting each value individually (e.g. LV = 120/5, a = 9). The post a wave period can also contributes important information about how ventricular muscle accommodates forces generated by filling but requires more complicated measurement. A mean value for ventricular pressure is physiologically meaningless and is not reported.

The a wave can be measured by physiological monitors for both left and right ventricles but because of the dominance of left heart catheterisation, only left ventricular EDP is generally evaluated in assessing ventricular performance, and right heart function is evaluated separately. The EDP may be elevated due to inadequate force of myocardial contraction (systolic dysfunction) or to inadequate relaxation in diastole (diastolic dysfunction).

Left ventricle and aorta

As the left ventricle contracts and left ventricular pressure exceeds that of the aorta, the aortic valve is forced open and blood is ejected from the ventricle. Aortic pressure begins to rise as soon as the aortic valve opens, when ventricular blood enters the aorta. Because the aortic valve is open there is continuity of flow between left ventricle and aorta, and pressure in the two chambers equalises. Thus aortic pressure follows and parallels left ventricular pressure during the ventricular systolic ejection period (Figure 14.4). Both pressures peak at midsystole then decline when the force of ventricular contraction diminishes. As these pressures fall, left ventricular pressure drops below aortic pressure and the aortic valve closes, ending the left ventricular ejection period and marking the beginning of diastole, called protodiastole. Specifically, protodiastole marks the time between the start of ventricular relaxation and the second heart sound caused by aortic valve closure.

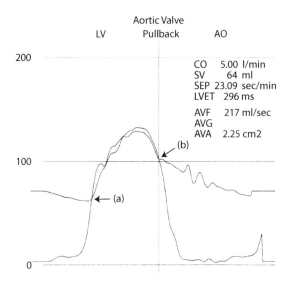

Figure 14.4 Simultaneous left ventricular and aortic pressures demonstrating point of opening of aortic valve when left ventricular pressure exceeds aortic pressure **(a)** and point of closure of aortic valve at the dichrotic notch **(b)** when ventricular pressure again falls below aortic pressure. The ventricular ejection period is the time interval between points a and b. Ventricular diastole begins at **(b)**.

Timing of valve movement

The dynamics of the system are such that valve movement on left and right sides is not in perfect synchrony. The aortic valve does not close instantly with the fall in left ventricular pressure. There is a very slight time lag during which its forward momentum continues to propel blood forward for a moment. Blood flow slows and even reverses in a rebound effect from elastic arterial recoil, causing the dichrotic notch or incisura in the arterial waveform (this phenomenon results in aortic valve closure slightly later than would be expected from a fall in pressure alone). Because of residual arterial tone, aortic pressure drops only gradually during ventricular diastole, until the next ventricular contraction again opens the aortic valve. A brief period of isovolumetric ventricular contraction ensues, which coincides with closure of both mitral and aortic valves. Aortic valve closure is easily recognisable as the dichrotic notch on aortic waveforms, although fluid-filled catheter systems can be affected by artefactual distortions which can introduce additional unidentifiable notches.

Pressure equalisation

As described, during the period of atrial drainage into the ventricles when atrioventricular valves (mitral and tricuspid) are open there is unrestricted flow between atria and ventricles. Haemodynamically, since blood is a fluid and exerts pressure equally in all directions, pressure equalises between the two cardiac chambers. This means that for a brief period during ventricular diastole pressure in the atrium (and hence in the pulmonary wedge trace) is identical to pressure in the ventricle (see Figure 14.5), as the atrioventricular valves (mitral and tricuspid) are both open during ventricular diastole. Pressure equalisation is best observed when pressures in both chambers are recorded simultaneously.

A similar situation exists between any two cardiac chambers separated by an open valve: Pressure in each chamber will momentarily equilibrate until the valve closes again. Thus aortic systolic pressure will be identical to the left ventricular systolic trace when the aortic valve is open and there is continuity between ventricle and aorta during the ventricular systolic ejection period (as shown in Figure 14.4).

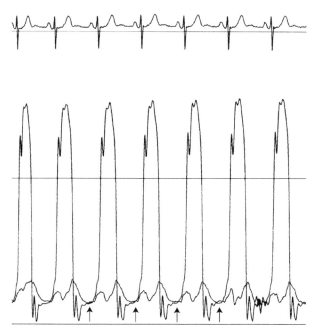

Figure 14.5 Synchrony between left ventricle and pulmonary wedge pressures measured simultaneously at the same magnification (0-200 mmHg). Note pressure equalisation when the mitral valve is open (arrows) prior to atrial systole.

The same applies to pulmonary artery and right ventricular systolic values, for the semilunar valves (aortic and pulmonary) are open during systole.

Pulmonary cycle

As with the left ventricle and aorta, the pulmonary valve opens when right ventricular pressure exceeds pulmonary artery pressure and closes when ventricular pressure again falls below pulmonary artery pressure. Pulmonary valve opening, which slightly precedes aortic valve opening, marks the beginning of the right ventricular systolic ejection period (which lasts until the pulmonary valve again closes). Apart from the slight asynchrony in timing of valve movement, right heart dynamics parallel those of the left side.

Isovolumetric contraction

Isovolumetric (or isovolumic or isometric) contraction is the period between closure of the atrioventricular valves (mitral and tricuspid) and opening of the semilunar valves (aortic and pulmonary), and represents a period of myocardial contraction marked by a sudden sharp increase in ventricular

pressure without change in ventricular volume (Figure 14.6). This occurs because, as ventricular contraction begins, both inlet and outlet ports to the ventricles are closed, which serves to build up pressure reserve in the ventricles. Myocardial contraction without this initial head of pressure would reduce propulsive velocity of blood flow, velocity of ventricular wall motion during contraction and the force of ventricular contraction. Consequently, blood is ejected forcefully from the ventricles when the semilunar valves first open. Both speed of propulsion and ventricular ejection pressure reach a peak during early systole then decline, although at different rates. Rate of change of pressure with respect to time (dP/dt) is another variable which can be recorded automatically by computer and is a measure of efficiency of myocardial contraction, particularly for the left ventricle.

Isovolumetric relaxation

Isovolumetric relaxation is the period between closure of the semilunar valves and opening of the atrioventricular valves and is the diastolic equivalent of isovolumetric contraction. Ventricular pressure continues to drop sharply following aortic and pulmonary

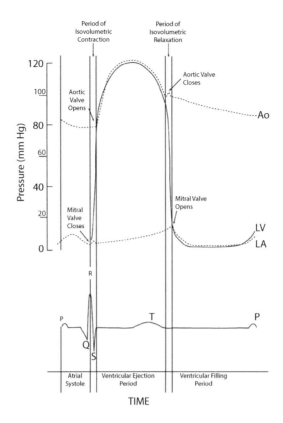

Figure 14.6 Superimposed left ventricular, aortic and left atrial pressures illustrating periods of ventricular and atrial systole and diastole in relation to valve opening and closure with the electrocardiogram. Note the periods of isovolumetric contraction and relaxation, when all four cardiac valves are closed.

valve closure at the end of the systolic ejection period, when mitral and tricuspid valves are also closed (Figure 14.6). Ventricular volume is unable to change and therefore remains constant while pressure drops to its diastolic value and myocardial muscles relax. When ventricular pressure drops below atrial pressure, mitral and tricuspid valves open and the atrial cycle begins again. These changes are clearly demonstrated by pressure-volume loops.

Complete cardiac cycle

The entire cardiac cycle can be summarised by a series of charts, as shown in Figure 14.7a and b. All events are synchronised with the electrocardiogram, which also serves as a means of timing cardiac events. Like all electrocardiogram recorders, modern computer monitors print paper at a selected rate which can be used to calculate timing of specific events such as ventricular ejection period or diastolic filling period.

Heart sounds

Valve motion causes a series of characteristic heart sounds that can be detected by auscultation or phonocardiography, as described in Figure 14.7b. The atrioventricular valves close with a loud slap at the very beginning of ventricular systole: This is called the first heart sound. The aortic and pulmonary valves close audibly when systole ends: This is called the second heart sound. To a certain extent the first and second heart sounds may be 'split', due to asynchronous closure of the mitral/tricuspid or aortic/pulmonary valves. This splitting is more marked on inspiration and is usually never wide (<0.03 seconds). Wide splitting of the second sound may occur in right bundle block, pulmonary stenosis, atrial septal defect, or anomalous pulmonary venous drainage (the last two causing fixed splitting). Paradoxical splitting of the second sound may occur in tetralogy of Fallot and truncus arteriosus.

Increased loudness of the first heart sound may be noted in mobile mitral or tricuspid stenosis, when the valve is pliable, a short PR interval, and during sinus tachycardia. A loud second sound may occur in systemic hypertension (aortic valve closure) or pulmonary hypertension (pulmonary valve closure).

A third or fourth heart sound is referred to as an added or extra sound, and these occur during diastole. The third heart sound is less distinct and represents the end of the rapid filling phase of the ventricular filling period in early diastole (just prior to the beginning of diastasis) and is thought to result from vibrations of the ventricular wall. The fourth heart sound occurs before the first and is caused by atrial systole into a poorly compliant left ventricle. Extra heart sounds are always abnormal, apart from the third which may be normal in children. The combination of an extra heart sound in a patient with tachycardia is called a gallop rhythm.

Interference with laminar blood flow across a valve, such as occurs with incomplete opening or closure of valve leaflets, can cause turbulence that may be identified as an audible heart murmur or a palpable vibration ('thrill'). Murmurs and thrills can be used by the cardiologist to detect turbulence arising from valve stenosis or incompetence (leaking) and are invaluable in diagnosing valve disease. Identifying heart sounds is a highly skilled craft of cardiology that requires considerable experience to perfect.

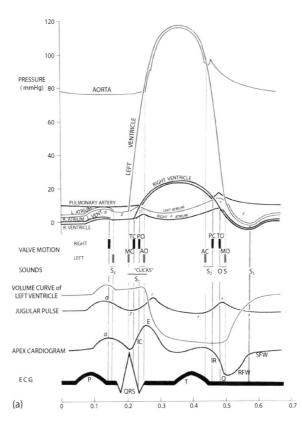

Figure 14.7 (a) Diagram of the cardiac cycle, showing the pressure curves of the great vessels and cardiac chambers, valvular events and heart sounds, left ventricular volume curve, jugular pulse wave, apex cardiogram (Sanborn piezo crystal), and the electrocardiogram. For illustrative purposes, the time intervals between valvular events have been modified. (*Abbreviations:* Valve motion – MC, mitral component of the first heart sound; MO, mitral valve opening; TC, tricuspid component of the first heart sound; TO, tricuspid valve opening; AC, aortic component of the second heart sound; AO, aortic valve opening; PC, pulmonic valve component of the second heart sound; PO, pulmonic valve opening; OS, opening snap of atrioventricular valves; Apex cardiogram – IC, isovolumic or isovolumetric (isochoric) contraction wave; IR, isovolumic or isovolumetric (isochoric) relaxation wave; O, opening of mitral valve; RFW, rapid filling wave; SFW, slow-filling wave. (*Continued*)

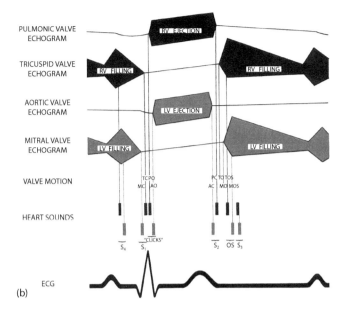

Figure 14.7 (Continued) **(b)** Timing of events in the cardiac cycle: Schematic presentation of the relationships between electrical and mechanical events and heart sounds during the cardiac cycle. The right atrium starts to contract before the left atrium but the left ventricle starts to contract before the right ventricle does; right ventricular ejection begins before left ventricular ejection and ends later than left ventricular ejection does. (*Abbreviations:* MC, mitral component of the first heart sound (S1); TC, tricuspid component of the first heart sound (S1); PO, pulmonic valve opening; AO, aortic valve opening; AC, aortic component of the second heart sound (S2); TO, tricuspid valve opening; TOS, tricuspid opening snap; MOS, mitral valve opening snap. Time intervals are not necessarily in proportion. (Reproduced with permission from Schlant et al., *Hurt's The Heart*, 8th ed. courtesy of McGraw-Hill Education.)

Left heart pressure recordings

Typical pressure recordings for a left heart (diagnostic) catheterisation are shown in Figure 14.8. Aortic and/or ventricular pressures are recorded prior to coronary angiography and ventriculography to obtain baseline values. Following ventriculography, pullback measurements from ventricle to aorta are routinely taken to note changes in EDP and to quantify the degree of aortic stenosis. (The illustration used in Figure 14.4 is a computer-generated overlay of ventricular and aortic pressure traces from two different heartbeats to illustrate absence of an aortic gradient on pullback.)

The following are key features to note with left heart pressures:

1. Systolic, diastolic and mean values are required for the aorta and other arteries.
2. Systolic and end-diastolic values are required for the left ventricle. An EDP of more than 15 mmHg is considered abnormal.

3. Note any difference in systolic pressure between ventricle and aorta on pullback. A patient with an intact aortic valve will have the same systolic value for both chambers.
4. It is physiologically impossible for aortic pressure to be greater than ventricular pressure on pullback. If this were noted it would be due to artefact, such as respiratory variations, pressure damping, calibration, or a sudden change in blood pressure. It is commonly seen if left ventricular pressure has not fully recovered from the negative inotropic effect of contrast, in which case the pullback should be delayed until pressure is stable.
5. An aortic systolic pressure lower than that of left ventricle indicates aortic stenosis.
6. Leaking valves are routinely evaluated by angiography rather than pressure. A wide pulse pressure is often associated with a leaking aortic valve. A large *v* wave is in the PAW trace is often associated with a leaking mitral valve.

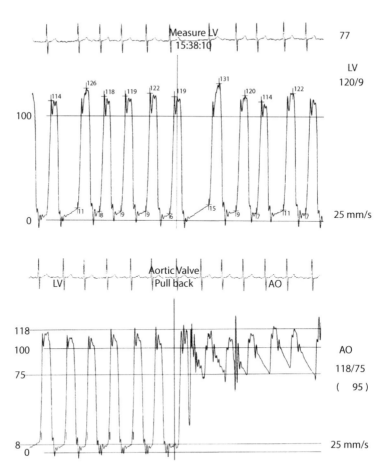

Figure 14.8 Left heart pressures taken during cardiac catheterisation. Pullback measurements from left ventricle (LV) to aorta (AO) following ventriculography determine presence or absence of aortic stenosis by identifying systolic pressure differences across the aortic valve. Even with atrial fibrillation, this patient clearly has similar systolic values for ventricle and aorta, indicating absence of aortic stenosis.

7. Current recommendations support echocardiography as the preferred method for evaluating aortic or mitral stenosis.

Aortic stenosis

Systolic differences between left ventricle and aorta caused by aortic stenosis can be readily evaluated on catheter pullback by comparing pressures obtained from the preceding ventricular beats with subsequent aortic beats. Severity of aortic stenosis is determined by the magnitude of the pressure difference across the aortic valve on pullback (Figure 14.9) and is referred to as a peak-to-peak gradient (i.e. the difference between systolic values of ventricle and aorta). Computerised systems will also calculate a mean aortic valve gradient, which is a measure

of the area bounded by the two curves when aortic and ventricular pressures are superimposed (Figure 14.10). In practice (as in Figure 14.10), the mean aortic valve gradient is obtained by superimposing selected aortic and ventricular beats on pullback, although there will always be minor differences in pressure, heart rate, systolic ejection and diastolic filling times with each individual beat. It is also possible to use double lumen catheters to record simultaneous left ventricular and aortic pressure tracings, permitting consecutive beat-by-beat evaluation of aortic stenosis.

Alternatively, aortic valve gradients can be obtained by simultaneously recording left ventricular pressure directly from the catheter in the left ventricle, and femoral artery pressure (in lieu of aortic pressure) from the side port of the groin

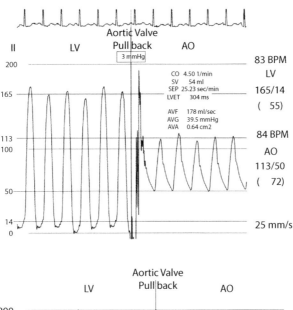

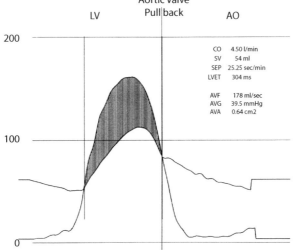

Figure 14.9 Pullback pressures (top) and overlapping pressures (bottom) from left ventricle (LV) and aorta (AO) from a patient with aortic stenosis. Note peak-to-peak gradient (52 mmHg), and mean gradient (39.5 mmHg) across the aortic valve. Size of gradient is directly related to severity of stenosis. The symbols and figures indicate automatically-derived computer calculations. Note the delayed rise in aortic systolic pressure (bottom) with aortic stenosis.

sheath (Figure 14.10a) prior to ventriculography. This permits accurate computerised measurement of an aortic valve gradient using pressures taken during the same heartbeat (Figure 14.10b) and eliminates potential problems from using two central catheters. Simultaneous ventricular and aortic (or femoral, or brachial) pressures from the same heartbeat can be corrected for time lag (by aligning aortic end-diastole with the upstroke of left ventricular pressure, as in Figure 14.10c) to obtain a true measure of the mean gradient

across the valve, provided additional correction is also made for slight pressure differences that can exist between femoral artery and aorta. This intrinsic difference (i.e. either the mean difference between femoral and aortic pressure, or simply the average systolic difference between the two pressures) can be detected following pullback, when aortic and femoral pressures are superimposed (Figure 14.10d). If femoral systolic pressure were higher than aortic, the intrinsic difference should be added to the mean valve gradient (or subtracted

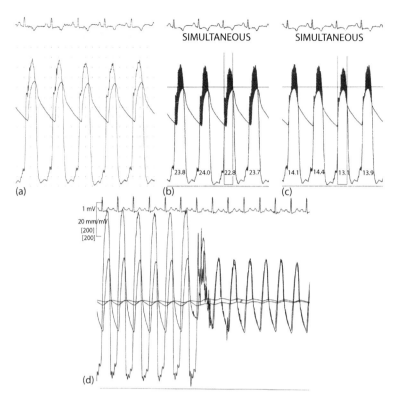

Figure 14.10 Simultaneous pressures from left ventricle and femoral artery from a patient with aortic stenosis. In **(a)** and **(b)**, the mean gradient across the valve is 23.2 mmHg. Figure **(c)**, which is corrected for the time lag between ventricle and femoral artery, shows that the actual mean gradient between left ventricle and femoral artery is 13.6 mmHg. In Figure **(d)**, left ventricular, aortic and femoral artery pressures recorded on pullback from left ventricle for another patient with aortic stenosis are shown. In this example aortic systole is 162 mmHg and femoral artery systole is 164 mmHg. As femoral systole is 2 mmHg higher than aortic systole, this intrinsic difference of 2 mmHg must be added to the mean aortic valve gradient (as measured between femoral artery and left ventricle). If femoral systole is less than aortic systole, then the intrinsic difference must be subtracted from the ventricular/femoral gradient. In this case the intrinsic difference is inconsequential but greater differences are commonly encountered. Scale is 0–200 mmHg.

if femoral pressure were lower than aortic). This procedure eliminates artefactual variations induced by superimposing measurements taken from separate heartbeats on pullback alone and is particularly helpful when the length of the cardiac cycle is variable, as in atrial fibrillation or with frequent premature beats.

Ultimately it is not the size of the gradient across the valve that determines prognosis and treatment of a stenotic valve but rather size of the opening across the valve, i.e. the valve area. Valve area is derived from the Gorlin formula, which depends on a number of variables such as heart rate, cardiac output and mean aortic valve gradient at the time of measurement. It follows that variations in any or all of these values will affect the derived value for aortic valve area. During right heart catheterisation, cardiac output is calculated prior to ventriculography, whereas the valve gradient is calculated by catheter pullback after ventriculography, when blood pressure, heart rate, peripheral vascular resistance and cardiac output can change unpredictably. Combining these variables indiscriminately in the Gorlin formula may yield unreliable results for aortic valve area.

Thus, simply by using an aortic valve gradient derived from the pressure difference between femoral artery and left ventricle, the cardiac output, valve gradient and heart rate can all be measured during the same steady state prior to ventriculography to yield accurate valve areas, within the limits of cardiac catheterisation.

The Gorlin formula for calculating aortic valve area is

$$A = \frac{CO/(SEP \times HR)}{VC \times \sqrt{G}} \qquad (14.1)$$

where CO = flow across the valve (cm³/min), SEP = mean systolic ejection period (sec/beat), HR = heart rate (bpm), VC = valve constant (44.3 for aortic valve) and G = mean valve gradient (mmHg). In practice, an abbreviation of this formula (A = CO (L/min)/√G) can be used to quickly calculate an approximate valve area, given the other variables cancel to a value of 1.0.

Right heart pressure recordings

For right heart catheterisation or combined left and right heart catheterisation, it is desirable to obtain baseline values by recording right atrium, right ventricle and pulmonary artery pressures

prior to ventriculography. The PAW pressure is taken by advancing the right heart catheter as far as possible until the catheter tip wedges firmly at the arterioles, effectively plugging flow and recording the reflected pressure from the left atrium. After the catheter is advanced to the wedge position, it is customary to record wedge pressure simultaneously with left ventricular EDP, usually on a magnified scale. Both transducers should be re-zeroed prior to this recording, ensuring both are at mid-chest level and set on the same gain. This is essential to accurately quantify possible mitral stenosis, as small errors in zeroing transducers or in catheter height may falsely indicate the presence of a significant mitral gradient.

Figure 14.11a and b illustrates a simultaneous tracing of pulmonary arterial wedge and left ventricular pressures for a patient with a normal mitral valve, where wedge pressure directly overlies ventricular diastolic pressure, indicating absence of mitral stenosis. PAW pressure is routinely measured as a substitute for left atrial pressure, introducing a time lag which as shown in Figure 14.12b is easily corrected by computer.

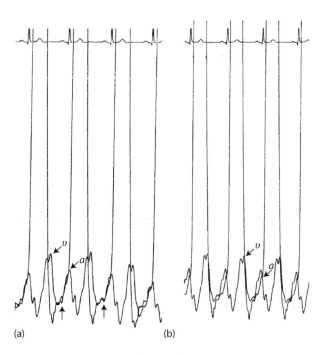

(a) (b)

Figure 14.11 Simultaneous pressure recordings from left ventricle and pulmonary wedge from a patient without mitral stenosis. Figure **(a)** is unedited. Note identical *a* wave values in both ventricle and pulmonary wedge, indicating absence of a mitral gradient. Note also the overlapping descent of the *v* wave in Figure **(b)** (which is corrected for time lag) with the downslope of the left ventricular waveform, and equilibration of both pressure traces during the period of mitral valve opening (vertical arrows).

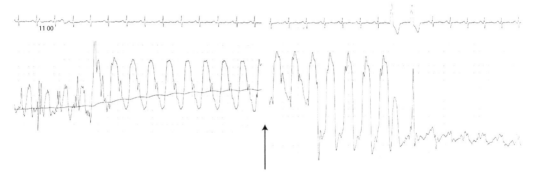

Figure 14.12 Typical pressure recording of right heart pressures from pulmonary wedge to pulmonary artery, then from pulmonary artery to right ventricle to right atrium. Note that mean wedge pressure cannot be higher than mean pulmonary artery pressure and is roughly the same as diastolic pulmonary artery pressure. Blood samples for Fick calculations can be collected from pulmonary artery and ventricle, then the right-side pullback is completed by withdrawing the catheter to right atrium.

A right heart pullback records the change in pressure from wedge position to pulmonary artery to right ventricle to right atrium (Figure 14.12). The right heart pullback can be interrupted to collect blood samples from left ventricle and pulmonary artery along with Douglas bag samples for calculations of cardiac output by the Fick method, or by thermodilution. It may be possible to calculate cardiac output for comparison by both methods. The Fick principle is considered more accurate, particularly for low output states, but only if correct procedures are followed (such as simultaneous collection of blood and respiratory gas samples). Convenience, ease of use and improved catheter design have resulted in a preference by many cardiologists for thermodilution over the Fick method to determine cardiac output. Thermodilution cardiac output measurements can also be repeated easily. Expected haemodynamic values for a resting adult are shown in Table 14.1.

The following are key features to note with right heart pressures:

1. Pulmonary arterial wedge pressure cannot be greater than pulmonary artery pressure.
2. Damping artefacts are commonly encountered. As a guide, mean wedge pressure is generally the same as diastolic pulmonary artery pressure.
3. For sinus rhythm, wedge pressure is biphasic, showing both *a* and *v* waves; for atrial fibrillation the *a* wave is technically absent.
4. Large *v* waves are expected with severe mitral insufficiency but are also seen with mitral stenosis or shunts.
5. As for aortic stenosis, pulmonary stenosis will show a systolic pressure gradient across the pulmonary valve on pullback.
6. Simultaneous tracings are not generally required for evaluating tricuspid stenosis. Elevated right atrial pressure relative to right ventricular EDP on pullback is sufficient.
7. Right heart pressures may be elevated in conditions such as primary or secondary pulmonary hypertension or pulmonary oedema.

Table 14.1 Expected haemodynamic values (mmHg) for a resting adult patient

	a	v	Mean	Systole	Diastole	Mean
RA	2–10	2–10	0–7			
RV				15–25	0–8	
PA				15–25	8–15	10–20
PAW	3–15	3–12	6–12			
LA	3–15	3–12	6–12			
LV				90–140	6–12	
AO				90–140	60–90	70–105

8. A fasting patient can be dehydrated and show falsely low right heart pressures, which may mask a pressure gradient characteristic of mitral stenosis; rehydration may be necessary.
9. Intravascular pressures cannot be negative. If so, transducers should be re-zeroed and reset at mid-chest level. Occasional overshoot may artefactually induce a negative pressure.
10. Movement of the catheter with each cardiac contraction or on pullback (catheter whip) may cause artefactual spikes or exaggerated waveforms to appear. There may be provision to compensate for this electronically by introducing low-frequency noise filters.

Pulmonary stenosis

Evaluation of pulmonary stenosis is similar to that for aortic stenosis. Absolute pressure values in the right ventricle or pulmonary artery are on a scale of approximately 20%–25% those in the left ventricle or aorta. A pulmonary valve gradient <20 mmHg is considered mild stenosis, while a pulmonary gradient >40 mmHg is considered severe. Systolic differences across a stenotic pulmonary valve are readily detected on right heart pullback, as for the aortic valve.

Mitral stenosis

The mitral valve is open during ventricular diastole, when ventricular pressure is low. Unlike systolic pressure gradients generated across the aortic valve, which can be much higher, pressure gradients across the mitral valve are very low and a simple pullback recording is inconclusive in diagnosing severity of mitral stenosis. To accurately measure mitral stenosis, left atrial and left ventricular pressure are simultaneously recorded to display the area bounded by the two curves. As with the mean aortic valve gradient, if cardiac output is known, a variation of the Gorlin formula is used to derive valve area.

The Gorlin formula for calculating mitral valve area is:

$$A = \frac{CO/(DFP \times HR)}{VC \times \sqrt{G}} \quad (14.2)$$

where CO = flow across the valve (cm³/min), DFP = mean diastolic filling period (sec/beat), HR = heart rate (bpm), VC = valve constant

(37.7 for mitral valve) and G = mean valve gradient (mmHg). As for the aortic valve, the abbreviation of this formula (A = CO (L/min)/√G) can be used to quickly calculate an approximate valve area.

Figure 14.13a and b show a simultaneous tracing of pulmonary artery wedge and left ventricular pressures for a patient with severe mitral stenosis, where wedge pressure is markedly elevated relative to left ventricular diastole. The area bounded by the two curves averages 19.9 mmHg in Figure 14.13a but reduces to 18.0 mmHg in Figure 14.13b when corrected for time lag. It is essential to measure ventricular and wedge pressures simultaneously as even small variations between different beats can introduce unacceptable errors. This is not a problem if left atrial pressure is measured directly by transseptal puncture. Individual beat variations are not as critical when dealing with the large values that can occur with aortic gradients. A mean gradient of 10 mmHg across a mitral valve is

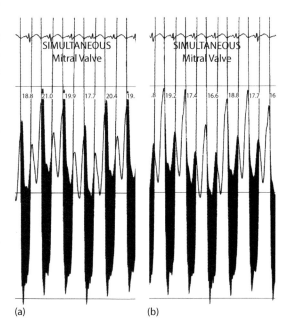

(a)   (b)

Figure 14.13 Left ventricle and pulmonary wedge pressures from a patient with mitral stenosis. Left atrial pressure is elevated relative to left ventricular diastolic pressure, causing a pressure gradient across the mitral valve, evident as the shaded area between the two waveforms. Figure (a) with a mean gradient of 19.9 mmHg is unedited, Figure (b) with a mean gradient of 18.0 mmHg is corrected for time lag by shifting the wedge trace to the left, so that the downstroke of the v wave overlies the downstroke of the ventricular trace.

considered to be moderate, whereas a mean gradient of 40 mmHg or a systolic gradient of 60 mmHg or more is severe across an aortic valve.

Tricuspid stenosis

This is relatively uncommon but is routinely checked with every right heart pullback. If required, a computer-generated overlay ('splice') of right atrial and ventricular pressures can be produced on a magnified scale for evaluation, using traces from separate heartbeats. Generally, however, tricuspid gradients are readily detected and quantifying their exact size is considered unnecessary (Figure 14.14).

Rhythmic pressure fluctuations

Inhalation and exhalation have a secondary effect on blood pressure. Negative intrathoracic pressure draws air into the lungs, increasing venous blood return to the right heart. There is also pooling of blood in the lungs and a corresponding fall in pulmonary artery pressure, with decreased pulmonary venous return to the left atrium, which in turn decreases left ventricular filling, thereby decreasing cardiac output and also lowering central arterial blood pressure. A positive intrathoracic pressure during exhalation causes a corresponding rise in pulmonary artery pressure that results in increased left ventricular filling with an increased cardiac output and an increase in systemic arterial volume and pressure. Thus, the relative systolic values of the PA and systemic arterial pressure parallel each other. These cyclic fluctuations in pressure waveforms can be reduced by asking patients to gently stop breathing mid-breath.

Other forms of cyclic pressure variations may occur. These are under control of the vasomotor centre of the medulla oblongata in the midbrain and are caused primarily by sympathetic neural regulation of vessel tone, resulting in arterial vasoconstriction and vasodilatation. The vasomotor centre may induce slow rhythmic changes in arterial tone, evident as cyclic arterial pressure fluctuations that occur at the same frequency as respiration (Traube-Hering waves), or independently of respiration and at a slower rate (Mayer waves).

Valve insufficiency

Unlike stenotic valves, an incompetent or leaking valve does not induce pressure gradients across adjacent chambers, although artefactual flow-related gradients can occur, and characteristic changes in pressure waveforms can be identified. Whether in the right or left heart, valvular insufficiency can generate volume and pressure overload in the corresponding ventricle, resulting in associated pathologies involving ventricular distension,

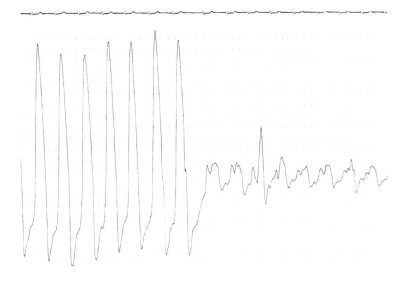

Figure 14.14 Pressure difference between right ventricular end-diastole and right atrium in a patient with tricuspid stenosis. Note elevation of right atrial pressure in this condition, clearly evident during simple catheter pullback. The exact value of the tricuspid gradient can be quantified by electronically overlapping right ventricular and atrial pressures (as in Figure 8–13b for mitral stenosis).

hypertrophy, and hypertension. Initial diagnosis of valve insufficiency relies primarily on a clinical evaluation with auscultation, angiography and echocardiography rather than on pressure readings alone. Colour Doppler echocardiography can quantify valve incompetence by measuring factors such as regurgitant flow and regurgitant fraction.

Interpretation of data

Correct diagnosis by cardiac catheterisation depends largely on accuracy of measuring instruments. Care must be taken to ensure accurate and regular calibration and maintenance of equipment by a reliable operator, as well as maintaining satisfactory laboratory standards. As with other diseases cardiac disorders are evaluated from a variety of tests, of which cardiac catheterisation is only one. Disputes can arise from artefacts which, despite high standards of practice, can cause unexpected errors to occur. With invasive cardiology, accurate interpretation of data relies as much on clinical assessment as on electronic data collection and interpretation.

FURTHER READING

Kern MJ, Sorajja P, Lim MJ. *The Cardiac Catheterization Handbook.* 6th ed. Philadelphia, PA: Elsevier; 2016. p. 492.

Klabunde R. *Cardiovascular Physiology Concepts.* 2nd ed. Philadelphia, PA: Lippincott Williams & Wilkins; 2011. p. 256.

Kovacs G, Avian A, Olchewski A, Olchewski H. Zero tolerance level for right heart catheterisation. *Eur Resp J.* 2013:42;1586–1594.

Levy MN, Pappano AJ, Berne RM. *Cardiovascular Physiology.* 9th ed. Philadelphia, PA: Mosby Elsevier; 2007. p.269.

Moscucci M, Grossman W. Blood flow measurement: Cardiac output and vascular resistance. In: Moscucci M, editor. *Grossman & Baim's Cardiac Catheterization, Angiography, and Intervention.* 8th ed. Philadelphia, PA: Wolters Kluwer/Lippincott Williams & Wilkins; 2014. pp. 245–260.

Ragosta M. *Textbook of Clinical Hemodynamics.* 2nd ed. Philadelphia, PA: Saunders Elsevier; 2008. p. 249.

15

Physiological interpretation of pressure waveforms

GEOFFREY S. OLDFIELD

INTRODUCTION

Interpretation of pressure waveforms involves careful and continued calibration of pressure transducers, physiological reporting devices and cardiac output modules. There may also be times when the accuracy of automatic equipment needs to be checked with manual methods. When interpreting data, consideration must be given to heart rate, cardiac rhythm, pressure scale, recording speed, the waveform of normal physiology related to the cardiac chamber being examined, the disease state under investigation, and the differential diagnosis. This chapter deals with the most common conditions likely to be encountered:

1. Pulsus alternans
2. Ventricular ectopy
3. Stenotic lesions:
   - Aortic stenosis
   - Mitral stenosis
   - Pulmonary stenosis
   - Tricuspid stenosis
   - Intra-ventricular pressure gradients

4. Regurgitant lesions:
   - Aortic
   - Mitral
   - Tricuspid
5. Left ventricular end diastolic pressure (LVEDP)
6. Pulmonary artery wedge (PAW) pressure, pulmonary capillary wedge (PCW) pressure and their relationship to pulmonary vein and left atrial (LA) pressures
7. Constrictive pericarditis, restrictive cardiomyopathy, cardiac tamponade
8. Nitrates

PULSUS ALTERNANS

This describes alternating strong and weak heart beats. Every second pulse is reduced in amplitude (Figure 15.1). It is recorded in aortic and left ventricular (LV) pressure tracings and indicates severe myocardial impairment from left ventricular damage. It may be seen in dilated cardiomyopathy, ventricular failure from systemic hypertension, ischaemic heart disease and aortic stenosis. When the alteration in pressure is greater than 20 mmHg it can be detected by palpation in the large arteries. Beats with the lower pressure wave have a lower pulse pressure and slower upstroke in the aortic tracing, whilst in the LV

tracing there is a delayed early relaxation phase. In patients with pulsus alternans in the LV trace there is usually no change in PAW pressure or in pulmonary artery (PA) pressure, although pulsus alternans may be seen simultaneously or independently in the right ventricular and PA traces.[1] If mitral regurgitation is present, alternating large v waves may be seen in the PAW trace, the large v wave corresponding to the higher aortic pressure.

The underlying mechanism for pulsus alternans was originally considered to be related to changes in contractility from inflow pressures, LVEDP and left ventricular volume (Frank Starling curves),[2] but is now believed to result from localised or patchy electromechanical dissociation in the myocytes resulting from variation in calcium movement in the sarcoplasmic reticulum of the myocytes.[3] The changes in traces associated with pulsus alternans may be augmented in aortic regurgitation or following administration of nitroglycerine, which decreases venous return.

Heart rate plays a role in determining the significance of pulsus alternans in heart failure. At heart rates of 50 bpm, it is an indicator of significant failure but if a tachycardia exists (>100 bpm) its significance decreases as heart rate increases. When not obvious, pulsus alternans may become prominent following an ectopic beat.[1,4]

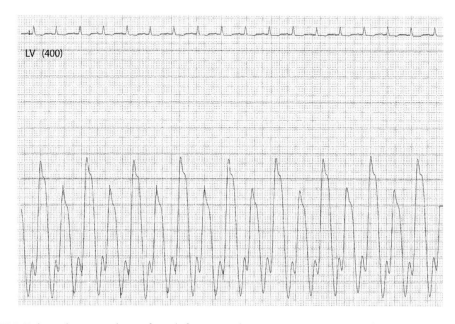

Figure 15.1 Pulsus alternans shown for a left ventricular pressure trace. Note the regular sequence of alternating strong and weak beats.

VENTRICULAR ECTOPY

In the normal heart, a ventricular ectopic beat shows a sharp fall in systolic pressure in the left ventricle and aorta, has a shortened diastolic filling period, and results in a prolonged diastolic filling period for the post ectopic beat. The post-ectopic beat itself has a slower dP/dt, as a result of reduced peripheral resistance and afterload that follow the prolonged diastolic post-ectopic period. In the absence of cardiac or peripheral vascular disease, this may also result in a reduction in LV systolic and aortic pressure during the post-ectopic contraction, in spite of a greater LV volume and force of myocardial contraction. In aortic stenosis or in the damaged heart with left ventricular failure, systolic pressure and dP/dt are enhanced or accentuated following an ectopic beat. This is due to an elevated afterload caused by high peripheral vascular resistance that prevents aortic run off, and increased inotropism from the post ectopic pause. Similarly, in valvular aortic stenosis, left ventricular pressure, aortic pressure, the aortic valve gradient and pulse pressure are all elevated following an ectopic beat.

With hypertrophic obstructive cardiomyopathy (HOCM), aortic pressure falls following a ventricular ectopic beat. This is the Brockenbrough effect (Figure 15.2). To assist with diagnosis, pressures may need to be recorded with an ectopic during the valsalva manoeuvre, which increases the LVEDP and potentiates the appearance of the Brockenbrough effect.[5] This occurs because the increased inotropic effect of the augmented LV filling is offset by an increase in LV outflow tract gradient. Thus, intraventricular pressures rise markedly but aortic pressure falls.

STENOTIC LESIONS

Aortic stenosis

This is one of the most common valve abnormalities requiring haemodynamic study in the adult in the western world. The most frequent cause is degenerative calcific aortic stenosis (AS) of a trileaflet valve. Bicuspid valves are occasionally seen uncalcified in young adults, while calcific bicuspid valves are seen from middle age onwards. There are a number of ways to evaluate the severity of AS with modern physiological recording equipment.

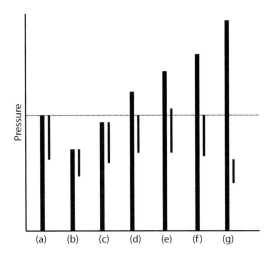

Figure 15.2 Examples of left ventricular and aortic pressure changes with ventricular ectopy. Heavy line represents ventricular pressure; thin line aortic pressure. (a) Normal sinus beat. (b) Ventricular ectopic beat. (c) Post-ectopic beat. (d) Sinus beat with aortic stenosis. (e) Post-ectopic beat with aortic stenosis. In valvular or membranous sub-valvular aortic stenosis, a post-ectopic beat shows potentiation of left ventricular and aortic pressures, with an increased gradient and increased aortic pulse pressure. (f) Sinus beat with hypertrophic obstructive cardiomyopathy (HOCM). (g) Post-ectopic beat with HOCM, showing ventricular potentiation and elevated pressure gradient. The dotted line represents an arbitrary normal systolic value.

1. Pullback from left ventricle to aorta: A pigtail or multi-purpose catheter is introduced into the left ventricle and withdrawn to the aortic root while recording pressures continuously. Traditionally ten consecutive left ventricular and aortic pressure traces are recorded. Manual or electronic superimposition of pressure traces is performed to calculate the gradient across the valve. The 'peak to peak' gradient measured by this and other techniques approximates the mean stenotic valve gradient.

   This technique should not be used in atrial fibrillation or if frequent ectopics are present, as waveforms with similar R-R intervals are required for manual calculation.

2. Simultaneous recording of LV and aortic pressures; this can be performed:

a. With a single femoral puncture using a double lumen catheter in which the distal lumen (with end and side holes) measures LV pressure and the proximal lumen (side holes) measures aortic pressure.

b. By using a Brockenbrough catheter to cross the inter-atrial septum and advancing into the left ventricle to measure pressure whilst simultaneously recording aortic pressure with a pigtail catheter.

c. Using two femoral punctures and two catheters, one in the LV, the other remaining in the aortic root (Figure 15.3a).

d. With a single femoral puncture, using a large sheath (e.g. a 6F pigtail catheter with a 7F sheath). The catheter is introduced into the left ventricle and the femoral/iliac arterial tracing recorded via a side port. This technique is not as accurate as with the preceding methods but is used in some laboratories. In pressure waveforms (LV and arterial) visualised with this technique, there is a time delay of some 40 msec in the upstroke of the aortic/iliac pressure trace compared with the LV trace (Figure 15.3b). Realignment can be performed electronically by some physiological recording equipment, but it has

been shown by Folland et al.[6] that only a slight (9 mmHg) over-estimation of aortic valve gradient is made if realignment is not performed.

If pressure traces are realigned an under-estimation of aortic valve gradient is made, as the iliac/femoral pulse wave has a slightly higher pressure (8–10 mmHg) and dP/dt of the upstroke than the central aortic root, caused by reflection of waveforms from the periphery. Whenever this technique is used a 'pullback' recording as described above should be performed following left ventricular interrogation. If a left ventriculogram is performed the catheter should be flushed carefully and the operator should wait a few minutes after the left ventriculogram for the haemodynamic effect of the contrast agent to wear off. The need for 'pullback' recording is to correlate the two techniques. Normally, femoral artery systolic pressure is greater than that of the aorta. Many elderly patients have co-existent peripheral vascular disease that dampens the iliac/femoral waveform, exaggerating the gradient between left ventricle and the femoral artery. Comparison with the pullback gradient makes this evident. Presence of coexistent aortic regurgitation precludes use of this technique, as it causes amplification of the peripheral pulses with

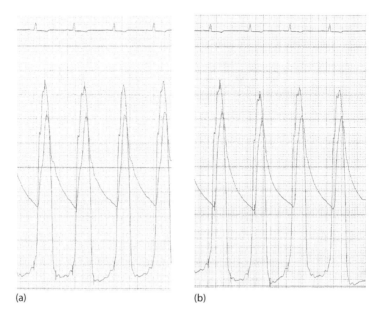

(a)   (b)

Figure 15.3 Simultaneous pressure traces in left ventricle and central aorta (a), and left ventricle and distal aorta (b) in a patient with aortic stenosis. The time lag of the distal aortic trace relative to the left ventricular trace is clearly evident in (b).

increased systolic pressure and increased pulse pressure, thus falsifying the gradient.

The abovementioned techniques essentially provide either a peak-to-peak gradient (Figure 15.4a) or a mean aortic valve gradient (Figure 15.4b). A third value, the instantaneous gradient, is measured by echocardiography (Figure 15.4c). As indicated, the peak of the aortic pressure trace is delayed with respect to the peak of the left ventricle (the slow rise in dP/dt in the aortic trace is due to outflow obstruction caused by aortic stenosis. It is this delay between the Ao and LV peaks that generates the difference between the peak-to-peak and instantaneous gradients.

The upstroke of the aortic pressure waveform varies between patients with normal valves and those with significant aortic stenosis. The anacrotic notch is a notch on the upstroke of the arterial pulse, indicating severe AS. As the severity of aortic stenosis increases, the anacrotic notch appears earlier on the upstroke of the aortic trace and the upstroke (dP/dt) in general slows. The anacrotic notch represents the point of maximal stroke volume and

maximal peak flow velocity. At the end of this point 80% of the blood has been ejected from the left ventricle. If aortic pressure is recorded peripherally, the anacrotic notch will be lower on the upstroke of the waveform than if recorded centrally.

Changes evident with aortic stenosis in the LV waveform are increased LVEDP and a prominent a wave. The former is related to the Frank Starling principle initially but may, in severe aortic stenosis, reflect LV failure. The force of atrial contraction is increased due to increase in LV work resulting from an increased LV mass, LV systolic pressure and prolonged systolic ejection period. The increased atrial a wave is often best seen in the LA or PAW traces and protects against pulmonary congestion in the face of increased ventricular compliance and failure. The peak of the left ventricular trace becomes rounded rather than flattened.

VARIANTS OF AORTIC STENOSIS

Aortic stenosis may be evident as valvular, subvalvular or supravalvular stenosis. If subvalvular, it

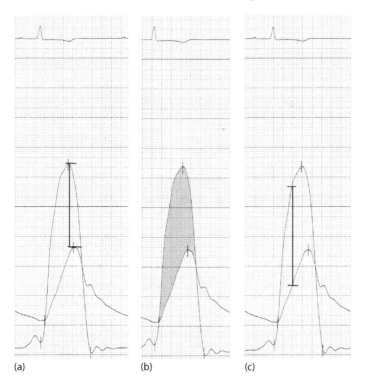

(a) (b) (c)

Figure 15.4 Simultaneous pressure traces of left ventricle and central aorta showing the three common methods for quantifying aortic stenosis. The peak-to-peak gradient (a) is measured by cardiac catheterisation. The mean aortic gradient (b) is calculated as the area between the two curves. The instantaneous gradient (c) is the value measured by echocardiography. The instantaneous gradient is greater than the peak-to-peak gradient, and both approximate the mean gradient.

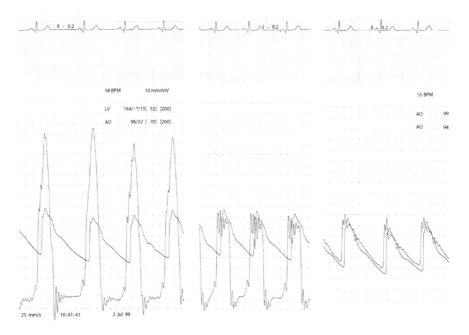

Figure 15.5 Simultaneous pressure traces of left ventricle and aorta, showing the presence of an intraventricular gradient during a continuous pullback recording from the ventricular apex to the aortic arch.

may be classified as membranous AS or as HOCM. Unlike the situation with the first two variants, simultaneous left ventricular and aortic traces do not diagnose subvalvular aortic stenosis. A pullback tracing from the LV apex to the arch of the aorta is required for this, as well as for detecting intraventricular gradients (Figure 15.5).

An ectopic can usually differentiate intraventricular gradients, including distinguishing HOCM from membranous subvalvular AS (Figure 15.6). The intraventricular gradient (HOCM) shows the distinctive Brockenbrough effect while subvalvular membranous AS shows the same haemodynamics as valvular AS.

With intracavity (or intraventricular) gradients occurring lower in the ventricle, the LV pressure waveform may have a 'bitten off' appearance that is due to catheter entrapment. Operators should be alert to this possibility.

At times other techniques such as a Valsalva manoeuvre or administration of nitroglycerine may be required for differentiation of the types of subvalvular aortic stenosis. In supravalvular aortic stenosis a slow withdrawal to the aortic arch using an end-hole catheter identifies the gradient as being above the valve. Techniques described above for AS can be used to obtain simultaneous recordings as required.

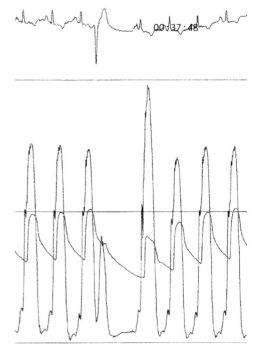

Figure 15.6 Simultaneous traces of pressure in left ventricle and femoral artery for a patient with hypertrophic obstructive cardiomyopathy (HOCM) showing accentuation of the pressure gradient on a post-ectopic beat (the Brockenbrough effect).

Note the Gorlin Formula for aortic stenosis[7] (see also Chapter 14):

$$AVA = \frac{CO /(SEP \times HR)}{44.3 \times \sqrt{AVG}} \quad (15.1)$$

where AVA = aortic valve area, CO = cardiac output (i.e. flow across the valve), SEP = systolic ejection period, AVG = aortic valve gradient, HR = heart rate. When cardiac output is calculated at the same time that pressure gradients are measured, aortic valve area can be calculated with this formula, an automatic process with modern physiological monitoring systems. If significant regurgitation is present with a leaking valve, valve area calculations are not valid, as CO is not equal to flow across the valve.

MITRAL STENOSIS

This is normally due to rheumatic fever although it may occasionally be due to degenerative calcific disease in some elderly patients. The hallmark pressure waveform finding of mitral stenosis occurs with the simultaneous recording of LVEDP and either LA or PAW pressure at the same gain setting (usually a scale of 0–40 mmHg) (Figure 15.7). In the normal patient the LV diastolic pressure and PAW/LA diastolic pressures overlap, but with mitral stenosis left atrial pressure is greater than LV diastolic pressure. The left atrial pressure waveform may be obtained directly by transeptal puncture using the Brockenbrough catheter. If recording LA and LVEDP simultaneously (via atrial septal puncture), the pressure traces should overlap exactly. Any variation in the 'a' wave pressure, even during early diastole, indicates some degree of stenosis. Note that when using PAW pressure and LVEDP these traces do not overlap in early diastole, even in the normal patient.

Many patients with mitral disease are in atrial fibrillation and the a wave is not present on LVEDP, PAW or LA recordings. When the patient with mitral stenosis remains in sinus rhythm there is a gradient between the a wave of the LV diastole and PAW or LA pressure. Thus, presence of an a wave gradient

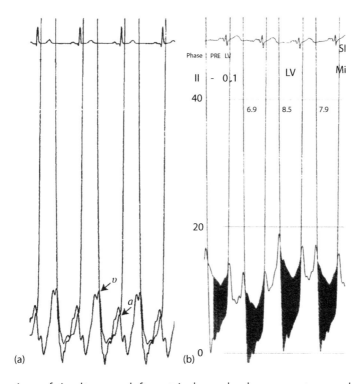

Figure 15.7 Comparison of simultaneous left ventricular and pulmonary artery wedge pressure (PAWP) for a patient with a normal mitral valve (a), and for one with a stenosed mitral valve (b). Note diastolic equalisation of pressures in (a) and elevation of PAWP pressure in (b). Shaded area represents diastolic pressure difference between the two curves, referred to as the mitral gradient.

(or if in atrial fibrillation an end diastolic gradient) is the haemodynamic hallmark of mitral stenosis.

The haemodynamics of mitral stenosis may be mimicked by those of an atrial myxoma, a benign atrial tumour arising from the left atrial wall. The tumour may encroach on the mitral valve and cause obstruction to left ventricular inflow. At times, it is difficult to differentiate atrial myxoma from mitral stenosis if not clinically suspected. However, differences occur in the pulmonary artery wedge pressure, where mitral stenosis has a slow y descent and atrial myxoma a normal y descent. Also of note is that in left atrial pressure tracings, both a and v waves in mitral stenosis are increased but the x wave is slow (decreased dP/dt).

Most patients with mitral stenosis present with dyspnoea on effort and these patients have elevated PAW pressures and, more importantly, elevated pulmonary capillary pressure which causes the symptoms. Pulmonary artery pressures are often only mildly elevated (passive pulmonary hypertension). At times these symptoms are replaced by listlessness and fatigue. Haemodynamically the latter patients have much higher PA pressures, higher pulmonary vein resistance and slightly higher PAW and LA pressures, with a much lower cardiac output. Such patients develop what Grossman refers to as 'second stenosis' from pulmonary vascular disease affecting distal arterioles and the capillary bed (active pulmonary hypertension).[8] The cause of these reactive changes is uncertain. The latter group shows clinically and on the electrocardiogram (ECG) the signs of pulmonary hypertension and right ventricular pressure overload. When the active pulmonary hypertension becomes severe, prognosis is worsened.

Note the Gorlin formula for mitral stenosis:

$$MVA = \frac{CO(DFP \times HR)}{37.7 \times \sqrt{MVG}} \qquad (15.2)$$

where MVA = mitral valve area, CO = cardiac output (i.e. flow across the valve), DFP = diastolic filling period, MVG = mitral valve gradient, HR = heart rate. As for aortic valve area, this calculation is automatically derived by modern physiological monitoring systems.

PULMONARY STENOSIS

Pulmonary stenosis in its various forms is the most common congenital anomaly in cardiology. A mean gradient between right ventricle (RV)

and PA of >5 mmHg is required to make such a diagnosis and is easily confirmed by catheter pullback. Calculation of valve area is made using the equivalent Gorlin formula for aortic stenosis. In the presence of left to right shunts, pulmonary stenosis is frequently present. A simplification of the Gorlin formula can be used to estimate the size of the gradient across the valve after correction of the shunt and determine the need for treatment of the valve stenosis. Using the abbreviated formula:

$$PVA = \frac{CO}{\sqrt{PVG}} \qquad (15.3)$$

where PVA = pulmonary valve area, PVG = pulmonary valve gradient, CO = cardiac output (i.e. flow across the valve). For example, for a given pulmonary valve area, if there is a 2:1 shunt, when the shunt is closed, flow across the pulmonary valve is halved, and the $\sqrt{PVG}$ is also halved. If the PVG is 80 mmHg, then $\sqrt{80} = 9$. So, if halving the shunt halves the pulmonary flow and the $\sqrt{PVG}$, then halving 9 gives 4.5, therefore the new mean gradient = $4.5^2 = 20$ mmHg. Thus, after closure of the shunt, the new mean PVG = 20 mmHg and intervention on the valve is not required. This simple calculation works well and provides a quick means of assessing the severity of pulmonary stenosis following shunt correction.

TRICUSPID STENOSIS

This complication is nearly always rheumatic but may rarely be seen in carcinoid tumour (although tricuspid incompetence is more frequent), tricuspid atresia in congenital heart disease and right atrial (RA) tumours and myxomas. It also results increasingly from stenosis of bioprosthetic valves implanted for prior tricuspid regurgitation. When due to rheumatic heart disease it is always associated with rheumatic mitral valve disease and often with rheumatic aortic valve disease.

The hallmark finding of tricuspid stenosis is a diastolic gradient across the tricuspid valve associated with a large a wave in the RA pressure trace when in sinus rhythm that is at times almost as high as the right ventricular (RV) systolic pressure, and a slow y descent on the RA pressure trace. However most of these patients are in atrial fibrillation at the time of catheterisation, so RA and RV traces both lack an a wave. As in mitral stenosis (see Figure 15.7), there is an end diastolic gradient, with the RA pressure trace well above that of end diastole on the RV trace. Systemic venous congestion (liver, gut, lower limbs) occurs early in tricuspid stenosis, with gradients as low as 5 mmHg, and cardiac output is substantially reduced at rest with little or no rise with exercise.

Exhalation reduces and may even abolish the gradient and so exercise, infusion of normal saline, deep inspiration or even atropine may be required to demonstrate the gradient. Adequate demonstration requires two catheters, one in the RA and the other in the RV or else a double lumen catheter. To calculate stenotic valve area the Gorlin and Gorlin formula is used as for mitral stenosis.

REGURGITANT LESIONS

Aortic regurgitation

This is leakage of blood from the ascending aorta into the LV during diastole and is usually progressive and chronic although at times may be sudden or acute. Forward blood flow is reduced by an amount equivalent to the regurgitant fraction. The degree or amount of regurgitation depends upon:

1. Size of the valve opening
2. Diastolic duration (filling period)
3. Diastolic aortic pressure

Initially, when mild, aortic regurgitation occurs in early diastole but as it becomes more severe the regurgitation progresses throughout diastole. LV filling in this instance is due to a combination of normal blood flow across the mitral valve and blood leaking from the aortic root (regurgitant fraction). Stroke volume, or flow across the aortic valve per heartbeat, is therefore not equivalent to the forward cardiac output (normal cardiac output = heart rate × stroke volume; cardiac output with aortic regurgitation = heart rate × stroke volume minus regurgitant fraction). Cardiac output with aortic regurgitation is thus a measure of effective systemic flow (i.e. forward flow minus regurgitant flow). Without aortic regurgitation, cardiac output is the same as forward flow, whether measured by Fick or thermodilution. It is not possible by cardiac catheterisation to quantify the regurgitant component.

Significant aortic regurgitation is said to exist when the leaking valve area is ≥ 0.5 cm^2.[8] It is associated with increased systolic LV pressure from increased stroke volume and low diastolic pressure in the aortic root (from regurgitation) giving a widened pulse pressure. When the heart starts to fail, the ejection fraction begins to fall and the left ventricular end diastolic and end systolic volumes rise. On echocardiography this is indicated by an increased LV internal diameter in systole of >5.4 cm. In severe chronic aortic regurgitation, the excessive regurgitant fraction leads to partial closure of the mitral valve (restriction of inflow orifice) owing to LV pressure exceeding LA pressure in mid diastole.[9] This may be seen on echocardiography and may cause a mitral diastolic murmur (Austin Flint murmur) even in the absence of mitral valve disease.

Acute versus chronic regurgitation

In acute aortic regurgitation, the ventricle is usually of normal or only slightly increased dimensions and systolic pressure and pulse pressure tend to be in the normal range. If severe, the LVEDP rises rapidly, causing a greater increase in left atrial pressure than occurs for a similar degree of chronic regurgitation. In chronic aortic regurgitation, simultaneous pressure recordings of LV and iliac via a femoral sheath show a much higher systolic pressure in the peripheral arterial trace than in the central aortic root pressure; this is further exaggerated in acute aortic regurgitation.

Presence of an atrial a wave in the aortic pressure trace in diastole has high specificity for acute aortic regurgitation.[10]

Mitral regurgitation

Mitral regurgitation is failure of the mitral valve to prevent retrograde blood flow from the LV to the LA during systole and may be acute or chronic. The mitral valve consists of a large anterior and smaller posterior leaflet and its integrity depends upon the mitral valve annulus, the *chordae tendinae* and the two papillary muscles. The commonest cause of chronic mitral regurgitation is rheumatic heart disease in underdeveloped or third world countries, whereas mitral valve prolapse and myocardial ischaemia are more frequent in the western world. Dilated cardiomyopathy is frequently associated with chronic mitral regurgitation and it is often difficult at presentation to determine whether the problem is mitral regurgitation leading to left ventricular failure, or cardiomyopathy with mitral regurgitation.

Acute mitral regurgitation occurs in infective endocarditis, acute myocardial ischaemia (often causing acute pulmonary oedema), flail mitral leaflets and rupture of *chordae tendinae* or papillary muscle (ischaemic). Some 'acute' causes may be considered to be more 'acute-on-chronic', e.g. a long-standing history of mild mitral valve prolapse with new-onset rupture of *chordae* or flail leaflet, or recurrent endocarditis.

One of the differentiating features of acute versus chronic mitral regurgitation is the chamber size, especially that of the LA. In acute mitral regurgitation, left atrial size is usually normal echocardiographically, as is the LV, although in the aging western population both left ventricular and left atrial size is influenced by other factors (e.g. hypertension) and may be slightly enlarged.

In chronic mitral regurgitation the left ventricle ejects blood antegradely into the high-pressure systemic circulation and retrogradely into the low pressure left atrium and pulmonary veins. The major determinant of regurgitation is the effective orifice size.

The hallmark pressure trace of mitral regurgitation is an increased v wave in the PAW pressure or LA trace which reflects LA filling in systole and early LA emptying (y descent) in early diastole. Grossman and others[8,11,12] suggest the v wave may be increased in any cause of LV failure, as the v wave reflects the pressure-volume relationship of the left atrium. Thus in chronic mitral regurgitation the atrium expands and the v wave increases only slightly over a long period, whereas in acute mitral regurgitation the v wave is much higher for the same degree of mitral regurgitation and the patient is more symptomatic. Other conditions that can affect this pressure-volume relationship are those that affect LA volume (large left to right shunt) and compliance (ischaemic or rheumatic fibrosis, infiltrative disease [amyloid, sarcoid, haemochromatosis]). Thus the factors affecting the v wave are:

1. The volume of blood entering the left atrium during ventricular systole from the pulmonary bed and that regurgitating from the left ventricle and the rate of filling
2. Left ventricular contraction
3. Systemic vascular resistance
4. Extra-cardiac compression
5. Cardiac rhythm

A v wave of at least twice the mean LA or PAW pressure indicates severe mitral regurgitation and if greater than three times the left atrial mean pressure then severe mitral regurgitation is almost certainly present.[8] As chronic mitral regurgitation progresses and regurgitant volume increases, the LA and left atrial appendage dilate, as does the LV. As the LV simultaneously empties into both aortic root and LA, factors which affect systemic vascular resistance either worsen or alleviate the regurgitant volume. This is the reason for use of vasodilatory agents (nitrates) and ACE inhibitors in providing symptomatic relief to patients with chronic mitral regurgitation.

In severe mitral regurgitation, or in acute or acute-on-chronic mitral regurgitation, the v wave may be seen in the PA pressure trace due to transmission through the pulmonary vascular bed, but owing to a delay in transmission, is seen in the descending limb of the PA pressure (Figure 15.8); severe mitral regurgitation with failing LV systolic

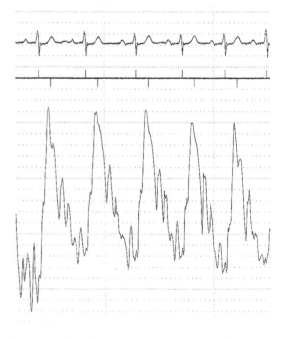

Figure 15.8 Pulmonary artery (PA) trace from a patient with severe mitral regurgitation, showing retrograde transmission of v waves (arrows) to the PA pressure trace.

functions may at times have a normal v wave due to the capacitance of the LA and decreased LV systolic pressure (LV pressure-volume loop).

As mentioned above, at presentation of a patient in cardiac failure with significant mitral regurgitation, it is at times difficult to determine whether the patient has severe mitral regurgitation and a failing left ventricle, or a dilated cardiomyopathy with moderate to severe mitral regurgitation due to stretching of the mitral valve annulus and chordae tendinae. Generally, if the cv wave is greater than 50 mmHg it relates to valvular pathology and the height of the v wave does not always correspond to the severity of mitral regurgitation. It may relate more to acuteness (see above). Others consider that if a separate c wave is present in the PAW tracing then incompetence is not severe.

Tricuspid regurgitation

Most commonly tricuspid regurgitation is due to right ventricular and tricuspid annular dilatation, often referred to as functional tricuspid regurgitation. Functional tricuspid regurgitation is due to pulmonary hypertension of any cause, most frequently mitral valve disease or severe left ventricular failure due to hypertensive heart disease, cardiomyopathy or chronic obstructive airways disease. Other causes include pulmonary stenosis and primary pulmonary hypertension.

Tricuspid regurgitation from valvular disease is most commonly seen in infective endocarditis, right ventricular infarction, tricuspid valve prolapse, rheumatic heart disease, trauma, Ebstein's anomaly and rarely carcinoid syndrome.

THE CV WAVE

No matter what the aetiology, regurgitation is associated with a large systolic wave in the right atrial pressure tracing. The systolic wave is best referred to as a cv wave as its timing precedes the onset of the usual v wave, although it has also been referred to as the S wave. In severe tricuspid regurgitation the S wave mirrors the RV pressure tracing. Grossman[8] considers that if RV systolic pressure is >60 mmHg then tricuspid regurgitation is functional, whereas if it is <40 mmHg, it is organic. Organic tricuspid regurgitation requires surgical intervention whereas functional tricuspid regurgitation may improve with medical treatment.

Pulmonary incompetence

Whereas pulmonary stenosis is always organic and mostly congenital, pulmonary incompetence is mostly functional due to high pulmonary artery pressures. Doppler echocardiography frequently shows physiological pulmonary regurgitation in 'normal' populations. However once PA pressure rises to >70 mmHg from any cause, pulmonary regurgitation becomes evident clinically (e.g. chronic obstructive airways disease, mitral valve disease, cardiomyopathy, primary pulmonary hypertension). Organic pulmonary regurgitation is most commonly seen in infective endocarditis, idiopathic pulmonary artery dilatation and rarely in carcinoid disease, where plaque formation leads to fibrosis and constriction of the valve and valve annulus.

LEFT VENTRICULAR END DIASTOLIC PRESSURE (LVEDP)

The diastolic filling period commences when the mitral valve opens and continues until the end of diastole when the mitral valve closes (see Figure 15.7). Note the following:

1. Early ventricular relaxation and dilatation causing low pressures
2. Rapid inflow through the mitral valve followed by
   - Slower mitral inflow
   - Left atrial contraction

Various disease processes affect the left ventricular diastolic wave pattern and LVEDP. The EDP is a relationship between pressure inflow across the mitral (and at times aortic) valve and the distensibility and compliance of the left ventricle itself. Distensibility and compliance are not the same thing. Distensibility (i.e. filling capacity) relates to the upward/downward movement (the systolic component) of the LV pressure volume curve where the slope remains unchanged, as can happen in angina pectoris and in treatment with nitroglycerine. Compliance (i.e. stiffness) involves the shape and slope of the LV pressure volume curve, so in these two conditions the slope remains the same but in angina the entire curve is displaced upwards, whereas with nitroglycerine it is displaced downwards.

Factors affecting LV distensibility

1. Intrinsic myocardial left ventricular problems such as:
   a. LV hypertrophy – includes myocyte hypertrophy and increased fibrosis
   b. Abnormal left ventricular wall structure with infiltration (amyloid, sarcoid, haemochromatosis, fibrosis ischaemia/infarct)
   c. Drug effects (hypercalcaemia, betablockers, calcium antagonists)
2. Extramyocardial problems such as: constrictive pericarditis, cardiac tamponade, external compression [tumour, pneumothorax, chronic lung disease (emphysema)], drug effects (e.g. nitroglycerine), right atrial pacing
3. Interaction of ventricles
   a. RV pressure overload (primary pulmonary hypertension)
   b. RV volume overload (large left to right shunt)

Effects of supine exercise

In normal patients there is little or no rise in LVEDP with exercise, and stroke work index rises. In the abnormal ventricle, even if LVEDP is 'normal' at onset of exercise, LVEDP will rise with exercise. The effect on stroke work index is variable and may fall or rise, while PA and PAWP increase with exercise. Pulmonary vascular resistance falls in the absence of cardiovascular disease and rises in the abnormal patient.[14]

Effects of right atrial pacing

This technique has been used in many laboratories as a diagnostic aid in coronary artery disease and valvular disease to assess the need for intervention. There are two techniques:

1. Fixed-rate pacing at rates of 120–160 per minutes for 10 minutes[15]
2. Incremental increases in heart rates of 2–3 minutes each until atrio-ventricular block or symptoms occur[16]

The LVEDP falls in normal patients and is related to a fall in end diastolic volume (stroke volume) but rises in abnormal hearts especially if myocardial ischaemia is induced. The rise in EDP may relate to changes in compliance secondary to contracture of the ischaemic segment of myocardium, or else impairment of segmental relaxation. Immediately post-pacing, abnormal ventricles respond with an abrupt increase in EDP relative to that of the normal population.

Post ventriculographic changes in LVEDP

The normal LV has an EDP of 3–12 mmHG. Following ventriculography, depending on the contrast used, there can be a small rise in EDP of 5–10 mmHg in normal patients. In patients with an abnormal left ventricle the rise can be as high as 20–23 mmHg. Injection of contrast causes decreased inotropy, reducing LV and aortic systolic pressure, decreasing the peripheral vascular resistance and resulting in peripheral vasodilation.

Nitrogylcerine

Vasodilation by nitroglycerine causes peripheral pooling of blood and a decrease in stroke volume and end diastolic pressure. Heart size may also decrease from a decreased stroke volume. A fourth heart sound, if present, may disappear and the v wave of mitral regurgitation decreases.

Constrictive pericarditis

The LVEDP in constrictive pericarditis (see below) has a typical dip and plateau or square root sign pressure pattern. In early diastole there is significant dip or drop in pressure. This is followed by a rapid rise in pressure from mitral inflow, then the pressure plateaus until atrial contraction at end diastole. The RVEDP and LVEDP in constrictive pericarditis are the same (see Figure 15.9).

Relationship of PAWP and PCP to pulmonary vein and LA pressure

When measuring right heart pressures, the PAWP measurement is generally taken as an approximation for LA pressure. This is possible because wedging a catheter in the PA blocks flow to the distal artery, causing the catheter tip to detect the LA pressure conducted retrogradely via the pulmonary veins.

It is necessary to draw a distinction between PAWP and PCP. The PAWP and PCP are often used interchangeably but incorrectly.[17,18]

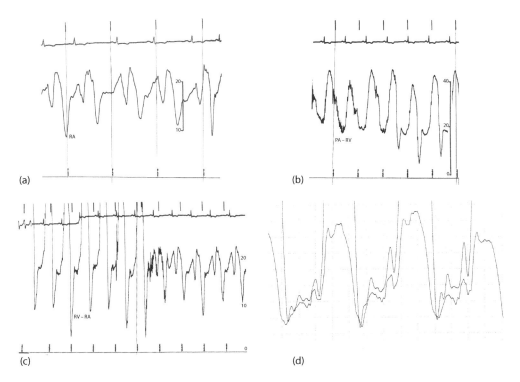

Figure 15.9 Right heart pressure traces from a patient with constrictive pericarditis. Note elevated atrial pressure in (a), with a characteristic 'M' pattern. There is also general equalisation of diastolic pressures, as shown in (b) for the pulmonary artery and right ventricle, and in (c) for the right ventricle and right atrium, and in (d) for right and left ventricles. Note also the 'dip and plateau' or 'square root' configuration in (d).

PAWP is the pressure measured by occlusion of the pulmonary arteries and may vary according to the site of occlusion. The site of venous pressure measured is the segment supplied by the occluded arterial vessel and is considered to be the point where a vein with no flow adjoins the veins with flow. The larger the artery occluded the larger the vein measured, i.e. the farther away from the capillary bed and the closer to the left atrium. The pressure recorded by a Swan-Ganz catheter is not the same as that recorded by a 5 F or 7 F Cournand catheter, where it is considered that the diameter of the vein measured is the same as that of the artery occluded. The PCP is the pressure at the capillary level, not the peripheral arterial or proximal venous level of the PAWP and is higher, forcing blood flow through to the left atrium.[19]

It is the PAWP that is generally measured during cardiac catheterisation and is taken as an approximation for LA pressure. This is because in most situations there is no flow across the mitral valve in end diastole; thus pressures in the LVEDP, LA and pulmonary vein (PV) equilibrate, particularly as there is little resistance to flow across the normal pulmonary veins into the normal heart in the horizontal plane (so normally PAWP = LA = LVEDP). It is this phenomenon that permits PAWP, or the PA occlusive pressure, to be used as an approximation for both LV diastole (EDP, or filling pressure) and for pulmonary venous pressure.

In some diseases the pulmonary veins are affected causing a rise in pulmonary vascular resistance. Here the PCP and pulmonary vein pressure are elevated even though the PAWP may be normal when measured by a Swan-Ganz catheter (a Cournand catheter showing a higher pressure), as in veno-occlusive disease, central pulmonary oedema, hypovolaemic shock or infusion of adrenergic agonists.[20–23] PAWP usually equates to left ventricular diastolic pressure and is a factor in determining the LV end diastolic volume (pre-load in the Frank-Starling equation). However, the LV end diastolic volume is determined by transmural ventricular distending pressure, which is the LVEDP minus the juxta-cardiac pressures and ventricular compliance. One of the commonest causes of variation in juxta-cardiac pressure is positive end expiratory pressure (PEEP) and severe emphysema.

Ventricular compliance is influenced most commonly by myocardial ischaemia and hypertension and less frequently by pericardial diseases. It should be noted that height of the catheter tip relative to the horizontal LA level can affect PCP measurements; the higher the position (particularly if an upper respiratory lobe is selected), the lower arterial and venous pressures become relative to alveolar pressure.

Importantly, PAWP does not always equilibrate with LVEDP. In some situations:

1. LA pressure inaccurately reflects LVEDP (mitral stenosis, *cor triatriatum*, severe mitral regurgitation, acute myocardial infarction, hypertension, hypertrophic cardiomyopathy and occasionally dilated cardiomyopathy).
2. The pulmonary vein pressure inaccurately reflects LA pressure (veno-occlusive disease, atrial myxoma, central pulmonary oedema, infusion of adrenergic agonists, large left to right shunts).
3. Pulmonary artery wedge pressure inaccurately reflects pulmonary vein pressure (large left to right shunts, high output heart failure [thyrotoxicosis], chronic obstructive airways disease, PEEP and artefacts).

If a large pulmonary artery is used to measure PAWP (via a Swan-Ganz catheter), more likely pulmonary alveolar pressure is most closely approximated (especially if an upper lobe artery is used, as this can cause collapse of the distal artery so neither the pulmonary capillary pressure nor the pulmonary vein pressure is measured). Loss of a or v waves or marked respiratory variation in the pressure trace indicates that the catheter is too proximal and needs to be repositioned appropriately.

CONSTRICTIVE PERICARDITIS

This is the result of a thickened fibrotic pericardium preventing appropriate diastolic filling of the left and right ventricles. As the pericardium consists of visceral and parietal portions these usually become fused and act as one. In third world countries tuberculosis is likely to be the commonest cause, but in the western world the most common cause is idiopathic,

followed by viral infection then other causes such as radiotherapy, chronic renal failure (especially dialysis patients), connective tissue disorders (rheumatoid arthritis, SLE), malignancy and surgery.[24-26]

The development of signs of constrictive pericarditis is often slow and easily missed until the late stage, when calcification of the pericardium may occur. Treatment involves surgical removal of the pericardium, although this may not be possible in patients where it is a late complication of coronary artery bypass grafting, when symptomatic treatment with diuretics may be tried initially.[27]

The constricting effect of the thickened fibrotic pericardium affects all chambers of the heart equally, impairing diastolic filling and causing a rise in diastolic pressures. When recordings of right and left ventricular pressures are made simultaneously on the same gain settings, and the diastolic portion of the traces should overlap exactly or within 5 mmHg. This diastolic equalisation of pressure may be evident across all cardiac chambers.

Due to other factors, however, such as coexistent mitral or tricuspid valve disease, atrial pressures may not always be equal. At times, if the patient has been aggressively treated with diuretics, mean atrial filling pressure may be low and the ventricular characteristics may be missing; thus when constrictive pericarditis is suspected and RA pressure is <12 mmHg, a rapid infusion of 1000 mL saline should be given. This elevates pressures, bringing right and left ventricular pressure traces into equilibrium, confirming the diagnosis in such cases.[28]

Atrial pressure traces show high pressures (≥15 mmHg) with rapid x and y descents (similar to ASD, restrictive cardiomyopathy) giving an M or W pattern (Figure 15.9). The a wave is elevated and particularly steep.

Atrial contraction occurs into a ventricle that will not expand further against pericardial constraint; this leads to a steep x descent, and a steep and deep y descent occurs as the atrium abruptly empties into the diastolic ventricle.

Normally on inspiration, intra-thoracic and intra-pericardial pressures fall, causing increased venous return to the right atrium, with a slight increase in right ventricular size. There is also a slight decrease in left ventricular size due to (a) decreased pulmonary venous return to LA from pooling of blood in the lungs and (b) a slight bulge from the interventricular septum into the LV. The consequent left ventricular changes can lead to a fall in systolic blood pressure of up to 10 mmHg. The opposite effect is observed with exhalation, with the net effect of normal breathing on systolic left and right ventricular pressures causing a decrease on inspiration and increase with exhalation over the course of the respiratory cycle. Normally, diastolic left and right ventricular pressures move separately and independently during breathing, while their relative systolic values vary in unison and parallel each other. This parallel systolic motion with breathing is called 'concordance', while opposite abnormal motion is termed 'discordance'.[29]

Inspiration with constrictive pericarditis leads to a paradoxical rise in RA mean pressures, exaggerating the y descent. This is clinically seen in the neck veins as a rise in JVP with a clear y descent, referred to as Kussmaul's sign, which is also seen in restrictive cardiomyopathy, right ventricular infarction and pulmonary embolism.

Kussmaul's sign in constrictive pericarditis is based on the fact that in these patients, negative intra-thoracic inspiratory pressure is not transferred through the thickened fibrotic pericardium to the intra-pericardial space and right ventricle, so blood flow through the right ventricle to the lungs remains constant (not increasing). This causes the increased systemic venous return to accumulate in the right atrium, seen in the neck as a rise in jugular venous pulse. As inspiration normally causes a decrease in LV stroke volume, the aortic component of the second heart sound (A2) occurs a little earlier, and P2 is delayed due to increased venous return of blood to the lungs. With constrictive pericarditis, on inspiration, because of fixed right-sided flow, P2 does not move and A2 occurs much earlier than expected as a result of the augmented decrease in LV stroke volume, thus causing the sudden wide splitting of A2/P2 with the first post-inspiratory beat.[30]

In the ventricular traces an 'early dip and plateau' or 'square root' configuration in diastole is apparent. The early dip is normal, but because of pericardial constraint the ventricles fill rapidly and ventricular filling stops abruptly in early diastole, causing a flat or plateau pattern on the pressure trace (Figure 15.9). On auscultation a 'pericardial knock' may be heard in early diastole, coinciding with the abrupt cessation of flow into the ventricles.

Another key feature of constrictive pericarditis is the presence of left and right ventricular systolic discordance. As with the right heart, the thickened pericardium prevents negative intrathoracic pressure on inspiration being transmitted to the LV, with reduced left ventricular filling that results in accumulation of blood volume in the RV. The net result of this exaggerated ventricular discordance is that with inspiration the LV systolic pressure falls to its minimum and RV systolic pressure to its highest level suggesting ventricular interdependence is present as a result of the pericardial constriction causing decreased LV filling and stroke volume and increased RV filling and stroke volume. Effects of breathing can also be detected in diastole, with a slight separation of LVEDP and PAW pressures on exhalation during simultaneous pressure recording.[31]

RESTRICTIVE CARDIOMYOPATHY

Restrictive cardiomyopathy may be caused by haemochromatosis, amyloid and metabolic storage diseases or may be idiopathic. At times, presentation may occur years before a diagnosis can be made histologically.

Differentiation from constrictive pericarditis can at times be very difficult. Clinical findings can be the same with tachycardia, raised systemic venous pressure with Kussmaul's sign, normal systolic contraction of the ventricles and reduced stroke volume. Whereas in constrictive pericarditis the myocardium is usually normal, in restrictive cardiomyopathy it is the myocardium itself which, due to infiltration of amyloid, iron or fibrosis, causes impaired diastolic filling. The LVEDP is usually higher than the RVEDP, rather than equivalent as in pericardial constriction. These pressures are exaggerated by exercise. Generally, in restrictive cardiomyopathy, pulmonary artery pressures are elevated (≥50 mmHg) and the EDP is usually less than one-third the right ventricular systolic pressure[32] (see Table 15.1).

Even careful examination of haemodynamics may not differentiate between constrictive pericarditis and restrictive cardiomyopathy. The most useful haemodynamic distinction between the two conditions may be the absence of ventricular interdependence, with separation of left and right ventricular diastolic pressures by more than 5 mmHg (LVEDP- RVEDP). The presence of ventricular systolic concordance is expected in restrictive heart disease where expiration causes both systolic ventricular pressures to rise on expiration and fall on

Table 15.1 Summary of basic haemodynamic differences between constrictive and restrictive pericarditis, where clinical signs are the same

Constriction	Restriction
LVEDP may be >1/3 systolic pressure	LVEDP usually <1/3 systolic pressure
Systolic pressure <50–60 mmHg	Systolic pressure >50–60 mmHg
Diastole equalises in all chambers (may need saline infusion)	Diastolic variation from chamber to chamber (pressures do not equalise with saline infusion)
Systolic ventricular discordance	No ventricular systolic discordance

inspiration, whereas in constriction the systolic pressure changes are discordant and on inspiration LV systolic pressure falls to its lowest pressure and RV systolic pressure rises to its maximum.

Cardiac, liver, rectal and skin biopsies are also helpful in diagnosing infiltration. In cases of amyloidosis, lupus erythematosus, radiation induced cardiac disease or heart transplantation with rejection, it may still be impossible to differentiate the two, as these diseases affect the myocardium and pericardium causing fibrosis/infiltration and may also cause substantial pericardial effusions. Cardiac MRI is a useful investigation to distinguish between myocardial and pericardial pathology.

CARDIAC TAMPONADE

This may be acute from trauma or cardiac rupture (ischaemic), or chronic from neoplasm, viral pericarditis, chronic renal failure or collagen vascular disorders. Haemodynamically, the pericardial collection of fluid, blood or pus causes a rise in intra-pericardial pressure that in turn restricts diastolic function. In acute form (trauma), only small amounts of fluid are necessary, whereas in chronic form (neoplasia, uraemia) the gradual rise in volume and pressure leads to stretch of the pericardium and a more gradual rise in intrapericardial pressures. Thus, much larger fluid volumes are seen before tamponade develops. The clinical consequences of a pericardial effusion therefore depend on the rate of fluid collection and the compliance of the pericardium. The fluid volume is not so important. In the author's experience 190 mL caused severe tamponade when the right ventricle was perforated during right ventricular biopsy for dilated cardiomyopathy, and over 1.2 litres was removed from a patient with idiopathic pericardial effusion with tamponade (presumed viral). Reddy et al.[33] have described three phases of cardiac tamponade, phase one showing pressure but not flow changes, phase two showing mild to moderate pressure and flow changes and phase three showing severe pressure and flow changes (see Table 15.2).

Patients with trauma causing tamponade with only small amounts of pericardial fluid frequently

Table 15.2 The three phases of cardiac tamponade

	PHASE 1	PHASE 2	PHASE 3
Intrapericardial pressure	<RA but RA is increased	Equal to RA but less than PAWP (both increased)	Equal to RA and PAWP
Pulsus paradoxus	Rarely seen	Occasionally seen	Always seen
Pressure/flow changes	Pressure changes only	Pressure/some flow	Severe pressure and severe flow changes
Effects of pericardiocentesis	1. ↓IPP, ↓RAP, ↓PAWP	1. ↓IPP, ↓RAP ↓PAWP	1. ↓IPP, ↓↓RAP ↓↓PAWP
	2. Minor reduction in the exaggerated inspiratory decrease in arterial systolic pressure	2. Large reduction in the exaggerated inspiratory decrease in arterial systolic pressure	2. Reversal to normal inspiratory decrease in systolic pressure
	3. No change in cardiac output	3. Slight increase in cardiac output	3. Marked increase in cardiac output

demonstrate Beck's triad[34] of (a) progressive elevation of jugular venous pulse, (b) progressive systemic arterial hypotension and (c) a small quiet heart. These patients require urgent surgical consultation. With the more chronic development of effusion and tamponade, intra-pericardial volumes are usually larger and percutaneous pericardiocentesis is appropriate if the echo free space is ≥10 mm.[35] Most units now introduce a pigtail catheter into the pericardial space, allowing (a) pressure measurement and (b) prolonged drainage to assess re-accumulation. Echocardiography is used in the diagnosis of pericardial effusion and tamponade. Right atrial and right ventricular diastolic collapse occurs through all phases of tamponade and so does not indicate severity. Ultrasound guidance is also commonly used during pericardiocentesis.

PULSUS PARADOXUS

Pulsus paradoxus is a non-specific finding. Initially described by Kussmaul in constrictive pericarditis but found in cardiac tamponade, severe emphysema and severe pulmonary embolism, the mechanisms vary.

As already mentioned, during normal inspiration, pooling of blood in the lungs during deep inspiration results in less blood flowing to the left side of the heart, and consequently less blood is pumped into the systemic circulation. If this fall in systolic pressure is >10 mmHg, it is called pulsus paradoxus. This is in fact a misnomer as pulsus paradoxus is simply an exaggeration of a normal physiological finding, not a paradox.

In tamponade, inspiration leads to a marked decrease in intra-pericardial pressure but is equally transmitted to both right and left ventricles. This causes increased venous return with an increase in right ventricular stroke volume, causing the interventricular septum to bulge into the left ventricle. Increased pooling of blood in the lungs results from decreased gradient from the pulmonary artery to the left ventricle (pulmonary vascular resistance) causing a substantial fall in left ventricular stroke volume and systolic pressure, with an associated decrease in pulse pressure.

In constrictive pericarditis, pulsus paradoxus is frequently seen only in one or two beats on inspiration. It occurs because the thickened, fibrotic pericardium prevents changes in intra-thoracic pressure being transferred to the intra-pericardial space and the cardiac chambers. Inspiration causes a fall in PAWP and PCP but not in LVEDP, which remains the same. Flow to LV decreases and stroke volume decreases, leading to a decreased systolic pressure. Intramural pressures do not alter throughout.

In severe emphysema and severe pulmonary embolism, pulsus paradoxus results from (a) transfer of significantly negative intra-thoracic pressures to the lungs, pulmonary artery and right heart so that the right ventricular stroke volume pools in the lungs, leading to a decrease in left ventricular stroke volume, (b) some transfer of the negative intra-thoracic pressure to the aorta and great vessels and (c) pulmonary hypertension, which may actually prevent an inspiratory increase in venous return transferring to the pulmonary artery and lungs.

NITRATES

These drugs are commonly used in the catheterisation laboratory and for ischaemic heart disease to prevent angina.

Nitroglycerine is a potent peripheral vasodilator (reducing preload), but is also an arterial and coronary dilator affecting both preload and afterload. Nitrates cause venous pooling, leading to decreased LVEDP, stroke volume and heart size. Arterial dilatation causes decreased arterial pressures and decreased systemic vascular resistance (afterload).

Cardiac output usually falls but may remain unchanged when significant cardiomegaly is present, and nitrates are administered. In the normal heart, LVEDP may fall to sub-optimal filling ranges, but in the enlarged heart, when LVEDP is significantly elevated, nitrates reduce the LVEDP moves to normal levels.

Mitral regurgitation

Administration of nitroglycerine reduces the degree of mitral regurgitation and in so doing, reduces the v wave of the PAWP. The reduction of mitral regurgitation is related to (a) reducing systemic arterial pressure (afterload) which also reduces the regurgitant fraction, (b) decreasing heart size and (c) improved myocardial perfusion with reduction of ischaemia and improvement in function of the mitral apparatus if the regurgitation is related to myocardial ischaemia affecting either papillary muscle or global myocardial function.

Clinically, with nitroglycerine the murmur of rheumatic mitral regurgitation or papillary muscle dysfunction becomes quieter or diminished, whereas that of mitral valve prolapse occurs earlier and may become pan-systolic.

Aortic regurgitation

With aortic regurgitation administration of nitrates reduces the regurgitant fraction with a decrease in systolic pressure (afterload). As a result of this, the regurgitation impinging upon the anterior leaflet of the mitral valve is lessened. Any Austin Flint murmur noted will soften or disappear. Contrary to this, because of decreased systemic vascular resistance in mitral stenosis, the gradient across the mitral valve increases and the diastolic rumble of mitral stenosis increases in intensity and duration. This is potentiated by accompanying tachycardia, increasing cardiac output and raising left atrial pressure.

Hypertrophic obstructive cardiomyopathy/idiopathic hypertrophic sub-aortic stenosis

In hypertrophic obstructive cardiomyopathy (HOCM), reduction in systemic arterial pressure by nitrates causes an increased gradient from left ventricle to aorta. There is also increased inotropism of the left ventricular outflow tract and tachycardia, caused by the nitrates which also cause an increase in intensity and duration of the murmur associated with HOCM. Similarly, in valvular aortic stenosis, the tachycardia associated with the nitrates increases the intensity of the aortic stenotic murmur.

REFERENCES

1. Hada Y, Wolfe C, Craige E. Pulsus alternans determined by biventricular simultaneous systolic time intervals. *Circulation.* 1982;65(3):617–626.
2. Gleason WL, Braunwald E. Studies on Starling's law of the heart: VI. Relationships between left ventricular end-diastolic volume and stroke volume in man with observations on the mechanism of pulsus alternans. *Circulation.* 1962;25(5):841–848.
3. Verheugt F, Scheck H, Meltzer RS, Roelandt J. Alternating atrial electromechanical dissociation as contributing factor for pulsus alternans. *Br Heart J.* 1982;48(5):459–461.
4. Hess OM, Surber EP, Ritter M, Krayenbuehl HP. Pulsus alternans: Its influence on systolic and diastolic function in aortic valve disease. *J Am Coll Cardiol.* 1984;4(1):1–7
5. Brockenbrough EC, Braunwald E, Morrow AG. A hemodynamic technic for the detection of hypertrophic subaortic stenosis. *Circulation.* 1961;23(2):189–194.
6. Folland ED, Parisi AF, Carbone C. Is peripheral arterial pressure a satisfactory substitute for ascending aortic pressure when measuring aortic valve gradients? *J Am Coll Cardiol.* 1984;4(6):1207–1212.
7. Gorlin R, Gorlin S. Hydraulic formula for calculation of the area of the stenotic mitral valve, other cardiac valves, and central circulatory shunts. *Am Heart J.* 1951;41(1):1–29.
8. Feldman T, Grossman W, Moscucci M. Profiles in vascular heart disease. In: Moscucci M, editor. *Grossman & Baim's Cardiac Catheterization, Angiography, and Intervention.* 8th ed. Philadelphia, PA: Lippingcott, William & Wilkins; 2014. p 943–969.
9. Mann T, McLaurin L, Grossman W, Craige E. Assessing the hemodynamic severity of acute aortic regurgitation due to infective endocarditis. *N Engl J Med.* 1975;293(3):108–113.
10. Godlewski KJ, Talley JD, Morris GT. Interpretation of cardiac pathophysiology from pressure waveform analysis: Acute aortic insufficiency. *Cathet Cardiovasc Diagn.* 1993;28(3):244–248; discussion 8–9.
11. Pichard AD, Kay R, Smith H, Rentrop P, Holt J, Gorlin R. Large V waves in the pulmonary wedge pressure tracing in the absence of mitral regurgitation. *Am J Cardiol.* 1982;50(5):1044–1050.
12. Fuchs RM, Heuser RR, Yin FC, Brinker JA. Limitations of pulmonary wedge V waves in diagnosing mitral regurgitation. *Am J Cardiol.* 1982;49(4):849–854.

13. Haskell RJ, French WJ. Accuracy of left atrial and pulmonary artery wedge pressure in pure mitral regurgitation in predicting left ventricular end diastolic pressure. *Am J Cardiol.*1988;61:136–141.

14. Khaja F, Parker JO, Ledwich RJ, West RO, Armstrong PW. Assessment of ventricular function in coronary artery disease by means of atrial pacing and exercise. *Am J Cardiol.* 1970;26(2):107–116.

15. Parker JO, Khaja F, Case RB. Analysis of left ventricular function by atrial pacing. *Circulation.* 1971;43(2):241–252.

16. Sowton G, Balcon R, Cross D, Frick M. Measurement of the angina threshold using atrial pacing: A new technic of the study of angina pectoris. *Cardio Vasc Res.* 1967;1:301–307.

17. Wiedemann H. Wedge pressure in pulmonary veno-occlusive disease. *N Engl J Med.* 1986;315(19):1233.

18. Holloway H, Perry M, Downey J, Parker J, Taylor A. Estimation of effective pulmonary capillary pressure in intact lungs. *J App Physiol: Resp Env Exer Physiol.* 1983;54(3):846–851.

19. Zidulka A, Hakim T. Wedge pressure in large vs. small pulmonary arteries to detect pulmonary venoconstriction. *J App Physiol.* 1985;59(4):1329–1332.

20. Shaffer A, Silber E. Factors influencing the character of the pulmonary arterial wedge pressure. *Am Heart J.* 1956;51(4):522–532.

21. Walston A, Kendall ME. Comparison of pulmonary wedge and left atrial pressure in man. *Am Heart J.* 1973;86(2):159–164.

22. Wiedemann HP, Matthay MA, Matthay RA. Cardiovascular-pulmonary monitoring in the intensive care (part I). *Chest.*1984;85:537–549.

23. O'Quin R, Marini JJ. Pulmonary artery occlusion pressure: Clinical physiology, measurement, and interpretation. *Am Rev Resp Dis.* 1983;128(2):319–326.

24. Cameron J, Oesterle SN, Baldwin JC, Hancock EW. The etiologic spectrum of constrictive pericarditis. *Am Heart J.* 1987;113(2):354–360.

25. Marsa R, Mehta S, Willis W, Bailey L. Constrictive pericarditis after myocardial revascularization: Report of three cases. *Am J Cardiol.* 1979;44(1):177–183.

26. Cohen MV, Greenberg MA. Constrictive pericarditis: Early and late complication of cardiac surgery. *Am J Cardiol.* 1979;43(3):657–661.

27. Ayzenberg O, Oldfield G, Stevens J, Beck W. Constrictive pericarditis following myocardial revascularization: A case report. 5th *Af Med J.* 1984;65(18):739–741.

28. Bush CA, Stang JM, Wooley CF, Kilman JW. Occult constrictive pericardial disease. Diagnosis by rapid volume expansion and correction by pericardiectomy. *Circulation.* 1977;56(6):924–930.

29. Geske JB, Anavekar NS, Nishimura RA, Oh JK and Gersh BJ. Differentiation of constriction and restriction complex cardiovascular hemodynamics. *JACC* 2016; 68: 2329–2347.

30. Beck W, Schrire V, Vogelpoel L. Splitting of the second heart sound in constrictive pericarditis, with observations on the mechanism of pulsus paradoxus. *Am Heart J.* 1962;64(6):765–778.

31. Doshi S, Ramakrishnan S, Gupta SK. Invasive hemodynamics of constrictive pericarditis. *Indian Heart J.* 2015;67(2):175–182.

32. Shabetai R, Fowler NO, Fenton JC. Restrictive cardiac disease: Pericarditis and the myocardiopathies. *Am Heart J.* 1965;69(2):271–280.

33. Reddy PS, Curtiss EI, Uretsky BF. Spectrum of hemodynamic changes in cardiac tamponade. *Am J Cardiol.* 1990;66(20):1487–1491.

34. Beck CS. Two cardiac compression triads. *JAMA.* 1935;104(9):714–716.

35. Krikorian JG, Hancock EW. Pericardiocentesis. *Am J Med.* 1978;65(5):808–814.

16

Measurement of cardiac output and shunts

MICHAEL P. FENELEY

INTRODUCTION

Cardiac output (CO) is a key indicator of cardiac performance and is used to derive other important haemodynamic variables, including the cardiac index, stroke volume and vascular resistance. These derived variables, together with additional findings from right heart catheterisation, are invaluable in establishing a diagnosis and in guiding therapy. The direct Fick method is considered the most accurate and precise method for determination of CO under steady-state conditions, but the intermittent bolus thermodilution method is a practical alternative. This chapter briefly describes various ways to determine CO and explains the methodology in determining CO by both the Fick and thermodilution methods, including clear examples of Fick CO and shunt calculations for evaluation of oximetry runs from a left-to-right shunt, a right-to-left shunt and a bidirectional shunt.

CARDIAC OUTPUT

CO is the total quantity of blood delivered to the systemic circulation per unit of time and is generally expressed in litres per minute (L/min). In the normal heart, systemic flow equals pulmonary flow. Normal CO at rest for a 70 kg adult is approximately 5 L/min. It is usual to normalise CO measurements for differences in body size by dividing the CO by the body surface area, yielding the cardiac index (L/min/M^2). Trained athletes are capable of increasing CO up to 6-fold at peak exercise. Maximal O_2 delivery to the tissues can be increased even further by increasing the amount of O_2 extracted by the tissues from each unit of blood: This is called the extraction reserve, which permits up to a 3-fold increase in O_2 extraction from the blood. When the 6-fold CO reserve is multiplied by the 3-fold extraction reserve, it can be seen that the body has the capacity to increase O_2 delivery to the tissues up to 18-fold above normal resting values.

Conversely, the minimum CO compatible with life is one-third the normal resting CO because below this level the extraction reserve is exhausted.

The Fick principle

CO is usually measured in the cardiac catheterisation laboratory by the Fick oxygen (O_2) method, which is a variation on the principle first stated by Adolph Fick: The amount (A) of any substance taken up or released by an organ is the product of the blood flow to the organ (Q) and the difference between the concentration of the substance in blood on the arterial (C_A) and venous (C_V) sides of the organ:

$$A = Q \times (C_A - C_V). \tag{16.1}$$

By rearranging Equation 16.1, it can be seen that blood flow through an organ can be determined by measuring the amount of any substance taken up or released by the organ and the arterio-venous (A-V) concentration difference of the substance:

$$Q = \frac{A}{C_A - C_V} \tag{16.2}$$

Fick oxygen method

This method of measuring CO applies the Fick principle to uptake of O_2 from the lungs. This method relies on the fact that under steady-state conditions, uptake of O_2 from the lungs into the blood (A) is equal to the uptake of O_2 from room air by the lungs. The A–V O_2 concentration difference across the lungs (C_A–C_V) is taken to be the difference between blood samples drawn from the pulmonary artery and the left ventricle (or pulmonary veins, or any systemic artery). Use of left ventricular or systemic arterial blood in place of pulmonary venous blood is a matter of sampling convenience. Doing so ignores the small contribution of bronchial and thebesian venous drainage (1.5%) but this involves minimal error. In the presence of a right-to-left shunt, however, (see below) systemic arterial O_2 concentration cannot be substituted for the true pulmonary venous O_2 concentration.

Two methods have been used commonly in cardiac catheterisation laboratories to measure O_2 uptake from room air by the lungs:

THE DOUGLAS BAG METHOD

In this method, a collection bag (the Douglas bag) attached to a mouthpiece via a 3-way valve is used to collect all of the patient's expired air over a precisely measured time period, usually 3 minutes. Prior to inserting the mouthpiece, the technician must ensure that a nose clip is correctly placed and that the patient's lips are firmly clasped over the mouthpiece so that all expired air passes through the mouthpiece. The 3-way valve should first be adjusted to permit the patient to breathe room air quietly for no less than 30 seconds before the valve is adjusted to direct the expired air into the bag, and the collection period begins. Because the lungs have a large reservoir capacity, the assumption of the method that O_2 uptake from room air is equal to O_2 uptake from the lungs to the blood is valid only under *steady-state* conditions. For this reason, it is important that the room be quiet and the patient's breathing pattern remain undisturbed throughout the collection period, ensuring there are no leaks in the system.

The amount (A in Equation 16.1) of O_2 taken in by the lungs is then calculated as the product of the volume (Q) of the expired air collected and the difference in O_2 concentration between room air and expired air. The volume of expired air is measured with a spirometer. The O_2 content of the samples of room air and expired air can be measured directly with a fuel-cell technique, or derived from measurements of the partial pressure of O_2 (pO_2) in the samples. The total amount of O_2 consumed during the 3-minute collection period is then divided by 3 to express the O_2 consumption (VO_2) in mL/min.

The other two factors in the Fick equation, O_2 content of arterial and mixed venous blood, are obtained by blood gas analysis. Modern haemoximeters use spectrophotometric analysis to determine the total Hb concentration of blood, expressed as g%, i.e. the amount of Hb in grams per 100 mL of blood. The O_2 content of blood is calculated from this value (see example below). First, the O_2 carrying capacity of blood is obtained as the product of the total Hb concentration and the O_2-binding affinity of blood, 1.36 (reported values for the O_2-binding affinity of blood vary from 1.34–1.39). Blood saturation is also measured directly by haemoximetry, and the O_2 content of blood is then calculated as the product of the O_2-carrying capacity of blood and the fractional blood saturation (i.e. the O_2 saturation expressed as a fraction). Leaving aside the potential measurement error of the total O_2 carrying capacity of blood, measurement of total blood Hb is inaccurate in the presence of abnormal Hb or if some Hb is bound to carbon monoxide (as in smokers).

Pulmonary blood flow is then calculated, according to Equation 16.2, by dividing the measured VO_2 by the A-V O_2 content difference. In the absence of a shunt, pulmonary blood flow is equal to the total CO.

POLAROGRAPHIC O_2 METHOD

This is an alternative to the older Douglas bag method of measuring VO_2. The patient is connected by a hood or face mask to a servo-controlled unit that maintains a unidirectional flow of air from the laboratory through the hood or mask and into the polarographic O_2 sensor. The flow rate is automatically adjusted to maintain the O_2 content of air detected by the sensor at a constant level. As a consequence of this design, the only variable determining the patient's VO_2 under steady-state conditions is the speed of the blower in the servo-control unit because the remaining determinants are constants. Metabolic carts using a VO_2 hood that provides an indirect Fick CO using breath-by-breath metabolic analysis are routinely used for cardiopulmonary exercise testing but are not generally used in the cardiac catheterisation laboratory.

Sample calculations: CO by the Fick method

An example of how to calculate CO by the Fick method is shown in the following. The following data were collected from a patient, and blood samples taken from the left ventricle (LV) and pulmonary artery (PA).

- Height: 152 cm; Weight: 50 kg; Age: 68 y Sex: Female.
- Body surface area (BSA): 1.45 m².
- VO_2: 200 mL/min.
- Hb: 12.5 g%.
- Body surface area is used to calculate cardiac index and other derived haemodynamic variables.
- Hb concentration is needed to calculate the O_2 carrying capacity of blood (O_2 capacity = Hb concentration × 1.36).

- O_2 saturation of arterial and mixed venous blood is used to calculate the O_2 content of each sample.
- The O_2 content is used to calculate the A-V O_2 content difference ($C_A - C_V$).

Height, weight, age and sex are used to determine surface area and to estimate VO_2 from morphometric charts or computed algorithms as an alternative to a Douglas bag collection but is less accurate. For this patient, for example, the assumed VO_2 was 165 mL/min and the measured value was 200 mL/min.

O_2 carrying capacity of blood: =
$$12.5 \times 1.36 = 17.0 \text{ mL/100 mL, or Vol\%}$$

LV saturation: 97.3%, therefore: LV O_2 content: =
$$17.0 \times 0.973 = 16.5 \text{ Vol\%}$$

PA saturation: 68.7%, therefore: PA O_2 content: =
$$17.0 \times 0.687 = 11.7 \text{ Vol\%}$$

A-V O_2 content difference ($C_A - C_V$): =
$$16.5 - 11.7 = 4.8 \text{ Vol\%}$$

A correction factor of ×10 is required to convert Vol% (mL/100 mL) to mL/L: Thus 4.8 Vol% (i.e. 4.8 mL of O_2/100 mL of blood) becomes 48 mL of O_2/L of blood).

CO, or Q, can then be calculated according to Equation (16.2):

$$CO = O_2 \text{ consumption}/C_A - C_V = 200 \text{ mL/min}/4.8 \text{ mL/L}$$
$$= 200 \text{ L}/48 \text{ min}$$
$$= 4.2 \text{ L/min}$$

Dividing CO by BSA gives the cardiac index:
$$4.2 \text{ L/min}/1.45 \text{ m}^2 = 2.9 \text{ L/min/m}^2$$

Indicator dilution methods

Thermodilution using a Swan-Ganz catheter has replaced the original dye dilution techniques, but the principle behind all indicator dilution methods is the same. These methods also rely on the Fick principle. In these methods, a specified amount of a substance (A) is injected as rapidly as possible at one point in the circulation and the concentration (C) of the substance is then measured continuously as a function of time (t) at some point downstream from the injection site. Figure 16.1 shows an example of the type of curve resulting from plotting continuous measurements of concentration over time at the downstream site. Because all of the substance injected (A) must pass the measurement site, blood flow rate can be calculated as a variation of Equation 16.2:

$$Q = \frac{A}{\int C(t)dt} \qquad (16.3)$$

where the denominator of Equation 16.3 is the integral of concentration with respect to time for the period of time that it takes for all of the substance injected to pass the measurement point *for the first time*. This integral is equivalent to the area under the curve indicated in Figure 16.1. Note that there is a second hump in Figure 16.1 that occurs because after all the injected substance passes the measurement point for the first time ('first pass'), it then recirculates and passes the measurement point again. It is important, therefore, to determine the area under the concentration-time curve only for that period of time corresponding to the first pass of the substance. This is done by converting the concentration-time curve to a logarithmic concentration scale, which permits linear extrapolation to be used to accurately define the time at which the first pass is completed, and these measurement operations are automated. One advantage of the

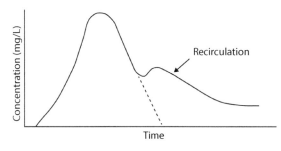

Time

Figure 16.1 Graph of concentration-time curve as measured by the indicator dilution technique for determination of cardiac output. Detection of indicator reaches a peak on its first pass, then declines. There is a smaller second hump, indicating detection of a second pass as the indicator recirculates. With thermodilution techniques, temperature is the indicator and there is no second pass. Dotted line indicates extrapolated estimate of the area under the curve for the first pass.

thermodilution technique is that there is essentially no recirculation of the injectate, which simplifies calculation of the area under the concentration-time curve.

In the indocyanine green method, a 1 mL sample (usual concentration 5 mg/mL) is injected into the pulmonary artery and blood withdrawn at a constant rate from the femoral artery (or any other systemic artery) and passed through a densitometer cuvette to generate the concentration-time curve. Dye dilution has now been replaced by thermodilution.

In the thermodilution method, the 'indicator' is a known volume (usually 10 mL) of a cold solution, such as 5% dextrose, which is injected at a proximal site, such as the right atrium. The temperature of the injectate is measured before injection. The temperature at the distal site, usually the pulmonary artery, is measured continuously with a thermistor on a Swan-Ganz catheter. The amount of' 'cold' injected (A in Equation 16.3) is the product of (a) volume of the injectate, (b) temperature difference between blood and injectate, and (c) the ratio of the products of specific gravity and specific heat of blood and injectate, respectively (this ratio is 1.08 for 5% dextrose). This calculated amount of 'cold' is then divided by the area under the temperature-time curve in the pulmonary artery (equivalent to the concentration-time area in the denominator of Equation 16.3) to yield the CO, which is inversely proportional to the area under the curve. The final value is usually multiplied by an empirical correction factor (0.825) to account for warming of the injectate in the catheter prior to injection.

Advantages of the thermodilution method over dye dilution techniques include not only the virtual absence of recirculation but also the simplicity of the 'cold' indicator, absence of the need for systemic arterial blood sampling and, consequently, the ease with which multiple measurements can be made. This last is an important advantage, as thermodilution CO determination should be based on at least three sequential measurements.

Bioimpedance cardiography

Non-invasive determination of CO is possible, for example, by means of echocardiography (see below) or by thoracic electrical bioimpedance (TEB), a form of electrical impedance plethysmography.

TEB can determine CO, stroke volume, systemic vascular resistance, thoracic fluid level, certain indices of myocardial contractility, and other haemodynamic parameters. A small alternating current is transmitted through the thorax. Sensors on the sides of the neck and chest detect changes in impedance along the aorta, recording changes in blood volume and flow with each heartbeat, while a pressure cuff on the upper arm automatically measures arterial blood pressure. TEB is a relatively new technology and is not widely used in the cardiac catheterisation laboratory. Nevertheless, it provides a viable alternative to right heart catheterisation for monitoring high-risk or critically ill candidates who require haemodynamic monitoring. Other non-invasive or minimally invasive methodologies are also available, each with its own advantages and disadvantages.

CARDIAC SHUNTS

A connection between a vessel or chamber that permits mixing of oxygenated arterial blood with desaturated venous blood, or vice versa, is called a shunt. In the cardiac catheterisation laboratory, cardiovascular shunts are quantified by an oximetry run, a collection of blood samples from various cardiopulmonary chambers and vessels from which to measure O_2 saturations. These saturations are used to localise the site of the shunt and to determine the size of the shunt. Shunts can occur from mixing of blood via a patent foramen ovale, an atrial or ventricular septal defect (Figure 16.2a), a patent ductus arteriosus, an A-V fistula, other congenital disorders or from intrapulmonary vascular or alveolar abnormalities (Figure 16.2b).

Shunt measurements are based on a variation of the Fick O_2 method discussed above. In the presence of an intracardiac shunt, the outputs of the left and right heart are no longer equal. In order to measure the size of the shunt, therefore, it is necessary to determine pulmonary blood flow (Q_P) and systemic blood flow (Q_S) separately. Pulmonary blood flow measurement is identical to the measurement described above for the CO determination by the standard Fick O_2 method: That is, VO_2 divided by the pulmonary A-V O_2 content difference before or after the shunt for each circuit. As noted above, the pulmonary venous O_2 content can be approximated from a left ventricular or systemic arterial blood sample provided there is no evidence of a right-to-left shunt, which would be suggested by a systemic O_2 saturation less than 95%. If a right-to-left shunt is suspected, a direct sample from one of the pulmonary veins (often possible in the presence of an atrial septal defect) should be used; otherwise, an assumed value for the pulmonary venous O_2 content can be calculated as the product of an assumed saturation of 98% multiplied by the O_2 carrying capacity of blood.

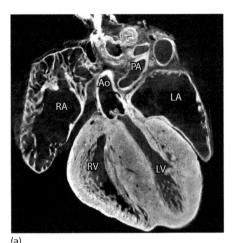 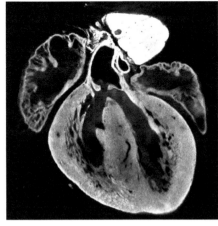

(a)

Figure 16.2 **(a)** Cross-section through the heart of a normal mouse embryo (left) and one with a developmental defect showing a septal defect across the high interventricular septum (right). (*Abbreviations:* RA, right atrium; RV, right ventricle; AO, aorta; PA, pulmonary artery; LA, left atrium; LV, left ventricle).

(Continued)

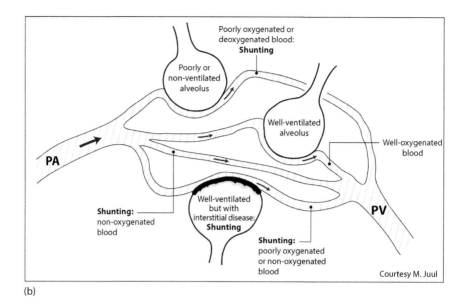

(b)

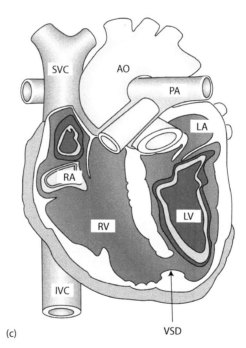

(c)

Figure 16.2 (Continued) **(b)** Example of possible shunting from intrapulmonary vascular or alveolar abnormalities. **(c)** Illustration of cardiovascular site selection of blood oximetry samples for evaluation of intracardiac shunts. Arrow points to a ventricular septal defect (*Abbreviations:* SVC, superior vena cava; IVC, inferior vena cava; RA, right atrium; RV, right ventricle; AO, aorta; PA, pulmonary artery; LA, left atrium; LV, left ventricle; VSD, ventricular septal defect). ([a] Courtesy of Hongjun Shi, Victor Chang Research Institute.)

Systemic blood flow in the presence of an intracardiac shunt is calculated by dividing the VO_2 by the systemic A-V O_2 content difference ($Qs = VO_2/$ systemic A-V O_2 content difference), which is the difference between the systemic arterial O_2 content and the mixed venous O_2 content *in the chamber immediately proximal to the shunt.* Pulmonary blood flow is obtained by dividing VO_2 by the pulmonary A-V O_2 content difference ($Qp = VO_2/$pulmonary A-V O_2 content difference), which is the difference between arterial O_2 content and mixed venous O_2 content *after* the shunt, usually taken as the pulmonary artery sample.

In order to localise the site of the shunt, an oximetry run is performed. This is done by placing an end-hole catheter in the right or left pulmonary artery. The catheter is then withdrawn in serial steps, taking sequential 2 mL heparinised blood samples for O_2 saturation and O_2 content measurements at each of the following sites: Right or left pulmonary artery, main pulmonary artery, right ventricular outflow tract, mid-right ventricle, right ventricular inflow tract, low, mid, and high right atrium, low superior vena cava (junction with right atrium), high superior vena cava, high inferior vena cava, and low inferior vena cava. Oximetry samples should also be taken from the left ventricle and any arterial site distal to the insertion of a possible ductus arteriosus into the aorta (usually the femoral artery). From these samples, it is possible to identify the site of a step-up that would occur in any chamber up to the pulmonary artery (Figure 16.2c).

In the event that a step-up occurs in the pulmonary artery, the average of the right ventricular blood samples should be used as the mixed venous O_2 content in the calculation of systemic blood flow because the right ventricle would be the chamber immediately proximal to the shunt. In the case of a left-to-right shunt through a ventricular septal defect (VSD), the step-up would occur in the right ventricle. The appropriate value for mixed venous O_2 content to be used in the calculation of systemic blood flow in the presence of a VSD would be the average of the right atrial measurements because the right atrium is the chamber immediately proximal to the shunt. In the case of a left-to-right shunt through an atrial septal defect, the step-up would occur in the right atrium. In this case, both the superior and inferior venae cavae are the sites proximal to the level of the shunt, so that the mixed venous O_2 content value to be used for the calculation of systemic blood flow should be the average of the measurements made in both venae cavae.

A problem arises in that although the heart receives 25% of its blood volume from the superior vena cava and 75% from the inferior vena cava, O_2 content of blood from the upper body is lower than that from the lower body due to differences in O_2 extraction by different organs. Renal stream saturations are typically higher than from the hepatic stream, and saturations are not evenly mixed until blood reaches the

right ventricle. It has been demonstrated empirically, however, that a sample of blood consisting of the three SVC samples and one IVC sample represents a true mixed venous saturation. Thus, the most accurate method of performing this averaging process is to add ¾ of the superior vena caval saturation value to ¼ of the inferior vena caval saturation.

The size of the shunt is reported as the Q_P to Q_S ratio, which is the ratio of pulmonary to systemic flow. This would involve using the Fick equation to calculate pulmonary and systemic flows individually, and the absolute value of the left-to-right shunt would be given by Q_P–Q_S in L/min. The shunt size is more commonly reported, however, not as an absolute value, but as the ratio Q_P/Q_S, according to the equation:

$$Q_P/Q_S = \frac{VO_2 / \text{Pulmonary A} - V\, O_2\, \text{Content Difference}}{VO_2 / \text{Systemic A} - V\, O_2\, \text{Content Difference}}$$

(16.4)

It is fortuitous, however, that because VO_2 is common to both numerator and denominator in Equation 16.4, this common value cancels out in the calculation: Thus, in order to determine shunt size as the Q_P/Q_S ratio, it is not necessary to measure VO_2. The size of the shunt can be calculated directly from oximetry data using saturation values alone, greatly simplifying the calculation into the equation:

$$Q_P/Q_S = \frac{\text{Systemic A} - V\, O_2\, \text{Content Difference}}{\text{Pulmonary A} - V\, O_2\, \text{Content Difference}}$$

(16.5)

Sample shunt calculations

NO SHUNT

When no shunt is present, there is no sudden step-up in any chamber, and saturations in the oximetry run do not vary significantly, as in the example shown in Table 16.1. No additional measurements or calculations are required to confirm this.

LEFT-TO-RIGHT SHUNT

A left-to-right -shunt is the most common type of shunt. Because VO_2 is eliminated from the equation, CO calculations are not necessary to determine whether a shunt is present or not. A blood oximetry run is sufficient, as demonstrated in the example shown in Table 16.2.

Table 16.1 Oximetry run from a patient without an intracardiac shunt

Site	O₂ saturation (%)	O₂ content (Vol%)
SVC1	69.5	12.5
IVC	68.2	10.3
HRA	67.9	10.3
MRA	69.8	10.5
LRA	66.7	10.1
RV	67.2	10.2
PA1	67.9	10.3
PA2	66.7	10.1
LV	96.5	14.6

Note: Hb = 10.5 g%; O₂ capacity = 14.3 Vol%; Measured O₂ consumption = 220 mL/min.
Abbreviations: SVC, superior vena cava; IVC, inferior vena cava; RA, right atrium; RV, right ventricle; PA, pulmonary artery; LV, left ventricle.

Table 16.2 Oximetry run from a patient with a left-to-right shunt, as shown by a sudden 'step up' in saturation at the level of the right atrium, indicating an atrial septal defect

Site	O₂ saturation (%)	O₂ content (Vol%)
SVC1	69.5	9.9
SVC2	67.5	9.7
IVC	75.8	10.8
RA	87.1	12.5
RV	87.1	12.5
PA1	86.8	12.4
PA2	87.2	12.5
PV	98.4	14.1
Arterial	97.9	14.0

Note: Hb = 10.5 g%; O₂ capacity = 14.3 Vol%; Measured O₂ consumption = 220 mL/min.
Abbreviations: SVC, superior vena cava; IVC, inferior vena cava; RA, right atrium; RV, right ventricle; PA, pulmonary artery; PV, pulmonary vein.

The key issue is to determine whether there is a sudden rise in saturation in a right heart chamber. In the above example, there is a sudden step-up in saturation in the RA sample, indicating a shunt (caused by flow of oxygenated left atrial blood into the right atrium across an atrial septal defect). The critical values in calculating the size of the shunt are taken as the arterial sample, and the venous samples before the shunt (venae cavae) and after the shunt (PA). An accurate measure of true

mixed venous blood (MV) saturation before the shunt is given by the average of 3 SVC and 1 IVC samples ([68.5 + 68.5 + 68.5 + 75.8/4] = 281.3/4 = 70.3%). In this example the average PA saturation is 87.0%, and the arterial saturation is 97.9%.

Here, the IVC saturation is higher than SVC, indicating the sample has come from the renal stream. If the IVC saturation is lower than SVC, the IVC sample has come from the hepatic stream and should be discarded. Typically, SVC saturation is lower than IVC. Taking the average of 3 SVC samples +1 IVC sample overcomes this sampling variability and provides a true mixed venous sample when right atrial saturation cannot be used, as above with an atrial septal defect.

The size of the shunt is reported as the Q_P to Q_S ratio, which as explained above, can be calculated directly from the PA and MV saturations. Thus:

$$\text{Pulmonary A-V Difference} = (\text{Arterial Saturation} - \text{PA Saturation}) = 97.9 - 87.0 = 10.9 \text{ Vol\%}$$

$$\text{Systemic A-V Difference} = (\text{Arterial Saturation} - \text{MV Saturation}) = 97.9 - 70.3 = 27.6 \text{ Vol\%}$$

The shunt ratio is reported as the ratio of the systemic A-V difference to the pulmonary A-V difference, which is (27.6/10.9), or 2.5:1. This means that 2.5 times more blood circulates through the right heart than the left.

A Q_P/Q_S ratio less than 1.5 indicates a small left-to-right shunt that may not warrant surgical intervention, but the threshold for intervention to close intracardiac shunts is becoming lower, particularly in the case of atrial septal defects, because of the availability of percutaneous closure methods.

BIDIRECTIONAL SHUNT

A bidirectional shunt means that blood flows simultaneously in both directions from the left heart to the right and from the right side to the left, either across an intracardiac defect or via separate communications. Calculation of bidirectional shunts is more complicated and depends on using the Fick equation to calculate both systemic flow and pulmonary flow separately, but *a third flow calculation is also necessary: The flow that would theoretically occur in the absence of the shunt*, which is called the Effective Blood Flow, EBF.

To calculate a bidirectional shunt, the Fick equation is applied three times to calculate Pulmonary

Blood Flow (PBF), Systemic Blood Flow (SBF) and EBF according to the following equations:

$$PBF = O_2 \, \text{Consumption}/\text{PV-PA } O_2 \, \text{Content}$$
$$SBF = O_2 \, \text{Consumption}/\text{LV-MV } O_2 \, \text{Content}$$
$$EBF = O_2 \, \text{Consumption}/\text{PV-MV } O_2 \, \text{Content}$$

A PV sample is difficult to obtain, and it is customary to assume a saturation of 98%. Note also the change in terminology from Q_p to PBF and from Q_s to SBF. Furthermore, unlike a simple left-to-right shunt calculation, a bidirectional shunt is expressed in terms of differences in absolute flow, instead of flow ratios:

- The left-to-right-shunt is the difference PBF–EBF
- The right-to-left shunt is the difference SBF–EBF

The following data (Table 16.3) from an oximetry run from a patient with Eisenmenger's syndrome demonstrate very low arterial and venous saturations in both systemic and pulmonary systems:

As for the previous example, IVC saturation is higher than SVC, and the average of 3 SVC samples + 1 IVC sample is representative of a true mixed venous sample before the shunt (MV). The sample after the shunt (PA) is the average of PA1 and PA2. Note that here LV saturation is well below 95%.

Table 16.3 Oximetry run from a patient with Eisenmenger's syndrome with a bidirectional shunt, indicated by a low saturation level in the left ventricle

Site	O_2 saturation (%)	O_2 content (Vol%)
SVC1	57.7	15.4
IVC	68.2	18.2
RA high	68.9	18.4
RA medium	71.3	19.0
RA low	69.9	18.7
RV	72.8	19.4
PA1	72.6	19.4
PA2	72.6	19.4
LV	87.9	23.5

Note: Hb, 19.6 g%; O_2 capacity, 26.7 Vol%; Measured O_2 consumption, 252 mL/min.
Abbreviations: SVC, superior vena cava; IVC, inferior vena cava; RA, right atrium; RV, right ventricle; PA, pulmonary artery; LV, left ventricle.

This example demonstrates how the above equations for PBF, SBF, and EBF are used to calculate cross-cardiac flows, from which to determine the size and direction of a bidirectional shunt. Thus, converting Vol% (mL/100 mL) to mL/L and applying the Fick equation using mixed venae cavae samples, and assuming a PV saturation of 98% with a PV content of 26.2 Vol%:

$$PBF = O_2 \, \text{Consumption}/\text{PV-PA } O_2 \, \text{Content}$$
$$= (252/262–194) = 252/68 = 3.7 \, \text{L/min}$$

$$SBF = O_2 \, \text{Consumption}/\text{LV-MV } O_2 \, \text{Content}$$
$$= (252/235–161) = 252/74 = 3.4 \, \text{L/min}$$

$$EBF = O_2 \, \text{Consumption}/\text{PV-MV } O_2 \, \text{Content}$$
$$= (252/262–161) = 252/101 = 2.5 \, \text{L/min}$$

The left-to-right-shunt is the difference PBF–EBF
$$= (3.7–2.5) = 1.2 \, \text{L/min}$$

The right-to-left shunt is the difference
$$SBF–EBF = (3.4–2.5) = 0.9 \, \text{L/min}$$

In this example, the patient has a left-to-right shunt of 1.2 L/min, with a smaller right-to-left shunt of 0.9 L/min.

RIGHT-TO-LEFT SHUNT

If a right-to-left shunt only is suspected, the possibility of a simultaneous left-to-right shunt must be excluded and the full range of calculations must also be undertaken, as for a bidirectional shunt.

With a right-to-left shunt, mixing occurs only into the systemic arterial side, so that arterial saturations are reduced without affecting right heart saturations. If arterial saturations are 90% or less, a right-to-left shunt should be suspected, and a bidirectional shunt should be considered.

In this example, only essential information is provided to permit calculations of flow:

Arterial O_2 Content = 18.5 Vol%

PV O_2 Content = 22.8 Vol%

MV O_2 Content = 10.6 Vol%

PA O_2 Content = 10.6 Vol%

O_2 Consumption = 385 mL/min

Given these data, and converting Vol% (mL/100 mL) to mL/L, the following calculations can be used to determine the shunt:

$$PBF = VO_2/PV\text{-}PA\ O_2\ Content = (385/228\text{--}106)$$
$$= 385/122 = 3.2\ L/min$$

$$SBF = VO_2/LV\text{-}MV\ O_2\ Content$$
$$= (385/185\text{--}106) = 385/79 = 4.9\ L/min$$

$$EBF = VO_2/PV\text{-}MV\ O_2\ Content = (385/228\text{--}106)$$
$$= 385/122 = 3.2\ L/min$$

The left-to-right shunt is the difference PBF–EBF
$$= (3.2\text{--}3.2) = 0\ L/min$$

The right-to-left shunt is the difference SBF–EBF
$$= (4.9\text{--}3.2) = 1.7\ L/min$$

As expected, with a pure right-to-left shunt there is no flow from the systemic to the pulmonary side, so the left-to-right flow is zero mL/min. This occurs because with no right-to-left shunt, MV and PA O_2 content are equal at 10.6 Vol%, and pulmonary blood flow is identical to the effective blood flow (3.2 L/min). In this example, there is a right-to-left shunt from the pulmonary to the systemic side of 1.7 L/min.

Echocardiographic and magnetic resonance imaging methods

It should be noted that it is rare for intracardiac shunts to be detected for the first time at cardiac catheterisation. Diagnosis of intracardiac shunts is now more commonly made by echocardiography. While it has been possible for many years to detect atrial septal defects by peripheral venous injection of agitated saline and observation of some of the resulting bubbles crossing to the left side of the heart, colour Doppler echocardiography has made the detection and localisation of intracardiac shunts a relatively straightforward procedure. Using this technique, the abnormal jet of blood flow across an atrial or ventricular septal defect or across a patent ductus arteriosus can be directly visualised. It is also possible to measure both the CO and the size of an intracardiac shunt using echocardiographic techniques. Total blood flow across any one of the four cardiac valves is equal to the product of the cross-sectional area of the open valve and the velocity-time integral of the blood flow crossing the valve. The cross-sectional area of the annulus of the aortic or pulmonary valve can be determined by two-dimensional echocardiography. It is usual to measure the diameter (D) of the annulus from the cross-sectional image of the valve, then calculate the area as $\Pi D^2/4$. The velocity of blood flow across the valve of interest is measured by the Doppler technique, and displayed as a function of time. The echocardiographic machine permits the area under the velocity-time curve for each systolic period (the velocity-time integral) to be determined automatically after the curve is traced. From the product of cross-sectional area and velocity-time integral measurements, the machine automatically calculates stroke volume. In the presence of a left-to-right intracardiac shunt, the ratio of pulmonary blood flow to systemic blood flow (Q_P/Q_S) is the same as the ratio of the pulmonary stroke volume to the systemic stroke volume and provides an estimate of the shunt size. Alternatively, Q_P and Q_S can be measured with great accuracy non-invasively using 2D phase-contrast cardiac magnetic resonance imaging (MRI).

SUMMARY

While shunt detection and calculations are based routinely on Doppler echocardiography, and phase-contrast cardiac MRI provides a non-invasive gold standard, catheter-based shunt calculations remain important in some situations, particularly for serial measurements in the intensive care setting and when a bidirectional shunt is suspected.

FURTHER READING

Armstrong W, Ryan, T. Haemodynamics. In: *Feigelbaum's Echocardiography*. 7th ed. Philadelphia, PA: Lippincott Williams & Wilkins; 2010. p. 217–240.

Davidson CJ, Bonow RO. Cardiac catheterization. *Heart Disease*. 9th ed. Philadelphia, PA: Saunders Elsevier; 2012. p. 383–405.

Geerts BF, Aarts LP, Jansen JR. Methods in pharmacology: Measurement of cardiac output. *British J Clin Pharmacol*. 2011;71(3):316–330.

Morton Kern M, Clinical Editor. Measurement of Cardiac Output in the Cath Lab: How Accurate is It?: Cath Lab Digest; 2014 Available from: https://www.cathlabdigest.com/articles/Measurement-Cardiac-Output-Cath-Lab-How-Accurate-It.

Moscucci M, Grossman W. Blood flow measurement: Cardiac output and vascular resistance. In: Moscucci M, editor. *Grossman & Baim's Cardiac Catheterization, Angiography, and Intervention*. 8th ed. Philadelphia, PA: Wolters Kluwer/ Lippincott Williams and Wilkins; 2014. p. 245–260.

Ragosta M. *Textbook of Clinical Hemodynamics E-Book* [Internet]. London, UK: Elsevier Health Sciences; 2017. Available from: https://www.elsevier.com/books/ textbook-of-clinical-hemodynamics/ ragosta/978-0-323-48042-0. 56 p.

Venkateshwaran S. Principle of Fick–utilities and limitations. *Kerala Heart J*. 2014;4(2).

17

Analysis and interpretation of Fick and thermodilution cardiac output determinations

GARY J. GAZIBARICH, JOHN EDWARD BOLAND AND LOUIS W. WANG

INTRODUCTION

In the modern cardiac catheterisation laboratory, cardiac output (CO) is predominantly determined using the Thermodilution method, while the direct or indirect Fick method may be preferable in certain situations, such as in severe tricuspid regurgitation, in low cardiac output states or in evaluating intracardiac shunts. In this chapter we discuss use of both methods and their practical application in the cardiac catheterisation laboratory. We use an example to show how to calculate CO by the direct Fick method and examine the underlying physiological principles. We also evaluate both methods and demonstrate our approach to systematically analyse complex thermodilution CO data sets in

conditions where there may be no steady-state (e.g. atrial fibrillation or intermittent pacing), or when CO measurements are inconsistent.

THE FICK METHOD

The two commonly-used methods for determination of cardiac output (CO) are the Fick method and Thermodilution method. Both methods require right heart catheterisation and are based on the original Fick principle, which states that if an indicator substance enters a flowing stream, its concentration at a point downstream is dependent on its concentration before its entry point and the rate of flow of the stream.[1] The Fick method uses a simple mathematical equation to calculate CO, yet the input data convey little understanding or appreciation of the basic underlying physiological principles involved in its application. Thus, although the direct Fick method is regarded as the most accurate method, it is an invasive procedure requiring dedicated equipment and technically demanding measurements that limits its use to highly specialised units such as the cardiac catheterisation laboratory or intensive care unit. It is thus becoming a lost art, and many practitioners would have difficulty in applying it.

The Fick principle

Assumptions of the Fick principle (with oxygen as the indicator substance):

1. The circulation is in a steady-state with equal pulmonary and systemic flows and no intracardiac shunt.
2. Correct anatomical sampling and analysis of blood samples.
3. Correct collection and analysis of the exhaled volume and gas fractions.

When the above assumptions are satisfied, the Fick method is universally accepted as the most reliable measure of CO,[2] and is more accurate than thermodilution during low CO states.[3]

The Fick equation

The Fick equation calculates the pulmonary blood flow required to replenish the oxygen consumed by cellular metabolism and is equal to the volume of oxygen diffusing from the lungs into the pulmonary capillaries per minute divided by the difference in arterial and mixed venous oxygen content, and is calculated as:

$$CO = \frac{VO_2}{CaO_2 - CMvO_2} \qquad (17.1)$$

where CO = Cardiac output (mL/min); VO_2 = Oxygen consumption (mL/min); CaO_2 = Arterial oxygen content (mL/100 mL blood), and $CMvO_2$ = Mixed venous oxygen content

(mL/100 mL blood). The difficulty arises in that none of these parameters can be measured directly and must be derived from other measured variables.

Direct Fick method

There are two main steps involved in calculating CO by the direct Fick method:

COLLECTION AND ANALYSIS OF ARTERIAL AND MIXED VENOUS BLOOD SAMPLES FOR CALCULATION OF OXYGEN CONTENT

An arterial blood sample is collected from the left ventricle, aorta or major systemic artery by left heart cardiac catheterisation or arterial puncture. A mixed venous blood sample is collected from the pulmonary artery by right heart catheterisation. Arterial and mixed venous blood samples are taken mid-way through the exhaled gas collection period (refer next section for collection of exhaled gases).

A blood gas analyser measures the haemoglobin concentration and oxygen saturation of blood samples and this information is used to calculate blood oxygen content.

Blood oxygen content is the total amount of oxygen carried in blood and comprises oxygen bound to haemoglobin plus oxygen dissolved in plasma, and is calculated as:

$$O_2 \text{ Content} = Hb \times 1.36 \times O_2 \text{ sat}\%/100 + 0.0031 \times PO_2 \qquad (17.2)$$

where O_2 Content (mL/100 mL blood), Hb = Haemoglobin concentration (g/100 mL blood), O_2 sat% = Percent oxygen saturation, 0.0031 = Solubility of oxygen in plasma (mL O_2/100 mL blood/mmHg), and PO_2 = Partial pressure of oxygen in blood (mmHg). The binding affinity of oxygen for haemoglobin has reportedly ranged from 1.34–1.39 mL O_2/g Hb.[4] 1.36 mL O_2/g Hb is used in this chapter.

The blood oxygen content calculation can be simplified if the dissolved oxygen is ignored (dissolved oxygen comprises only about 1.5% of the total blood oxygen content[5] to:

$$O_2 \text{ content} = Hb \times 1.36 \times O_2 \text{ sat}\%/100 \qquad (17.3)$$

Table 17.1 Calculation of the oxygen content difference between arterial and mixed venous blood (CaO_2–$CMvO_2$) using the haemoglobin concentration (Hb), percent arterial oxygen saturation ($SaO_2\%$) and percent mixed venous oxygen saturation ($SMvO_2\%$)

Hb concentration	13.3 g/dL
$SaO_2\%$	98.1
$SMvO_2\%$	66.9
CaO_2 content (= Hb × 1.36 × $SaO_2\%$/100)	13.3 × 1.36 × 98.1/100 = 17.8 mL/100 mL
$CMvO_2$ content (= Hb × 1.36 × $SMvO_2\%$/100)	13.3 × 1.36 × 66.9/100 = 12.1 mL/100 mL
CaO_2–$CMvO_2$	17.8–12.1 = 5.7 mL/100 mL

Note: The value 1.36 indicates the volume of oxygen bound to each gram of Hb, and 5.7 mL/100 mL indicates that 5.7 mL of oxygen was extracted by the tissues from every 100 mL of blood.

The haemoglobin concentration (Hb), percent arterial oxygen saturation ($SaO_2\%$) and percent mixed venous oxygen saturation ($SMvO_2\%$) are directly measured and are used to calculate arterial oxygen content (CaO_2) and mixed venous oxygen content ($CMvO_2$). A worked example of how to calculate CaO_2–$CMvO_2$ (the denominator in Equation 17.1) is shown in Table 17.1.

COLLECTION AND ANALYSIS OF EXHALED VOLUME AND GAS FRACTIONS FOR CALCULATION OF VO_2

Traditionally, resting exhaled gases are collected for several minutes in a Douglas bag under ambient pressure, ambient temperature and saturated water vapour conditions (ATPS). A sample of exhaled gas is taken from the Douglas bag and analysed for the percent exhaled oxygen ($FEO_2\%$) and percent exhaled carbon dioxide ($FECO_2\%$) using gas analysers. Exhaled volume is then measured by emptying the Douglas bag through a volume meter, such as a wet-sealed spirometer or gas meter. Minute volume (VE L/min, ATPS) can be calculated by dividing the exhaled volume (L) by the gas collection period (min).

Oxygen consumption (VO_2) is normally expressed under standard temperature (0°C), standard pressure (760 mmHg) and dry gas conditions (STPD), and calculated as:

$$VO_2 \text{ (L/min, STPD)} = \text{True } O_2 \text{ Difference}$$
$$\times \text{ VE (L/min, ATPS)} \times \text{‘ATPS to STPD’ Factor}$$
$$= \text{True } O_2 \text{ Difference} \times \text{VE (L/min, STPD)} \qquad (17.4)$$

where True O_2 difference is the fraction of oxygen consumed from each litre of exhaled air in one minute, and when breathing room air is calculated as:

True O_2 Difference = $0.265 - 1.265 \times FEO_2 - 0.265 \times FECO_2$ (see Appendix 1 for derivation).[6] 'ATPS to STPD' factor is the volume conversion factor from ATPS to STPD conditions and can be calculated or obtained from published tables.

For practical applications, VO_2 (mL/min, STPD) can be calculated using either of two different equations:

$$VO_2 \text{ (mL/min, STPD)} = \text{True } O_2 \text{ Difference}$$
$$\times \text{ VE (L/min, STPD)} \times 1000 \qquad (17.5)$$

$$VO_2 \text{ (mL/min, STPD)} = O_2\% \text{ Difference}$$
$$\times \text{ VE (L/min, STPD)} \times 10 \qquad (17.6)$$

where $O_2\%$ Difference = $0.265 \times FEN_2\% - FEO_2\%$

Traditionally, cardiac technicians prefer equation (17.5) because it permits easier operation with a handheld calculator. A worked example of VO_2 calculations using Equations (17.4) and (17.5) is shown in Tables 17.2 and 17.3. The $O_2\%$, $CO_2\%$ and $N_2\%$ in exhaled gas varies from patient to patient (see Table 17.4).

VO_2 data can also be calculated breath-by-breath using modern computerised lung function testing systems. These sophisticated systems provide accurate, real-time data but require calibration and are expensive, which usually limits their use to research studies.

It is generally accepted that the accuracy of the Fick method is approximately 10%.[1]

Table 17.2 Calculation of oxygen consumption (VO_2, mL/min) for a 73 year old male patient who was at rest and exhaled 20 L of air into a Douglas bag over two minutes at a barometric pressure of 762 mmHg and ambient temperature of 20°C

Demographics	Patient Height: 165 cm, Weight: 88 kg, Age: 73 years, Sex: Male
Minute volume	VE (L/min, ATPS) = Exhaled Volume (L, ATPS)/Collection Period (min) = 20.0/2.0 = 10.0 VE (L/min, STPD) = VE (L/min, ATPS) × 'ATPS to STPD' factor = 10.0 × 0.9120 = 9.12
True O_2 difference	= 0.265−(1.265 × FEO$_2$%/100)−(0.265 × FECO$_2$%/100) = 0.265−1.265 × 18.3/100−0.265 × 2.3/100 = 0.02741
O_2% difference	= (0.265 × FEN2%−FEO2%) × 9.12 × 10 = (0.265 × (100−18.3−2.3)−18.3) × 9.12 × 10 = 2.741
VO_2	Using equation (17.5) = True O_2 difference × VE (L/min, STPD) × 1000 = 0.02741 × 9.12 × 1000 = 250 mL/min Using equation (17.6) = O_2% difference × VE (L/min, STPD) × 10 = 2.741 × 9.12 × 10 = 250 mL/min

Note: A sample of collected gas was analysed and showed a FEO$_2$% = 18.3 and FECO$_2$% = 2.3. ATPS to STPD conversion factor = 0.9120, obtained from published tables. [ATPS = ambient temperature (20°C), barometric pressure (762 mmHg) and saturated with water vapour (17.5 mmHg at 20°C); STPD = standard temperature (0°C), standard pressure (760 mmHg) and dry gas; FEO$_2$% = percent exhaled oxygen gas; FECO$_2$% = percent exhaled carbon dioxide gas; FEN$_2$% = percent exhaled nitrogen gas = 100−FEO$_2$%−FECO$_2$%].

Table 17.3 Cardiac Output calculation by the direct Fick method using CaO_2, $CMvO_2$ and VO_2 data from Tables 17.1 and 17.2

Cardiac Output	= VO_2/(CaO_2 − $CMvO_2$) = (250 mL O_2/min)/(17.8 − 12.1) mL O_2/100 mL blood = 250/5.7 × O_2 content blood volume = 43.9 × 100 mL/min = 4390 mL/min = 4.4 L/min

Note: This calculation shows that 43.9 units of blood were required to supply the body with the oxygen it consumed (250 mL/min), where 1 unit of blood equals 100 mL CaO_2 and $CMvO_2$ are expressed in mL O_2/100 mL blood, and VO_2 in mL O_2/min. O_2 content blood volume = Volume of blood used in CaO_2 and $CMvO_2$ determinations is 100 mL.

Table 17.4 Example of the composition of inhaled gases (Room Air) and exhaled gases from two patients undergoing cardiac catheterisation with Douglas bag collection by the direct Fick method

	Inhaled gases Room Air	Exhaled gases Patient 1	Exhaled gases Patient 2
$O_2\%$	20.93	18.3	18.6
$CO_2\%$	0.03	2.3	1.4
$N_2\%$	79.04	79.4	80.0
TOTAL	100.0	100.0	100.0

Note: Only oxygen and carbon dioxide participate in alveolar gas exchange; nitrogen and trace amounts of other gases do not. When the percent oxygen ($O_2\%$) and percent carbon dioxide ($CO_2\%$) of gas samples are measured, the percent of nitrogen and trace amounts of other gases (labelled as $N_2\%$) can be calculated as '$100 - O_2\% - CO_2\%$' for both inhaled and exhaled gases. Patient 1 is the same patient used in Table 17.2.

Indirect Fick method

An alternative to the direct Fick is the indirect Fick method, where one or more variables in the Fick equation is estimated rather than measured. VO_2 is estimated from nomograms involving basal metabolic rate or formulae based on patient height, weight, age and sex.[7] The disadvantage of the indirect Fick method is that it can introduce potentially large errors into the Fick calculation.[8,9] In the example in Table 17.2, a predicted VO_2 of 230 mL/min can be obtained from nomograms for a patient height (165 cm), weight (88 kg), age (73 years) and sex (Male). Using the predicted VO_2 for this patient (230 mL/min), CO would be 4.0 L/min (= 230/5.7 × 100 = 4035 mL/min = 4.035 L/min) instead of 4.4 L/min obtained from the direct Fick method. A difference of 0.4 L/min (<10%) can be tolerated but greater differences are common, particularly in obese patients.[9]

Modern cardiac catheterisation laboratory monitoring systems and even cellular phone applications can derive VO_2 or CO using actual or assumed data. Two commonly used equations for estimating VO_2 are the Lafarge-Mettienen and the Bergstra et al. equations, which correct for factors such as heart rate, age, or sex.[7] Although not recommended, it is possible to assume additional factors for individual patients, e.g. $SaO_2\%$ can be estimated by pulse oximetry and

$CaO_2 - CMvO_2$ can be assumed as 5 mL/100 mL in healthy patients and 3 mL/100 mL in critically ill patients.[10] Inserting these assumed values into the Fick equation introduces greater error and should be avoided. There is no widely accepted technique of estimating $SMvO_2\%$ non-invasively.

Limitations and reliability of the Fick method

Blood analysis: Potential sources of error with the Fick method arise from inaccuracies in analysis of blood samples by oximetry, either from sampling variations due to improper blood collection, streamlining of flow through the cardiac chambers, unknown congenital defects, or possible haemoglobin abnormalities.[1]

Steady-state conditions: The Fick method assumes a steady metabolic state during the period of blood and lung gas collection, which may not always be the case.

VO_2 differences: In low-output states the arterio-venous oxygen difference is greater, and the more accurate is the calculation of VO_2. Thus, inaccuracies may arise in conditions with very high CO where the arterio-venous oxygen difference is low.

Assuming VO_2: Using the indirect Fick method and applying an assumed VO_2 in the Fick equation can introduce considerable error.[8,9]

Valvular regurgitation

The Fick method estimates forward blood flow from the left ventricle based on differences in oxygen saturation between pulmonary and systemic arteries, and is not affected by backwards or regurgitant flow that would occur in the presence of aortic, mitral or tricuspid valve insufficiency. This backwards flow reduces the overall net forward output (net flow = forward minus backward flow) but has no effect on oxygen saturation and therefore does not affect the Fick calculation.

THERMODILUTION METHOD

Given pulmonary flow equals systemic flow in the normal heart, it is possible to measure CO by thermodilution in the pulmonary artery. The thermodilution method is now more commonly performed in the cardiac catheterisation laboratory than the direct or indirect Fick method. Thermodilution also relies on the Fick principle with a specified amount of thermal indicator (A) injected rapidly at one point in the circulation and the concentration (C) of the indicator then measured continuously as a function of time (t) at some point downstream from the injection site. Assuming all of the indicator (A) passes the measurement site, blood flow can be calculated by a modification of the Stewart-Hamilton equation:

$$Q = A/\int C(t)dt \qquad (17.7)$$

where the denominator is the integral of concentration with respect to time for the period of time taken for all the indicator to pass the measurement point for the first time. The integral of this first pass represents the area under the washout curve. Correct application of the thermodilution technique calls for at least three rapid injections of a 10 mL bolus of cold saline (at room temperature, or no less than 10°C below body temperature).

Limitations and reliability of the thermodilution method

Loss of indicator: Loss of thermal indicator can result in a falsely elevated thermodilution CO. If some indicator entering the circulation is lost, or if a smaller volume than the predetermined amount is injected, the reduction in heat transfer can lead to a smaller change in blood temperature, resulting in a smaller area under the curve and overestimation of CO.

Indicator temperature: Theoretically, the greater the difference between injectate and body temperature, the more accurate the thermodilution CO is likely to be. The actual effect on CO measurement, although variable, is not significant.

Transient lowering of heart rate during cold indicator injection: The heart rate can transiently lower during cold indicator injection, which can potentially reduce the measured thermodilution CO.

Cyclic changes in CO: Spontaneous or mechanical ventilation affect the actual CO, with stroke output variations, particularly in the right ventricle. For these reasons there is more variance in thermodilution measurements and therefore repeated, multiple measurements are recommended.

Valvular regurgitation

The thermodilution method, by its very nature, calculates forward flow in the pulmonary artery. Its precision is compromised by tricuspid (but not by mitral or aortic) regurgitation, and it fails to quantify regurgitant flow across an incompetent tricuspid valve. As a cold saline bolus is injected into the right atrium, the effect of tricuspid insufficiency and associated backwards flow is to reduce the transient cooling of surrounding blood, resulting in a smaller change in distal temperature and a prolonged thermodilution curve. As CO is inversely related to the temperature change (and to the area under the curve), the calculated CO is reduced. Thus, severe tricuspid regurgitation is associated with underestimation of thermodilution CO.[11]

THE GORLIN EQUATION

The simplified Gorlin equation[12] requires total blood flow (forward CO plus regurgitant flow) to accurately derive cardiac valve areas. Since the Fick and thermodilution methods both measure only forward flow, using these in the Gorlin equation may provide inaccurate estimates of cardiac valve area in cases of severe tricuspid or mitral regurgitation.

INTRACARDIAC SHUNTS

Shunt calculations are not accurate with thermodilution, as estimation of CO in the pulmonary artery is affected by left-to-right or right-to-left blood flow across an anatomical defect. In the presence of an intracardiac shunt, outputs from the left and right heart are no longer equal, and the pulmonary blood flow (Qp) and systemic blood flow (Qs) must be determined separately. With a simple left-to-right shunt the shunt is expressed as the shunt ratio (Qp/Qs).

With a bi-directional shunt (combined left-to-right and right-to-left shunts) the effective blood flow (Qeff, the theoretical flow that would naturally occur without the shunt) must also be calculated (see Chapter 16). All these flows can be calculated by the direct Fick method using the following equations:

$$Qp = VO_2/(CpvO_2 - CpaO_2) \qquad (17.8)$$

$$Qs = VO_2/(CsaO_2 - CvO_2) \qquad (17.9)$$

$$Qeff = VO_2/(CpvO_2 - CvO_2) \qquad (17.10)$$

Where VO_2 = oxygen consumption, $CpvO_2$ = oxygen content of pulmonary venous blood, $CpaO_2$ = oxygen content of pulmonary arterial blood, $CsaO_2$ = oxygen content of arterial blood, and CvO_2 = venous oxygen content of blood collected from the chamber (right ventricle, right atrium or vena cavae for left-to-right shunts) immediately proximal (before) the shunt.[13]

The left to right shunt equals Qp − Qeff and the right-to-left shunt equals Qs − Qeff.

CLINICAL EXAMPLES OF THERMODILUTION STUDIES

To accurately assess a patient's resting cardiac function, CO measurements should be performed in a short time interval (preferably within 5 minutes), under steady-state resting conditions and without compromising patient safety and comfort. Current guidelines recommend reporting CO as the average of at least three measurements.[14,2] The precision of triplicate CO measurements ranges from 10%–20% of the average CO.[2]

Imprecise CO determinations are more likely under non-steady-state conditions, as with arrhythmias like atrial fibrillation or intermittent pacing, or with a restless or non-compliant patient. It is not always possible to perform additional measurements to match CO values because of patient safety concerns e.g. potential volume overload in patients with severe pulmonary hypertension. The challenge is to provide the clinician with relevant data to guide patient therapy when the assumed measurement conditions are not satisfied.

Our approach to analysing CO data builds on current guidelines in order to improve the accuracy and precision of the reported CO for variable or complex CO data sets. We demonstrate our approach using thermodilution CO data collected in cases from a variety of clinical conditions, including atrial fibrillation, intermittent pacing and tricuspid regurgitation. CO data are shown in Table 17.5. A summary of our approach is presented below, followed by analysis of cases.

We typically record between three and five technically acceptable CO measurements and report the average CO from three representative CO values. The representative CO values are assumed to be the values closest to the average CO, with other values treated as outliers. Excluding outliers from data analysis increases the precision of the reported CO values.

According to our systematic approach, only three measurements are required when all CO values are within 10% of the average CO for the first three measurements (Repeatability Range).

For three measurements, the reported CO is the average CO from the first three measurements (Mean First 3) for both the current guidelines and our approach (see Case 1). When at least one of the CO values in the first three measurements lies outside the Repeatability Range (see Cases 2–7) then one or two additional measurements are recorded.

If four measurements are recorded, the CO value furthest from the Mean First 3 is excluded, and the Revised CO is the average CO from the remaining three measurements (see Case 4).

If five measurements are recorded, the smallest and largest CO values are excluded, and the Revised CO is the average CO from the remaining three measurements (see Cases 2, 5, 7).

Table 17.5 Analysis of bolus thermodilution cardiac output (CO) data in 7 patients undergoing pulmonary artery catheterisation for various clinical conditions

Case	HR	Recorded CO data (L/min)	Mean first 3 (L/min)	Repeatability Range (L/min)	Revised CO (L/min)
1.	52	**3.84**,[a] **3.80, 3.75**	3.80	3.42–4.18	3.80 (n = 3)
2. AF	75–96	5.54, **6.70, 6.72**, 6.73, 5.72	6.32	5.69–6.95	6.38 (n = 5, Range 5.72–6.72)
3. Pacing	60	2.93, 3.61 paced	n/a	n/a	3.27 (n = 2, Range 2.93–3.61)
	22	1.52 un-paced	n/a	n/a	1.52 (n = 1)
	22–55	2.56, 2.40 mixed	n/a	n/a	2.48 (n = 2)
4.	86–90	**5.75**, 6.26, 4.63, **5.86**	5.55	4.99–6.10	5.96 (n = 4)
5.	64	**2.7, 2.8**, 3.3, 3.3, 2.5	2.93	2.64–3.23	2.93 (n = 5, Range 2.7–3.3)
6. TR	49	3.3, 4.2, **3.8**	3.77	3.39–4.14	3.77 (n = 3, Range 3.3–4.2)
7.	98–106	6.7, 3.9, 4.5, 4.1, 4.5	5.03	4.53–5.54	4.37 (n = 5)

[a] Bold text denotes CO values for measurements 1–3 that lie within the Repeatability Range.

Abbreviations: HR, heart rate (beats/min); Recorded CO data, Technically acceptable CO data for up to 5 measurements; Mean First 3, Reported CO using current guidelines and is equal to the average CO from the first 3 measurements; Repeatability Range, Range of CO values within 10% of the Mean First 3; Revised CO, Reported CO using our approach and is equal to the average CO from representative measurements (i.e. middle values of the data set); n, number of measurements recorded; Range, modified CO data range reported for inconsistent CO values (i.e. Representative CO values >10% difference from the Revised CO); AF, atrial fibrillation; TR, tricuspid regurgitation. Refer to text for further details.

If only one, two or more inconsistent CO measurements are recorded, all measurements are averaged to obtain the Revised CO (see Cases 3, 6).

For all cases, we report the number of measurements recorded (n) as a guide to the precision of the final measurement. For inconsistent CO values, we also report the modified CO data range (i.e. smallest and largest CO values used to calculate the Revised CO).

Case 1: This case represents the ideal situation where three consecutive measurements were performed within two minutes, and all CO values were in the Repeatability Range. Mean First 3 and Revised CO were both calculated as the average CO from the three measurements and equal to 3.80 L/min.

Case 2: With atrial fibrillation, measurement of CO may be associated with a variable number of measurements, and some operators calculate the reported CO as the average CO from all measurements. For Case 2, the average CO from the five measurements was equal to 6.28 L/min. Using our approach, Mean First 3 was 6.32 L/min and only two measurements were in the Repeatability

Range. Two additional measurements were recorded. The lowest and highest CO values (5.54 from trial 1 & 6.73 from trial 4, respectively) were excluded, and the Revised CO (6.38) was the average CO from the remaining three measurements (CO values 6.70, 6.72 & 5.72). Given the inconsistent CO values used to determine the Revised CO (i.e. CO = 5.72 was −10.3% from the Revised CO), the Range 5.72–6.72 L/min was added to the report.

For this case, the reported CO using all measurements (6.28), Mean First 3 (6.32), and Revised CO (6.38) were similar. Our approach also reported the modified CO data range to flag the inconsistent CO data set.

Case 3: Intermittent pacing from a permanent pacemaker allowed paced, unpaced and mixed measurements to be recorded. In this situation, all CO values were useful to the clinician. For pacing at HR = 60 bpm, the Revised CO (3.27) was obtained from two inconsistent CO values (2.93 and 3.61 which were 10.4% from the Revised CO) and the Range 2.93–3.61 L/min was added to the report. For unpaced, the Revised CO (1.52) was obtained from one trial. For mixed pacing, the

Revised CO (2.48) was obtained from two measurements with consistent CO values of 2.56 and 2.40 L/min. Mean First 3 was not applicable.

Case 4: Using our approach, Mean First 3 was 5.55 L/min and only one CO value was in the Repeatability Range. One additional trial was recorded. On data review, trial 3 (CO value 4.63) was excluded, and the Revised CO (5.96) was the average CO from measurements 1, 2 and 4 with consistent CO values of 5.75, 6.26 and 5.86 L/min.

Mean First 3 was 0.42 L/min lower than the Revised CO. Given the CO value for trial 3 was much lower than the other measurements, this suggested that Mean First 3 underestimated the true CO.

Case 5: This was a pre-operative assessment with a wide range of CO values. The reported CO may influence suitability for surgery and careful consideration was given on the selection of the reported CO. Using our approach, Mean First 3 was 2.93 L/min and only two measurements were in the Repeatability Range. Two additional measurements were recorded. The average CO from all 5 measurements was 2.92 L/min. The lowest and highest CO values (2.5 from trial 5 & 3.3 from trial 4, respectively) were excluded, and the Revised CO (2.93) was the average of the remaining three measurements (CO values 2.7, 2.8 & 3.3). Given the inconsistent CO values (CO= 3.3 was +12.5% from the Revised CO), the Range 2.7–3.3 L/min was added to the report.

On data review, it appeared the true CO may be somewhere within the range of 2.50–3.30 L/min. No significant difference in reported CO was evident among averaging all five measurements (2.92), Mean First 3 (2.93) and Revised CO (2.93). This case demonstrated the difficulty in finding a single representative CO value when there was a wide scatter in CO values, and any reported CO close to the mid-range CO (2.9) was considered reasonable. Our approach reported the modified CO data range in order to assist with surgical considerations for this patient.

Case 6: These values were obtained for a patient with mild tricuspid insufficiency, where the thermodilution method may underestimate the true CO. Using our approach, Mean First 3 was 3.77 L/min and only one trial was in the Repeatability Range.

No additional measurements were recorded. Revised CO (3.77) was the average of all three measurements (CO values 3.3, 4.2 and 3.8). Given the inconsistent CO values (CO = 3.3 was −12.4% from the Revised CO), the Range 3.3–4.2 L/min was added to the report.

There was no difference in the reported CO for the Mean First 3 and Revised CO. Our approach reported the modified CO data range for the inconsistent CO data set.

Case 7: Using our approach, Mean First 3 was 5.03 L/min and no CO values were in the Repeatability Range. Two additional measurements were recorded. The average CO of all five measurements was 4.74 L/min. The lowest and highest CO values (3.9 from trial 2 and 6.7 from trial 1, respectively) were excluded, and the Revised CO (4.37) was the average of the remaining three measurements with consistent CO values of 4.5, 4.1 and 4.5 L/min.

On data review, the average CO using all five measurements was 0.37 L/min higher than our approach. Given the CO for trial 1 appeared much larger than any other trial, the average CO for all 5 measurements presumably overestimated the true CO. Since Mean First 3 included trial 1 it also overestimated the true CO. Note that such a disparity between consecutive samples is not uncommon and may be due to sudden changes in heart rate or rhythm, or other factors such as patient discomfort.

The preceding cases demonstrate the difficulty of adhering to strict guidelines and that following our systematic approach in the analysis of inconsistent CO data sets provides valuable scientific and clinical information. In all situations the challenge is to provide the most accurate and precise data to assist the clinician in guiding therapy.

SUMMARY

The direct Fick method remains the gold standard for accurate CO determination. Yet, practical constraints such as time, personnel training and expertise, availability of instrumentation, patient comfort and immediate results favour use of thermodilution. Advantages of thermodilution over Fick are its comparative simplicity, repeatability, low cost and ease of use, and ability to conduct pre- and post-interventions in clinical studies, whereas the Fick method is preferable to evaluate flow in intracardiac shunts, in severe tricuspid incompetence and in low output states. Understanding the principles and limitations behind these methods is essential for the correct calculation and interpretation of right heart investigations. Our systematic analysis for thermodilution studies provides a practical guide to enhance current guidelines in the reporting of CO for inconsistent CO data sets.

APPENDIX

Derivation of True O_2 difference. True O_2 difference is the fraction of oxygen consumed from each litre of exhaled air in one minute.

Glossary

VIN_2 inhaled volume of nitrogen (and trace amounts of other inert gases)

VEN_2 exhaled volume of nitrogen (and trace amounts of other inert gases)

FIN_2 dry gas fraction of inhaled nitrogen (and trace amounts of other inert gases)

FEN_2 dry gas fraction of exhaled nitrogen (and trace amounts of other inert gases)

VI inhaled volume

VE exhaled volume

FIO_2 dry gas fraction of inhaled oxygen = 0.2093 = 20.93%

$FICO_2$ dry gas fraction of inhaled carbon dioxide = 0.0003 = 0.03% (assumed as 0 in calculations)

FEO_2 dry gas fraction of exhaled oxygen

$FECO_2$ dry gas fraction of exhaled carbon dioxide

VO_2 (vol) volume of oxygen consumed

VIO_2 volume of inhaled oxygen

VEO_2 volume of exhaled oxygen

According to the law of conservation of mass, the volumes of inhaled and exhaled nitrogen (and other inert gases) are equal, and can be mathematically expressed as:

$$VIN_2 = VEN_2. \qquad (17.11)$$

$$FIN_2 \times VI = FEN_2 \times VE. \qquad (17.12)$$

Solve (17.12) for VI

$$VI = (FEN_2/FIN_2) \times VE. \qquad (17.13)$$

The sum of the inhaled and exhaled dry gas fractions equals 1 (water vapour is removed prior to gas analysis), and can be mathematically expressed as:

$$FIO_2 + FICO_2 + FIN_2 = 1. \qquad (17.14)$$

$$FEO_2 + FECO_2 + FEN_2 = 1. \qquad (17.15)$$

Solving (17.14) and (17.15) for FIN_2 and FEN_2, respectively:

$$FIN_2 = 1 - FIO_2 - FICO_2. \qquad (17.16)$$

$$FEN_2 = 1 - FEO_2 - FECO_2. \qquad (17.17)$$

Substituting (17.16) and (17.17) in (17.13):

$$VI = [(1 - FEO_2 - FECO_2)/(1 - FIO_2 - FICO_2)] \times VE. \qquad (17.18)$$

Volume of oxygen consumed = inhaled oxygen volume − exhaled oxygen volume, and can be mathematically expressed as:

$$VO_2 \text{ (vol)} = VIO_2 - VEO_2. \qquad (17.19)$$

$$VO_2 \text{ (vol)} = FIO_2 \times VI - FEO_2 \times VE. \qquad (17.20)$$

Substituting (17.18) in (17.20):

$$VO_2 \text{ (vol)} = FIO_2 \times [(1 - FEO_2 - FECO_2)/(1 - FIO_2 - FICO_2)] \times VE - FEO_2 \times VE. \qquad (17.21)$$

$$VO_2 \text{ (vol)} = \{FIO_2 \times [(1 - FEO_2 - FECO_2)/(1 - FIO_2 - FICO_2)] - FEO_2\} \times VE. \qquad (17.22)$$

Assuming $FICO_2 = 0$, (17.22) simplifies to:

$$VO_2 \text{ (vol)} = \{FIO_2 \times [(1 - FEO_2 - FECO_2)/(1 - FIO_2)] - FEO_2\} \times VE. \qquad (17.23)$$

$$VO_2\ (vol) = \{FIO_2/(1-FIO_2) \times$$
$$[(1-FEO_2-FECO_2)- $$
$$(1-FIO_2) \times$$
$$FEO_2]\} \times VE. \qquad (17.24)$$

$$VO_2\ (vol) = \{1/(1-FIO_2) \times$$
$$[(FIO_2-FIO_2 \times FEO_2-FIO_2$$
$$\times FECO_2)-FEO_2 + FIO_2 \times$$
$$FEO_2]\} \times VE. \qquad (17.25)$$

$$VO_2\ (vol) = \{1/(1-FIO_2) \times$$
$$(FIO_2-FIO_2 \times FECO_2$$
$$-FEO_2)\} \times VE. \qquad (17.26)$$

Rearranging terms in (17.26):

$$VO_2\ (vol) = \{(FIO_2-FEO_2-$$
$$FIO_2 \times FECO_2)/$$
$$(1-FIO_2)\} \times VE. \qquad (17.27)$$

True O_2 difference is the mathematical expression in curly brackets in (17.27):

$$True\ O_2\ difference = (FIO_2-FEO_2-$$
$$FIO_2 \times FECO_2)/$$
$$(1-FIO_2). \qquad (17.28)$$

Substituting $FIO_2 = 0.2093$,
$$and\ 1-FIO_2 = 1-0.2093 =$$
$$0.7907\ in \qquad (17.29)$$

$$True\ O_2\ difference =$$
$$(0.2093-FEO_2-0.2093 \times$$
$$FECO_2)/0.7907. \qquad (17.30)$$

$$True\ O_2\ difference =$$
$$[0.2093/0.7907]-$$
$$[FEO_2/0.7907]-$$
$$[0.2093 \times FECO_2/$$
$$0.7907]. \qquad (17.31)$$

$$True\ O_2\ difference =$$
$$0.265-[1.265 \times$$
$$FEO_2]- [0.265 \times$$
$$FECO_2]. \qquad (17.32)$$

REFERENCES

1. Moscucci M, Grossman W. Blood flow measurement: Cardiac output and vascular resistance. In: Moscucci, M, editor. Grossman & Baim's Cardiac Catheterization, Angiography, and Intervention, 8th ed. Philadelphia, PA: Wolters Kluwer/ Lippincott Williams and Wilkins; 2014. p. 245–260.
2. Geerts BF, Aarts LP, Jansen JR. Methods in pharmacology: Measurement of cardiac output. Br J Clin Pharmacol. 2011;71(3):316–330.
3. van Grondelle A, Ditchey RV, Groves BM, Wagner WW Jr, Reeves JT. Thermodilution method overestimates low cardiac output in humans. Am J Physiol. 1983;245(4):H690–H692.
4. Lumb AB. The oxygenation of blood. In: Andrew B. Lumb, editor. Nunn's Applied Respiratory Physiology. 5th ed (p. 264). Oxford, UK: Butterworth-Heinnemann; 2006. p. 687.
5. Cotes J, Chinn D, Miller M. The oxygenation of blood. Lung function: Physiology, Measurement and Application in Medicine, 6th ed. 2006:258–274.
6. Gregory I. The oxygen and carbon monoxide capacities of foetal and adult blood. J Physiol. 1974;236(3):625–634.
7. Bergstra A, Van Den Heuvel A, Zijlstra F, Berger R, Mook G, Van Veldhuisen D. Validation of fick cardiac output calculated with assumed oxygen consumption: A study of cardiac output during epoprostenol. Neth Heart J. 2004;12(5):208–213.
8. Narang N, Gore MO, Snell PG, Ayers CR, Lorenzo S, Carrick-Ranson G, et al. Accuracy of estimating resting oxygen uptake and implications for hemodynamic assessment. Am J Cardiol. 2012;109(4):594–598.
9. Narang N, Thibodeau JT, Levine BD, Gore MO, Ayers CR, Lange RA, et al. Inaccuracy of estimated resting oxygen uptake in the clinical setting. Circulation. 2013;129(2):203–210.
10. Reske AW, Costa EL, Reske AP, Rau A, Borges JB, Beraldo MA, et al. Bedside estimation of nonaerated lung tissue using blood gas analysis. Crit Care Med. 2013;41(3):732–743.
11. Martin B, Jan P, Jan H. Effect of the degree of tricuspid regurgitation on cardiac output measurements by thermodilution. Intensive Care Med. 2002;28(8):1117–1121.

12. Hakki AH, Iskandrian AS, Bemis CE, Kimbiris D, Mintz GS, Segal BL, et al. A simplified valve formula for the calculation of stenotic cardiac valve areas. *Circulation.* 1981;63(5):1050–1055.

13. Grossman W, Moscucci M. Shunt detection and quantification. In: Moscucci M, editor. *Grossman & Baim's Cardiac Catheterization, Angiography, and Intervention*, 8th ed. Philadelphia, PA: Wolters Kluwer/Lippincott Williams and Wilkins; 2014. p. 261–271.

14. Galiè N, Humbert M, Vachiery JL, Gibbs JS, IL, Torbicki A, et al. Guidelines for the diagnosis and treatment of pulmonary hypertension: The task force for the diagnosis and treatment of pulmonary hypertension of the European Society of Cardiology (ESC) and the European Respiratory Society (ERS), endorsed by: Association for European Paediatric and Congenital Cardiology (AEPC), International Society of Heart and Lung Transplantation (ISHLT). *Eur Heart J.* 2016;37(1):67–119.

18

Pressure-volume loops: Background theory with practical examples

PANKAJ JAIN AND CHRISTOPHER S. HAYWARD

INTRODUCTION: BACKGROUND

Otto Frank was one of the first physiologists to apply muscle physiology to the heart in a systematic way.[1] Because geometric differences in fibre orientation compared to isolated muscle strips makes assessment of individual fibre shortening difficult, Frank recognised that the description of cardiac function in simple terms of time-varying parameters such as pressure or volume was inadequate. Studying the frog ventricle, Frank described cardiac chamber or pump function in terms of simultaneous pressure (P) and volume (V)—*independent of time*. Such pressure-volume (P-V) relationships were initially referred to as 'work' diagrams, referring to the work performed by the heart on the blood.[2] Once difficulties in the continuous measurement of ventricular volume were overcome[2,3] (pressure recordings having been mastered earlier),

a new era of cardiovascular physiology based on the analysis of P-V loops began.[4–9]

As seen in Figure 18.1, the P-V loop is performed anti-clockwise. Starting at the onset of contraction (or end-diastole, A) pressure can be seen to increase with little change in volume. This phase (AB) corresponds to left ventricular isovolumic contraction. At 'B' the aortic valve opens and cardiac ejection commences. There is dominant decrease in volume with a small variable increase in left ventricular pressure. The shape of the loop during ejection is dependent on the interaction of cardiac ejection with arterial characteristics.[11] At 'C', the end of systole, the left ventricle starts to relax with a rapid fall in pressure and little change in volume (CD, isovolumic relaxation). At 'D' the left ventricle starts to fill until atrial systole ('E') occurs, completing left ventricular filling and the cardiac cycle.

DEFINITION OF SYSTOLIC FUNCTION USING P-V LOOPS

From a series of variably preloaded P-V loops, three related indices of chamber function can be derived. They are the end-systolic P-V relationship (ESPVR), the preload recruitable stroke work relationship (PRSWR), and the dP/dt_{max}-end-diastolic volume (EDV) relationship. Each is derived from simultaneous, continuous measurement of pressure and volume during alteration in cardiac loading conditions by decreasing preload (usually by occlusion of the inferior vena cava[12–15]), or increasing afterload (usually pharmacologically by phenylephrine). IVC occlusion has the advantage that a large, rapid change in loading conditions can be achieved before sympathetic reflex responses are evident. It has been shown that methods that increase afterload are associated with a reflex increase in contractility.[12,16–18]

Continuous left ventricular volumes may be obtained using a conductance catheter,[12,13,19] from ultrasonic crystals deriving volume from orthogonal pairs of crystals,[20] from radionuclide ventriculography,[21] magnetic resonance imaging, or three-dimensional echocardiography. By obtaining such on-line recordings, ESPVRs have been extensively used to define inotropic effects of drugs[14,22–26] and ischaemia,[27–29] as well as the effects of ventricular remodelling in cardiomyoplasty.[30]

Derivation of the end-systolic P-V relationship

The ratio of simultaneous pressure and volume defines the elastance (the inverse of compliance, or stiffness) of the ventricle. It can be shown that this increases to a maximum during systole and then decreases to a low value during diastole.[8] If cardiac function is examined in terms of ventricular elastance, end-systole may be defined as the point at which elastance reaches a maximum.[31] This corresponds to point 'C' on the P-V loop diagram shown in Figure 18.1.

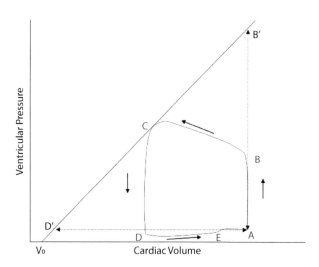

Figure 18.1 Schematic of generation pressure-volume (P-V) loops and an idealised end-systolic P-V relationship (ESPVR). The P-V cycle is performed anticlockwise. Isovolumic contraction begins at 'A' and continues until 'B' when the aortic valve opens and cardiac ejection commences. Following end-systole, 'C', there is a period of isovolumic relaxation, (CD). At 'D' the left ventricle starts to fill until atrial systole ('E') occurs, completing left ventricular filling and the cardiac cycle. AB` and AD` represent hypothetical P-V trajectories generated by isometric and isotonic contractions respectively. The line B`CD` represents the idealised ESPVR. (Modified from Sagawa, K. et al., *Cardiac Contraction and the Pressure-Volume Relationship*, New York, 1988.)

The distinction of end-systole from end-ejection may not be great under normal conditions, but does become significant in situations of elevated afterload, as may occur with aging or hypertension.[31,32] The linear ESPVR is then calculated from a series of end-systolic points under varying load (Figure 18.2).[7-9,33]

The slope of the line is termed the end-systolic elastance (Ees) and the extrapolated intercept, V_0, the volume at zero pressure. An increase in Ees has been interpreted as an increase in ventricular chamber performance,[34] an increase in contractility,[4,35] and an increase in preload sensitivity.[36] One problem with the ESPVR is that it is sensitive to ventricular size.[6,34,37] To account for this, various normalising techniques have been suggested, including normalising to left ventricular mass,[38] end-diastolic volume,[6] or body surface area.[4,21,33] Many commentators, however, are not satisfied that current normalisation techniques have achieved their aim.[37] The ESPVR differs from preload recruitable stroke work (PRSW, discussed subsequently) in this respect.[28,39]

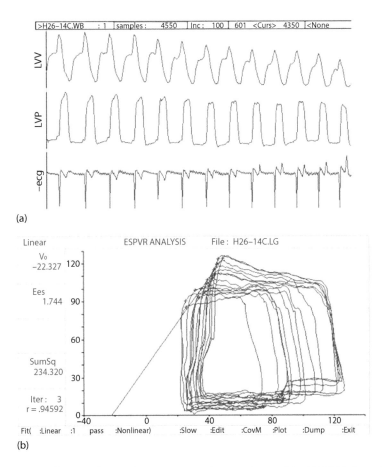

(a)

(b)

Figure 18.2 Derivation of the end-systolic pressure-volume relationship (ESPVR) from inferior vena caval (IVC) occlusion using pressure-volume analysis software. The raw data (a) shows a gradual decrease in both left ventricular pressure (LVP) and volume (LVV). The ESPVR is calculated by linear regression of the end-systolic points ($r = 0.95$ in this study). The gradual decrease in the size of loops during IVC occlusion is seen in (b).

Preload-recruitable stroke work relationship (PRSWR)

PRSWR is the relationship between stroke work and end-diastolic volume, and an extension of the Frank-Starling concept.[20,40,41] The PRSWR is highly linear. Stroke work will increase in a linear fashion with increased preload when preload is defined by end-diastolic volume rather than filling pressure. The non-linear relationship between stroke work and end-diastolic pressure (EDP) reflects the non-linearity of the relationship between EDP and end-diastolic volume.[20] The degree to which stroke work increases with end-diastolic volume (the slope of the relation, often termed M_{SW}) is dependent on the contractility of the ventricle[20] and is independent of heart rate and size.[39] The independence from size contrasts with ESPVR, and allows better comparison of subject responses to the same intervention.[28]

A major advantage of PRSWR is that there is a much greater percentage change in stroke work than end-systolic pressure for any given change in preload (EDV) due to IVC occlusion.[42] This gives the relationship better reproducibility and it tends to be more robust than the ESPVR or the dP/dt_{max}-end-diastolic relationship.[39,42,43] A possible downside of this finding is that some investigators have found M_{SW} to be less sensitive than Ees in responding to inotropic changes,[40,44,45] but this finding is not universal.[46] A limitation of PRSWR is that it does not distinguish diastolic from systolic dysfunction.[34] This is particularly a problem in conditions with steep end-diastolic P-V relationships such as hypertrophy and ischaemia and may complicate assessment of systolic function.[40]

Single beat estimation of ESPVR and PRSW

One of the greatest difficulties with both ESPVR and PRSW is that they traditionally rely on systematic alteration of loading conditions, most effectively achieved invasively by transient balloon occlusion of the inferior vena cava.[47] However, non-invasive techniques to generate load-independent indices of contractility

have been developed.[48,49] One method derives non-invasive, single-beat ESPVR from non-invasive blood pressure, echocardiographically derived stroke volume, ejection fraction and an estimated normalised end-diastolic elastance. This method has been shown to correlate well with invasively obtained values,[49] and does not require prior calculation of V_0. Its basis lies in the finding that under different loading as well as inotropic conditions the normalised elastance-time curve is remarkably stable,[50,51] which adds circumstantial evidence to the suggestion that the P-V loop is a macrostructural representation of cellular and subcellular machinery. Alternative mechanisms for derivation of single beat elastance have been proposed, including mathematical estimation of the isovolumic pressure for a single ejecting beat based on a curve-fitting algorithm.[52,53]

A method to determine non-invasive, single-beat estimation of the PRSWR has also been developed.[54] In contrast to the ESPVR method described above in which the volume-axis intercept is not required, this method relies on echocardiographic measurement of baseline epicardial and myocardial volumes to estimate V_{0-SW}, the theoretical volume at which there is zero stroke work. It should also be noted that in this method, stroke work is estimated as the product of stroke volume and mean ejection pressure rather than the area enclosed by the P-V loop, obviating the need for determination of diastolic pressures. Nevertheless, it has been shown in conscious dogs to be both sensitive to alterations in inotropy and insensitive to loading conditions.[54]

dP/dt_{max}-EDV relationship

While dP/dt_{max} is preload-dependent, it is largely independent of afterload. To account for this, a further index incorporating preload was derived. This dP/dt_{max}-end-diastolic volume is derived from the same P-V loops and based on the time-varying elastance model used in the derivation of ESPVR.[55] Because dP/dt_{max} occurs during isovolumic contraction, it provides a conceptual framework to understand left ventricular performance during early systole. Nevertheless, while the relation is sensitive to changes in inotropic state, it suffers from much greater variability than either ESPVR or PRSWR[39,42,43] and is rarely reported independently.

DEFINITION OF DIASTOLIC FUNCTION USING PRESSURE-VOLUME LOOPS

Just as the onset and duration of diastole has generated controversy,[56] accurate quantification of intrinsic diastolic left ventricular function has also been controversial.[57] While diastole was initially considered to be entirely passive, it is now accepted as an energy-dependent process,[58] particularly in its early part. More than systole, it is dependent on factors extrinsic to the left ventricle, including the pericardium, respiration and, via septal interaction, the right ventricle.[59–61] Because of this, drug effects on diastolic function may be mediated by effects on the venous system, altering preload and thus the degree of pericardial constraint and ventricular interaction, rather than any direct effect on left ventricular relaxation.[62]

End-diastolic pressure-volume relationship

Simple indices of passive ventricular performance have been used to demonstrate chamber stiffness. The simplest of these is diastolic chamber compliance or dV/dP.[58] It has been shown that this relationship is non-linear.[61] As the ventricle fills, therefore, the slope of this relation increases. This relation of EDP and volume across a range of filling pressures defines the end-diastolic P-V relationship (EDPVR).[61,63,64] Meaningful comparison of results for compliance, even in the same individual, can therefore only be made at the same diastolic pressure. As a result of atrial contraction, curve fitting to the entire duration of diastole may be inaccurate.[65] Because of this, clinical studies using EDPVR use the portion of diastolic filling prior to atrial contraction.[26,28,66,67]

The entire EDPVR is complex and dependent on cardiac and non-cardiac factors, as mentioned above. Viscosity or elasticity of the heart

is only one of the variables. Marked changes in the slope of the EDPVR in response to haemodynamic interventions may be explained by factors extrinsic to the left ventricle.[59,62,68] Some authors have suggested that passive characteristics of the left ventricle may only be altered acutely by active ischaemia.[69]

Figure 18.3 shows derivation of the end-systolic and EDP-volume relationships as well as the PRSWR. The linearity of ESPVR, EDPVR and PRSWR is easily appreciated within physiological changes in volume.

PRESSURE-VOLUME AREA (PVA) AND VENTRICULAR ENERGETICS

A further benefit of assessment of left ventricular function using P-V loops is the ability to determine ventricular energetics[20,70–72] and efficiency.[73,74] Figure 18.4 shows the derivation of ventricular energy expenditure derived from P-V loops.[75] From this it can be seen that the end-systolic point (C), the end-systolic volume (D), and the ESPVR define potential energy of contraction. It is independent of the shape of the P-V trajectory. The external mechanical work is defined by the P-V loop (ABCD). The combination of the potential and external mechanical energy defines the PVA, which is closely correlated with energy consumption of the left ventricle.[75]

The recognition that the heart performs work in ejecting blood is fundamental to the understanding of ventricular energetics. Since early this century, attempts have been made to quantify this work, in an effort to define the efficiency and energetic cost of cardiac contraction. In 1932, Katz calculated total work from the potential and kinetic energy of blood leaving the heart based on the mean ventricular pressure and volume of blood ejected.[76] It has since been shown that the total mechanical energy of contraction of the heart can be described by the area defined within a closed P-V loop.[75] This is made up of both the area inside the loop (defining external work of the heart), as well as the area circumscribed by the ESPVR (defining the potential energy of contraction), as in Figure 18.4.

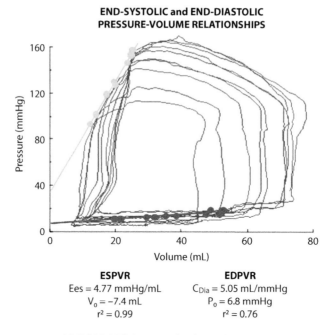

END-SYSTOLIC and END-DIASTOLIC
PRESSURE-VOLUME RELATIONSHIPS

ESPVR	EDPVR
E_{es} = 4.77 mmHg/mL	C_{Dia} = 5.05 mL/mmHg
V_0 = −7.4 mL	P_0 = 6.8 mmHg
r^2 = 0.99	r^2 = 0.76

PRELOAD RECRUITABLE STROKE WORK RELATIONSHIP

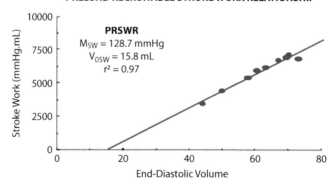

PRSWR
M_{SW} = 128.7 mmHg
V_{0SW} = 15.8 mL
r^2 = 0.97

Figure 18.3 Example of load-independent indices for one subject. The derivation of end-systolic pressure-volume relationship (ESPVR) and end-diastolic volume relationship (EDPVR) are shown from the end-systolic and end-diastolic points overlying the pressure-volume loops. The preload recruitable stroke work relationship (PRSWR) is derived from the stroke work (area within the loop) and end-diastolic volume for the corresponding loop.

The significance of this finding is the recognition that the myocardial oxygen consumption/beat is linearly correlated with this P-V area.[70] This empirical relation between energy consumption and contraction has been verified by other investigators.[11,71,77,78] The surprising constancy of this relation suggests a fundamental physical phenomenon of chemo-mechanical energy transduction.[72,79] Furthermore, the ratio of stroke work to PVA can be considered a measure of LV mechanical efficiency, analogous to myocardial efficiency, which is traditionally defined as the ratio of myocardial oxygen consumption to external work.[80]

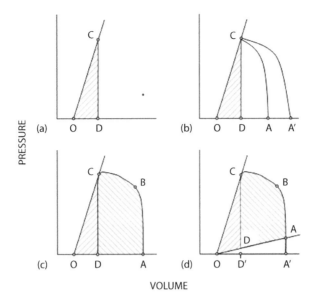

Figure 18.4 Derivation of pressure-volume (P-V) area and relation to ventricular energetics. **(a)** Mechanical potential energy at end-systole (DCO), defined by the end-systolic PV relationship (OC). **(b)** This area (DCO) is independent of trajectory of contraction (DC, AC or A'C). **(c)** External mechanical work in an ejecting contraction (ABCD). **(d)** P-V area (ABCD+DCO). Note: ADO represents the end-diastolic PV relationship. (Adapted from Suga, H., Am. J. Physiol., 236, H498, 1979.)

PRESSURE-VOLUME STUDY PROTOCOL

P-V studies are usually performed at the completion of routine left heart catheterisation in appropriate patients. The 6 French (Fr) femoral arterial sheath is exchanged for an 8.5 Fr arterial sheath and a 9 Fr femoral venous sheath inserted. An 8 Fr volume catheter (Webster 7212-08, Webster Lab Inc) is then inserted to the ventricular cavity under fluoroscopic control. Following electrical calibration, a 2 Fr Millar pressure micromanometer (SPC-360, Millar Instruments, Houston TX) is passed through the volume catheter to rest at its tip. Once catheters are in position, simultaneous pressure and volume data are displayed on-line and recorded. Volume calibration is performed off-line using a radio-opaque sphere of known diameter. Alternative methods include determination of cardiac output by thermodilution (obtained by right ventricular catheterisation) for calibration of the measured

stroke volume from the ventriculogram. Because the ventricular catheter remains in situ for approximately 30–40 minutes, a slow pressurised heparin infusion (2500 units sodium heparin in 500 mL 5% Dextrose) is attached via an arterial pressure bag and Tuohy-Borst adaptor.

Manipulation of Loading Conditions: A 35 mm vena caval balloon catheter (Cordis 530000A-15565, Cordis Corporation, Miami FL) is used for acute preload reduction. The balloon catheter is passed to the right atrium under fluoroscopic guidance. Inferior vena caval balloon occlusion (IVCBO) is performed by brief inflation of vena caval balloon (for 8–10 seconds or until ventricular ectopy occurred) with 30–35 mL of carbon dioxide in the right atrium, and then gently withdrawing the catheter to lodge in the mouth of the inferior vena cava. The load-independent indices ESPVR, PRSWR and EDPVR are calculated from IVCBO data. Runs with changes in heart rate of >10% during IVCBO are excluded.

Two main sets of data are recorded using P-V measurements. Continuous pressure and volume data sets in a stable rhythm (10–20 beats) are collected for 'steady-state' analysis. The second set of data involves preload reduction with continuous recording during reducing pressure and volume. An example of the generation of ESPVR by inferior vena caval occlusion in a single subject is shown in Figure 18.2. The ESPVR is determined by linear regression of the end-systolic points as described above. An iterative procedure is performed from the linear regression of the lines using an initial estimate of V_0 of 0 mL. Subsequent iterations are performed until errors are minimised.[12,81]

End-diastolic relationships are determined from two EDP/EDV points on each P-V loop. The points chosen are those immediately prior to the a-wave and a second point at 10% of the filling volume earlier in the same loop.[67] By examining diastole prior to atrial contraction, this best reflects passive diastolic properties of the left ventricle. A linear model is assumed for EDPVR, as this is simpler and has been shown to be as valid as more complex exponential regression models.[28] Although the slope of the regression describes an elastance, the results are usually reported as the inverse, chamber compliance, C_{Dia}.[62] The equation for diastolic compliance is therefore $V = C_{Dia} \cdot P + V_{oDia}$, where V_{oDia} is the volume axis intercept. Previous studies have shown that a linear description of diastolic compliance is simpler and fits data just as well as exponential curves.[28]

CLINICAL RELEVANCE OF INFORMATION DERIVED FROM PRESSURE-VOLUME LOOPS

One of the strengths of P-V analysis is that information is available on systolic and diastolic ventricular function, as well as its interaction with the arterial tree. The effect of inotropes, exercise, and pericardial disease on ventricular filling and stroke volume may also be easily understood. Figure 18.5a shows the effect of a change in inotropy on the P-V loop. A positive inotrope (in isolation) increases stroke work with a small associated increase in stroke volume, whereas a negative inotrope can be seen to decrease stroke volume. These effects are independent of end-diastolic volume, which in this

simplified model remains constant. In cardiomyopathic states (with intrinsically lower contractility and therefore lower Ees), the response is to increase end-diastolic volume to maintain stroke volume. The reflex sympathetic response in cardiac failure increases both contractility (Ees) and heart rate in an attempt to maintain cardiac output. In response to exercise, with increased sympathetic tone, increased stroke volume is maintained in the face of an increase in heart rate by increasing contractility. In patients without contractile reserve (who are already under sympathetic stimulation due to cardiomyopathy), the heart is unable to respond in this manner, limiting stroke volume and thereby exercise tolerance.

The effect of a decrease in diastolic compliance (increase in passive diastolic stiffness), as may be found in states of left ventricular hypertrophy or ischaemia, is to increase the ventricular filling pressure required to achieve the same volume. This can occur in the absence of systolic dysfunction, as shown in Figure 18.5b. Pericardial constriction imposes a similar limitation on ventricular filling.

Perhaps the most significant haemodynamic breakthrough that P-V loop analysis allows is integration of information concerning arterial function with that concerning the left ventricle. This integration is termed ventriculo-vascular coupling. Other methods used to characterise ventricular function are implicitly dependent on arterial function, as ventricular ejection has long been recognised to depend on the afterload imposed on it by the arterial tree.[82–84] As arterial impedance, commonly accepted as the most appropriate method of determining afterload,[84–86] requires invasively obtained aortic pressure and flow, it is not commonly measured. Effective arterial elastance (Ea) derived from P-V loops incorporates much of the information available from the aortic impedance spectrum, and is considered as a reasonable alternative to the definition of afterload.[25,87–89] A major benefit of this arterial elastance is that it is expressed in the same units, and is defined by the same method as ventricular elastance, allowing an obvious and direct introduction into the concept of ventriculo-arterial coupling,[90] defined simply as the ratio of arterial to ventricular elastance. It has been demonstrated that maximal stroke work is achieved when this ratio approaches unity.[90]

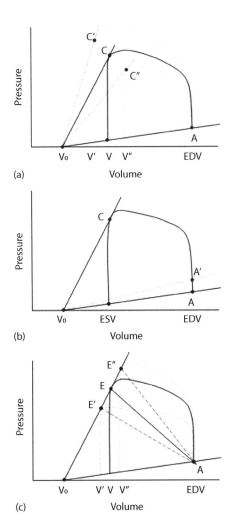

(a)

(b)

(c)

Figure 18.5 (a) Effects of changes in inotropic status on stroke volume. In the absence of a change in arterial function or end-diastolic volume (EDV), an increase in contractility results in an increase in stroke volume (EDV-V'). In cardiomyopathy or under the influence of a negative inotrope (EDV-V''), the stroke volume is decreased. End-systolic pressure can also be seen to change in a similar fashion (C', C'' respectively) assuming no change in heart rate. (b) An impairment of diastolic function, shown as an increase in the slope of the end-diastolic volume relationship (AV$_o$→A'V$_o$), results in a significant rise in end-diastolic pressure in response to a small change in EDV. Stroke volume is not affected. (c) If arterial properties change, stroke volume is affected, even in the absence of changes in contractility. Stroke volume falls (EDV-V'') in response to an increase in arterial elastance (AE→AE'') and increases (EDV-V') if arterial elastance falls (AE→AE').

The effect of an isolated change in arterial stiffness as expressed by arterial elastance is shown in Figure 18.5c. Reduction in arterial elastance results in increased stroke volume, reduced PVA and increased mechanical efficiency, as defined by the stroke work to PVA ratio, without altering ventricular elastance.[80] It can be seen that stroke volume is therefore sensitive to arterial compliance (Ea) in addition to contractile state (Ees). Numerous drug studies have used this fact to compare and contrast ventricular with vascular effects.[91-93] The effects of arterial properties on ventricular stroke volume, energy consumption and mechanical efficiency are of particular importance in the management of the failing heart, in which the Ea:Ees ratio is increased above 1.[94] In this setting, use of nitroglycerine to 'unload' the failing heart not only results in increased stroke volume, but also results in restoration of Ea:Ees towards 1, optimising stroke work, and an increased stroke work to PVA ratio, optimising mechanical efficiency.[92]

EFFECTS OF STRUCTURAL HEART INTERVENTIONS ON THE PRESSURE-VOLUME LOOP: TWO ILLUSTRATIVE EXAMPLES

The effects of structural heart interventions on ventricular function can be easily appreciated when represented in the form of P-V loops. In Figure 18.6a, simulated P-V loops demonstrate the effect of insertion of a continuous, axial-flow transvalvular cardiac assist device (Impella, Abiomed, Danvers MA) for an acutely failing left ventricle. Continuous cardiac assistance results in loss of the isovolumic contraction and relaxation periods, with the P-V loop approaching a triangular shape. As a result, left ventricular chamber size continues to reduce well beyond the point of maximum elastance, reflecting increased discordance between the elastance-based and ejection-based definitions of end-systole. There is reduction in both left ventricular end-diastolic volume and pressure without a significant change in the diastolic P-V relationship. The P-V area is reduced, reflecting reduced myocardial oxygen consumption.

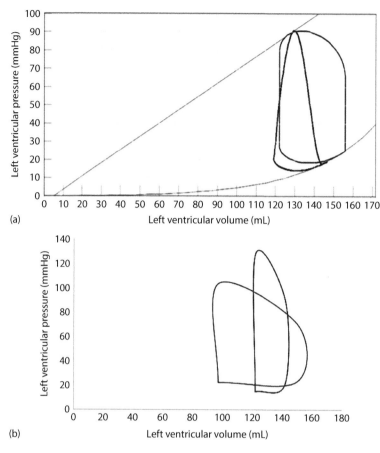

(a)

(b)

Figure 18.6 (a) Effect of transvalvular continuous-flow microaxial left ventricular support (Impella) on the left ventricular P-V loop in acute heart failure. Wide loop = unsupported left ventricle; thin loop = post-initiation of support with a 5 L/min device. (b) Effect of transcatheter mitral valve replacement (Tendyne) on the left ventricular pressure-volume loop in a patient with severe mitral incompetence. Wide loop = pre-deployment; thin loop = one-minute post-deployment. ([a] Adapted from Burkhoff, D., HARVI: Cardiovascular Physiology & Hemodynamics. Part II. Advanced physiological concepts. Version 2.0.0. Mobile application software. 2012. Updated 2014. https://itunes.apple.com/gb/app/harvi/id568196279?mt=8. Accessed 30 November 2017; [b] Adapted from Namasivayam, M., J. Am. Coll. Cardiol., 67, 1032, 2016; Modified from Katz, L.N., Am. J. Physiol., 99, 579, 1932.)

Figure 18.6b illustrates the immediate effect of transcatheter mitral valve replacement (Tendyne, Abbott Vascular, Santa Clara, CA, USA) in a patient with severe mitral incompetence. Resolution of mitral incompetence results in acutely increased afterload, reflected in increased effective arterial elastance, and it should be noted that this is likely due to reduced shunting of blood into the low-resistance left atrium rather than due to any change in the arterial vasculature. This is accompanied by increased end-systolic volume, decreased ejection fraction, mildly increased PVA and reduced stroke work to PVA ratio.

ACKNOWLEDGEMENT

Dr Jain is supported by an NHMRC Postgraduate Research Fellowship.

REFERENCES

1. Frank O. On the dynamics of cardiac muscle. Am Heart J. 1959;58(3):467–478.
2. Katz AM, Katz LN, Williams FL. Registration of left ventricular volume curves in the dog with the systemic circulation intact. Circ Res. 1955;3(6):588–593.

3. Baan J, van der Velde ET, de Bruin HG, et al. Continuous measurement of left ventricular volume in animals and humans by conductance catheter. *Circulation.* 1984;70(5):812–823.

4. Grossman W, Braunwald E, Mann T, McLaurin LP, Green LH. Contractile state of the left ventricle in man as evaluated from end- systolic pressure-volume relations. *Circulation.* 1977;56(5):845–852.

5. Katz LN. The Lewis A. Conner Memorial Lecture: The performance of the heart. *Circulation.* 1960;21(4):483–498.

6. Sagawa K. The ventricular pressure-volume diagram revisited. *Circ Res.* 1978;43(5):677–687.

7. Sagawa K, Suga H, Shoukas AA, Bakalar KM. End-systolic pressure/volume ratio: A new index of ventricular contractility. *Am J Cardiol.* 1977;40(5):748–753.

8. Suga H, Sagawa K. Instantaneous Pressure-volume relationships and their ratio in the excised, supported canine left ventricle. *Circ Res.* 1974;35(1):117–126.

9. Suga H, Sagawa K, Shoukas AA. load independence of the instantaneous pressure-volume ratio of the canine left ventricle and effects of epinephrine and heart rate on the ratio. *Circ Res.* 1973;32(3):314–322.

10. Sagawa K, Maughan L, Suga H, Sunagawa K. *Cardiac Contraction and the Pressure-Volume Relationship.* New York: Oxford University Press; 1988.

11. Kelly RP, Tunin R, Kass DA. Effect of reduced aortic compliance on cardiac efficiency and contractile function of in situ canine left ventricle. *Circ Res.* 1992;71(3):490–502.

12. Kass DA, Yamazaki T, Burkhoff D, Maughan WL, Sagawa K. Determination of left ventricular end-systolic pressure-volume relationships by the conductance (volume) catheter technique. *Circulation.* 1986;73(3):586–595.

13. McKay RG, Aroesty JM, Heller GV, Royal HD, Warren SE, Grossman W. Assessment of the end-systolic pressure-volume relationship in human beings with the use of a time-varying elastance model. *Circulation.* 1986;74(1):97–104.

14. McKay RG, Miller MJ, Ferguson JJ, et al. Assessment of left ventricular end-systolic pressure-volume relations with an impedance catheter and transient inferior vena cava occlusion: Use of this system in the evaluation of the cardiotonic effects of dobutamine, milrinone, posicor and epinephrine. *J Am Coll Cardiol.* 1986;8(5):1152–1160.

15. Van Fossen D, Fontana ME, Unverferth DV, Walker S, Kolibash AJ, Bashore TM. Safety and efficacy of inferior vena caval occlusion to rapidly alter ventricular loading conditions in idiopathic dilated cardiomyopathy. *Am J Cardiol.* 1987;59(9):937–942.

16. Baan J, van der Velde ET, Steendijk P. Ventricular pressure-volume relations in vivo. *Eur Heart J.* 1992;13(Suppl E):2–6.

17. Burkhoff D, de Tombe PP, Hunter WC, Kass DA. Contractile strength and mechanical efficiency of left ventricle are enhanced by physiological afterload. *Am J Physiol.* 1991;260(2 Pt 2):H569–578.

18. Freeman GL, Little WC, O'Rourke RA. The effect of vasoactive agents on the left ventricular end-systolic pressure-volume relation in closed-chest dogs. *Circulation.* 1986;74(5):1107–1113.

19. Burkhoff D, van der Velde E, Kass D, Baan J, Maughan WL, Sagawa K. Accuracy of volume measurement by conductance catheter in isolated, ejecting canine hearts. *Circulation.* 1985;72(2):440–447.

20. Glower DD, Spratt JA, Snow ND, et al. Linearity of the Frank-Starling relationship in the intact heart: The concept of preload recruitable stroke work. *Circulation.* 1985;71(5):994–1009.

21. McKay RG, Aroesty JM, Heller GV, et al. Left ventricular pressure-volume diagrams and end-systolic pressure-volume relations in human beings. *J Am Coll Cardiol.* 1984;3(2):301–312.

22. Cheng CP, Noda T, Nordlander M, Ohno M, Little WC. Comparison of effects of dihydropyridine calcium antagonists on left ventricular systolic and diastolic performance. *J Pharmacol Exp Ther.* 1994;268(3):1232–1241.

23. Feldman MD, Pak PH, Wu CC et al. Acute cardiovascular effects of opc-18790 in patients with congestive heart failure:

Time- and dose-dependence analysis based on pressure-volume relations. *Circulation*. 1996;93(3):474–483.

24. Herrmann HC, Ruddy TD, William Dec G, William Strauss H, Boucher CA, Fifer MA. Inotropic effect of enoximone in patients with severe heart failure: Demonstration by left ventricular end-systolic pressure-volume analysis. *J Am Coll Cardiol*. 1987;9(5):1117–1123.

25. Kass DA, Grayson R, Marino P. Pressure-volume analysis as a method for quantifying simultaneous drug (amrinone) effects on arterial load and contractile state in vivo. *J Am Coll Cardiol*. 1990;16(3):726–732.

26. Nussbacher A, Arie S, Kalil R, et al. Mechanism of adenosine-induced elevation of pulmonary capillary wedge pressure in humans. *Circulation*. 1995;92(3):371–379.

27. Kass DA, Marino P, Maughan WL, Sagawa K. Determinants of end-systolic pressure-volume relations during acute regional ischemia in situ. *Circulation*. 1989;80(6):1783–1794.

28. Kass DA, Midei M, Brinker J, Maughan WL. Influence of coronary occlusion during PTCA on end-systolic and end- diastolic pressure-volume relations in humans. *Circulation*. 1990;81(2):447–460.

29. Thormann J. The influence of clinical intervention on pressure-volume relationships-the conductance (volume) technique. *Eur Heart J*. 1992;13(Suppl E):69–79.

30. Kass DA, Baughman KL, Pak PH, et al. Reverse remodeling from cardiomyoplasty in human heart failure: External constraint versus active assist. *Circulation*. 1995;91(9):2314–2318.

31. Suga H. End-systolic pressure-volume relations. *Circulation*. 1979;59(2):419–420.

32. Nishioka O, Maruyama Y, Ashikawa K, et al. Effects of changes in afterload impedance on left ventricular ejection in isolated canine hearts: Dissociation of end ejection from end systole. *Cardiovasc Res*. 1987;21(2):107–118.

33. Sagawa K. The end-systolic pressure-volume relation of the ventricle: Definition, modifications and clinical use. *Circulation*. 1981;63(6):1223–1227.

34. Kass DA, Maughan WL. From 'Emax' to pressure-volume relations: A broader view. *Circulation*. 1988;77(6):1203–1212.

35. Cohen-Solal A, Dahan M, Guiomard A, et al. [Effects of aging on left ventricle-arterial coupling in man]. *Arch Mal Coeur Vaiss*. 1993;86(8):1095–1097.

36. Chen CH, Nakayama M, Nevo E, Fetics BJ, Maughan WL, Kass DA. Coupled systolic-ventricular and vascular stiffening with age: Implications for pressure regulation and cardiac reserve in the elderly. *J Am Coll Cardiol*. 1998;32(5):1221–1227.

37. Mirsky I. An appraisal of ventricular and myocardial function variables based on the elastance concept. *J Am Coll Cardiol*. 1989;14(2):354–356.

38. Suga H, Hisano R, Goto Y, Yamada O. Normalization of end-systolic pressure-volume relation and emax of different sized hearts. *Jpn Circ J*. 1984;48(2):136–143.

39. Takeuchi M, Odake M, Takaoka H, Hayashi Y, Yokoyama M. Comparison between preload recruitable stroke work and the end-systolic pressure-volume relationship in man. *Eur Heart J*. 1992;13(Suppl E):80–84.

40. Foëx P, Leone BJ. Pressure-volume loops: A dynamic approach to the assessment of ventricular function. *J Cardiothorac Vasc Anesth*. 1994;8(1):84–96.

41. Kass DA, Beyar R, Lankford E, Heard M, Maughan WL, Sagawa K. Influence of contractile state on curvilinearity of in situ end- systolic pressure-volume relations. *Circulation*. 1989;79(1):167–178.

42. Feneley MP, Skelton TN, Kisslo KB, Davis JW, Bashore TM, Rankin JS. Comparison of preload recruitable stroke work, end-systolic pressure-volume and dPdtmax-end-diastolic volume relations as indexes of left ventricular contractile performance in patients undergoing routine cardiac catheterization. *J Am Coll Cardiol*. 1992;19(7):1522–1530.

43. Rahko PS. Comparative efficacy of three indexes of left ventricular performance derived from pressure-volume loops in heart failure induced by tachypacing. *J Am Coll Cardiol*. 1994;23(1):209–218.

44. Little WC, Cheng CP, Mumma M, Igarashi Y, Vinten-Johansen J, Johnston WE. Comparison of measures of left ventricular contractile performance derived from pressure-volume loops in conscious dogs. *Circulation.* 1989;80(5):1378–1387.

45. Starling MR. Responsiveness of the maximum time-varying elastance to alterations in left ventricular contractile state in man. *Am Heart J.* 1989;118(6):1266–1276.

46. Kass DA, Maughan WL, Guo ZM, Kono A, Sunagawa K, Sagawa K. Comparative influence of load versus inotropic states on indexes of ventricular contractility: Experimental and theoretical analysis based on pressure-volume relationships [published erratum appears in Circulation 1988;77(3):559]. *Circulation.* 1987;76(6):1422–1436.

47. Starling MR, Montgomery DG, Walsh RA. Load dependence of the single beat maximal pressure (stress)/volume ratios in humans. *J Am Coll Cardiol.* 1989;14(2):345–353.

48. Karamanoglu M, Falkin D, Feneley M. Totally non-invasive pressure-area measurements of left ventricular contractility during non-invasive preload reduction in humans. *J Am Coll Cardiol.* 1996;27(2):49–50.

49. Chen CH, Fetics B, Nevo E, et al. Noninvasive single-beat determination of left ventricular end-systolic elastance in humans. *J Am Coll Cardiol.* 2001;38(7):2028–2034.

50. Senzaki H, Chen CH, Kass DA. Single-beat estimation of end-systolic pressure-volume relation in humans: A new method with the potential for noninvasive application. *Circulation.* 1996;94(10):2497–2506.

51. Shishido T, Hayashi K, Shigemi K, Sato T, Sugimachi M, Sunagawa K. Single-beat estimation of end-systolic elastance using bilinearly approximated time-varying elastance curve. *Circulation.* 2000;102(16):1983–1989.

52. Shih H, Hillel Z, Thys D. A61 Validation of a new real-time single-beat method to determine left ventricular contractility in humans. *Anesthesiology.* 1997;87(Supplement):61A.

53. Takeuchi M, Igarashi Y, Tomimoto S, et al. Single-beat estimation of the slope of the end-systolic pressure-volume relation in the human left ventricle. *Circulation.* 1991;83(1):202–212.

54. Karunanithi MK, Feneley MP. Single-beat determination of preload recruitable stroke work relationship: Derivation and evaluation in conscious dogs. *J Am Coll Cardiol.* 2000;35(2):502–513.

55. Little WC. The left ventricular dP/dt$_{max}$-end-diastolic volume relation in closed- chest dogs. *Circ Res.* 1985;56(6):808–815.

56. Brutsaert DL, Rademakers FE, Sys SU. Triple control of relaxation: Implications in cardiac disease. *Circulation.* 1984;69(1):190–196.

57. Glantz SA. Computing indices of diastolic stiffness has been counterproductive. *Fed Proc.* 1980;39(2):162–168.

58. Grossman W. Diastolic properties of the left ventricle. *Ann Int Med.* 1976;84(3):316.

59. Alderman EL, Glantz SA. Acute hemodynamic interventions shift the diastolic pressure-volume curve in man. *Circulation.* 1976;54(4):662–671.

60. Shirato K, Shabetai R, Bhargava V, Franklin D, Ross J. Alteration of the left ventricular diastolic pressure-segment length relation produced by the pericardium. Effects of cardiac distension and afterload reduction in conscious dogs. *Circulation.* 1978;57(6):1191–1198.

61. Janicki JS, Weber KT. Factors influencing the diastolic pressure-volume relation of the cardiac ventricles. *Fed Proc.* 1980;39(2):133–140.

62. Kass DA. Diastolic compliance of hypertrophied ventricle is not acutely altered by pharmacologic agents influencing active processes. *Ann Int Med.* 1993;119(6):466.

63. Noble MIM, Milne ENC, Goerke RJ, et al. Left ventricular filling and diastolic pressure-volume relations in the conscious dog. *Circ Res.* 1969;24(2):269–283.

64. Templeton GH, Ecker RR, Mitchell JH. Left ventricular stiffness during diastole and systole: The influence of changes in volume and inotropic state. *Cardiovasc Res.* 1972;6(1):95–100.

65. Gaasch WH, Cole JS, Quinones MA, Alexander JK. Dynamic determinants of letf ventricular diastolic pressure-volume relations in man. *Circulation*. 1975;51(2):317–323.

66. Hayward CS, Kalnins WV, Rogers P, Feneley MP, Macdonald PS, Kelly RP. Effect of inhaled nitric oxide on normal human left ventricular function. *J Am Coll Cardiol*. 1997;30(1):49–56.

67. Liu CP, Ting CT, Yang TM, et al. Reduced left ventricular compliance in human mitral stenosis. Role of reversible internal constraint. *Circulation*. 1992;85(4):1447–1456.

68. Pak PH, Maughan WL, Baughman KL, Kass DA. Marked discordance between dynamic and passive diastolic pressure-volume relations in idiopathic hypertrophic cardiomyopathy. *Circulation*. 1996;94(1):52–60.

69. Rankin JS, Arentzen CE, Ring WS, Edwards CH 2nd, McHale PA, Anderson RW. The diastolic mechanical properties of the intact left ventricle. *Fed Proc*. 1980;39(2):141–147.

70. Khalafbeigui F, Suga H, Sagawa K. Left ventricular systolic pressure-volume area correlates with oxygen consumption. *Am J Physiol*. 1979;237(5):H566–569.

71. Takaoka H, Takeuchi M, Odake M, Yokoyama M. Assessment of myocardial oxygen consumption (Vo2) and systolic pressure-volume area (PVA) in human hearts. *Eur Heart J*. 1992;13(suppl E):85–90.

72. Suga H. Ventricular energetics. *Physiol Rev*. 1990;70(2):247–277.

73. De Tombe PP, Jones S, Burkhoff D, Hunter WC, Kass DA. Ventricular stroke work and efficiency both remain nearly optimal despite altered vascular loading. *Am J Physiol*. 1993;264(6 Pt 2):H1817–1824.

74. van den Horn GJ, Westerhof N, Elzinga G. Optimal power generation by the left ventricle. A study in the anesthetized open thorax cat. *Circ Res*. 1985;56(2):252–261.

75. Suga H. Total mechanical energy of a ventricle model and cardiac oxygen consumption. *Am J Physiol*. 1979;236(3):H498–505.

76. Katz LN. Observations on the external work of the isolated turtle heart. *Am J Physiol -- Legacy Content*. 1932;99(3):579.

77. Nozawa T, Cheng CP, Noda T, Little WC. Relation between left ventricular oxygen consumption and pressure- volume area in conscious dogs. *Circulation*. 1994;89(2):810–817.

78. Starling MR, Mancini GB, Montgomery DG, Gross MD. Relation between maximum time-varying elastance pressure-volume areas and myocardial oxygen consumption in dogs. *Circulation*. 1991;83(1):304–314.

79. Gibbs CL, Chapman JB. Cardiac mechanics and energetics: Chemomechanical transduction in cardiac muscle. *Am J Physiol*. 1985;249(2 Pt 2):H199–206.

80. Starling MR. Left ventricular-arterial coupling relations in the normal human heart. *Am Heart J*. 1993;125(6):1659–1666.

81. Kass DA, Md MM, Phd WG, Brinker Fsca JAM, Maughan WL. Use of a conductance (volume) catheter and transient inferior vena caval occlusion for rapid determination of pressure-volume relationships in man. *Catheter Cardiovasc Diag*. 1988;15(3):192–202.

82. Sonnenblick EH, Downing SE. Afterload as a primary determinat of ventricular performance. *Am J Physiol*. 1963;204:604–610.

83. Elzinga G, Westerhof N. Pressure and flow generated by the left ventricle against different impedances. *Circ Res*. 1973;32(2):178–186.

84. Milnor WR. Arterial impedance as ventricular afterload. *Circ Res*. 1975;36(5):565–570.

85. Nichols WW, Pepine CJ, Geiser EA, Conti CR. Vascular load defined by the aortic input impedance spectrum. *Fed Proc*. 1980;39(2):196–201.

86. Noble MIM. Left ventricular load, arterial impedance and their interrelationship. *Circ Res*. 1979;13(4):183–198.

87. Kelly RP, Ting CT, Yang TM, et al. Effective arterial elastance as index of arterial vascular load in humans. *Circulation*. 1992;86(2):513–521.

88. Latham RD, Rubal BJ, Sipkema P, et al. Ventricular/vascular coupling and regional arterial dynamics in the chronically hypertensive baboon: Correlation with cardiovascular structural adaptation. *Circ Res*. 1988;63(4):798–811.

89. Sunagawa K, Maughan WL, Burkhoff D, Sagawa K. Left ventricular interaction with arterial load studied in isolated canine ventricle. *Am J Physiol*. 1983;245(5 Pt 1):H773–H780.

90. Sunagawa K, Maughan WL, Sagawa K. Optimal arterial resistance for the maximal stroke work studied in isolated canine left ventricle. *Circ Res*. 1985;56(4):586–595.

91. Freeman GL. Improved cardiac performance secondary to dobutamine: The role of ventricular-vascular coupling. *J Am Coll Cardiol*. 1990;15(5):1136–1137.

92. Haber HL, Simek CL, Bergin JD, et al. Bolus intravenous nitroglycerin predominantly reduces afterload in patients with excessive arterial elastance. *J Am Coll Cardiol*. 1993;22(1):251–257.

93. Kameyama T, Asanoi H, Ishizaka S, Sasayama S. Ventricular load optimization by unloading therapy in patients with heart failure. *J Am Coll Cardiol*. 1991;17(1):199–207.

94. Ishihara H, Yokota M, Sobue T, Saito H. Relation between ventriculoarterial coupling and myocardial energetics in patients with idiopathic dilated cardiomyopathy. *J Am Coll Cardiol*. 1994;23(2):406–416.

95. Burkhoff D. HARVI: Cardiovascular Physiology & Hemodynamics. Part II. Advanced physiological concepts. Version 2.0.0. Mobile application software. 2012. Updated 2014. https://itunes.apple.com/gb/app/harvi/id568196279?mt=8. Accessed 30th November 2017.

96. Namasivayam M, Feneley M, Hayward C, et al. Safety of mitral valve replacement in severe systolic heart failure: first intra-operative evaluation of left ventricular contractile performance during off-bypass, transcatheter mitral valve replacement. *J Am Coll Cardiol*. 2016;67(13):1032.

19

The electrocardiogram in ischaemic heart disease

GEOFFREY S. OLDFIELD AND DENNIS L. KUCHAR

INTRODUCTION

The electrocardiogram (ECG) underpins almost every aspect of cardiology, and mastering the skills of ECG interpretations remains a core learning objective for medical students, nurses, technicians and other paramedical staff. A clear understanding of the ECG is absolutely necessary for monitoring patients undergoing a variety of procedures, and is critical for the diagnosis of many cardiac pathologies. Monitoring and identifying arrhythmias requires an appreciation of cardiac anatomy, the electrical conduction system, and ischaemic abnormalities. This chapter describes the basic components of the cardiac conduction system and reviews the standard methods for obtaining and interpreting a 12-lead ECG, with emphasis on the characteristics of ischaemia, infarction and specific arrhythmias.

ELECTRICAL ACTIVATION OF THE HEART

Anatomy

The electrical system of the heart consists of specialised muscle fibres. These are unrecognisable from contractile muscle by the naked eye and require histochemical techniques to be recognised. The components of this system are the sino-atrial (SA) node, the inter-nodal pathways, the atrio-ventricular (A-V) node, the Bundle of His and the Purkinje system (Figure 19.1). It is interesting that the discovery of the various parts of the pathway was in reverse order of activation, commencing with Purkinje in 1845 and finishing with Keith & Flack discovering the sinus node in 1907.

The S-A node is the primary cardiac pacemaker and is found high in the right atrium, just anterolateral to its connection with the superior vena cava (SVC). It is approximately 25 mm in length and is richly supplied with autonomic nerve fibres and blood vessels. It is connected to the A-V node by three internodal tracts—the anterior, middle and posterior internodal tracts. The anterior tract passes anteriorly and to the left of the superior vena cava, entering the anterior inter-atrial band, which

splits into two parts, the first passing to the left atrium (Bachmans' Bundle), the second descending anteriorly in the inter-atrial septum to the A-V node. The middle internodal tract runs in the inter-atrial septum to the A-V node, while the posterior internodal tract terminates with most of its fibres bypassing the proximal and middle portions of the AV node to enter the distal portion.

The AV node is approximately $6 \times 3 \times 2$ mm in size and lies in the right atrium, on the right side of the inter-atrial septum, in front of the opening of the coronary sinus above the attachment of the septal cusp of the tricuspid valve. The distal "tail" of the A-V node is contiguous with the Bundle of His, which is approximately 20×3 mm. It bifurcates early into "branching" and "penetrating" segments. The branching segments arise immediately distal to the A-V node in the proximal His Bundle. It branches proximally to form the posterior fibres of the left bundle branch, then divides to form the anterior fibres of the left bundle branch and the right bundle branch.

The "penetrating" branch runs through the central fibrous structure and has no contact with myocardium. The right main bundle runs down the right side of the interventricular septum towards the apex. Initially it lies deep in the endocardium and has only a few branches, but on reaching the moderator band its free edge runs inwards to the base of the anterior papillary muscle of the right ventricle, where it branches to supply the whole of the right ventricular endocardium. The left main bundle emerges on the left side of the interventricular septum (IVS), just below the non-coronary cusp of the aortic valve and passes down the septum, sending branches into the septum until about a third of the way down the IVS. Here it breaks into posterior and anterior branches that pass the postero-medial and antero-lateral papillary muscles, where it branches to form the complex Purkinje network of fibres supplying the left ventricular endocardium.

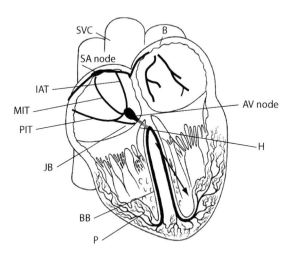

Figure 19.1 The electrical system of the heart. SVC, superior vena cava; LA, left atrium; B, Bachman's bundle of the anterior internodal tract; IAT, interatrial bundle of anterior internodal tract; MIT, middle internodal tract; PIT, posterior internodal tract; JB, James' bypass fibres; His, common bundle of His; BB, bundle branches; P, Purkinje network.

Mode of activation of myocardium

The normal impulse originates in the S-A node and passes longitudinally through the atria as a "wavefront", initially activating the right atrium in a rightwards and anterior direction. This is followed by activation of the left atrium, in a left and posterior direction. The "wavefront" is rapid, travelling longitudinally and contiguously at approximately 1000 mm/second throughout the atrial muscle.

The impulse arrives at the A-V node via the specialised internodal pathway, where it is delayed due to decremented conduction. The earliest sub-endocardial depolarisation is detected simultaneously on the left central side of the interventricular septum, and on the high anterior and infero-apico-septal regions. The wave of depolarisation then spreads transversely from endocardium to epicardium through the thickness of the left and right ventricular walls. The epicardial depolarisation is detected first on the right antero-apical region, followed by the anterior and posterior para-septal regions of the left ventricle. The lateral wall and basal septum are activated last. The Purkinje system extends to varying depths into the sub-endocardial layer in each individual, penetrating up to 3–4 mm into the free ventricular walls from the endocardium. Activation of the sub-endocardial layer (which is electrically silent) is not recorded on the surface electrocardiogram (ECG). It was originally theorised by Sodi-Pallares[1–4] that the island of Purkinje tissue acted as a "closed polarised island" where activation from the many Purkinje fibres spreads outwards in a "spherical" manner through the myocardium. It was not until activation reached the endocardium that the "closed islands" opened and net activation began to spread to the epicardium so a positive potential would be recorded (Figure 19.2). Sodi-Pallares referred to the (electrically silent) Purkinje ridge sub-endocardial layer as the "electrical sub-endocardial surface". The

thickness or depth of this sub-endocardial layer is highly variable. Durrer[5] and others subsequently showed the complete sequence of ventricular activation of the heart.

On the ECG, when the wave of depolarisation moves towards a positive pole, the deflection is positive; when it moves away from the positive pole, or towards a negative pole, the deflection is negative. In an isolated muscle strip, depolarisation (an advancing wave of positive charge) and repolarisation (a wave of negative charge) both take place from the endocardium to epicardium. The result of this is that the polarity of repolarisation in the muscle strip is the opposite to that of depolarisation.

In the intact human heart, however, depolarisation also takes place from endocardium to epicardium but repolarisation takes place in the opposite direction, from epicardium to endocardium. Hence, polarity of repolarisation is the same as for depolarisation. A small number of individuals, however, especially athletes, may have their repolarisation process as in the isolated muscle strip, so in these individuals T wave inversion may be seen in many leads, particularly the precordial leads.

Thus, depolarisation begins on the left side of the interventricular septum and spreads outwards through the free walls of the ventricles. From an electrocardiographic point of view, the ventricles consist of three muscle masses, the interventricular septum and the free walls (muscle masses) of the right and left ventricles (Figure 19.3a).

The standard surface-recorded ECG is the sum of the potential electrical forces recorded in

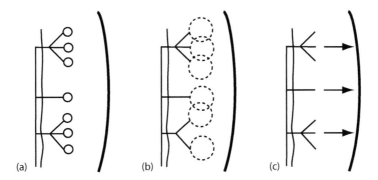

Figure 19.2 Diagrammatic representation of Sodi-Pallares' "electrical endocardial surface" concept. Electrical activation arrives at the endocardial surface via the Purkinje fibres. At first, activation is restricted to closed polarised spheres, or "closed islands" (a). The spheres coalesce and open to the endocardium (b), forming a progressive electrical wavefront spreading outwards and transversely (c) through the ventricular free wall.

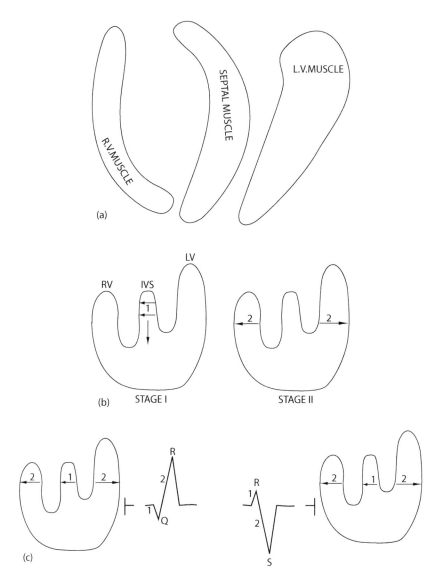

Figure 19.3 **(a)** The ventricle may be considered electrographically as three separate muscle masses, as shown. **(b)** Activation of ventricular muscle proceeds first from the interventricular septum (IVS) **(1)**, then spreads across the rest of the muscle mass **(2)**. RV, right ventricle; LV, left ventricle. Arrows indicate direction of signal. **(c)** The size of the electrical potential depends on the thickness of each of the three muscle masses. As the left ventricular wall mass is considerably thicker than that of the right ventricle, its signal is correspondingly stronger and overrides that of the right ventricle on the ECG trace. Arrows and numbers indicate sequence and direction of signal.

various planes. Activation of the interventricular septum occurs first (stage 1) and is followed by activation of the rest of the muscle mass (stage 2) (Figure 19.3b).

Because the mass of the left ventricle (LV) is much greater than that of the right ventricle (RV), the electrical potential from the LV overrides that of the RV on surface ECG electrodes (Figure 19.3c).

STANDARD ECG LEADS AND ELECTROCARDIOGRAPHIC INTERPRETATION

Einthoven's triangle (Figure 19.4a) is derived from leads placed on the right and left wrists and the left ankle. The standard ECG is made up of 12 leads: Three standard bipolar leads I, II and III derived from

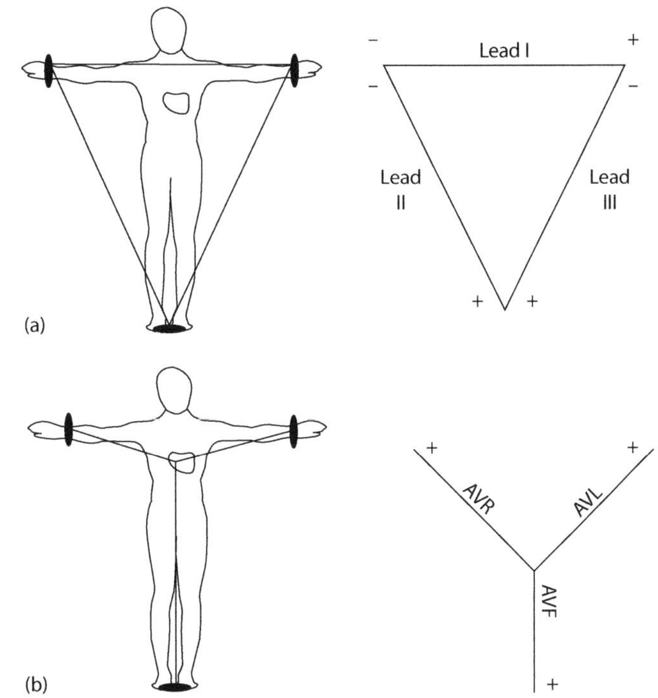

Figure 19.4 (a) Einthoven's triangle, showing the three lines of reference derived from the limb leads. (b) Three additional lines of reference formed from the augmented limb leads.

Einthoven's equilateral triangle, plus three augmented extremity leads, which are uni-polar leads and are prefixed with the letter "a", plus six chest "V" leads.

The augmented uni-polar leads on the arms and legs are seen as an extension of the torso and record actively from each peripheral electrode (Figure 19.4b). Following is a brief description of the 12 basic ECG leads:

I – Lead I connects the left and right wrists.
II – Lead II connects the right arm and left ankle.
III – Lead III connects the left arm and left ankle.
aVR – The right arm augmented unipolar lead effectively records conduction from the right shoulder.
aVL – The left arm augmented unipolar lead records conduction from the left shoulder.
aVF – The left leg augmented unipolar lead records conduction from the left thigh.
V1 – This lead is placed on the 4th right intercostal space, 2.5 cm from the midline of the sternum.
V2 – This lead is placed on the 4th left intercostal space, 2.5 cm from the middle of the sternum.
V3 – This lead is placed halfway between V2 and V4.
V4 – This lead is placed on the 5th left intercostal space in the mid-clavicular line.

V5 – This lead is placed on the anterior axillary line at the same level as V4.
V6 – This lead is placed on the mid-axillary line at the same level as V5.

The standard and augmented unipolar leads are orientated through the frontal or coronal plane of the body, whereas the precordial unipolar or V leads are orientated through the horizontal body plane. The Hexagonal reference system is an amalgamation of the orientation of the standard bipolar and augmented unipolar leads, placed through a central point of the heart, and is used to calculate the electrical axis of the heart (Figure 19.5).

PQRST complex

The PQRST complex is a recording of the electrical cardiac activity detected by skin electrodes. The P wave represents atrial activation, the QRS complex represents ventricular depolarisation, and the T wave represents ventricular repolarisation. Atrial repolarisation can occasionally be seen as a "ta" wave interposed in the QRS complex, but is generally lost in the stronger T wave.

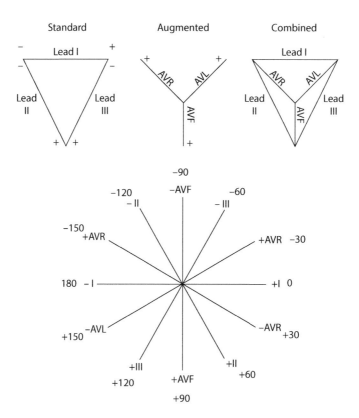

Figure 19.5 Amalgamation of the standard and augmented limb leads to form the hexagonal reference system in the frontal plane.

The PR interval (or PQ interval) represents the time from onset of atrial depolarisation to that of ventricular depolarisation, where the impulse has travelled through the atria and down the specialised internodal pathway to the A-V node. It then traverses the His Bundle, the three bundle branches, the left posterior, left anterior and right tracts, and the Purkinje system, finally activating the electrical endocardial surface of the Sodi-Pallares system.

QRS complex

The QRS complex is the net resultant electrical potential generated from ventricular depolarisation as seen by the appropriate surface electrode. Activation in the ventricle commences in the left side of the interventricular septum and spreads to the right and left surface, then activates the ventricle. Activation proceeds in the anterior and posterior regions adjacent to the septum (the resultant is electrically neutral) and then traverses the apical and lateral walls of both ventricles. The last areas activated are the lower portion of the interventricular septum and the low posterior wall adjoining it.

QRS interval

This is usually 0.06–0.10 ms in adults, tends to last longer in men and should be measured from the widest QRS complex, usually found in the mid precordial leads.

QRS axis

Axis is the direction of the dominant line of electrical excitation through the heart. It lies between −30° to +90° in adults and −30° to +110° in children and adolescents. A slight variation can occur in the same individual from time to time. Axis determines whether conduction is affected by factors such as infarction and hypertrophy and can be judged roughly by inspecting the direction of the R waves in leads I to III. Figure 19.6a shows examples of normal axis, left axis deviation and right axis deviation. To obtain a more accurate assessment

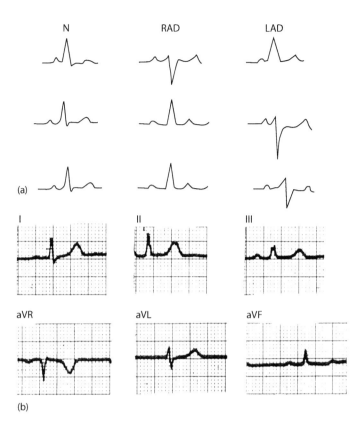

Figure 19.6 **(a)** Direction of the QRS complex is determined by the axis of the heart. At left is its appearance with a normal axis (N), in the middle is its appearance with right axis deviation (RAD), and at right is its appearance with left axis deviation (LAD). **(b)** Example of QRS direction with an axis rotated to +60°.

the hexagonal system may be used. First, the ECG lead with the greatest deflection (tallest R wave), represents the major direction of electrical axis. This is compared with the most equiphasic leads where the R and S deflections are equal. The electrical axis lies at 90° to this lead, and in the direction of the lead with the tallest R wave.

Figure 19.6b illustrates an example. In this case the lead with the tallest positive R wave is lead II, so the major direction of electrical axis is in this direction, which is +60°. The most equiphasic lead is aVL (the axis of aVL is −30°). The electrical axis of the heart lies at 90° to the aVL lead and in the direction of lead II, which is +60°.

MYOCARDIAL INFARCTION AND ISCHAEMIA

The hallmark of myocardial infarction is the development of pathological Q waves. These are waves greater than 0.04 seconds in width and more than 1/3 the height of the R wave, or complete loss of the R wave with replacement by a Q wave. Q waves are present when 40% or more of the transmural thickness of the myocardial wall is infarcted or necrotic (Figure 19.7).

Necrotic or scar tissue is electrically inactive so that an electrical "window" appears when an electrode is placed over the infarct. In Figure 19.7, the interventricular septum and right ventricular free wall are recorded from the electrode facing the left ventricular free wall. When cardiac tissue is ischaemic or injured, it becomes electrically negative, whereas the adjacent normal tissue remains positively charged. As a consequence, a negative current of injury is recorded from the injured surface by an electrode facing it (as in Figure 19.7), and a continuous positive current is recorded by an electrode facing the normal tissue adjacent to the injured tissue (as in Figure 19.8a).

In widespread sub-endocardial ischaemia or unstable angina, the whole endocardium is

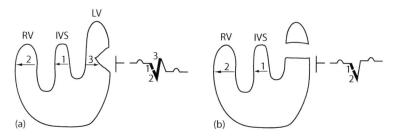

Figure 19.7 (a) An electrode placed over an infarcted segment of myocardium (3) records the current in regions (1) and (2) as moving away from the electrode, i.e. segment (3) is transparent electrically, hence forming pathological Q waves (a positive charge moving away from a positive electrode records a negative deflection on ECG). The illustration in (b) depicts a transmural infarct with only a QS complex. There is no R wave.

negatively charged. The ECG shows widespread varying ST depression due to an elevated baseline resulting from the continuous positive current (Figure 19.8b) transmitted from the normal tissue adjacent to the injured tissue. The changes occur because the continuous current related to injury affects the resting electrical baseline, but with depolarisation the true electrical baseline is re-assumed.

Myocardial infarction, however, is not usually an all-or-nothing situation. The region involved in necrosis usually contains patches of injured, ischaemic or even normal tissue. Adjacent to the most damaged portion is a surrounding area of injured tissue, and adjacent to that is ischaemic tissue (Figure 19.9).

The site of infarction relates to the coronary artery involved. Extended infarction relates to the position of the coronary lesion, such that the more proximal the lesion, generally the more extensive the infarction (taking into consideration other mitigating factors such as use of thrombolytic therapy, the extent of the luminal thrombotic occlusion, the presence or absence of diabetes mellitus, degree of collateralisation and other factors). Anterior

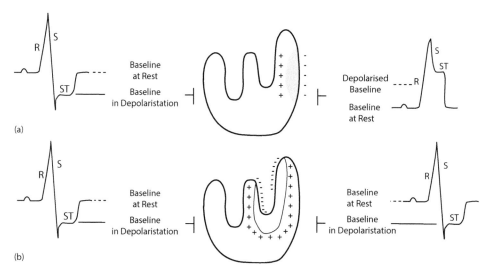

Figure 19.8 (a) Depiction of an ECG tracing of a myocardial infarct, where an electrode facing a region of infarction registers ST elevation, and an electrode away from the infarction registers ST depression ('reciprocal' change in ST level). (b) This shows an ECG tracing in myocardial ischaemia without infarction and is more widespread. An electrode over the ischaemic region and another one away from it both record ST segment depression.

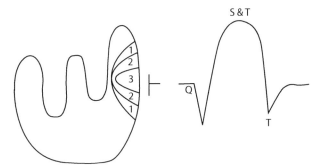

Figure 19.9 Appearance of QRS complex with a Q wave caused by an infarct. At left is the infarcted region in wall of ventricle (1 = ischaemia, 2 = injury, 3 = necrosis).

infarction usually involves the left anterior descending artery, inferior infarction usually involves the right coronary artery and posterior infarction involves the area usually supplied by the left circumflex artery. However, there are variations to this. If a diagonal branch of the left anterior descending artery occludes, T wave inversion is usually seen only in left anterior descending territory. A distal left anterior descending artery occlusion causing apical infarction usually involves T wave inversion in the apico-lateral leads. The proximal circumflex branches, when occluded, are often electrocardiographically silent on a standard ECG. To diagnose these, chest leads V7 to V12 are used. These are at the same level as lead V6 and 2 inches (5 cm) apart, coursing posteriorly around the chest.

Following is a summary of the major infarction patterns, and their association with the coronary blood supply and corresponding ECG changes.

Anterior infarction: Involves the left anterior descending artery and/or its major branches, with changes in leads V2-V4.

Septal infarction: Involves the proximal left anterior descending artery and its septal branches, with changes in leads V2-V3.

Apical infarction: Associated with rsR pattern in leads V4-V5.

High lateral infarction: Involves the obtuse marginal branch of circumflex, e.g. intermediate artery or a very proximal diagonal branch of the left anterior descending artery, with changes in leads I and aVL.

Lateral infarction: Involves the distal diagonal branches of the left anterior descending artery, distal circumflex or distal right coronary artery branches, with changes in leads V5-V6.

Inferior infarction: Usually involves the right coronary artery, but occasionally the circumflex (when dominant, in about 10% of cases) supplies the inferior surface (usually supplied by the posterior descending artery); changes in leads II, III and aVF.

Inferior infarction can show some variation in ECG pattern such that:

a. Sometime after the event Q waves may only be seen in III/aVF, whereas acutely they were present in all inferior leads; this indicates that the infarct is infero-basal, affecting the proximal portion of the inferior left ventricular wall and the interventricular septum.

b. ST depression may be noted at the same time in leads V1-V4, which is usually a mirror image of ST elevation in the posterior leads. This implies extension of the infarct upwards along the posterior wall due to:

1. A right coronary artery with numerous postero-lateral branches extending up the posterior wall of the heart, or

2. The circumflex artery is dominant, supplying the posterior descending branch (PDA).

There may be co-existing ST changes in V5-V6 due to involvement of the lateral wall, from a postero-lateral branch or a large PDA running to the apex.

Atrial infarction is unusual and occurs in the context of a large ventricular infarction. It is diagnosed by elevation of the PR segment, at times with a change in P wave morphology. In **acute pericarditis** there may be depression of the PR segment.

ABNORMAL RHYTHMS ASSOCIATED WITH MYOCARDIAL INFARCTION

Sinus node abnormalities

SINUS BRADYCARDIA

This may be due to:

a. Ischaemia of the SA node, causing local acidosis depressing nodal automaticity or elevation of adenosine causing a negative inotropic effect, or
b. Intense vagal stimulation which can be reversed by the administration of atropine. Bradycardia is up to three times more common in infero-posterior infarction, compared to anterior infarct. It is most likely to occur early in acute infarction (<3 hours) and is associated with a higher incidence of ventricular fibrillation, possibly as ventricular threshold is reduced with a bradycardia or because ventricular ectopics may be precipitated by long R-R intervals.

SINUS TACHYCARDIA

This is usually due to left ventricular failure but may be due to fever, coexistent pericarditis, anxiety, pulmonary embolus and other ailments. When sinus tachycardia is present there is usually a higher incidence of AV block 1° (first degree), 2° (second degree) and 3° (third degree) AV block.

SINUS ARREST

This is a rare occurrence (and is often due to S-A exit block) and occurs in inferior infarction with occlusion of the right coronary artery very proximally.

Atrial dysrrhythmias

ATRIAL ECTOPICS

These are very common in acute myocardial infarction and are due to either atrial ischaemia or atrial distension arising from heart failure with elevated LV diastolic pressure.

ATRIAL FIBRILLATION

This occurs in up to 10% of patients with acute myocardial infarction or with cardiac failure. It may be co-existent in patients with atrial disease or with damage from ischaemia, hypertension, pericarditis, chronic airways disease or other ailments. Atrial flutter and atrial tachycardia are very rare in acute myocardial infarction, when it may cause haemodynamic impairment due to rapid ventricular response. It may be treated with amiodarone (with intravenous loading), or judicious use of beta-blockers or electrical cardioversion.

Ventricular and nodal (junctional) rhythms

NODAL ESCAPE RHYTHM

These are inherently escape rhythms that occur when there are periods of sinus arrest, sinus bradycardia or abnormalities of impulse conduction with S-A block or A-V block. These rhythms are reasonably frequent in acute myocardial infarction, particularly inferior infarction as this is often associated with disorders of the S-A node causing sinus arrest, sinus bradycardia or S-A block. Nodal escape rhythm usually occurs at a rate of 50–60 beats per minute. Faster rates of AV nodal rhythm (which has automaticity) are the same as the causes of sinus tachycardia.

VENTRICULAR ECTOPIC BEATS

These occur in virtually all patients with acute myocardial infarction and they are of little prognostic significance, although it is considered that those arriving from the left ventricle are more likely to precipitate ventricular fibrillation. In the past there have been recommendations for pharmacological suppression of ventricular ectopy, but controlled trials have shown that doing so has not prevented ventricular fibrillation. Most coronary units now do not prophylactically suppress these ectopics.

VENTRICULAR TACHYCARDIA

Ventricular tachycardia consists of a series of three or more consecutive ventricular ectopic beats that occur at a rate faster than the underlying sinus rhythm. 3–10 escape beats are common in the first 36 hours after an acute myocardial infarction and are of little prognostic significance. However, rapid polymorphic ventricular tachycardia in the first 36 hours following infarction is of prognostic significance. Patients with a torsades de pointes

(TDP) pattern should have attention paid to the pro-arrhythmic effects of existing anti-arrhythmic therapy. TDP is also associated with the use of phenothiazines, tricyclic anti-depressants, erythromycin based anti-histamines, hypokalaemia and hypomagnesaemia. When polymorphic ventricular tachycardia is due solely to the myocardial infarction it usually responds well to anti-arrhythmic therapy.

IDIOVENTRICULAR TACHYCARDIA

This is frequently seen in acute myocardial infarction and often occurs following thrombolytic therapy, when re-perfusion of the coronary artery involved takes place. This rhythm rarely results in ventricular fibrillation and does not usually require treatment. However, because of loss of the atrial contraction, cardiac output can be significantly impaired by up to 20%, causing symptomatic hypotension and cardiac failure. Under these circumstances it should be treated with either anti-arrhythmic drugs or atropine.

VENTRICULAR FIBRILLATION

Prevention of death from dysrrhythmia is one of the major aims in acute coronary care. Ventricular fibrillation is often induced by electrolyte abnormalities and is more common the more extensive the myocardial infarction. The incidence decreases from 5% to −7% of patients with acute myocardial infarction in the early 1970s to <2% in the late 1980s. This is partly due to use of beta-blockers in acute myocardial infarction, and more vigorous and effective treatment of cardiac failure and correction of electrolyte imbalances. Clinical trials have shown that ventricular premature beats are unreliable predictors of the development of ventricular fibrillation.

CONDUCTION DISTURBANCES IN ACUTE MYOCARDIAL INFARCTION

1° Atrio-ventricular block

This is a delay in conduction of the P wave from the SA node to the AV node and is evident as a prolonged PQ interval. It is seen in inferior infarction involving the AV node, where it is a benign finding, and less frequently in anterior infarction with septal involvement causing distal conduction delay. In this situation it indicates a far more extensive infarction.

2° Atrio-ventricular block

There are two main types:

Mobitz Type I, or Wenckebach block, is a progressive lengthening of the PQ interval with a subsequent "dropped" QRS beat. The mechanism is similar to that of 1° AV block. It is common to see a patient's rhythm progress from 1° AV block to Wenkebach block and then back, although Wenkebach block may be present for some time (>24 hours) before reverting to 1° block. The QRS complex usually remains narrow except in the presence of anterior infarction, when left anterior hemiblock or right bundle branch block may develop. In this situation the course may be more complicated.

Mobitz Type II block is evident as one or more "dropped" QRS beats following failure of a P wave to conduct to the AV node. It is due to ischaemia of the septal infra-nodal conduction pathway in anterior infarction and may be associated with a narrow or wide QRS complex. In the latter, due to bundle branch block, the prognosis is poor. Mobitz Type II may progress to 3° AV block and require temporary pacemaker insertion.

3° Atrio-ventricular block

This is complete conduction failure of propagation of impulse from atrium to ventricle and results in ventricular standstill, evident as a prolonged flat ECG signal. It may occur in inferior or anterior myocardial infarction. The mechanisms differ and have different prognostic implications. In inferior infarction it is the result of necrosis or ischaemia of the AV node (with or without vagal stimulation) and may progress from 1° AV block to 2° AV block (Mobitz Type I) to 3° AV block. Usually it is benign and haemodynamics are maintained, although a temporary pacemaker may at times be required. In anterior myocardial infarction the prognosis is much poorer due to the extensive nature of the infarct. Rather than having a gradual onset as in inferior infarction it may be of abrupt onset with major haemodynamic impairment. A temporary pacemaker is usually required to maintain haemodynamics and often a permanent pacemaker is required if the patient survives. Due to the large amount of left ventricular impairment associated with an anterior myocardial infarction and heart block, an implantable defibrillator may be indicated to prevent subsequent death.

Hemiblock

Left anterior hemiblock may occur in antero-septal infarction and is of little significance unless right bundle branch block also develops. In this situation (bi-fascicular block) high grade AV block (Mobitz Type II or 3° AV block) may develop requiring a temporary pacemaker implantation.

Bundle branch block

This is failure of either the right or left bundle branch to conduct and is seen as a widened QRS complex. When occurring in the context of acute myocardial infarction it usually indicates extensive infarction with significant haemodynamic impairment.

PSEUDO-INFARCT PATTERNS ON STANDARD ECG

These are cardiac conditions where the standard resting ECG may be confused with an ischaemic pattern. Following is a brief description of the various types encountered.

Wolff–Parkinson–White syndrome

The delta wave can mimic Q waves in the inferior, lateral and posterior leads, mimicking infarction patterns.

Hypertrophic cardiomyopathy

This can occur with or without obstruction of the left ventricular outflow tract and is associated not only with cardiac failure but also with ventricular dysrrhythmias, and at times, atrial dysrhythmias. The resting ECG can show Q waves due to hypertrophy and also ST/T wave changes mimicking hyperacute infarction (ST elevation), old infarction (Q waves) or ischaemia (ST/T changes).

Chronic obstructive airways disease and right ventricular hypertrophy

These conditions may be associated with weak R wave development in the inferior and early precordial leads ('poor R wave progression'), mimicking old infarction.

Pulmonary emboli

This may be associated with T wave changes due to right ventricular strain suggesting ischaemia. At times, Q waves may develop in lead III, suggesting old infarction. If chronic recurrent pulmonary emboli occur, then right ventricular hypertrophy with clockwise precordial rotation and slow R wave development in V1–V4 may result, suggesting old antero-septal myocardial infarction.

Thoracic cage deformity

This condition, especially *pectus excavatum*, which causes flattening or compression of the heart with movement to the left, causes slow R wave development in leads V1-V4, suggesting anterior infarction.

Miscellaneous

A list of additional conditions that demonstrate pseudo-Infarct patterns on standard ECG are listed in Table 19.1, and Figure 19.10 shows some examples of pseudo-infarct patterns on ECG.

Figure 19.10a shows a pseudoinfarct pattern in Wolff–Parkinson–White syndrome. There is a Q wave in the inferior leads which is produced by pre-excitation of the posteroseptal left ventricle.

Figure 19.10b shows the ECG pattern in Brugada syndrome: This shows ST elevation in the precordial leads V_1 and V_2, which can be confused with an anteroseptal myocardial infarction.

Figure 19.10c shows the ECG pattern in hyperkalaemia: There are extensive ST segment changes and underlying heart block due to this metabolic abnormality.

The ECG in Figure 19.10d is from a patient with Q waves in leads III and aVF consistent with an old inferior infarction, Q waves in leads I, V_3 and a small RSR in V_4. She has had a previous antero-apicoseptal infarction and the RSR in V_4 indicates apical aneurysm. There are ST/T wave changes in leads I, aVL, V_5 and V_6 consistent with lateral ischaemia.

The ECG in Figure 19.10e shows this patient has atrial fibrillation and right bundle branch block but there is a small Q wave in leads V_1–V_3 as well as a Q wave in III and aVF. This patient has had

Table 19.1 Conditions that present pseudo-infarct patterns on the electrocardiogram

Cardiomyopathy	• Dilated • Hypertrophic • Takotsubo
Infiltrative cardiac disease	• Amyloid • Sarcoid • Haemochromatosis • Scleroderma • Primary and secondary cardiac tumours
Pericardial disease	• Acute pericarditis • Infective • Trauma • Post infarction
Myocarditis	
Myocardial injury/contusion	
Congenital heart disease	• Fallot's tetralogy • Primum ASD • Congenital coronary anomalies
Left ventricular hypertrophy	
Hyperkalaemia	
Cerebrovascular accident/Subarachnoid haemorrhage	
Kawasaki disease	
Pulmonary disease	• Emphysema • Spontaneous pneumothorax • Pulmonary embolus • Left sided thoracic cage deformity • Marked pectus excavatum
Neurological diseases	• Muscular dystrophy • Friedreich's ataxia
Cardiac rhythm/electrical disturbances	• Left bundle branch block • Stokes Adams with giant T wage inversion • Post tachycardia ST/T wave inversion • Pacemaker-induced T wave changes

previous inferior infarction and in the presence of right bundle branch block, also shows a previous septal infarction.

The ECG in Figure 19.10f was taken from a patient who presented to hospital with severe central pre-cordial chest pain, and was found to have normal coronary arteries. A subsequent ventilation quellum (VQ) scan showed massive pulmonary embolus. Her T wave changes in leads I, aVL, V_1–V_6 could easily be mistaken for myocardial ischaemia.

REFERENCES (HISTORICAL)

1. Sodi Pallares D, Rodriguez MI, Bisteni A. Electrocardiographic diagnosis of left bundle branch block complicated by myocardial infarct. *Arch Inst Cardiol Mex.* 1952;22(1):1–48.
2. Sodi-Pallares D, Bisteni A, Medrano GA, Cisneros F. The activation of the free left ventricular wall in the dog's heart; in normal conditions and in left bundle branch block. *Am Heart J.* 1955;49(4):587–602.

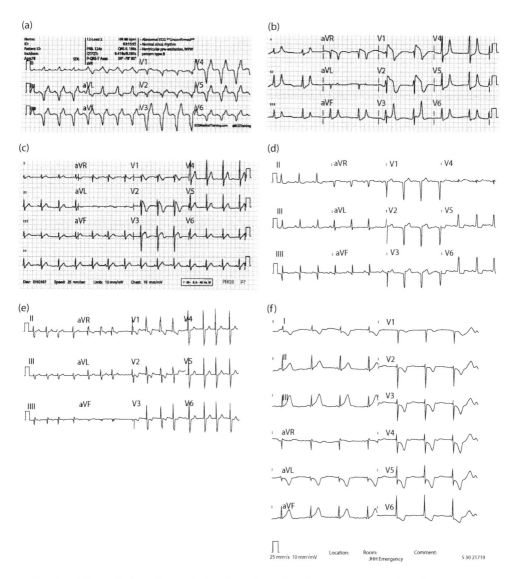

Figure 19.10 (a–f) Compilation of sample ECG tracings showing various pseudo-infarct patterns. See text for description.

3. Sodi-Pallares D, Estandia A, Soberon J, Rodriguez MI. The left intraventricular potential of the human heart. II. Criteria for diagnosis of incomplete bundle branch block. *Am Heart J*. 1950;40(5):655–679.
4. Sodi-pallares D, Medrano GA, De Micheli A, Testelli MR, Bisteni A. Unipolar QS morphology and Purkinje potential of the free left ventricular wall. *Circulation*. 1961;23(6):836–846.
5. Durrer D, van Dam RT, Freud GE, Janse MJ, Meijler FL, Arzbaecher RC. Total excitation of the isolated human heart. *Circulation*. 1970;41(6):899–912.

FURTHER READING

Garcia TB. 2014. *Introduction to 12 Lead ECG: The Art of Interpretation*. 2nd ed. Burlington, MA: Jones & Bartlett Learning, p. 536.
Hampton JR, Hampton J. 2019. *The ECG Made Easy*. Elsevier Health Sciences, p. 240.
Morris F, Brady WJ, Camm J. 2009. *ABC of Clinical Electrocardiography*. 2nd ed. Boston, MA: Blackwell Publishing, p. 112.
Wesley K. 2016. *Pocket Guide to Huszar's Basic Dysrhythmias and Acute Coronary Syndromes*. 4th ed. St. Louis, MO: Elsevier Mosby Jems, p. 524.

20

Recognition of common arrhythmias

NICHOLAS P. KERR AND RAJESH N. SUBBIAH

INTRODUCTION

Rapid recognition and accurate diagnosis of common cardiac arrhythmias are critical skills for personnel working in a cardiac catheterisation centre. Life-threatening bradyarrhythmias and tachyarrhythmias may occur in percutaneous coronary and structural cardiac procedures as well as during invasive electrophysiology and cardiac electronic device implantation. This chapter focuses on the recognition and diagnosis of common arrhythmias. Important aspects of the causation, management and pitfalls of arrhythmia are briefly addressed. However, a comprehensive coverage of the mechanisms, diagnosis and management of arrhythmias is beyond the scope of the chapter. Arrhythmias occurring in the setting of acute myocardial infarction are covered specifically due to their common occurrence during primary percutaneous coronary intervention. Life-threatening arrhythmias leading to haemodynamic instability should be managed according to Advanced Cardiac Life Support algorithms.

BRADYARRHYTHMIAS AND CONDUCTION DISEASE

Sinus node dysfunction

Sinus bradycardia is present when the sinus rate is less than 60 bpm (Table 20.1). It may be physiological when it occurs in situations of elevated parasympathetic tone, as in athletes and during sleep, or may be pathological in association with medications, metabolic derangement or intrinsic sinus node disease. Most cases are transient and are managed by treating the underlying cause. Specific treatment for acute sinus bradycardia is rarely required, but may include the use of atropine, isoprenaline or temporary pacing.

Table 20.1 Common causes of sinus bradycardia

Increased parasympathetic nervous system
   activity
   - Athletes
   - Sleep
   - Vasovagal (cardioinhibitory) or carotid
     sinus hypersensitivity mediated
   - Inferior myocardial infarction
   - Obstructive sleep apnoea
   - Raised intracranial pressure
Medications
   - Beta-blockers
   - Calcium channel blockers
   - Digoxin
   - Antiarrhythmic medications (amiodarone,
     flecainide)
   - Ivabradine
Metabolic
   - Hypoxia
   - Sepsis
   - Hypothyroidism
   - Hypothermia
   - Hypoglycaemia
Intrinsic sinus node disease

When the sinus node is unable to generate a heart rate that meets the physiological demands of an individual, sick sinus syndrome is the most likely cause (Figure 20.1a). It manifests as periods of unprovoked sinus bradycardia, sinoatrial pauses or arrest, paroxysms of sinus bradycardia, or pauses following atrial tachyarrhythmias ('tachy-brady' syndrome) and chronotropic incompetence with exercise intolerance. Chronotropic incompetence is defined as failure to achieve 70% of age-predicted maximum heart rate during exercise and is an often-overlooked cause of breathlessness and exercise intolerance. Sinus node fibrosis is the most common cause of sick sinus syndrome in the absence of reversible factors such as medications and hypothyroidism. If a reversible cause cannot be found and corrected, permanent pacing is indicated for symptomatic patients.

Atrioventricular conduction disease

Impaired atrioventricular (AV) conduction is classified as first, second or third degree (complete) block (Figure 20.1b). First degree AV block is diagnosed when the PR interval is prolonged to greater than 200 ms, with all atrial impulses conducted to the ventricles with a 1:1 relationship. In second degree AV block, there is failure of conduction of some atrial impulses to the ventricles. There are two main types of second-degree AV block: Wenckebach (Mobitz I) and Mobitz II.

In Wenckebach (Mobitz I) second degree AV block, there is progressive PR interval prolongation until a non-conducted atrial beat occurs, giving a 'group beating' pattern on the electrocardiogram (ECG). The block is usually at the AV node level and may be secondary to ischaemia, inflammation (myocarditis), increased parasympathetic nervous system activity or drugs. Classically, the absolute increase in PR interval decreases with subsequent beats so that the RR intervals shorten prior to the blocked beat. The pause following block is less than twice the proceeding RR interval. Wenckebach block typically improves with manoeuvres that increase AV nodal conduction (exercise, atropine) and may worsen with manoeuvres that impair AV nodal conduction (carotid sinus massage). Wenckebach block is often intermittent and asymptomatic, and rarely requires treatment.

In Mobitz II second degree AV block there are intermittently blocked atrial beats with a constant PR interval. The block is generally below the level of the AV node in the His-Purkinje system. Causes include ischaemia, degenerative disease of the conduction system, infiltrative disease, and inflammation. In contrast to Wenckebach AV block, manoeuvres that increase the sinus rate and improve AV nodal conduction (exercise, atropine) may worsen conduction in Mobitz II block, as the vulnerable distal conduction system is exposed to a higher rate of input impulses and has a greater probability of failing to conduct them. Conversely, manoeuvres that slow AV nodal conduction (carotid sinus massage) may improve Mobitz II block by 'protecting' the distal conduction system. Mobitz II AV block has a higher rate of progression to complete heart block, and treatment with a permanent pacemaker is likely to be required once reversible causes have been excluded.

Second degree AV block commonly occurs in a 2:1 pattern with every second atrial impulse failing to conduct to the ventricles. Without at least two consequently conducted beats occurring prior to block, it is not possible to classify this pattern as Wenckebach or Mobitz II block, because there is no opportunity to observe the PR prolongation that occurs in Wenckebach pattern. Additional ECG and clinical criteria are needed to make the distinction between an AV nodal and infranodal mechanism of 2:1 block. ECG evidence favouring an infranodal mechanism may include the presence of another defect of distal conduction, for example bundle branch block or intraventricular conduction delay. Observing Wenckebach or Mobitz II block at other times in the same patient may also help to determine the level of block. Occasionally, in 2:1 AV block the PP intervals containing QRS completes are shorter than the PP intervals not containing QRS complexes. This is called ventriculophasic sinus arrhythmia. High-grade AV block refers to failure of two or more consecutive atrial beats to conduct to the ventricles.

In third degree (complete) AV block, there is no AV conduction, and there is complete dissociation of atrial and ventricular activity. If underlying sinus rhythm is present, complete AV block is diagnosed when (1) there is dissociation of P waves and QRS complexes, (2) there are more P waves than QRS complexes and (3) a regular QRS escape rhythm is present. The escape rhythm may be narrow if it arises from the AV junction, or wide if it arises from the ventricles. If there is failure of an escape rhythm to emerge when complete heart block occurs suddenly, the ECG may show a series of P waves without any ventricular activity (QRS complexes). This is called ventricular standstill.

AV dissociation alone does not imply complete heart block. It is possible for a subsidiary pacemaker to usurp the sinus node, for example, when there is sinus bradycardia and a competing junctional rhythm at a faster rate. Isorhythmic AV dissociation occurs when there is AV dissociation and the junctional and sinus rates are closely matched. Complete heart block may also be diagnosed when there is atrial fibrillation (AF) associated with a regularised slow ventricular rate, but not when there is a junctional rhythm and retrograde atrial activation.

Complete heart block may occur intermittently with an abrupt and unexpected change from 1:1 AV conduction to complete heart block, often with a period of ventricular standstill. This pattern may be due to block at the AV node (vagal AV block) or infranodal level. In the latter case, it is called paroxysmal AV block.[1] It is important to make the distinction between intermittent vagal AV block and paroxysmal AV block because paroxysmal

AV block is associated with unheralded syncope and a risk of sudden cardiac death. ECG clues that vagal AV block is the mechanism include PP and PR prolongation prior to block and sinus acceleration on resolution of block. In contrast, paroxysmal AV block is often preceded by tachycardia or initiated by an atrial or ventricular premature beat (Figure 20.1b).

Cardiac procedures are an important iatrogenic cause of AV block. Aortic or mitral valve replacement surgery is often accompanied by transient AV block related to periprocedural oedema. In aortic valve surgery, the infranodal conduction system is more likely to be damaged and the likelihood of requiring permanent pacing is higher. In mitral valve surgery, block is more commonly at the AV nodal level, is more likely to recover and a longer waiting period is usually applied before deciding to implant a permanent pacemaker. Complete heart block occurs in approximately 5% of patients following transcatheter aortic valve implantation. Pre-existing conduction disease, especially right bundle branch block (RBB), mitral annular calcification and a narrow left ventricular outflow tract predict this complication. AV block is more common with self-expanding implanted aortic valves compared with balloon-expandable versions.[2]

Regardless of the cause, acute management of AV block involves identifying and correcting reversible factors, and if there is haemodynamic instability or symptomatic bradycardia, supporting the patient with isoprenaline or temporary pacing while it is determined if permanent pacing is required.

Intraventricular conduction disturbances

Abnormalities of intraventricular conduction are commonly seen. They include left and right bundle branch block, isolated fascicular blocks (hemiblock), bifascicular block and non-specific intraventricular conduction delay (Figure 20.1c).

RBBB produces an rSR' pattern in lead V_1 and a wide, slurred S wave in leads I and V_6. The frontal plane axis is usually normal. Left bundle branch block (LBBB) produces a QS or rS pattern in V_1, and a broad, slurred, monophasic R wave in leads I, aVL and V_6. There may be left axis deviation, or the axis may be normal. When the QRS duration is greater than 120 ms, the bundle branch block is complete. Incomplete bundle branch block occurs when the same patterns are present but the QRS duration is 110–120 ms. Bundle branch blocks cause secondary abnormalities in repolarisation that manifest as displacement of the ST segment and T wave in the opposite direction to the major QRS deflection (i.e. the ST-T changes are discordant in direction to the QRS complex). Non-specific intraventricular conduction delay refers to QRS widening or abnormal fractionation that does not fit the patterns of typical left or right bundle branch block.

Bundle branch block can be chronic or intermittent. Transient rate-related bundle branch blocks may occur during tachycardia or sudden heart rate acceleration. This is also referred to as rate-related aberrancy. Ashman's phenomenon is a specific pattern of aberrant conduction, in which

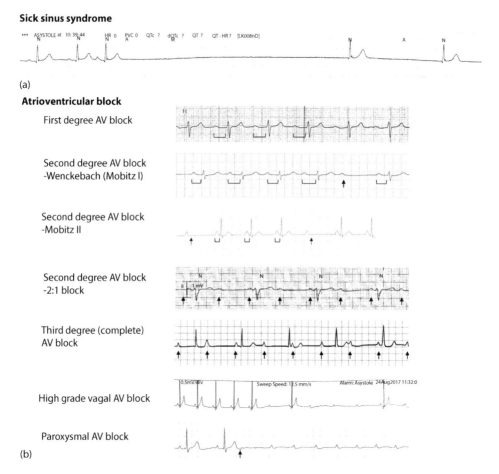

Figure 20.1 Bradyarrhythmias and conduction disease. **(a) Sick sinus syndrome.** There are two beats of sinus rhythm followed by an atrial premature complex (APC). The APC depolarises the sinus node causing a sinus pause of over 5 seconds after which a junctional escape rhythm emerges. **(b) Atrioventricular (AV) block.** First-degree AV block with a constant PR interval of 300 ms and preserved 1:1 AV conduction. Second-degree Wenckebach block with gradual PR interval prolongation prior to a blocked beat (arrow). Second-degree Mobitz II block with constant PR interval prior to blocked beats (arrows). Second-degree 2:1 AV block. There are twice as many P waves (arrows) as QRS complexes. Third degree (complete) heart block. There is AV dissociation, more P waves (arrows) than QRS complexes and a regular narrow complex escape rhythm. Note that the second P wave occurs at the same time as the T wave from the preceding QRS complex and is superimposed on it. Intermittent vagal AV block with sinus slowing prior to 2:1; then high-grade AV block. Paroxysmal AV block triggered by an APC (arrow). Note there is sinus acceleration during the period of complete heart block with ventricular standstill. *(Continued)*

Intraventricular conduction disease

Left bundle branch block (LBBB)

Right bundle branch block (RBBB)

1st degree AV block, Left anterior fascicular block & RBBB

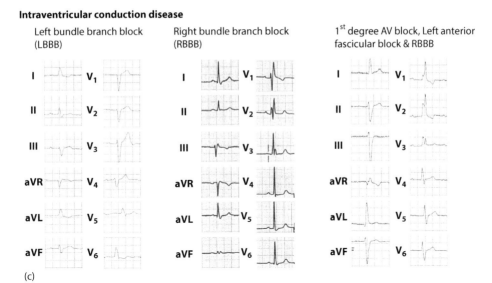

(c)

Figure 20.1 (Continued) Bradyarrhythmias and conduction disease. **(c) Intraventricular conduction disease.** Left bundle branch block with QRS duration of 150 ms, QS complex in lead V$_1$, wide slurred monophasic R waves in leads I, aVL and V$_6$. The axis is normal. Right bundle branch block (RBBB) with a QRS duration of 140 ms, RSR' in lead V$_1$, slurred S wave in leads I and V$_6$. The axis is normal. Note that in V$_1$, the initial r wave is of lower amplitude than the secondary R' wave, consistent with typical RBBB appearance. Complete RBBB associated with left axis deviation (positive QRS in lead I, negative QRS in leads II and III) is due to left anterior fascicular block. This combination is called bifascicular block. Note first degree AV block (PR prolongation) is also present in this example.

a wide QRS beat occurs when a short R-R interval is preceded by a long R-R interval. The wide QRS beat most often has a right bundle branch block morphology. Ashman's phenomenon often occurs in AF where the aberrantly conducted QRS complex may be misinterpreted as a premature ventricular complex. Transient bradycardia-dependent bundle branch blocks also occur but are relatively rare. While tachycardia-related aberrancy may be physiological or pathological (such as with coronary ischaemia), transient bradycardia-dependent bundle branch block is always pathological and signifies that underlying conduction disease is present.

Hemiblock

Hemiblock refers to conduction block in either of the two fascicles of the left bundle branch. Isolated left anterior fascicular block causes left axis deviation without QRS widening, while left posterior fascicular block causes right axis deviation. Left anterior fascicular block occurs about ten times more frequently than left posterior fascicular block

because the left anterior fascicle is a fine cord of conduction tissue that is more fragile than the broad sheet-like posterior fascicle. Hemiblock should only be diagnosed when there is no other cause for axis deviation. For example, left anterior fascicular block cannot be diagnosed when left axis deviation is present due to Q waves of previous inferior infarction, and left posterior fascicular block should not be diagnosed when right axis deviation is present due to right ventricular hypertrophy.

The combination of left anterior or posterior fascicular block with right bundle branch block is called bifascicular block. While isolated hemiblock is of little clinical significance, in bifascicular block all AV conduction is dependent on the single remaining fascicle, indicating a severe degree of intraventricular conduction disease and a high risk of progression to complete heart block. When bifascicular block is associated with PR prolongation (first degree AV block), the conduction disturbance is even more severe. This pattern is sometimes called 'trifascicular' block. That term should be avoided because one of the fascicles is not entirely blocked, but conducting with delay.

Similarly, it is confusing to refer to isolated left bundle branch block as 'bifascicular' block, or the combination of left bundle branch block and first-degree AV block as 'trifascicular' block.

SUPRAVENTRICULAR TACHYARRHYTHMIAS

Sinus tachycardia

Sinus tachycardia is defined as sinus rhythm at a rate greater than 100 bpm. Causes include pain, fever, hypovolaemia, hypoxia, anaemia, anxiety, decompensated heart failure, pulmonary embolism, hyperthyroidism and medications (e.g. beta-adrenoreceptor agonists). Management always involves identifying and treating reversible causes. Some patients have a rare condition called inappropriate sinus tachycardia. It typically affects young women and is defined as a resting heart rate of greater than 100 bpm, with a mean heart rate greater than 90 bpm over 24 hours. It is often associated with highly symptomatic palpitations. Reversible causes of sinus tachycardia and atrial tachycardia must be excluded. Beta-blockers, calcium channel blockers or ivabradine may be used to treat inappropriate sinus tachycardia, but sinus node modification by catheter ablation should generally be avoided.

Atrial premature complexes

Atrial premature complexes (APCs) are the most common rhythm abnormality detected during extended ECG monitoring. They may occasionally be experienced as palpitations but are generally asymptomatic. The ECG diagnosis is made when a P wave occurs prior to the next expected sinus beat. The P wave morphology is usually atypical of a sinus beat and reflects the location of the ectopic focus from where the beat originated. Most APCs are conducted with a longer PR interval, but occasionally the PR interval may be shorter if the focus is near the AV node. A very early APC may find the AV node refractory and not conduct to the ventricle, creating a short pause. In fact, blocked APCs are the commonest cause of pauses. An aberrantly conducted APC may be misdiagnosed as a ventricular premature complex if the preceding P wave is superimposed on the T wave and not noticed.

Atrial fibrillation

AF is the most common sustained arrhythmia. It is characterised by very rapid and disorganised electrical activity in the atria, which when conducted to the ventricles typically results in a rapid and irregular ventricular response. A fast irregular ventricular rate may cause palpitations, breathlessness and exercise intolerance. The rapid and disorganised atrial activity results in loss of atrial mechanical function. Loss of atrial mechanical contribution to ventricular preload contributes to symptoms, but more importantly, the absence of atrial contraction predisposes to formation of thrombus within the left atrium and left atrial appendage that may embolise to cause stroke or other thromboembolic events. The ECG in AF shows a lack of organised atrial activity with irregular fibrillatory waves with a flat isoelectric baseline, as well as irregularly irregular QRS complexes (Figure 20.2a).

AF is classified, based on duration, into paroxysmal (self-terminating, usually <48 hours), persistent (sustained longer than 7 days or terminated after treatment), and long-standing persistent (sustained for greater than 1 year). Permanent AF is long-standing persistent AF where the decision has been made to forgo attempts to restore sinus rhythm. AF is also classified as valvular AF or non-valvular AF. Valvular AF is associated with rheumatic mitral valve disease, or aortic or mitral valve replacement or repair. Risk factors for recurrent AF include increasing age, hypertension, ischaemia, valvular heart disease, heart failure and cardiomyopathy, hyperthyroidism, obstructive sleep apnoea and obesity. The term 'lone AF' was previously used to describe AF occurring in younger patients (<60 years old) without clinical or echocardiographic evidence of associated cardiac disease.

Up to 50% of acute AF episodes have a reversible cause (Table 20.2). Patients with acute AF who are haemodynamically unstable should be treated with urgent cardioversion. Stable patients with new or recent-onset AF are initially treated with rate-control medications (beta-blockers, calcium channel blockers or digoxin) and then anticoagulated with subcutaneous low molecular weight heparin, intravenous unfractionated heparin or direct oral anticoagulants (DOACs). Spontaneous reversion to sinus rhythm occurs in half to two-thirds of

Table 20.2 Common causes of acute episodes of atrial fibrillation

Cardiac
- Decompensated heart failure
- Myocardial ischaemia or infarction
- Cardiac surgery

Respiratory
- Pulmonary embolism
- Exacerbation of chronic lung disease
- Pneumonia

Metabolic
- Sepsis
- Post-operative state
- Thyrotoxicosis

Drugs
- Alcohol
- Cocaine
- Amphetamines
- Caffeine

patients with acute AF within 24 hours. If the episode does not terminate spontaneously, pharmacological or direct-current (DC) cardioversion can be attempted. Anticoagulation must be initiated prior to cardioversion and continued for at least 4 weeks, regardless of whether pharmacological or DC cardioversion is used. If the episode of AF is known to be less than 48 hours duration and the risk of stroke is low, cardioversion may be performed immediately without transoesophageal echocardiography. If the episode of AF is greater than 48 hours duration or of unknown duration, or the risk of stroke is high, transoesophageal echocardiography must be performed prior to cardioversion to exclude left atrial appendage thrombus. Alternatively, anticoagulation may be continued for at least 3 weeks prior to performing cardioversion in the absence of transoesophageal echocardiography.

Continuation of oral anticoagulation with warfarin or DOAC in the long-term is based on the risk of stroke as determined by the CHA_2DS_2-VASc score (see Chapter 12) for patients with non-valvular AF. Patients with a CHA_2DS_2-VASc score of 2 or more are recommended to have long-term anticoagulation and should be considered on an individual basis for males with a CHA_2DS_2-VASc score of 1. All patients with valvular AF require long term anticoagulation, generally with warfarin.

Recurrent AF may be managed with rate-control or rhythm-control strategies. Detailed discussion of these approaches is beyond the scope of this chapter. The options for rate control include medications such as beta-blockers, calcium channel blockers and digoxin or, as a last resort, AV node ablation and permanent pacemaker implantation. Pharmacological rhythm control can be attempted with antiarrhythmic medications such as flecainide, sotalol or amiodarone. Flecainide should not be used to treat AF without co-administration of an AV node blocking medication (see below). Rhythm control for AF can also be achieved with catheter or surgical ablation procedures.

Atrial flutter

Atrial flutter refers to a macro re-entrant arrhythmia involving the atrial myocardium. The most common form is 'typical' atrial flutter, with a circuit rotating in a counter clockwise (or less commonly, clockwise) direction in the right atrium around the tricuspid valve annulus. The narrowest part of the circuit is a zone of tissue called the cavotricuspid isthmus, which is bounded anteriorly by the tricuspid annulus and posteriorly by the inferior vena cava. When this isthmus is targeted for ablation, typical atrial flutter can be successfully cured in most cases.

Macro re-entrant left atrial flutter and non-cavotricuspid isthmus-dependent right atrial flutters occur less commonly and are generally arise after catheter ablation or surgical procedures that create scars in the atria that act as anatomic barriers that allow re-entry to occur.

Typical cavotricuspid isthmus-dependent flutter has an average atrial rate of 300 bpm and is most often conducted with 2:1 AV block, producing a ventricular response of 150 bpm. Higher ratios of AV block (e.g. 4:1 block) or variable AV block are commonly seen in the presence of AV conduction disease or AV node-blocking medications. When there is atrial conduction disease, or when antiarrhythmic medications are administered, the atrial rate can slow to <200 bpm increasing the probability of very rapid 1:1 ventricular response with severe haemodynamic effects. The risk of 1:1 AV conduction is especially prominent with the class Ic antiarrhythmic drug flecainide, which slows the atrial rate without inhibiting AV nodal conduction. For this reason, flecainide should not be given to patients with atrial flutter (or AF that may 'organise' into atrial flutter) without co-administration of an AV node blocking medication.

Typical counter clockwise cavotricuspid isthmus-dependent right atrial flutter produces a characteristic ECG pattern with 'saw-tooth' negative flutter waves in the inferior leads (II, III and aVF, reflecting activation of the interatrial sputum in an inferior-to-superior direction) and a small positive flutter wave in V_1. The less-common clockwise form produces the 'mirror-image' of this pattern, with an undulating positive wave in the inferior leads and a negative wave in lead V_1. Right atrial flutter generally has a positive wave in lead I and aVL, reflecting activation of the left atrium in a right-to-left direction. Left atrial flutter is more likely to show negative flutter waves in I and aVL, and concordance between the flutter wave direction in the inferior leads and V_1 (i.e. negative-negative or positive-positive). None of these patterns is completely specific and the associations are less robust in the presence of extensive atrial fibrosis, where typical counter clockwise flutter may show an atypical ECG pattern and, conversely, left atrial flutters may have a pattern reminiscent of typical right atrial flutter. A common pitfall in ECG interpretation is misdiagnosing 'coarse' AF as atrial flutter. The appearance in lead V_1 may mimic atrial flutter waves due to relatively uniform activation of the right atrial appendage and free wall. The distinction is made by noting a lack of complete uniformity of flutter waves within each lead throughout the ECG (Figure 20.2a).

The treatment of typical atrial flutter closely mirrors that of AF with rate-control, rhythm-control and anticoagulation, but atrial flutter is generally more difficult to control pharmacologically and easier to ablate than AF.

Multifocal atrial tachycardia is an uncommon irregular atrial rhythm seen most often in patients with advanced pulmonary disease. The ECG diagnosis is made when at least three different P-wave morphologies are present. It is distinguished from AF by the presence of a flat isoelectric baseline between P waves.

Paroxysmal supraventricular tachycardia

Paroxysmal supraventricular tachycardia (SVT) refers to episodic supraventricular tachyarrhythmias other than atrial flutter and AF that have a re-entrant or focal mechanism. The most common types are atrioventricular nodal re-entrant tachycardia, atrioventricular re-entrant tachycardia and (focal) atrial tachycardia (Figure 20.2b). They generally manifest as regular narrow complex tachycardia (NCT) with a 1:1 AV relationship, but may also present as a regular wide complex tachycardia (WCT) due to rate-related aberrancy or pre-excitation.

Atrioventricular nodal re-entrant tachycardia

Atrioventricular nodal re-entrant tachycardia (AVNRT) is the most common paroxysmal SVT. It affects women more often than men, and typically presents from age 10 to 40 years but can also present in old age. AVNRT occurs in individuals with dual AV nodal physiology. This implies the presence of a slow AV nodal pathway (with a slow conduction velocity but a long refractory period) and a fast AV nodal pathway (with a fast conduction velocity but a short refractory period). The pathways are functionally connected by upper and lower common pathways. Tachycardia is usually initiated by an atrial premature beat that blocks in the fast pathway (due to its short refractory period) and then conducts antegrade through the slow pathway. If the fast pathway has recovered from refractoriness by the time the impulse has reached the lower common pathway, it may conduct retrograde back up the fast pathway to re-enter the atrium. The circuit is complete when the impulse continues antegrade over the slow AV node pathway. The ECG at the onset of tachycardia often shows an APC with long PR interval due to conduction over the slow pathway. AVNRT usually produces a regular narrow complex tachycardia. The rate can be highly variable, from 120 to 250 bpm. It is classified as a short RP tachycardia. Due to small size of the re-entrant circuit in the AV node region, there is near-simultaneous atrial and ventricular activation. A retrograde P wave (negative P wave in leads II, III, aVF) is usually seen at end of the QRS complex and can cause pseudo-RBBB appearance in lead V_1. At other times, the P waves may not be visible at all as they are 'buried' within the QRS complex. The most common symptoms are episodes of rapid palpitations. Due to near-simultaneous atrial and ventricular activation, contraction of the atria may occur against closed AV valves. This may cause a sensation of neck palpitations, the 'frog' sign[3] and syncope from hypotension due to reflex activation of carotid sinus baroreceptors. Acute termination of AVNRT can often be achieved with vagal manoeuvres (VALSALVA manoeuvre or carotid sinus massage) or with bolus intravenous adenosine. Long-term management options include pharmacological therapy with beta-blockers and calcium channel blockers, often with the addition of flecainide (in those with a structurally normal heart and without significant conduction disease). Radiofrequency ablation of the AV node slow pathway region is highly effective for preventing recurrent AVNRT but is associated with a 1 in 200 risk of permanent AV block requiring a permanent pacemaker due to the proximity of the two pathways.

Atrioventricular re-entrant tachycardia

Atrioventricular re-entrant tachycardia (AVRT) is the second commonest cause of paroxysmal SVT. AVRT is more common in males than females and generally presents at a younger age than AVNRT. It occurs in patients with an accessory AV pathway (also called bypass tract) that allows AV (and/ or VA) conduction via another route than the normal AV node-His Purkinje system. Accessory pathways may conduct in both antegrade and retrograde directions, retrograde only, or uncommonly, antegrade direction only. When capable of conducting antegrade, accessory pathways cause pre-excitation pattern on the ECG. This occurs as conduction proceeds over the accessory pathway to activate the ventricles at another site earlier than conduction over the AV node. Pre-excitation on the ECG is manifest as a short PR interval, a wide QRS complex and a slurred onset to QRS called a 'delta wave'. When the ECG shows pre-excitation, the accessory pathway is said to be a manifest bypass tract. If the accessory pathway can only conduct in the retrograde direction, it is called a concealed bypass tract. Occasionally, there is no evidence of pre-excitation at rest but at increased sinus rates, more activation occurs over the accessory pathway so that pre-excitation becomes apparent. This is called a latent pathway. Patients with manifest pre-excitation and paroxysmal SVT have Wolff–Parkinson–White (WPW) syndrome.

In the absence of symptoms, a patient with an ECG appearance of pre-excitation is said to have WPW pattern.

Accessory pathways can be located anywhere on left (mitral) or right (tricuspid) AV valve rings. The commonest site is a left lateral pathway (lateral mitral annulus). This pathway causes a positive delta wave in lead V_1, negative delta wave in leads I and aVL and positive delta wave in the inferior leads. The second most common location is a right posteroseptal pathway, which gives a negative delta wave in lead V_1, usually transitioning to a positive QRS complex and delta wave in lead V_2. The delta waves are negative in inferior leads and usually positive in leads I and AVL (Figure 20.2c). Mid-septal, anteroseptal and right free wall are less-common sites for accessory pathways.

Accessory pathways can participate in three main types of tachycardia, (1) orthodromic AVRT, (2) antidromic AVRT and (3) as a bystander in another type of SVT such as atrial tachycardia or AF. In orthodromic AVRT, the tachycardia wavefront conducts antegrade over the AV node to the ventricles, then retrograde via the accessory pathway from the ventricle to the atrium and then antegrade over the AV node to complete the circuit. This typically causes a NCT unless there is rate-related bundle branch block. A retrograde P wave is usually present in the ST segment, making it a short RP tachycardia but with a longer RP interval than AVNRT (RP interval usually >80 ms).

In antidromic AVRT, which is about 10 times less common than orthodromic AVRT, the circuit direction is reversed, with conduction antegrade down the accessory pathway to the ventricle, then retrograde via the AV node to the atrium. The ECG shows a regular WCT with maximal pre-excitation pattern.

An accessory pathway may also be present as a bystander during another SVT, producing a WCT with pre-excitation pattern. This situation (along with antidromic AVRT) is called pre-excited tachycardia. A clinically important scenario is pre-excited AF, which produces an irregularly irregular WCT that may be mistaken for VT. Some accessory pathways can enable very fast antegrade conduction if they have a short refractory period and produce AF with an extremely rapid ventricular response, which may rarely degenerate into ventricular fibrillation (VF). Hence, a small proportion of patients with Wolff–Parkinson–White are at risk of sudden cardiac death.

Caution must be exercised in treating patients with pre-excited tachycardia with any medications that block AV node conduction. During pre-excited AF, they may cause preferential conduction down the accessory pathway at very rapid rates and precipitate VF and are contraindicated in this situation. Acute treatment of orthodromic AVRT is similar to AVNRT with vagal manoeuvres and adenosine, which may be used with a

defibrillator on standby. Pre-excited tachycardia may be treated with class Ic antiarrhythmic drugs (e.g. flecainide) which block conduction in the accessory pathway. If there is any doubt as to whether a pre-excited tachycardia is VT, it is safer to perform DC cardioversion. Long-term treatment for symptomatic patients includes antiarrhythmic drugs such as flecainide or ablation of the accessory pathway. Occasionally, asymptomatic patients with pathways capable of very rapid conduction have the pathway ablated to reduce risk of sudden cardiac death.

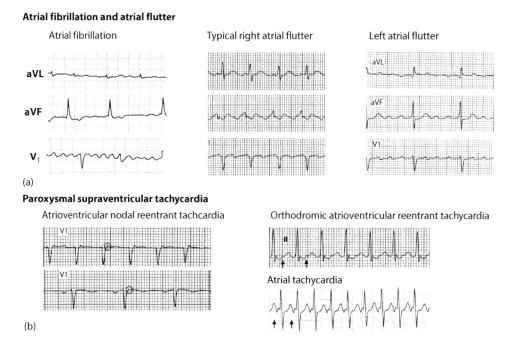

(a)

(b)

Figure 20.2 Supraventricular tachyarrhythmias. (a) **Atrial fibrillation and atrial flutter.** Atrial fibrillation with a controlled ventricular response. Disorganised fibrillation waves are present disturbing the isoelectric baseline. The appearance in lead V1 may sometime mimic atrial flutter (see text). Typical atrial flutter with 2:1 AV block. Underlying atrial rate is typically 300 bpm giving a ventricular rate of 150 bpm when there is 2:1 AV block. In this case, the atrial rate is 242 bpm and the ventricular rate is 121 bpm. The slower flutter rate may be due reduced atrial conduction velocity from scar or antiarrhythmic medications. Typical atrial flutter has negative 'saw-tooth' waves in the inferior leads, and positive flutter waves in leads I and V1. Left atrial flutter in a patient with previous lung transplantation. The flutter waves are positive in the inferior lead and in V1, but negative in lead I indicating a flutter circuit originating in the left atrium. (b) **Paroxysmal supraventricular tachycardia (pSVT)** presents as a regular narrow complex tachycardia (NCT) with a 1:1 AV relationship. In atrioventricular nodal reentrant tachycardia (AVNRT, the most common type of pSVT), there is a very short RP interval with a small positive deflection immediately after the QRS complex, giving a pseudo-RBBB appearance. The absence of this deflection in the sinus rhythm ECG confirms it is a P wave (circles). Orthodromic AVRT utilising a retrograde conducting accessory pathway causes a short RP tachycardia but the P wave is typically located in the ST segment with a longer RP interval than AVNRT. Atrial tachycardia usually causes a long RP tachycardia with a non-sinus rhythm P wave preceding the QRS complex.

(Continued)

Wolff-Parkinson-White syndrome

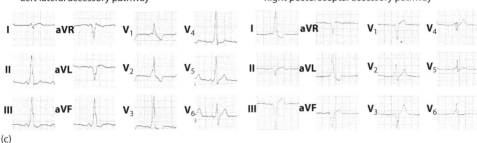

(c)

Response of narrow complex tachycardia to vagal manoeuvers and adenosine

Atrial flutter with high grade AV block following IV adenosine

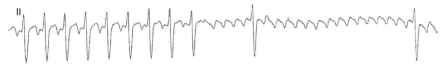

Termination of paroxysmal SVT following Valsalva manoeuver

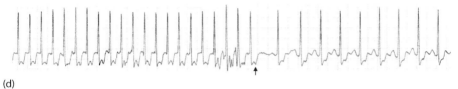

(d)

Figure 20.2 (Continued) Supraventricular tachyarrhythmias. **(c) Wolff–Parkinson–White syndrome (WPW)** occurs due to the present of an antegrade conducting accessory pathway that pre-excites the ventricles during sinus rhythm giving a short PR interval and a wide QRS complex with a slurred onset (delta wave). The commonest WPW pattern due to a left lateral accessory pathway has a positive delta wave in lead V1 and the inferior leads and negative delta wave/QRS complex in leads I and aVL. The next most common pattern due to a right posteroseptal accessory pathway has a negative delta wave/QRS complex in V1 with a transition to a positive delta wave in V2. The delta waves are negative in the inferior leads. **(d) Response of NCT to vagal manoeuvres and adenosine.** Initially this example of atrial flutter appears to have a 1:1 AV relationship but administration of IV adenosine increases the degree of block unmasking the underlying atrial flutter waves. pSVT terminates to sinus rhythm in response to a vagal manoeuvre (twice normal paper speed). The last event in the arrhythmia is a retrograde P wave (arrow) suggesting termination of a reentrant arrhythmia by block of antegrade conduction in the AV node. This pattern of termination is unlikely with atrial tachycardia.

Atrial tachycardia

Between 5% and 15% of cases of paroxysmal SVT are due to atrial tachycardia (AT, also called focal atrial tachycardia). AT is a regular atrial rhythm with a constant rate of greater than 100 bpm originating from an ectopic atrial focus other than the sinus node. These ectopic foci cluster at certain anatomic structures within the atria. The majority of atrial tachycardias originate in the right atrium along the tricuspid annulus or the crista terminalis. Left atrial tachycardias predominantly arise in or around the pulmonary veins. The P wave axis and morphology during AT can be helpful in localising the site of origin.[4] Atrial tachycardia occurs more commonly in older patients and those with structural heart disease or chronic pulmonary disease than AVNRT or AVRT. It is also seen with states of catecholamine excesses, chronic alcohol abuse and digoxin toxicity. The ECG during AT usually shows a P wave of non-sinus morphology just prior to QRS (long RP tachycardia) unless first degree AV block is also present, in which case it may follow the QRS complex (short RP tachycardia). Initial therapy for symptomatic patients should be with a beta-blocker or calcium channel blocker prior to a trial of antiarrhythmic drug therapy with flecainide, amiodarone or sotalol. Catheter ablation of the ectopic focus is recommended for patients who are refractory to medical therapy.

DIAGNOSIS OF NARROW COMPLEX TACHYCARDIA

Diagnosing the mechanism of NCT is generally straightforward if a systematic approach is used. An abrupt onset and offset argues against sinus tachycardia. The first step in diagnosing NCT is to determine if it is regular or irregular. Irregularly irregular NCT is due to AF, multifocal atrial tachycardia or atrial flutter with variable AV block. In AF, there will be no organised P waves and there may be fibrillatory atrial activity. Multifocal atrial tachycardia will show three different P wave morphologies, varying PR intervals and an isoelectric baseline between P waves. Atrial flutter demonstrates uniform rapid atrial activity often at 300 bpm without an isoelectric segment in some leads.

If the NCT is regular, the next step is to identify P waves, if present. If no P waves can be identified, the atrial activity is likely hidden within the QRS and the most likely diagnosis is AVNRT. If P waves are present with a 1:1 relationship, the tachycardia should be classified at a short RP tachycardia if the RP interval is less than half the RR interval, or a long RP tachycardia if the RP intervals is longer than half the RR interval. Short RP tachycardia is most likely to be typical AVNRT if the RP interval is <80 ms and more likely orthodromic AVRT if the RP interval is short but greater than 80 ms. Less commonly, atrial tachycardia with first degree AV block can cause a short RP tachycardia. The commonest cause of a long RP NCT is (focal) atrial tachycardia. The other main causes are an atypical form of AVNRT (with antegrade conduction via the fast pathway and retrograde conduction over the slow pathway) and orthodromic AVRT with a slow retrograde conducting accessory pathway.

If there is a 2:1 or higher relationship of P waves to QRS complexes, atrial flutter or atrial tachycardia with AV block is likely. If the rate is very close to 150 bpm and there appears to be a 1:1 AV relationship, it is important to look for an extra P wave of atrial flutter, as atrial flutter with 2:1 AV block commonly occurs at this rate.

The response to vagal manoeuvres and adenosine can be very helpful in the diagnosis of SVT. Slowing of the ventricular rate is often seen with sinus tachycardia, AF, atrial flutter, and atrial tachycardia. Occasionally, a higher degree of AV block in response to vagal manoeuvres or adenosine will unmask flutter waves that were hidden or produce atrial tachycardia with 2:1 block, which excludes AVRT. Re-entrant SVT, including AVNRT and AVRT generally show no response or terminate abruptly in response to vagal manoeuvres or adenosine. Abrupt termination following adenosine is not pathognomonic of re-entrant SVT, as up to 20% of focal atrial tachycardias may terminate with adenosine. If the tachycardia terminates and the last event is a P wave, it is much more likely to be AVNRT or AVRT. If atrial tachycardia terminates with a P wave, there would have to be simultaneous termination and block in the AV node, an unlikely coincidence (Figure 20.2d).

VENTRICULAR TACHYARRHYTHMIA

Ventricular premature contractions

Ventricular premature complexes (VPCs) are wide-complex early beats that originate from an ectopic site within either ventricle. The QRS usually has a slow initial onset due to slow cell-to-cell conduction through the ventricles away from the site of origin. VPCs occasionally arise from specialised conduction tissue or Purkinje fibres, in which case they may have a relatively narrow QRS morphology with rapid initial activation. VPCs often occur in repetitive patterns. Ventricular bigeminy refers to single VPCs alternating with conducted sinus beats, while trigeminy refers to a VPC following two sequential conducted sinus beats. VPCs are described as unifocal if they display a uniform, constant morphology, or multifocal if VPCs of two or more different morphologies are present. Two successive VPCs are referred to as a couplet. Three or more VPCs in a row is, by definition, VT if they occur at a rate greater than 100 bpm.

VPCs are usually followed by a fully compensatory pause, meaning the PP interval between the sinus beats on either side of the VPC is twice the basic sinus PP interval. If a VPC is early enough it may conduct retrogradely and reset sinus node to produce a non-compensatory pause. VPCs that fail to block the subsequent sinus beat from conducting through the AV node and activating the ventricles are termed interpolated VPCs.

Most VPCs do not require treatment and, in the absence of structural heart disease, do not appear to have prognostic significance. However, a high burden of VPCs (>20%–40% of heart beats are VPCs) can cause a reversible cardiomyopathy called VPC-induced cardiomyopathy. Suppression of the VPCs with antiarrhythmic medications or catheter ablation can often reverse the cardiomyopathy. It should be noted, however, that antiarrhythmic drugs such as flecainide and sotalol, which slow conduction and/or increase the dispersion of refractoriness, can increase risk of polymorphic ventricular arrhythmias and sudden cardiac death in patients with cardiomyopathy.

Monomorphic ventricular tachycardia

VT is defined as three of more consecutive ventricular beats at a rate greater than 100 bpm. VT is defined as non-sustained if it terminates spontaneously within 30 seconds, and sustained if it lasts longer than 30 seconds or requires cardioversion to terminate. There are two main patterns of VT: monomorphic and polymorphic VT (see below). In monomorphic VT, each QRS complex has a uniform morphology from beat to beat. The rate is generally regular, but some irregularity may be seen, particularly at the onset of tachycardia (Figure 20.3a).

Common causes of monomorphic VT (MMVT) are listed in Table 20.3. MMVT most often occurs in patients with structural heart disease such as prior myocardial infarction or cardiomyopathy. MMVT in the setting of prior myocardial infarction is also called scar-related VT. VT in patients with prior MI is associated with increased mortality and treatment with an implantable cardioverter-defibrillator (ICD) is usually required especially if there is accompanying LV systolic dysfunction. Because the mechanism of scar-related VT is re-entry, these arrhythmias are often amenable to overdrive pace-termination by the ICD (anti-tachycardia pacing, ATP). Recurrent post-infarction VT may be suppressed with antiarrhythmic drugs such as amiodarone or mexiletine. Another option is to use catheter ablation to destroy critical components of the VT re-entrant circuit, or to modify the VT scar substrate on the endocardial surface of the left ventricle.

Table 20.3 Common causes of monomorphic ventricular tachycardia

Monomorphic ventricular tachycardia in the presence of structural heart disease
• Previous myocardial infarction (scar)
• Non-ischaemic dilated cardiomyopathy
• Bundle branch reentrant ventricular tachycardia
• Hypertrophic cardiomyopathy
• Arrhythmogenic right ventricular cardiomyopathy
• Acute or prior myocarditis
• Infiltrative cardiomyopathy, especially cardiac sarcoidosis
• Congenital heart disease, especially following operative repair of tetralogy of Fallot
Monomorphic ventricular tachycardia in the absence of structural heart disease
• Right (or left) ventricular outflow tract ventricular tachycardia
• Left ventricular fascicular ventricular tachycardia

The QRS morphology and axis during VT can be used as an aid to localise the site of origin of post infarction VT. There are various published algorithms for this purpose.[5,6] If the VT has a RBBB appearance in lead V_1, then the site of origin is in the left ventricle. If lead V_1 shows a negative or LBBB pattern, then the origin is either in the right ventricle or the left ventricular septum. If the frontal plane axis is superiorly directed (i.e. QRS predominantly negative in the inferior leads) the VT origin is likely from the inferior wall, while an inferior axis (i.e. positive in the inferior leads) points to a superior origin usually on the anterior wall. If the axis is rightward (i.e. negative QRS in leads I and aVL) then the origin is likely to be in the lateral LV wall, while a leftward axis (positive in I and aVL) is more consistent with a septal origin. The QRS vector in leads aVR and V_4 can be used to localise the VT origin on the basal-apical axis of the LV. Since V_4 overlies the LV apex, a negative QRS in this lead suggests an apical origin of VT. A negative QRS in aVR and positive QRS in V_4 (and across the other praecordial leads) points to a basal origin near the mitral valve annulus. Since scar-related VT often arises in or around sites of previous infarction, the location of Q waves on the ECG and the location of scar on echocardiographic or cardiac magnetic resonance imaging studies also aids VT localisation.

Similar principles can be used to localise the site of origin in other types of monomorphic VT. VT in the setting of non-ischaemic dilated cardiomyopathy (DCM) is more likely to have an intramural or epicardial origin than post-infarction VT, which is more likely to endocardial, making ablation of non-ischaemic DCM more difficult. ECG clues to an epicardial origin of VT include a very broad QRS complex during VT, with very slow, slurred initial activation, and presence of QS complexes in lead I or the inferior leads.

A rare but important type of MMVT is bundle branch re-entrant VT, which is seen in patients with baseline His-Purkinje conduction disease and cardiomyopathy. The ECG during VT characteristically shows a typical LBBB pattern, often very similar to the sinus rhythm ECG. The circuit in bundle branch re-entrant VT involves antegrade conduction over the right bundle branch, transseptal conduction and retrograde conduction up the left bundle branch to the His bundle and then antegrade down the right bundle branch to complete the circuit. This is an important diagnosis to make as it can be easily cured by targeting the right bundle branch for ablation.

Arrhythmogenic right ventricular cardiomyopathy (ARVC) is a potentially lethal structural cardiomyopathy that presents with MMVT. The diagnosis can be difficult to make because patients may present with VT or sudden cardiac arrest prior to overt structural cardiomyopathy being evident on imaging studies. VT in ARVC has a LBBB pattern in lead V_1, indicating an origin in the right ventricle. There are usually multiple VT morphologies, often with different frontal plane axes. The sinus rhythm 12-lead ECG frequently has important characteristic features, including an incomplete RBBB pattern and epsilon wave (terminal notch in the QRS representing delayed conduction into the right ventricular outflow tract (RVOT) as well as T-wave inversions in the right praecordial leads. Cardiac magnetic resonance imaging to evaluate for ARVC should be performed in any patient without apparent structural heart disease with a VT morphology suggesting an origin in the RV. Management of patients with ARVC and VT requires an ICD, with antiarrhythmic mediations, and occasionally epicardial VT ablation used to control recurrent VT episodes.

Monomorphic VT may occur in patients without structural heart disease. The two most common syndromes are idiopathic right ventricular outflow tact (RVOT) VT and idiopathic left ventricular fascicular VT. RVOT ventricular arrhythmias represent a spectrum from frequent VPCs, repetitive salvos of non-sustained VT, to episodes of sustained VT often occurring on exertion. The ECG during VT has a LBBB pattern in V_1 with an inferior axis (tall R waves in the inferior leads). In general, RVOT VT does not require ICD implantation and has a low risk of sudden cardiac death once a detailed workup to exclude coronary and other structural heart disease (especially ARVC and cardiac sarcoidosis) has been completed. Many patients are successfully treated with beta-blockers or antiarrhythmic medications, but some require ablation in the RVOT, which usually has a high success rate. More recently, it has been recognised that many outflow tract VTs have a left-sided origin, often in the aortic cusps. A left-sided origin is suggested by an earlier praecordial R/S transition with a dominant R wave appearing in lead V_3 or earlier, compared to V_4 or later in VT originating from the RVOT.

Idiopathic LV fascicular VT typically presents at age 20–40 in patients without structural heart disease. The mechanism is thought to be re-entry with antegrade conduction over the left posterior fascicule of the left bundle branch, and retrograde conduction over abnormal Purkinje tissue in the most common form. The ECG during VT shows a RBBB-pattern left superior axis, which is often narrow and frequently mistaken for SVT with RBBB aberrancy. Fascicular VT characteristically terminates in response to acute treatment with intravenous verapamil. Oral verapamil to prevent recurrence is less effective, and many patients require ablation.

Polymorphic ventricular tachycardia

In polymorphic VT, the QRS morphology varies from beat to beat. It is seen in association with several cardiac ion channelopathies, including long QT syndrome, catecholaminergic polymorphic VT (CPVT) and Brugada syndrome, but may also occur in acute ischaemia and cardiomyopathy (Figure 20.3b). When polymorphic VT occurs in the setting of long QT syndrome it is called torsades de pointes, with the onset of VT following a characteristic long-short sequence of RR intervals.

Table 20.4 Causes of QT prolongation

Congenital long QT syndrome: Potassium, sodium, calcium channelopathies

Drugs
- Antiarrhythmic medications: class Ia (procainamide, disopyramide), class III (amiodarone, sotalol)
- Psychiatric medications: antipsychotics (phenothiazine, haloperidol, atypical antipsychotics), lithium, SSRIs, tricyclic antidepressants
- Antimicrobials: macrolides, quinolones, antifungal 'azoles', pentamidine, atovaquone, atazanavir
- Others: antiemetics (droperidol, $5HT_3$ antagonists), alfuzosin, methadone, ranolazine

Electrolyte disturbances
- Hypocalcaemia
- Hypokalaemia
- Hypomagnesaemia

Autonomic dysfunction
- Intracerebral haemorrhage
- Stroke
- Carotid endarterectomy
- Neck dissection

Miscellaneous
- Coronary artery disease
- Cardiomyopathy
- Bradycardia
- High-grade atrioventricular block
- Hypothyroidism
- Hypothermia
- Bundle branch blocks

Abbreviation: SSRI, selective serotonin reuptake inhibitors.

Torsades de pointes may occur with either congenital or acquired QT prolongation (Table 20.4). The risk is proportional to the degree of QT prolongation with a substantially increased risk once the QT interval is prolonged to greater than 500 ms. Acute treatment includes correction of reversible causes of QT prolongation and may require shortening the QT interval by increasing heart rate with isoprenaline or temporary pacing.

Brugada syndrome is associated with pseudo-RBBB pattern with down-sloping ST-elevation and T-wave inversion in leads V_1-V_3, and a risk of VF

and sudden cardiac death. It typically affects young males with arrhythmic events often occurring at night and in association with bradycardia. It has a genetic predisposition and approximately 30% of individuals have mutations in the cardiac sodium channel alpha subunit gene (*SCN5A*).

Catecholaminergic polymorphic VT (CPVT) is an inherited arrhythmia syndrome caused by intracellular calcium overload. The resting ECG during sinus rhythm is normal. Children and adolescents with CPVT present with exercise-induced ventricular arrhythmias, including polymorphic VT, VF and bidirectional VT. Bidirectional VT involves beat-to-beat alternation of QRS axis during VT. It may also occur with digoxin toxicity, acute ischaemia, myocarditis and other rare cardiac ion channel disorders.

DIAGNOSIS OF WIDE COMPLEX TACHYCARDIA

The differential diagnosis of WCT is listed in Table 20.5. The most common cause of WCT is VT, accounting for 80% of cases. However, SVT conducted with aberrancy (either fixed bundle branch block or rate-dependent bundle branch block), SVT conducted via an accessory pathway or ventricular paced tachycardia also cause WCT. In addition, an electrical or motion artefact on the ECG can commonly mimic WCT (Figure 20.3c).

Distinguishing the different causes of WCT, particularly differentiating VT from SVT with aberrancy, is a common clinical problem. A history of myocardial infarction, heart failure or left ventricular dysfunction is the best clinical predictor that WCT is VT. Since VT is the most common cause of WCT and potentially life-threatening, the index of suspicion for VT should be high in all patients. When there is diagnostic uncertainty or in an emergency it is best to treat WCT as VT.

Classic ECG features that favour the diagnosis of VT over SVT with aberrancy are listed in Table 20.6. AV dissociation (independent P waves, capture or

Table 20.5 Differential diagnosis of wide complex tachycardia

Ventricular tachycardia
Supraventricular tachycardia with aberrancy
Pre-excited tachycardia
Ventricular paced tachycardia
Artefact

fusion beats) when identified generally proves VT. However, a 1:1 AV relationship does not exclude VT due to the possibility of 1:1 retrograde VA conduction during VT. AV dissociation can also be difficult to identify at rapid rates. When the QRS during WCT is very wide (>140 ms in RBBB-type or >160 ms in LBBB-type) or when there is extreme axis deviation ('northwest' axis, 180°–270°, negative QRS complex in lead 1 and lead II/III), VT is more likely. When the QRS morphology has a typical bundle branch block pattern, SVT with aberrancy is suggested. An atypical RBBB-pattern with initial R wave > R' or a broad monophasic R wave in V_1 or an R wave greater than S wave in V_6 suggests VT. An atypical

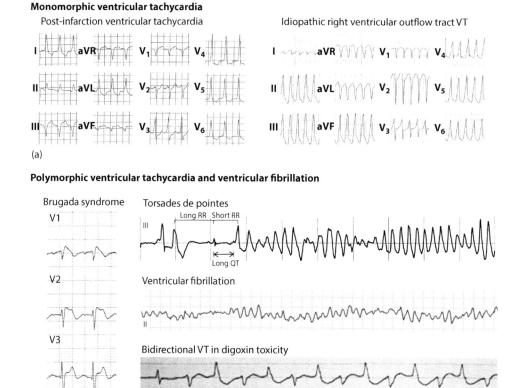

(a)

(b)

Figure 20.3 Ventricular tachyarrhythmias. (a) Monomorphic ventricular tachycardia (MMVT). The QRS complexes are of uniform morphology in MMVT. Most cases of MMVT occur in patients with structural heart disease, e.g. post myocardial infarction. A minority of MMVT occurs in the absence of structural heart disease, e.g. idiopathic right ventricular outflow tract (RVOT) tachycardia. The 12-lead ECG can be used to localise the likely origin of MMVT (see text for explanation). This example of post infarction VT is probably exiting scar to activate the basal inferoseptal left ventricle. The prominent positive R waves in the inferior leads, along with LBBB appearance in V1 and negative QRS in aVR and aVL are characteristic of idiopathic RVOT VT. (b) Polymorphic ventricular tachycardia and ventricular fibrillation may occur in the setting of inherited ion channel disorders such as congenital long QT syndrome and Brugada syndrome. Brugada syndrome has a characteristic ECG pattern of incomplete RBBB and down-sloping ST-elevation to an inverted T wave in the right chest leads (V1-V3). Long QT syndrome is associated with torsades de pointes polymorphic VT. Onset of torsades is typically following a long-short RR interval sequence with the initiating VPC often falling on the preceding T wave (R on T). Ventricular fibrillation is characterised by chaotic ventricular activation and causes loss of cardiac output typically resulting in death in the absence of prompt defibrillation. Bidirectional VT in which the QRS axis and morphology alternate from beat-to-beat may occur in digoxin toxicity or catecholamingeric polymorphic ventricular tachycardia.

(Continued)

Differential diagnosis of wide complex tachycardia

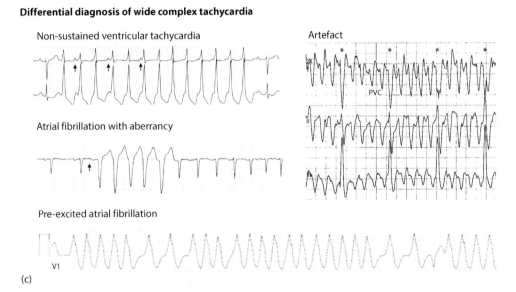

Non-sustained ventricular tachycardia

Atrial fibrillation with aberrancy

Pre-excited atrial fibrillation

Artefact

(c)

Figure 20.3 (Continued) Ventricular tachyarrhythmias. (c) Differential diagnosis of wide complex tachycardia (WCT) is a common clinical problem (see text). Ventricular tachycardia is the most common cause of WCT. This example of non-sustained VT shows one beat of sinus rhythm, initiation of NSVT with a VPC without a preceding P wave and AV dissociation with dissociated P waves (arrows) due to ongoing sinus rhythm during VT. The PR interval in the sinus rhythm beat following termination of NSVT is longer than that preceding tachycardia due to concealed retrograde penetration of VT wavefronts into the AV node. The example of atrial fibrillation (AF) with aberrancy shows sinus rhythm for two beats followed by five beats of WCT that transitions into an irregular narrow complex tachycardia (AF). There is a P wave (arrow) superimposed on the T wave preceding the first beat of wide complex tachycardia. The WCT is irregular like the atrial fibrillation. These observations make it more likely that a single tachycardia is responsible for the narrow and WCT. Pre-excited atrial fibrillation results in an irregularly-irregular WCT. Fast antegrade conduction over an accessory pathway may result in extremely rapid ventricular rates that may degenerate into ventricular fibrillation. AV node blocking medications are contraindicated in this situation. Motion artefact may mimic a wide complex tachycardia. This is case intrinsic QRS complexes (*) at 70 bpm are seen underlying the non-physiological artefact signals.

Table 20.6 Classic electrocardiogram features for distinguishing ventricular tachycardia from supraventricular tachycardia with aberrancy

Atrioventricular dissociation
Capture and fusion beats
Very wide QRS complex (>140 ms in RBBB-type, >160 ms in LBBB-type)
QRS complex atypical for bundle branch block
RBBB-type: R > r' or wide monophasic R in V1, S > r in V6
LBBB type: onset to nadir >60–100 ms in V1, Q wave in V6
Concordance (QRS in all praecordial leads with same pattern/direction)

Abbreviations: LBBB, Left bundle branch block; RBBB, Right bundle branch block.

LBBB-pattern suggesting VT has onset of QRS to nadir of greater than 100 ms or notching on the down-slope in V_1 or a Q wave in V_6. Concordance of the QRS complex direction across the praecordial leads (all positive or all negative) is a traditional criterion for VT. The absence of concordance does not exclude VT. Positive concordance may also be seen in pre-excited SVT. Negative concordance implies activation originating from near the LV apex, which is unusual in SVT and suggests the WCT is VT.

There are several limitations to these criteria. QRS bundle-branch morphology does not allow for the differentiation between VT and pre-excited tachycardia, as activation of the ventricle at the point of insertion of the accessory pathway is indistinguishable from VT arising from the same site. For the same reason, morphology criteria cannot differentiate between ventricular-paced tachycardia and VT. Certain rare forms of VT that use the specialised conduction system e.g. bundle branch reentrant tachycardia or left ventricular fascicular tachycardia have a QRS morphology that can be difficult to distinguished from SVT with aberrancy. SVT with very rapid rate e.g. atrial flutter with 1:1 conduction may produce very bizarre patterns of aberrancy that look like VT.

ARRHYTHMIAS DURING ACUTE MYOCARDIAL INFARCTION

Tachyarrhythmias and bradyarrhythmias arising from the ventricles and atria may complicate the course of acute myocardial infarction. The incidence is highest early after the onset of symptoms. Many serious arrhythmias, including VF, may develop prior to hospitalisation. Infarction-related arrhythmias arise from disturbances in myocyte transmembrane electrochemical gradients and slowed conduction velocity in ischaemic myocardium and are further promoted by electrolyte disturbances and autonomic nervous system imbalances. The ensuing tachycardia or bradycardia may have serious haemodynamic consequences, as infarct-related left ventricular dysfunction leads to a relatively fixed stroke volume with heart rate changes, leading to exaggerated reduction in cardiac output. Atrial arrhythmias may have marked haemodynamic effects in ST-elevation myocardial infarction (STEMI) due to increased dependence on atrial contribution to ventricular preload. VF is the major cause of sudden cardiac death in the setting of STEMI. Prompt recognition and treatment of this complication constitutes a major advance in the management of these patients.

Ventricular tachyarrhythmias

In the modern era of early reperfusion therapy, the presence of frequent and complex ventricular ectopy has poor sensitivity and specificity for predicting the occurrence of VF.[7] Suppression of ventricular ectopy following myocardial infarction with class I antiarrhythmic drugs may increase the risk for fatal bradycardic and asystolic events, and has been shown to increase the risk of death.[8] Beta-blockers should be administered to all patients post myocardial infarction when not otherwise contraindicated.

Accelerated idioventricular rhythm may be observed following STEMI and typically occurs during the first 2 days. While it often occurs following reperfusion, it also occurs in patients without reperfusion, and is therefore not a reliable marker that reperfusion has occurred. Accelerated idioventricular rhythm does not affect prognosis and does not routinely require treatment.

VT (sustained or non-sustained) occurs in approximately 25% of patients within the initial 7 days following AMI. VF is the most frequent mechanism of sudden cardiac death, with most VF episodes occurring within the first 48–72 hours after the onset of symptoms. Ventricular tachyarrhythmias are treated by correcting serum potassium to 4.5–5.0 mmol/L and magnesium to 1.0 mmol/L. Early beta-blocker use reduces the incidence of VF. Unstable VT or VF requires urgent electrical cardioversion and administration of intravenous amiodarone or lignocaine. Hypoxia, hypotension, acid-base and electrolyte disturbances should be corrected, and urgent revascularisation undertaken. Early ventricular arrhythmias are associated with an increased in-hospital mortality but an excellent long-term survival in patients who survive to discharge. Patients with VT or VF >48 hours after reperfusion without reversible cause have increased short and long-term mortality and electrophysiology study and/or ICD implantation should be considered before discharge.

Bradyarrhythmias

Bradycardia and AV block occur more frequently in patients with inferior and posterior infarction. Infarction in these territories elicits a reflex parasympathetic response (Bezhold-Jarisch reflex) due to activation of myocardial C-fibres by ischaemic mediators.[9] In contrast, bradycardia and AV block in the setting of anterior infarction indicates extensive tissue damage, portends a worse prognosis and is more likely to lead to the need for a permanent pacemaker.

Isolated sinus bradycardia occurs commonly early during STEMI, especially in inferior myocardial infarction. Severe sinus bradycardia associated with hypotension or marked QT-prolongation and high-grade ventricular ectopy may need to be treated with atropine, isoprenaline, or temporary pacing, in addition to urgent revascularisation.

Table 20.7 Typical features of atrioventricular block occurring in association with inferior compared to anterior myocardial infarction

	Inferior infarction	Anterior infarction
Site of block	Intranodal	Infranodal
Coronary artery lesion	Right coronary artery (90%), Left circumflex artery (10%)	Left anterior descending artery (septal perforators)
Pathogenesis	Excessive parasympathetic activity, ischaemia/infarction	Ischaemia/infarction
Predominant patterns of AV block	First degree, Mobitz type I second degree, complete heart block	Intraventricular conduction block and bundle branch block, Mobitz II second-degree, complete heart block
Features of escape rhythm	Narrow-complex escape rhythm, rate 45–60 bpm, ventricular stand-still uncommon	Wide complex escape rhythm rate often <30 bpm, moderate-high risk of ventricular stand-still
Duration of high-grade AV block	Usually transient (2–3 days)	Usually transient, but higher risk of persistent AV and/or intraventricular block
Prognosis	Favourable, permanent pacemaker rarely required	Unfavourable, as indicative of extensive infarction

Source: Dreifus, L.S. et al., J. Am. Coll. Cardiol., 18, 1–13, 1991.
Abbreviation: AV, atrioventricular.

Infarction may produce conduction block at any point in the conduction system, but the pattern and features of block differ characteristically between inferior and anterior myocardial infarction (Table 20.7).

Supraventricular tachyarrhythmias

Sinus tachycardia occurs due to augmented sympathetic activity associated with anxiety, persistent ischaemic pain, fever, pulmonary embolism, hypovolaemia, drugs (e.g. noradrenaline, adrenaline, dobutamine) and is especially common with left ventricular dysfunction in anterior infarction. Reversible causes should be treated. However, use of beta-blockers for sinus tachycardia due to left ventricular dysfunction is contraindicated, as it may precipitate pump failure.[7]

AF and atrial flutter are associated with increased mortality and risk of stroke in patients with STEMI. The loss of atrial contribution to left ventricular filling and increased ventricular rate can cause severe reduction of cardiac output. Beta-blockers should be administered in the absence of contraindications. Digoxin and amiodarone are appropriate if AF occurs in STEMI associated with heart failure or significant left ventricular dysfunction. Patients with recurrent episodes of AF during admission with acute myocardial infarction should be treated with anticoagulant medications, even if sinus rhythm is present at the time of discharge.[7]

REFERENCES

1. Lee S, Wellens HJJ, Josephson ME. Paroxysmal atrioventricular block. Heart Rhythm. 2009;6(8):1229–1234.
2. Roten L, Wenaweser P, Delacretaz E, Hellige G, Stortecky S, Tanner H, et al. Incidence and predictors of atrioventricular conduction impairment after transcatheter aortic valve implantation. Am J Cardiol. 2010;106(10):1473–1480.
3. Contreras-Valdes FM, Josephson ME. "Frog sign" in atrioventricular nodal reentrant tachycardia. N Engl J Med. 2016;374(15):e17.

4. Kistler PM, Roberts-Thomson KC, Haqqani HM, Fynn SP, Singarayar S, Vohra JK, et al. P-wave morphology in focal atrial tachycardia: Development of an algorithm to predict the anatomic site of origin. *J Am Coll Cardiol*. 2006;48(5):1010–1017.

5. Kuchar DL, Ruskin JN, Garan H. Electrocardiographic localization of the site of origin of ventricular tachycardia in patients with prior myocardial infarction. *J Am Coll Cardiol*. 1989;13(4):893–900.

6. Miller JM, Jain R, Dandamudi G, Kambur TR. Electrocardiographic localization of ventricular tachycardia in patients with structural heart disease. *Card Electrophysiol Clin*. 2017;9(1):1–10.

7. O'Gara PT, Kushner FG, Ascheim DD, Casey DE, Chung MK, de Lemos JA, et al. 2013 ACCF/AHA guideline for the management of ST-elevation myocardial infarction: A report of the American College of Cardiology Foundation/American Heart Association Task Force on Practice Guidelines. *J Am Coll Cardiol*. 2013;61(4):e78–e140.

8. Echt DS, Liebson PR, Mitchell LB, Peters RW, Obias-Manno D, Barker AH, et al. Mortality and morbidity in patients receiving encainide, flecainide, or placebo. The Cardiac Arrhythmia Suppression Trial. *N Engl J Med*. 1991;324(12):781–788.

9. Esente P, Giambartolomei A, Gensini GG, Dator C. Coronary reperfusion and Bezold-Jarisch reflex (bradycardia and hypotension). *Am J Cardiol*. 1983;52(3):221–4.

10. Dreifus LS, Fisch C, Griffin JC, Gillette PC, Mason JW, Parsonnet V. Guidelines for implantation of cardiac pacemakers and antiarrhythmia devices. A report of the American College of Cardiology/American Heart Association Task Force on Assessment of Diagnostic and Therapeutic Cardiovascular Procedures (Committee on Pacemaker Implantation). *J Am Coll Cardiol*. 1991;18(1):1–13.

Formation and progression of atherosclerosis

SIDDHARTH J. TRIVEDI AND BRIAN J. NANKIVELL

INTRODUCTION

Atherosclerosis is one of the most prevalent fatal diseases in Western populations, causing one half of all deaths. Atherosclerosis is the chronic, pathologic process of muscular arteries where degenerate material containing macrophages, lipids, connective tissue, calcium and debris accumulates within its inner layer to form an atheromatous plaque. Plaques develop in the aorta, cerebral, carotid, renal and intra-abdominal and peripheral arteries, in addition to the coronary circulation where they constitute the principal disease process of patients undergoing cardiac catheterisation.

These lesions begin in childhood and advance with aging. Early disease is characterised by thickened tunica intima and xanthoma accumulation, which later progresses to more complex plaques composed of pathological intimal thickening, early and late fibroatheromas with a variety of thin fibrous caps, ruptured plaques, healed rupture and fibrotic calcified plaques. Initial atheroma formation is asymptomatic, but as further progression occurs over time, symptoms can manifest as acute coronary syndrome, stroke, or other vascular events.

PATHOGENESIS OF ATHEROMATOUS PLAQUE

Early fatty streaks and plaque initiation

The first phase in atherosclerosis begins with focal intimal thickening and accumulation of foam cells, extracellular matrix, and smooth muscle cells.[1] Subtle alterations of the monolayer of endothelial cells of the tunica intima, which line the inner arterial surface,[2] can result from injurious stimuli including hypertension, dyslipidaemia, or pro-inflammatory mediators (Figure 21.1a). Plaque can form in areas of increased vascular turbulence near arterial branches, which suggests shear stress as an initiating factor. Upregulated adhesion molecules can trap circulating monocytes on their surfaces, which then enter the intimal layer and ingest and retain low-density lipoprotein (LDL) particles (Figure 21.1b). Proteoglycans within the intimal layer can trap extracellular lipoproteins. This process of intracellular and extracellular lipid deposition produces 'fatty streaks', which are regarded as the earliest precursor of plaque.[3]

Fatty streaks contain mixtures of monocyte-derived macrophages with endocytosed oxidised LDL particles, platelets, lymphocytes, mast cells, and extracellular matrix. Lipid-laden macrophages, termed 'foam cells', can release multiple inflammatory cytokines, chemokines and growth factors, including MCP-1, ICAM-1, GM-CSF, CD40 ligand, interleukin (IL)-1, IL-3, IL-6, IL-8, and IL-18, and TNFα. Some plaque macrophages may also function as antigen-presenting dendritic cells. Microvesicles, which later calcify, may transition some fatty streaks into atherosclerotic plaques.[4] As plaque forms and grows, smooth muscle cells from the tunica media (middle arterial wall layer) become activated, proliferate and migrate to the intima, responding

to platelet-derived growth factor (Figure 21.1c). These cells produce the extracellular matrix molecules, including collagen and elastin, forming the fibrous cap that covers the developing atheromatous plaque.[2] Apoptotic foam cells release extracellular lipids that cannot be efficiently cleared and accumulate with cellular debris, forming the lipid-rich necrotic core of the plaque.[5]

Later plaque progression and clinical events

Atheromatous plaque can undergo several potential outcomes. Some remain unchanged, some rupture, whereas others involute, with calcification and fibrosis characteristic of mature (and often stable) plaque. Fibrous cap atheromas are plaques with a distinct lipid core covered by a fibrous cap: composed of a relatively acellular dense collagen and/or contain abundant smooth muscle cells. A fibrous plaque results from a fatty streak with increased connective tissue and smooth muscle cells filled with lipids and a deeper extracellular lipid pool. More advanced plaques contain a necrotic lipid-rich core and calcified areas.[6] Growing atherosclerotic plaques develop their own microvascular network to supply oxygen and nutrients, which originates

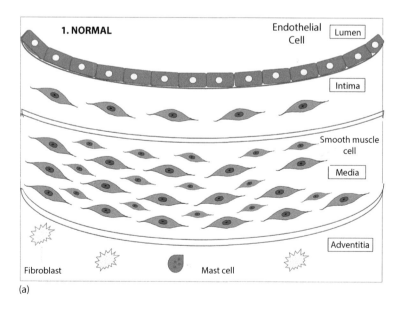

(a)

Figure 21.1 **(a)** Stages in the formation of atherosclerotic plaques. The normal artery consists of three layers: the tunica intima (the inner layer lined by a single layer of endothelial cells in contact with blood), the tunica media (the middle layer containing smooth muscle cells and extracellular matrix) and the outer tunica adventitia (composed of mast cells, microvessels, and nerve endings). *(Continued)*

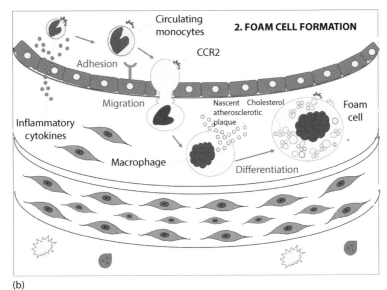

(b)

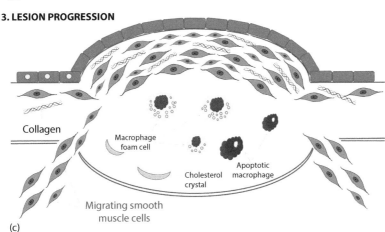

(c)

Figure 21.1 (Continued) **(b)** Early atherosclerosis is characterised by adhesion of blood leucocytes to the activated endothelium, then migration of these bound leucocytes into the intima and differentiation of monocytes into macrophages and their uptake of lipids, resulting in foam cells. **(c)** Further plaque progression results from migration of smooth muscle cells from the media to the intima, with further proliferation of these cells, and increased synthesis of extracellular matrix including collagen. Dead cells can accumulate in the central region of the plaque, called the necrotic core. Cholesterol crystals and microvessels can also form. *(Continued)*

from the adventitia and extends into the medial and thickened intimal layers.[7] The normal vasa vasorum network is a network of micro-vessels supplying the outer arterial wall. Disruption of thin-walled plaque vessels results in haemorrhage within the plaque substance and contributes to progression of disease.[7]

Similarly, the symptoms caused by atherosclerotic plaques are varied. Gradual flow-limiting stenoses can lead to distal tissue ischaemia, or local thrombus formation can occlude arterial blood flow, or embolise and lodge in a distal vessel (Figure 21.1d). Paradoxically, vascular thrombosis does not always occur at the most severely narrowed plaques. Instead, thrombi occur after physical plaque disruption, commonly from fracture of its fibrous cap, which then exposes pro-coagulant material of the plaque's core to blood coagulation proteins, triggering thrombosis.[2] Ruptured plaques typically comprise lesions with thin, collagen-poor fibrous

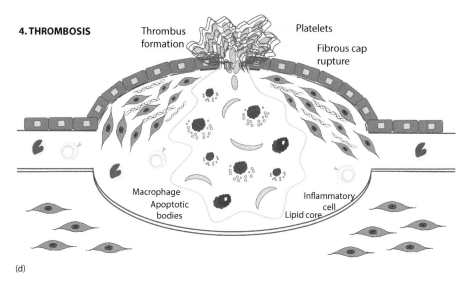

Figure 21.1 (Continued) **(d)** Thrombosis occurs when the plaque's fibrous cap ruptures, enabling contact between blood coagulation proteins and plaque tissue factor, potentially extending the thrombus into the arterial lumen and causing occlusion or limitation in blood flow.

caps containing few muscular cells but numerous macrophages. These inflammatory cells hasten disruption by releasing collagenolytic enzymes that can degrade structural collagen of the cap and shoulder regions, and accelerate the death of smooth muscle cells that generate arterial collagen.[8] Plaque macrophages also produce the procoagulant tissue factor that renders the lipid core thrombogenic. Thus, inflammation plays a key role in the pathogenesis of atherosclerosis: infiltrating inflammatory cells interact with intrinsic arterial cells (smooth muscle and endothelium), promoting lesion formation and subsequent complications.

A summary of the morphological classification of atherosclerotic lesions is described in Table 21.1 and depicted in Figure 21.2.

Table 21.1 Classification of atherosclerotic lesions based on morphology

Type of lesion	Key features
Nonatherosclerotic intimal lesions	
• Intimal thickening	Smooth muscle cells accumulate in the absence of lipid, macrophages foam cells, and thrombosis
• Intimal xanthoma	Superficial accumulation of foam cells without a necrotic core, fibrous cap, or thrombosis
Progressive atherosclerotic lesions	
• Pathological intimal thickening	Plaque rich in smooth muscle cells, with proteoglycan matrix and extracellular lipid
• Fibroatheroma	Macrophage infiltration, loss of matrix and cellular debris with an overlying fibrosis cap
• Intraplaque haemorrhage or plaque fissure	Large necrotic core with haemorrhage, communicates with the lumen through a fissure
• Thin-cap fibroatheroma	A thin, fibrous cap infiltrated by macrophages and lymphocytes, with rare or no smooth muscle cells

(Continued)

Table 21.1 (*Continued*) Classification of atherosclerotic lesions based on morphology

Type of lesion	Key features
Lesions with acute thrombi	
• Plaque rupture	Thin-cap fibroatheroma with cap disruption. Thrombosis is present and may be occlusive
• Plaque erosion	Occurs on pathological intimal thickening or on a fibroatheroma. Occlusive thrombus may be present
• Calcified nodule	Eruptive (shedding) of calcified nodule with an underlying fibrocalcific plaque with no necrosis
Healed lesion	
• Healed plaque rupture or erosion	Composed of smooth muscle cells, proteoglycans, collagen, and calcium

Source: Yahagi, et al. *Nat. Rev. Cardiol.*, 13, 79–98, 2016.

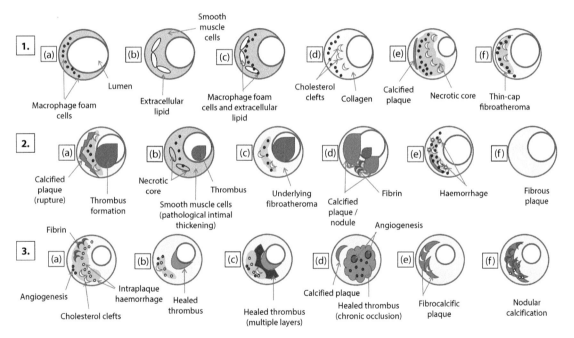

Figure 21.2 Progression of atherosclerosis in the arterial lumen—from nonatherosclerotic intimal lesions to progressive atherosclerosis to lesions with acute thrombi to complications of haemorrhage/thrombosis with healing and stabilisation. Initial pathology relates to changes in the intima (**1a**), followed by pathological intimal thickening (**1b,c**), fibroatheroma formation (**1d,e**), and thinning of the cap (**1f**). Lesions with acute thrombi can occur in the context of rupture (**2a**), erosion (**2b,c**), and calcified nodule (**2d**). Plaque fissure (**2e**) and fibrous plaque (**2f**) can also occur. Complications of haemorrhage/thrombosis (**3a**) include single (**3b**) or multiple (**3c**) layer healing, chronic total occlusion (**3d**), fibrocalcific plaque (**3e**) and nodular calcification (**3f**).

AETIOLOGICAL RISK FACTORS OF ATHEROSCLEROSIS

Multiple risk factors are involved in the pathogenesis of atherosclerosis. These include endothelial dysfunction, dyslipidaemia, inflammatory and immunologic factors, plaque rupture and smoking. Clinicians attempt to mitigate further vascular disease in patients with coronary events by secondary risk factor treatment, such as lipid control and cessation of smoking. The endothelium is the biologic interface that forms a unique and thrombo-resistant layer between blood and potentially thrombogenic subendothelial tissues. It also plays a major regulatory role: modulating vascular tone, cellular growth, local haemostasis and inflammation throughout the circulatory system. Endothelial vasodilator dysfunction is the first step in the formation of atherosclerosis, mediated by release of the vasodilator substance, endothelium-derived nitric oxide.[9] Endothelial dysfunction correlates with many traditional risk factors for atherosclerosis, including hypercholesterolemia, hypertension, cigarette smoking, and diabetes. A summary of clinical risk factors that cause endothelial dysfunction, along with interventions that help improve endothelial dysfunction, is presented in Table 21.2.

Dyslipidaemia

Lipid abnormalities are central to the development of atherosclerosis,[10] especially high levels of LDL cholesterol. Oxidation of LDL increases macrophage uptake, and cholesterol accumulates within foam cells and the lipid core of atherosclerotic plaque. Cholesterol-laden foam cells develop mitochondrial dysfunction, apoptosis and necrosis, with a resultant release of cellular proteases, inflammatory cytokines, and prothrombotic molecules.[11] In contrast to LDL, high-density lipoprotein (HDL) molecules display anti-atherogenic properties that include reverse cholesterol transport, maintenance of endothelial function and protection against thrombosis. Cardiovascular risk inversely relates to plasma HDL-cholesterol levels.

Hypertension and smoking

Hypertension is a major risk factor for atherosclerosis due to increased arterial wall tension, potentially leading to disturbed repair processes and aneurysm formation.[12] Cigarette smoking is another important risk factor that affects all phases of atherosclerosis, ranging from endothelial dysfunction to acute thrombotic clinical events. Cigarette smoke impairs endothelial-dependent vasodilation, increases the levels of multiple inflammatory markers[13] and accelerates LDL oxidation. Cigarette smoking reduces the availability of platelet-derived nitric oxide, decreases platelet sensitivity to exogenous nitric oxide (which may increase their activation and adhesion), increases fibrinogen level, and decreases fibrinolysis.[14]

Diabetes mellitus

Diabetes-related dyslipidaemia is atherogenic, and includes elevated triglycerides, low HDL

Table 21.2 Factors that cause and interventions that improve endothelial dysfunction

Factors associated with endothelial dysfunction	Interventions that improve endothelial function
Older age	L-arginine
Male gender	Antioxidants
Family history of ischaemic heart disease	Smoking cessation
Smoking	Cholesterol lowering
Increased serum cholesterol	ACE inhibitors
Low serum HDL cholesterol	Exercise
Hypertension	Mediterranean diet
Increased serum homocysteine	
Diabetes mellitus	
Obesity	
High-fat diet	

cholesterol, and small/dense LDL particles. Hyperinsulinemia also precedes the development of arterial diseases. Type 2 diabetes and atherosclerosis have similar pathophysiologies, with increased MCP-1 and IL-6 cytokines, which contribute to inflammation.[15] Overall, the risk increase conferred by type 2 diabetes mellitus is due to accelerated progression of pre-existing atherosclerosis towards clinical cardiovascular events. Diabetic coronary disease frequently comprises both lipid-rich plaque, and diffuse and distal coronary disease within the small arteries that is not suitable for stenting.

Circulating and vascular molecules

Several circulating and local substances are molecular risk factors for atheroma. Increased plasma concentrations of angiotensin II promote the development and severity of atherosclerosis, and modulate proliferation of vascular smooth muscle cells and generation of extracellular matrix.[16] Adhesion molecules such as ICAM-1 and VCAM-1 are cell surface glycoproteins that facilitate leucocyte adherence to endothelium, and are induced at endothelial sites of inflammation. Present at low levels on normal endothelium, expression of ICAM-1 and VCAM-1 are both increased in atherosclerotic lesions.[17] Endothelin-1 is a potent vasoconstrictor that induces vascular smooth muscle cell proliferation, stimulating their migration and growth. Oxidised LDL also stimulates its production and enhances its vasoconstrictor effects.[18] Inflammation plays a crucial role in atherosclerosis pathogenesis. Macrophages that have taken up oxidised LDL release multiple inflammatory substances, cytokines, and growth factors.[19] Tissue factor is the primary initiator of coagulation and is present in advanced atherosclerotic plaque and, along with enhanced platelet activity, provokes thrombosis following plaque rupture. Tissue factor also contributes to atherosclerosis via coagulation-dependant and coagulation-independent mechanisms.[20]

Genetic and environmental associations

Many genetic factors can contribute to the complex pathophysiological processes that occur in atherosclerosis. Genetic polymorphisms can occur in genes responsible for the pathways of lipid metabolism, inflammation and thrombogenesis. Hence, individuals and their families display differing propensity for developing coronary artery disease. Family history of early cardiovascular events is important clinical information to stratify risk. Chronic infection with certain pathogens, such as Chlamydia pneumoniae, cytomegalovirus, coxsackie B virus and Helicobacter pylori may contribute to the pathogenesis of atherosclerosis. Furthermore, the total pathogen burden, i.e. the number of pathogens to which an individual has been exposed, may be an important risk factor for atherosclerosis. There are a number of mechanisms by which chronic infection could act, including direct vascular injury and induction of a systemic inflammatory state. Most of this evidence is associative, rather than causal.

CLINICOPATHOLOGICAL OUTCOMES

Flow characteristics of atheroma

Atheroma frequently occurs at the site of bends, branches and bifurcations of arteries, suggesting that altered flow and shear stress contributes to atherosclerosis development. Disturbed flow can alter endothelial cell function and disrupt the atheroprotective role of the normal endothelium. Atherosclerosis generally does not cause symptoms until the severity of stenosis exceeds 70%–80% of the luminal diameter of the artery. Angina pectoris develops from reduced coronary blood flow to the myocardium.

Plaque erosion and rupture

Progression of atherosclerotic plaque thus involves two distinct clinical outcomes: a chronic process leading to gradual and progressive luminal narrowing, and an acute scenario of rapid luminal vascular obstruction from plaque haemorrhage and/or luminal thrombosis. Acute coronary and cerebrovascular syndromes (e.g. unstable angina, myocardial infarction, sudden death, and stroke) are typically secondary to plaque rupture or erosion, leading to acute thrombosis. Plaque rupture or erosion may also occur silently, without symptoms. Recurrent asymptomatic rupture and thrombosis of plaque, followed by wound healing, may contribute to progressive atherosclerosis,

Table 21.3 Clinical effects of plaque in different arterial systems

Arterial system	Haemodynamic impairment	Plaque rupture (± vessel thrombosis)
Cerebral	Vertebrobasilar ischaemia	Transient ischaemic attack ('ministroke'), cerebrovascular accident ('stroke')
Coronary	Exertional angina (exertional chest pain)	Unstable or crescendo angina, acute myocardial infarction
Renal	Renovascular hypertension	Ischaemic atrophy, renal infarction
Mesenteric	'Mesenteric angina' (abdominal pain after food)	Acute bowel infarction
Lower limb	Intermittent claudication	Acute vascular insufficiency of the leg, gangrene
Onset of symptoms	Slow and gradual	Sudden
Vascular impairment	Transient	Permanent
Organ damage	Nil	Infarction

associated with increased plaque burden, greater luminal stenosis, and pathological arterial remodelling. The clinical effects of plaque in different arterial systems is presented in Table 21.3.

ABNORMAL ATHEROSCLEROSIS SYNDROMES

Forms of accelerated arteriopathies include restenosis following percutaneous coronary intervention with stenting, coronary transplant vasculopathy, and atherosclerosis in chronic kidney disease patients.

Coronary stent restenosis

When an arterial vessel is injured by angioplasty, it reacts by initiating a healing inflammatory response. After a successful initial procedure, coronary stents may fail to maintain vessel patency due to restenosis. Reduction of luminal diameter of the stent following implantation occurs due to neointimal tissue proliferation associated with macrophage accumulation and extensive neovascularisation. This neointimal proliferation can be focal or distributed uniformly along the length of the stent.[21] Intracoronary stent restenosis is now much less common with the drug-eluting stents, compared to bare metal stents.

Cardiac allograft vasculopathy

Cardiac allograft vasculopathy (CAV) is an unusual pattern of arterial abnormalities that occur within the cardiovascular system of a transplanted human heart, and is an important cause of recipient death beyond the first year after cardiac transplantation. CAV is a pan-arterial disease characterised by diffuse, concentric and longitudinal intimal hyperplasia of the coronary arteries, and concentric medial disease of the microvasculature.[22] In contrast, traditional atherosclerosis is focal, noncircumferential, asymmetrical, and most often is observed proximally in the epicardial vessels. Both immunologic and nonimmunologic factors are implicated in CAV, but further research is needed. mTOR inhibitors are anti-fibrotic immunosuppressive agents (e.g. everolimus and sirolimus) that suppress both transplant rejection and limit progression of CAV.

Chronic kidney disease

Patients with chronic kidney disease and end-stage renal failure are at increased risk for developing cardiovascular disease, related to accelerated vascular disease and several traditional and non-traditional risk factors for cardiovascular disease. Traditional risk factors (hypertension, smoking, diabetes, dyslipidaemia, and older age) appear to be more important risk factors during the earlier stages of renal failure. Non-traditional risk factors include uraemic toxins, anaemia, elevated cytokine levels, increased calcium load, abnormalities in bone mineral metabolism, and/or an increased inflammatory-poor nutrition state. The pathology is characterised by diffuse fibrosis and calcification in the medial and adventitial arterial layers.

SUMMARY

Atherosclerosis, a chronic disease involving arterial walls, is a leading cause of death and loss of productive life years worldwide. Atherosclerotic lesions typically form over years to decades, and are characterised by the progressive accumulation of fatty streaks, macrophages, and various fibrous elements in the intimal layer of the artery. Despite the chronicity of atherosclerosis, thrombotic complications—the most dreaded clinical consequences of this disease—occur suddenly, and often without warning. Optimal management of cardiovascular risk factors may attenuate the incidence and progression of atherosclerotic disease. Preventive treatments include lifestyle modification, cessation of smoking, diabetic, lipid, and blood pressure control, as well as antiplatelet therapy to limit atheroma development and stabilise plaque. Clinically significant lesions with haemodynamic compromise, including exertional angina or acute coronary syndrome, require percutaneous coronary intervention or coronary artery bypass grafting.

REFERENCES

1. Davies MJ, Woolf N, Rowles PM, Pepper J. Morphology of the endothelium over atherosclerotic plaques in human coronary arteries. *Br Heart J.* 1988;60(6):459–464.

2. Libby P, Ridker PM, Hansson GK. Progress and challenges in translating the biology of atherosclerosis. *Nature.* 2011;473(7347):317–325.

3. Tabas I, Williams KJ, Boren J. Subendothelial lipoprotein retention as the initiating process in atherosclerosis: Update and therapeutic implications. *Circulation.* 2007;116(16):1832–1844.

4. Kockx MM, De Meyer GR, Muhring J, Jacob W, Bult H, Herman AG. Apoptosis and related proteins in different stages of human atherosclerotic plaques. *Circulation.* 1998;97(23):2307–2315.

5. Tabas I. Macrophage death and defective inflammation resolution in atherosclerosis. *Nat Rev Immunol.* 2010;10(1):36–46.

6. Stary HC, Chandler AB, Dinsmore RE, Fuster V, Glagov S, Insull W, Jr., et al. A definition of advanced types of atherosclerotic lesions and a histological classification of atherosclerosis. A report from the Committee on Vascular Lesions of the Council on Arteriosclerosis, American Heart Association. *Circulation.* 1995;92(5):1355–1374.

7. Kolodgie FD, Gold HK, Burke AP, Fowler DR, Kruth HS, Weber DK, et al. Intraplaque hemorrhage and progression of coronary atheroma. *N Engl J Med.* 2003;349(24):2316–2325.

8. Libby P. Molecular and cellular mechanisms of the thrombotic complications of atherosclerosis. *J Lipid Res.* 2009;50(Suppl):S352–S357.

9. Kitta Y, Obata JE, Nakamura T, Hirano M, Kodama Y, Fujioka D, et al. Persistent impairment of endothelial vasomotor function has a negative impact on outcome in patients with coronary artery disease. *J Am Coll Cardiol.* 2009;53(4):323–330.

10. Steinberg D, Witztum JL. Oxidized low-density lipoprotein and atherosclerosis. *Arterioscler Thromb Vasc Biol.* 2010;30(12):2311–2316.

11. Tabas I. Consequences of cellular cholesterol accumulation: Basic concepts and physiological implications. *J Clin Invest.* 2002;110(7):905–911.

12. Yusuf S, Hawken S, Ounpuu S, Dans T, Avezum A, Lanas F, et al. Effect of potentially modifiable risk factors associated with myocardial infarction in 52 countries (the INTERHEART study): Case-control study. *Lancet.* 2004;364(9438):937–952.

13. Bermudez EA, Rifai N, Buring JE, Manson JE, Ridker PM. Relation between markers of systemic vascular inflammation and smoking in women. *Am J Cardiol.* 2002;89(9):1117–1119.

14. Barua RS, Ambrose JA, Saha DC, Eales-Reynolds LJ. Smoking is associated with altered endothelial-derived fibrinolytic and antithrombotic factors: An in vitro demonstration. *Circulation.* 2002;106(8):905–908.

15. Park YM, R Kashyap S, A Major J, Silverstein RL. Insulin promotes macrophage foam cell formation: Potential implications in diabetes-related atherosclerosis. *Lab Invest.* 2012;92(8):1171–1180.

16. Potter DD, Sobey CG, Tompkins PK, Rossen JD, Heistad DD. Evidence that macrophages in atherosclerotic lesions contain angiotensin II. *Circulation.* 1998;98(8):800–807.

17. Iiyama K, Hajra L, Iiyama M, Li H, DiChiara M, Medoff BD, et al. Patterns of vascular cell adhesion molecule-1 and intercellular adhesion molecule-1 expression in rabbit and mouse atherosclerotic lesions and at sites predisposed to lesion formation. *Circ Res.* 1999;85(2):199–207.

18. Mathew V, Cannan CR, Miller VM, Barber DA, Hasdai D, Schwartz RS, et al. Enhanced endothelin-mediated coronary vasoconstriction and attenuated basal nitric oxide activity in experimental hypercholesterolemia. *Circulation.* 1997;96(6):1930–1936.

19. Berliner JA, Navab M, Fogelman AM, Frank JS, Demer LL, Edwards PA, etal. Atherosclerosis: Basic mechanisms. Oxidation, inflammation, and genetics. *Circulation.* 1995;91(9):2488–2496.

20. Hasenstab D, Lea H, Hart CE, Lok S, Clowes AW. Tissue factor overexpression in rat arterial neointima models thrombosis and progression of advanced atherosclerosis. *Circulation.* 2000;101(22):2651–2657.

21. Komatsu R, Ueda M, Naruko T, Kojima A, Becker AE. Neointimal tissue response at sites of coronary stenting in humans: Macroscopic, histological, and immunohistochemical analyses. *Circulation.* 1998;98(3):224–233.

22. Tuzcu EM, De Franco AC, Goormastic M, Hobbs RE, Rincon G, Bott-Silverman C, et al. Dichotomous pattern of coronary atherosclerosis 1 to 9 years after transplantation: Insights from systematic intravascular ultrasound imaging. *J Am Coll Cardiol.* 1996;27(4):839–846.

23. Yahagi K, Kolodgie FD, Otsuka F, Finn AV, Davis HR, Joner M, et al. Pathophysiology of native coronary, vein graft, and in-stent atherosclerosis. *Nat Rev Cardiol.* 2016;13(2):79–98.

22

Basic pharmacology of cardiac drugs

TERENCE J. CAMPBELL

INTRODUCTION

The pharmacology of cardiac drugs is an immense topic and reducing its components to a single chapter is a challenging task. This chapter presents a broad overview of a wide spectrum of cardiac drugs, classified into the following main groups: (1) Sympathomimetic Agents (including adrenaline, noradrenaline, metaraminol, isoprenaline, dopamine, dobutamine), Sympatholytic Agents (including alpha- and beta-blockers), Centrally acting Hypotensive Agents (including alpha-methyldopa, clonidine), Calcium Antagonists (including verapamil, diltiazem, nifedipine, other dihydropyridines), Angiotensin Converting Enzyme (ACE) Inhibitors, Angiotensin-II Antagonists, Nitrovasodilators, Diuretics, Cardiac Glycosides, Antiarrhythmics, Antithrombins, and Thrombolytics. Antiplatelet agents and Novel Oral Anticoagulants are discussed in separate chapters and are only briefly mentioned. This extensive list provides a useful and practical summary for the novice on the use and actions of many types of drugs and provides a general understanding of their clinical application in cardiology.

SYMPATHOMIMETIC AGENTS

Adrenergic receptors and the cardiovascular system

Catecholamines and other sympathomimetic agents exert most of their inotropic (force-increasing) and chronotropic (rate-increasing) effects on the myocardium via beta-adrenergic receptors. Alpha adrenoceptor stimulation is capable of producing a positive inotropic effect (about 10% of that seen in response to beta adrenoceptor stimulation).

The β1-adrenoreceptor subtype is responsible for the cardiac inotropic and chronotropic effects of catecholamines. There is now good evidence for the involvement of β2-adrenoreceptors in mediating the positive inotropic effects of adrenaline in the human atrium, and to a lesser extent in the human ventricle. The involvement of the β2-receptor appears to be most important in the sinoatrial node, less so in atrial myocardium and even less so in ventricle, although the relative importance of the β2 receptor appears to increase in patients with chronic heart failure.

The extracardiac effects of alpha- and beta-receptor stimulation of relevance to cardiovascular pharmacology include the well-known vasodilating effect of β2-adrenergic stimulation. This is most marked in the arterial bed within skeletal muscle. Both alpha1- and alpha2-receptor subtypes appear to mediate vasoconstriction in most arterial systems, with the coronary and cerebral circulations being relatively spared. The actions of alpha-receptor stimulation to promote platelet aggregation may also be of cardiovascular relevance.

At least one other receptor group needs to be considered in the present context. These are the dopamine receptors, which are traditionally subdivided into D1 and D2. The D1-receptor, the receptor of relevance to the present discussion, mediates vasodilatation, particularly in the renal and splanchnic beds, via the enhanced formation of cyclic AMP. The D2-receptor is also found in the pituitary gland.

Specific agents

The relative activities of the main sympathomimetic agents in clinical use for treatment of cardiovascular disorders at present are listed in Table 22.1. This table is an approximate guide to relative activities only, and not to quantitative accuracy.

ADRENALINE

Also known as epinephrine, and produced endogenously mainly in the adrenal medulla, this compound is a potent stimulator of both alpha and beta adrenergic receptors and its effects on target organs are complex. Bolus intravenous injections of large amounts (0.5–1.5 mg) tend to produce rapid increases in systolic blood pressure with lesser increases in diastolic pressure. This effect is due to a combination of vasoconstriction (alpha effect), increased contractility and heart rate (β1 and β2 effects), and vasodilatation in skeletal muscle vasculature (β2 effect). With a large bolus, the first two actions tend to predominate, and hypertension is produced. Frequently, the direct tachycardia is replaced by an indirect reflex-mediated bradycardia in response to the increase in intra-arterial pressure.

Intravenous infusion of adrenaline at 5–30 mcg per minute tends to produce an increase in systolic blood pressure with a decrease in diastolic

Table 22.1 Complexity of catecholamine activity in the cardiovascular system

Receptor	α	β1	β2	Dopaminergic
Actions	Vasoconstrictor Inotropic	Inotropic Chronotropic	Inotropic Chronotropic Vasodilator	Splanchnic and renal vasodilator (+Vasoconstrictor and inotropic in high doses)
Noradrenaline	++++	++	0	0
Adrenaline	+++	+++	++	0
Isoprenaline	0	++++	++++	0
Dopamine	0 to +++	++	0	++++
Dobutamine	+ to ++	+++	+++	0

pressure, and generally some increase in heart rate. As the rate of infusion is increased, there is a growing tendency for the vasoconstrictor (alpha) effect to predominate over vasodilatator (β2) and for the diastolic pressure to rise also. Myocardial oxygen consumption and blood lactate concentrations tend to rise considerably. Blood flow to skeletal muscles and the splanchnic bed tends to increase. There is no significant constriction of cerebral arterioles seen and, because of the increased pressure, cerebral blood flow tends to increase. Conversely, renal blood flow tends to fall considerably although there is a corresponding increase in filtration fraction, and glomerular filtration rate (GFR) is only slightly altered. In the presence of background nonselective beta-blockade, only vasoconstriction and increases in systolic and diastolic pressure are seen with adrenaline.

NORADRENALINE

Also known as norepinephrine, this compound is approximately as potent as adrenaline at stimulating β1-receptors. It is a little less potent than adrenaline on alpha-receptors and has very little action on β2-receptors. Consequently, intravenous infusion (approximately 10 mcg/min) tends to produce increases in both systolic and diastolic pressures.

There is commonly a reflex slowing of the heart rate in response to the hypertension. Blood flow tends to be reduced to the kidney, liver and skeletal muscle. Glomerular filtration rate (GFR) is initially maintained quite well but falls at higher doses. Coronary blood flow tends to increase. Both adrenaline and noradrenaline are rapidly destroyed in the body.

METARAMINOL (ARAMINE)

Metaraminol (or Aramine) is a powerful and fairly selective alpha adrenergic agonist. It leads to widespread vasoconstriction via its alpha receptor effect. There is relative sparing of the coronary arteries and cerebral arteries because these have few alpha-receptors. It is, therefore, useful for elevating blood pressure without placing undue strain on myocardial or cerebral blood supply. It must be given by intravenous injection or infusion.

ISOPRENALINE

Also known as isoproterenol, this substance is a potent non-selective beta-adrenergic agonist with negligible alpha-adrenergic effects. Intravenous infusion into humans normally lowers the peripheral resistance via the β2-adrenergic vasodilating effects of this agent. Mean and diastolic blood pressures fall, although systolic blood pressure may remain unchanged or even rise due to the concomitant inotropic and chronotropic actions of the drug on the heart. Renal blood flow falls in normotensive humans but generally increases in initially hypotensive patients as a result of an increase in cardiac output and reversal of reflex renal vasoconstriction. Its duration of action is very brief and it is normally administered by intravenous infusion.

DOPAMINE

This is the metabolic precursor of noradrenaline and adrenaline.

Table 22.1 indicates the complex actions of dopamine in the cardiovascular system. Low-dose infusion predominantly leads to D1 (dopaminergic) stimulation resulting in vasodilatation in the renal, mesenteric and coronary beds. This commonly results in an increase in renal blood flow, GFR and urine flow. These effects are typically seen at infusion rates of 1.5–5 mcg/kg/min.

As the infusion rate of dopamine is increased, positive inotropic and chronotropic effects mediated by beta-receptors are increasingly apparent. Dopamine also has the ability to release noradrenaline from nerve endings and this contributes to its actions. Systolic and mean blood pressure tend to rise. Diastolic blood pressure may increase slightly.

At very high infusion rates alpha1-adrenergic vasoconstrictor effects appear and eventually overcome the dopaminergic vasodilating action, resulting in further increases in blood pressure and eventually a reduction in blood flow to vital organs including the kidneys. Combination therapy with dobutamine, which has vasodilating properties, can help to overcome this tendency to cause vasoconstriction and lead to additive inotropic effects (see below).

DOBUTAMINE

This agent bears some resemblance to dopamine structurally and exerts its effects via both alpha- and beta-adrenergic receptors. It does not release noradrenaline from sympathetic nerve endings nor stimulate dopaminergic receptors. At therapeutic rates of infusion (2.5–15 mcg/kg/min), dobutamine tends to produce an increase in contractility with relatively less increase in heart rate than seen with other beta-stimulants such as isoprenaline. At the same time, the total peripheral resistance and the pulmonary vascular resistance tend not to change much and in fact may fall leading to a reduction in systemic and pulmonary venous pressures. This is due to a balance between the alpha1-receptor mediated vasoconstrictor actions and the β2-receptor mediated vasodilating effect. Consequently cardiac output rises with little change in peripheral resistance. Dobutamine also increases coronary blood flow secondary to a decrease in coronary vascular resistance mediated by β2-receptors. In the presence of beta-blockade, the cardiac effects are largely obliterated, and the net result is a largely alpha1-receptor mediated increase in peripheral resistance. Dobutamine is rapidly broken down enzymatically with a half-life of about 2 minutes.

SYMPATHOLYTIC AGENTS

Alpha-adrenergic blocking agents

Alpha-blocking agents are currently used only to a limited extent in cardiology. Prazosin is the most important, and the only example discussed in detail herein. Alpha-blocking agents can be alpha1-selective (e.g. prazosin), alpha2-selective (e.g. yohimbine), or nonselective (e.g. phentolamine and phenoxybenzamine). Nonselective alpha-blockers are basically unsuccessful as antihypertensive agents because of the reflex tachycardia with which they are associated. Phenoxybenzamine is still used in the management of phaeochromocytoma, but the only common cardiovascular application of alpha-blocking agents is the use of prazosin, either for hypertension or as an afterload-reducing agent in cardiac failure.

For most alpha-adrenergic antagonists, the fall in blood pressure produced by vasodilatation is opposed by baroreceptor reflexes causing increases in heart rate and cardiac output. This effect is more marked if the antagonist also blocks alpha2-receptors on peripheral sympathetic nerve endings. These presynaptic alpha2-receptors normally inhibit excessive release of noradrenaline. Their blockade leads to enhanced release of noradrenaline, resulting in increased stimulation of post-synaptic β1-receptors, further amplifying the tachycardia.

PRAZOSIN

Prazosin produces most of its effects by blocking alpha1-adrenergic receptors in arterioles and veins. This leads to a reduction in peripheral vascular resistance and also to venodilatation, which can reduce preload and venous return to the heart. There is generally little or no reflex tachycardia.

Beta-adrenergic blocking agents

There are large numbers of these agents currently available and their pharmacology is well covered in standard textbooks. The following is a brief outline of a very large topic, in an attempt to highlight points of major importance to the practice of cardiology.

Beta-blockers were first introduced in 1962 for treatment of arrhythmias and angina, but were soon found to have antihypertensive properties as well. The mechanism of the antihypertensive effect is still essentially unexplained. All beta-blockers are competitive inhibitors of beta-receptors, and structurally similar to catecholamines.

'Cardio-selective' (i.e. β1-selective) blockers such as metoprolol and atenolol have theoretical advantages over nonselective blockers such as propranolol in patients with peripheral vascular disease, diabetes or asthma. In practice no beta-blocker is absolutely safe in asthmatics.

The more lipophilic beta-blockers such as propranolol are probably more prone to cause central nervous system disturbances (such as bad dreams) than the more hydrophilic drugs such as atenolol.

Beta-blockers are generally well absorbed from the gut (90%+), but some (e.g. metoprolol and propranolol) undergo extensive first-pass metabolism. The half-lives of propranolol and metoprolol are 2–3 hours in acute usage but this may rise to about 6 hours with chronic use. The half-life of atenolol is about 8 hours. Water-soluble compounds such as atenolol tend to be eliminated in urine with minimal metabolism and hence have longer half-lives in renal disease. Lipid-soluble compounds are generally metabolised by the liver and because beta-blockers reduce hepatic blood flow, they tend to increase their own half-lives in chronic use.

Serious side effects include bronchospasm and acute left ventricular failure, both of which may be life threatening. Postural hypotension is not a problem, since the innervation of the alpha-receptor is intact. Peripheral vascular disease may be aggravated due to the reduction in blood flow and possibly also due to increased exercise tolerance associated with reduced angina pectoris. 'Minor' side effects may occur. Abdominal discomfort sometimes occurs with large doses of propranolol. A degree of weakness and lethargy can be present and this may interfere with exercise tolerance, particularly for vigorous sports. Central nervous system disturbances are common, mostly reduced sleep requirement and disturbed sleep with or without dreams, which may be bizarre or frightening. Depression may also be a problem. Impotence occurs in about 1%–3% of males on long-term beta-blockers. Despite concerns, there is little evidence that beta-blockade causes significant problems in most patients with diabetes mellitus. Beta-blockers may, however, mask the adrenergic symptoms of hypoglycaemia. Beta-blockers tend to have complex effects on plasma lipids. This is particularly true of beta-blockers without intrinsic sympathomimetic activity, which may reduce high density lipoprotein (HDL) cholesterol while elevating low density lipoprotein (LDL) cholesterol and triglycerides modestly. Total cholesterol may not change. These altered lipid concentrations may detract from some beneficial effects of the drug in the long-term.

It seems likely that the major antiarrhythmic and anti-anginal effects of beta-blockers relate directly to their antagonism to the actions of catecholamines, but as noted above, their mechanism of action in hypertension is unclear. The acute intravenous administration of propranolol, for example, usually causes a decrease in heart rate and cardiac output, but a reflex increase in peripheral resistance with little change in blood pressure. If blood pressure does fall, it is usually not for several hours after the administration of the agent and seems to result from a late reduction in peripheral resistance. It has been postulated that the mechanism is mediated via the central nervous system, but this seems unlikely in view of the fact that the less lipid-soluble beta-blockers appear to be as equally effective as antihypertensive agents as the more lipid-soluble compounds. Beta-blockade significantly inhibits release of renin and this mechanism may well be of particular relevance in patients with high renin hypertension. It has also been postulated that at least part of the antihypertensive action of beta-blocking drugs might be due to presynaptic beta-blockade resulting in inhibition of catecholamine release. Another popular theory is that beta-blockers somehow reset baroreceptors.

Combined alpha- and beta-blockade (labetalol)

This agent, which is of some value in the treatment of hypertension, is both an alpha1-receptor blocker and a nonselective beta-blocker. Its beta-blocking potency is three to seven times greater than its alpha-blocking action.

Beta-blockers recommended for chronic heart failure

A number of beta-blockers are now recommended for long-term management of chronic heart failure. These are bisoprolol, carvedilol, metoprolol succinate and nebivolol. As noted above, these agents share the potential to worsen acute heart failure and so should be introduced after careful stabilisation with more traditional therapies first. While any advantage of these drugs over older beta-blockers is probably marginal, they do have the advantage of being licensed for heart failure and of being available in a range of tablet sizes that allow starting at very low doses and increasing slowly over weeks to months, as is often necessary.

CENTRALLY ACTING ANTIHYPERTENSIVE AGENTS

This is an old term which is generally applied to two agents, alpha-methyldopa and clonidine. They act predominantly as agonists on central alpha2-receptors, producing a reduced sympathetic outflow from the brainstem and consequent reduction in blood pressure.

Alpha-methyldopa

It is now known that alpha-methyl-noradrenaline (a metabolite) actually has significant agonist activity and the major mechanism of action of alpha-methyldopa is thought to be due to this metabolite, which subsequently stimulates central alpha2-receptors.

A fall in arterial pressure lasting some 6–8 hours after the administration of oral or intravenous alpha-methyldopa is associated with a reduction in vascular resistance, with either no change or some decrease in heart rate and stroke volume. Plasma concentrations of noradrenaline and renin secretion both fall. These reflect the reduced sympathetic tone induced by this agent.

Clonidine

This compound has a very similar mechanism of action to methyldopa. As with methyldopa, clonidine decreases the plasma concentration of noradrenaline and renin. Also as with methyldopa, an unfavourable side effect profile has seen clinical use of clonidine fall markedly in the last decade.

CALCIUM ANTAGONISTS

A common fallacy concerning these important drugs is to think of them as a homogeneous group with only minor differences in dosage, kinetics, and side effects. There are in fact quite major differences between the calcium antagonist drugs. By far the most important distinction from a clinical point of view is between the dihydropyridines (nifedipine and related compounds) and the other two pharmacological groups, represented by verapamil and diltiazem (see below). It is therefore potentially quite misleading to refer to calcium antagonists as being useful or not being useful for a given clinical condition, without specifying the particular family of calcium antagonists indicated.

Calcium channels are found in a wide variety of tissues throughout the body, and it is therefore not surprising that calcium antagonists exhibit a large number of beneficial or potentially harmful effects. Of major relevance to cardiovascular pharmacology are the effects of these agents on myocardium and vascular smooth muscle. The other actions of calcium antagonists are well covered in standard text books and are not further discussed here.

Tissue selectivity

While there are calcium channels in all types of muscle, those in skeletal muscle do not play a major role in triggering contraction. Organic calcium channel antagonists therefore tend to exhibit clinical effects only on cardiac and smooth muscle. Furthermore, there are major differences between calcium antagonists in terms of their relative selectivity for myocardium and for vascular smooth muscle. For example, on a scale that rates verapamil as having roughly equal effects on both muscle types, diltiazem exhibits approximately nine times more effect on vascular smooth muscle than on myocardium, nifedipine approximately twenty times more vascular selectivity, and felodipine (another dihydropyridine) is over one hundred times more vascular-selective.

The vascular-relaxing effects of calcium antagonists tend to be predominantly seen in arteries and arterioles and not on the venous side of the circulation. This is because the former contains a higher proportion of smooth muscle, the tone of which is modulated by calcium channels, whereas veins depend more on neurogenic and humoral influences. It follows from this that the vasodilating actions of calcium antagonists tend to be seen predominantly as a reduction in cardiac afterload, with little effect on preload.

VERAPAMIL

Verapamil is a synthetic papaverine-like molecule. It is the only member of the phenylalkylamine family in widespread clinical use.

Verapamil exerts approximately balanced effects on myocardium and vascular smooth muscle, so that in therapeutic doses its negative inotropic effects tend to be balanced by a decrease in afterload, and the negative chronotropic effects balanced by reflex increases in sympathetic tone. In patients with abnormal hearts, however, verapamil is quite capable of provoking cardiac failure or significant bradycardia.

Verapamil has a number of clinical applications including therapy for hypertension, angina pectoris and a small but important sub-group of tachyarrhythmias in which part of the re-entrant circuit is calcium channel dependent (classically intra-nodal supraventricular tachycardia). More controversial applications of this agent include its use as a possible cardioprotective agent after myocardial infarction, and as therapy for pulmonary hypertension.

Side effects of verapamil include depression of contractility and heart rate already mentioned above, constipation due to gastrointestinal smooth muscle relaxation which can be particularly troubling to the elderly, non-specific tiredness, headache related to vasodilatation and occasionally an irritating pruritis of uncertain aetiology. Verapamil also interacts with digoxin and may produce a marked increase in serum levels of this drug.

DILTIAZEM

This is the only example of the benzothiazepine family in clinical use. The clinical applications of diltiazem are rather similar to those of verapamil, except that its role in treating angina pectoris is relatively greater, its use in hypertension (at least to date), relatively less and its application as an intravenous antiarrhythmic agent has not been widespread.

The side effects are mostly predictable, being due either to vasodilatation (resulting in headache or flushing and occasionally hypotension), or from depression of the SA or AV nodes (resulting in bradyarrhythmias or heart block). Diltiazem has less propensity for negative inotropic effects than verapamil, but has certainly demonstrated an ability to provoke or worsen cardiac failure in patients with abnormal myocardium. Diltiazem, like verapamil, may elevate plasma digoxin concentrations 20%–60% when these agents are co-administered orally.

NIFEDIPINE

This is the prototype of a number of agents from the dihydropyridine family in clinical use today. Others include nimodipine, amlodipine and felodipine. It is used for the management of angina pectoris, coronary artery spasm and hypertension. More recently it has been investigated as a cardioprotective agent in myocardial infarction and for its possible ability to reverse atherosclerosis.

As mentioned above, the dihydropyridines are basically pure vasodilators in therapeutic doses. Nifedipine is less vascular-selective than some other members of this family, but considerably more so than either verapamil or diltiazem. It does not commonly produce clinically significant negative inotropic or chronotropic effects, but there are reports of this occurring in patients with initially abnormal ventricles.

Because dihydropyridines act via their effects on arterioles and arteries but not veins, nifedipine markedly reduces peripheral resistance and cardiac afterload, but has no significant effect on preload.

The major side effects of nifedipine relate to its vasodilating properties and include headache, flushing and ankle oedema. In addition to this, the reduction in peripheral resistance produced by nifedipine frequently leads to symptomatic increases in sympathetic tone, which may be associated with palpitations or sweating. This increase in sympathetic tone as a reflex response to the direct action of nifedipine can act as a counteracting influence to the beneficial effects of this agent in myocardial ischaemia. This can lead to worsening rather than improvement in symptoms when the indication is angina pectoris, and has led to the widespread recommendation that nifedipine be combined with a beta-blocker for this application.

The main clinical uses for nifedipine are for myocardial ischaemia, particularly angina pectoris (and particularly if coronary artery spasm is thought to be playing a role), and for hypertension.

OTHER DIHYDROPYRIDINES

As mentioned above, those in clinical use include nimodipine, amlodipine and felodipine. Apart from the relatively experimental use of nimodipine for treatment of cerebral artery spasm in patients with subarachnoid haemorrhage, by far the major use of these agents is as anti-hypertensive drugs.

Amlodipine has a long half-life allowing once or twice daily dosage and making it attractive for treating hypertension. Calcium channel blockers are generally regarded as contra-indicated in patients with heart failure. This may change in the future as new data become available.

ANGIOTENSIN CONVERTING ENZYME (ACE) INHIBITORS

This group of compounds has revolutionised our thinking about the pharmacotherapy of cardiac failure and hypertension since captopril was introduced in the mid 1970s. In parallel with this, understanding of the renin-angiotensin system has widened markedly in recent years. The classical concept of the renin-angiotensin (R-A) system has been expanded to fit in with growing evidence of a number of local R-A systems within individual organs or tissues, including the heart. In the simplest formulation, renin is released from the juxtaglomerular apparatus of the kidney in response to a perceived reduction in renal perfusion pressure, hyponatraemia, or an increase in sympathetic tone. Renin splits the inactive peptide angiotensin I from its precursor protein angiotensinogen. Classically this occurs in the circulation, and the intravascular angiotensin I is then converted by angiotensin converting enzyme into the active peptide angiotensin II. This converting enzyme is traditionally thought to reside in the endothelium, particularly in the pulmonary circulation. Angiotensin II acts via a specific receptor to produce a large number of effects on various end organs. These include constriction of smooth muscle, particularly vascular smooth muscle, an increase in sympathetic tone (probably mediated by a presynaptic mechanism), the release of the salt- and water-retaining hormone aldosterone from the adrenal cortex, direct stimulation of the thirst centre in the hypothalamus, release of vasopressin from the posterior pituitary, which in turn produces water retention and further vasoconstriction, increased myocardial contractility and possibly hypertrophy of myocardium and vascular smooth muscle. Angiotensin II has other less well understood actions including a role in blood pressure control within the brain itself. Angiotensin converting enzyme is also a 'kininase', and as such is responsible for the degradation of a number of circulating vasodilating substances, particularly bradykinin. The clinical importance of this latter function is still under debate.

Side effects

The reported incidence of adverse effects with low dose captopril or enalapril is less than 10% in trials with large numbers of patients.

There are three particular adverse reactions that do appear to be 'class-specific' for all the ACE inhibitors. The first is hypotension, particularly after the first dose of drug. This is seen particularly in patients who are volume and salt-depleted. In addition, it seems to be less of a feature with the longer acting ACE inhibitors than with the short acting captopril. The second is the development of a cough, which may not begin until sometime after the commencement of treatment and is dry, irritating and persistent. The true incidence is uncertain with reports ranging from 0.2% to 10% (in the last published study the incidence was 14.6% of 109 women and 6% of 100 men). The cough almost invariably resolves within 2 weeks of discontinuation of ACE inhibitor therapy. Related to this side effect, though much less common, is angioneurotic oedema. As with cough, no predisposing factors have been identified. Angio-oedema usually, but not invariably, occurs within several days of initiation of therapy. When there is symptomatic involvement of the tongue, glottis or larynx, as evidenced by respiratory distress, prompt subcutaneous administration of adrenaline has been recommended as laryngeal obstruction can occur. It is thought that both cough and angio-oedema may be related to high levels of bradykinin in patients on ACE inhibitors.

The third adverse reaction attributable to ACE inhibitors is an acute deterioration in renal function. This overlaps to some extent with the hypotensive reaction discussed above, although that is not the only mechanism. Angiotensin has a number of effects on the glomerulus, one of which is to maintain vasoconstriction of the efferent arteriole. In many patients with cardiac failure in particular, this vasoconstrictor effect is essential to maintaining adequate glomerular filtration pressure. Patients with bilateral renal artery stenosis are particularly sensitive to this side effect.

As with most new antihypertensive compounds, there is very limited experience in the use of ACE inhibitors to treat hypertension or heart failure in pregnancy. It is well established however that captopril is quite toxic to the foetus in sheep, and for this reason ACE inhibitors in general should be avoided if there is any question of pregnancy.

In summary, ACE inhibitors are an extremely useful group of agents for treating hypertension and cardiac failure. Considerable care needs to be exercised in those with renal dysfunction, the elderly and those with a history of reactions to other ACE inhibitors. The drug should not generally be given in pregnancy. With these provisos, ACE inhibitors provide a useful once daily treatment for a large number of patients with mild to moderate hypertension. The addition of a single dose of thiazide diuretic has been shown to have a considerable synergistic effect, and provides effective antihypertensive therapy in the majority of patients with mild to moderate hypertension.

ANGIOTENSIN-II ANTAGONISTS

These agents have somewhat similar actions to the ACE inhibitors but are different in their mechanism of action. They directly antagonise the angiotensin II receptor. In fact the available agents (that include Irbesartan, candesartan and several others) all antagonise exclusively the AT_1 angiotensin receptor and have no effect on the AT_2 receptor. ACE inhibitors on the other hand decrease stimulation of both receptor types and also lead to increased circulating levels of vasodilating, nitric oxide-releasing substances such as bradykinin. This means that angiotensin-II antagonists, because they do not raise bradykinin levels, cause much less cough than do ACE inhibitors.

NITROVASODILATORS

The organic nitrates nitroprusside and related compounds have recently been designated as nitrovasodilators. These drugs have been used for clinical management of angina pectoris since soon after nitroglycerine was first synthesised in 1846, but their basic mechanism of action has only been elucidated in the last few years. Their detailed chemistry and pharmacology is well covered in standard textbooks and will not be discussed here.

The most commonly used examples are nitroglycerine (or glyceryl trinitrate), isosorbide dinitrate, isosorbide mononitrate and sodium nitroprusside.

It should be noted that the nitrovasodilators act on all smooth muscle. Bronchial smooth muscle and the muscles of the biliary tract, gastrointestinal tract (including the oesophagus), ureter and uterus may also be affected. Thus, 'angina' due to biliary or oesophageal spasm may also be relieved by nitrates.

Even when chest pain is truly due to myocardial ischaemia, the mechanisms by which nitrates relieve this pain are at least three-fold: The commonest effect seen with low-dose nitrovasodilators (especially sublingual and transcutaneous use) is preload reduction due to venodilatation. This can relieve ischaemia by reducing myocardial oxygen demand. Direct dilatation of the coronary arteries is a second important action of these agents. They are not, however, specific coronary artery dilators, and at doses in which this effect is seen, they also act to dilate other large arteries. It has recently been recognised that by reducing arterial wave reflection, this mechanism may lead to a significant reduction in afterload, the magnitude of which may be underestimated by monitoring effects on systolic blood pressure recorded in the brachial or radial arteries. Finally, in high doses (generally only seen with intravenous administration), nitrates produce arteriolar dilatation, leading to a reduction in peripheral resistance, which by reducing afterload, may also contribute to relief of ischaemia. This last effect can also lead to unwanted falls in blood pressure, and possibly in coronary perfusion.

Nitroprusside, unlike the organic nitrates (e.g. glyceryl trinitrate and isosorbide), breaks down spontaneously in blood to produce nitric oxide. It nonselectively dilates arteries, arterioles, veins and venules, unlike nitroglycerine, which appears to dilate only vessels greater than about 200 μm in diameter. Smaller vessels apparently lack the metabolic machinery required to break the nitrates down to release nitric oxide. This difference probably explains the observation that nitroprusside can result in redistribution of blood flow away from ischaemic myocardium in patients with coronary artery disease, whereas nitroglycerine appears to do the opposite, mainly by dilating collateral vessels.

Nitrate tolerance

Continuous administration of organic nitrates leads to rapid development of drug tolerance in most patients. In the case of intravenous administration of nitrates, this can generally be overcome simply by increasing the infusion rate. There is good evidence that development of tolerance to transcutaneous nitrate can be largely prevented by the practice of a nitrate-free interval of 10–12 hours per day, most commonly during the night. Similarly, it has been shown that tolerance to the clinical effects of isosorbide mononitrate develops with twice daily dosage but not when the drug is given once daily as recommended.

Toxicity and side effects

Most side effects from use of nitrovasodilators are predictable on the basis of their effects on smooth muscle. Headache is by far the commonest and may be quite severe, although it varies from patient to patient. Postural hypotension and even syncope are relatively frequent. These relate mainly to reductions in preload with a consequent fall in cardiac output rather than to a reduction in afterload. Patients with myocardial ischaemia or cardiac failure frequently have a high initial preload, and hence are less subject to this problem than normal volunteers taking nitrates.

DIURETICS

Diuretics are agents that increase production of urine by the kidneys. They comprise a large and heterogeneous group of compounds, of which only the more clinically important groups are discussed here. Comprehensive reviews are available in standard textbooks.

Benzothiadiazides

These are commonly referred to as the 'thiazide' diuretics.

At a normal glomerular filtration rate (approximately 125 mL/min) the total extracellular fluid volume is filtered every 100 minutes. Normally well over 99% of this is reabsorbed by the renal tubules. This reabsorption is largely achieved by active transport of electrolyte and other solutes, first into the tubular cell and then from the tubular cell into the extracellular fluid.

By far the most important electrolyte in the present discussion is the sodium ion. Essentially there is only one way of extruding sodium ions from the tubular cell into the extracellular fluid. This is via the Na-K-ATPase pump. There are at least five different mechanisms for reabsorbing sodium from the tubular filtrate into the tubular cell. These include passive diffusion down an electrochemical gradient, sodium entry coupled to an organic solute, sodium-hydrogen exchange, electroneutral co-transport of a sodium, a potassium and two chloride ions, and finally electroneutral co-transport of a sodium ion with a chloride ion. The first three mechanisms are seen in the proximal convoluted tubule, the first mechanism also in the late part of the proximal tubule, the fourth mechanism in the thick ascending limb of the loop of Henle, the fifth mechanism in the distal convoluted tubule, and the first and third mechanisms also in the distal tubule and collecting duct.

Potassium undergoes reabsorption in the proximal tubule and thick ascending limb of the loop of Henle, and secretion in the distal tubule. While the majority of filtered potassium is reabsorbed proximally, this fraction is relatively invariant, and the main physiological changes in potassium loss through the kidney are attributable to distal secretory mechanisms. One of the determinants of an increased rate of secretion of potassium distally appears to be the volume of unreabsorbed glomerular filtrate flowing through the distal tubule. Hence drugs such as thiazide diuretics, whose main effect is to decrease sodium reabsorption, can indirectly lead to increased loss of potassium as well.

The major site of action of the thiazides is the proximal part of the distal convoluted tubule, where they block the electroneutral sodium chloride co-transport mechanism (the fifth mechanism listed above). As 90% of filtered sodium has already been reabsorbed by this point, the maximal amount of sodium excretion that can be produced by thiazide diuretics is modest compared with that achieved by some other types of diuretics. Furthermore the thiazide-induced increase in flow through tubular segments distal to the early part of the distal tubule stimulates a modest amount of potassium secretion.

Thiazides also lead to enhanced proximal reabsorption and possibly decreased distal secretion of uric acid, and hence can elevate serum uric acid levels. In addition to this, and in contrast to the loop diuretics discussed below, thiazides decrease the renal excretion of calcium ions via a direct effect on the early part of the distal tubule. Thiazides increase the excretion of magnesium ions.

Loop diuretics

These agents are also called 'high-ceiling' diuretics because the peak diuretic effect they produce is far greater than that seen with other agents. Their main site of action is the thick ascending limb of the loop of Henle, hence their more common label. The agents to be discussed under this heading include furosemide (or frusemide), ethacrynic acid and bumetanide. Unlike the thiazides, these three agents have little in common in terms of chemical structure, although both furosemide and bumetanide are sulphonamides and weak inhibitors of carbonic anhydrase.

As noted above, the loop diuretics act primarily to inhibit electrolyte reabsorption in the thick ascending limb of the loop of Henle. They act at the tubular luminal phase to inhibit the Na-K-2Cl co-transport mechanism. They also tend to produce a rapid onset, short-lived increase in renal blood flow which is accompanied by increased excretion of prostaglandins and kinins by the kidney. Parenterally administered frusemide also causes a rapid increase in venous capacitance, which occurs before the diuretic effect, and results in a decrease in cardiac preload and left ventricular filling pressures, which may contribute to the early response seen in patients with pulmonary oedema.

The majority of clinical side effects experienced with loop diuretics relate to fluid and electrolyte imbalances produced by the main renal tubular actions of these agents. These actions include hyponatraemia, alkalosis, and contraction of the extracellular space.

Aldosterone antagonists

The archetype of this class of drugs is spironolactone. This is a steroid compound which competitively antagonises the actions of mineralocorticoids such as aldosterone. Aldosterone receptors are found in a number of tissues apart from the kidney, including salivary glands and colon. The major renal effect of aldosterone is to increase sodium reabsorption in the late distal tubule and collecting duct, in exchange for secretion of potassium (or hydrogen) ions. Because of the weak oestrogen-like effect of aldosterone, gynaecomastia (often painful) is a recognised side effect. Eplerenone is a newer aldosterone antagonist, less prone to gynaecomastia but also more expensive than spironolactone.

The aldosterone antagonists are commonly used in concert with thiazide or other diuretics in the treatment of fluid retention or hypertension. Spironolactone is frequently added to other diuretics as a means of preventing excessive potassium loss and used in management of primary (rare) or secondary hyperaldosteronism. Spironolactone has been shown to be of benefit added to other therapies in severe chronic heart failure. The mechanism is not entirely clear but may relate to an anti-fibrosis effect obtained by inhibiting aldosterone. The role of eplerenone in heart failure is also promising.

Other potassium-sparing diuretics

The two agents to be discussed under this heading are triamterene and amiloride. While these share some of the properties of spironolactone, they are not chemically related, nor are they mineralocorticoid antagonists. Both agents have some natriuretic activity of their own but are most frequently used for their ability to reduce potassium loss due to other diuretics.

The main mechanism of action appears to be inhibition of electrogenic reabsorption of sodium by cells in the distal tubule and collecting duct.

CARDIAC GLYCOSIDES

There are more than 500 known cardiac glycosides. Squill was in use some 3000 years ago, and digitalis was used in Wales in the thirteenth century. In 1955, Na-K ATPase inhibition was demonstrated and postulated to be its mechanism of action.

Drugs that have been used clinically include digoxin and digitoxin, which both come from the foxglove plant (Digitalis), and ouabain and strophanthidin from the squill plant (Strophanthus). Ouabain was once available in Australia for intravenous use only. It was thought to have a shorter onset of action than digoxin. Digitoxin is still available in the USA but not in Australia. It has 100% oral bioavailability and a half-life of nearly 1 week. Its major advantage is that it is metabolised by the liver rather than being excreted unchanged by the kidneys. Hence dosage adjustment is less of an issue in patients with renal failure on this compound.

Clinical pharmacology of digoxin

Digoxin is now the only cardiac glycoside in clinical use in Australia. It can be given intravenously or orally. It can also be administered intramuscularly, but this is painful. The dosage has to be adjusted carefully in renal disease. Approximately 10% of humans have a bacterium in their gut that can metabolise digoxin. If such a patient is stable on a given dose of digoxin and is then commenced on antibiotics that suppress this gut bacterium, it is possible that the digoxin level may rise as a result.

There are a number of clinically important drug interactions concerning digoxin. Administration of quinidine to a patient already on digoxin leads to an increase in the plasma concentration of digoxin in nearly all cases. This increase is usually of the order of 50%–150% and begins to appear within hours. A number of other agents, particularly other antiarrhythmic drugs, produce similar but usually less dramatic increases in digoxin concentrations. These include verapamil, amiodarone, propafenone and diltiazem. In addition to these drug interactions, digitalis toxicity is in general more common in patients with low levels of potassium or magnesium.

Mechanisms of action

The mechanisms by which digitalis in general and digoxin in particular exert their effects are traditionally divided into 'direct' and 'indirect'. Understanding of both of these has increased significantly in recent years although there are still a number of gaps in our knowledge.

The direct effects of digitalis are now believed to be mediated largely through two mechanisms. The first of these involves direct binding to and inhibition of the membrane-bound Na-K-ATPase molecule. The second effect of digitalis is to increase the slow inward calcium current (iCa) during the action potential.

Partial inhibition by digoxin of the ATPase molecule on myocardial cells leads to an increase in intracellular sodium concentration. This causes a reduction in calcium excretion from the cell via the sodium-calcium exchange mechanism. This in turn causes an increased level of calcium within the cell and a positive inotropic effect. Furthermore, the stoichiometry of the situation is such that a very small rise in intracellular sodium concentration (approximately 1 mM) can lead to a doubling of tension development by the myocardium.

Digitalis markedly increases vagal tone and can affect sympathetic tone. Enhancement of vagal activity typically tends to cause a decrease in the sinus rate and an increase in the effective refractory period of the atrioventricular node. The main effect on ordinary atrial fibres is a shortening of their action potential duration and hence of their refractory period.

Because of their relative paucity of vagal innervation, it has traditionally been considered that the indirect, vagally mediated effects of digitalis were of little relevance to the His-Purkinje system and to ventricular myocardium, except possibly in situations of digitalis toxicity where the high sympathetic tone may play a role in provoking arrhythmias. There is emerging evidence, however, that binding of digoxin to vagal afferent fibres from ventricular myocardium may play a role in reduction of the high background sympathetic tone seen in patients with cardiac failure. Withdrawal of sympathetic tone and consequent vasodilatation and afterload reduction may well be one of the more important mechanisms of action of digitalis in cardiac failure. While there is some evidence for symptomatic benefit for digoxin on top of optimal medical therapy in heart failure, there is also concern that no mortality gain has been demonstrated and there is some evidence of decreased survival in some studies, so its use is declining steadily at this time.

Haemodynamic effects

If digoxin is given to a normal volunteer it causes both a positive inotropic effect due to drug action on the myocardium, and an increase in afterload due to the increased tone in blood vessels. A patient with cardiac failure, however, is in a different situation. As mentioned above, one of the characteristics of cardiac failure from the very early stages is a marked increase in sympathetic tone. Digoxin administration results in a withdrawal of this abnormally enhanced sympathetic tone. Thus when a patient with cardiac failure is given digoxin, he gets the benefit of the positive inotropic effect as well as the withdrawal of sympathetic tone, which more than compensates for the direct tendency for digoxin to increase afterload. Afterload falls and the cardiac output increases.

ANTIARRHYTHMIC DRUGS AND RELEVANT ELECTROPHYSIOLOGY

A brief summary of the Vaughan Williams classification is given in Table 22.2 (and in Table 22.1). Further consideration of each class follows.

Clinical pharmacology of antiarrhythmic drugs

CLASS IA DRUGS: QUINIDINE, PROCAINAMIDE, DISOPYRAMIDE

Quinine has been prescribed for palpitations since the eighteenth century. It was largely replaced for this purpose by its *d*-isomer, quinidine, after the work of Wenckebach and Frey from 1914 to 1918. The use of procainamide stems from observations by Mautz in 1936 which showed that procaine increased the threshold to electrical stimulation of ventricular muscle. Further studies led to its replacement by procainamide, which exhibited similar properties but has a much longer duration of action. The antiarrhythmic properties of disopyramide were described in animals in 1962, and a clinical trial was reported in 1963.

In the clinical electrophysiology laboratory, these drugs produce very similar effects. Hence, it is not surprising that all three compounds are useful in the treatment and prophylaxis of a variety of atrial and ventricular arrhythmias, though there is a tendency to reserve procainamide for the latter.

All three have been used successfully for reversion of, and prophylaxis against, atrial flutter and fibrillation. If administered as the sole therapy for these arrhythmias, each of these drugs may produce an acceleration of the ventricular rate. This is due, in part, to a drug-induced reduction in atrial rate, and hence reduction in repetitive concealed conduction into the A-V node. As well as this, quinidine and disopyramide, and (to a much lesser extent) procainamide, exhibit vagolytic activity that can accelerate conduction through the A-V node. For this reason, they are normally administered in conjunction with digitalis for treatment of atrial flutter and fibrillation.

Supraventricular tachycardia of the intranodal type is most commonly and successfully treated with verapamil which blocks the A-V nodal limb of the re-entrant circuit. The IA drugs, however, can be used with moderate success for this arrhythmia. They can also be quite useful in supraventricular tachycardias caused by an accessory atrioventricular connection (as in Wolff–Parkinson–White Syndrome). In these cases, the drugs act by slowing conduction in part of the circuit to the point of block.

Class IA drugs are often effective in suppressing ventricular ectopic beats by their effect on automaticity. The widespread recognition of their potential for "proarrhythmic" effects and the advent of implantable cardioverter-defibrillators has seen their use largely disappear in recent years.

IB DRUGS: LIGNOCAINE, MEXILETINE, TOCAINIDE

Lignocaine is the oldest and best-known of this group (it was synthesised in 1946). Because of extensive first-pass metabolism in the liver, lignocaine must be administered parenterally. It achieved widespread acceptance as first line pharmacological therapy for serious ventricular arrhythmias in acute myocardial infarction, but is

Table 22.2 Clinical pharmacology of antiarrhythmic drugs

	Drug	Action
Class I	Quinidine, procainamide disopyramide, lignocaine tocainide, mexiletine, etc.	Block fast sodium current, shorten repolarisation period, reduce conduction
Class II	Beta blockers	Block effects of catecholamines
Class III	Amiodarone, sotalol	Lengthen action potential duration
Class IV	Verapamil, diltiazem	Calcium antagonists

used much less often than in the past because of concerns about proarrhythmia and the availability of amiodarone and various device therapies.

Central nervous system side effects are not uncommon with lignocaine. These include paraesthesiae (often perioral), mental changes, tremor, convulsions and coma.

Mexiletine and tocainide are chemically very similar to lignocaine. They share the advantage of being effective when given by mouth but are now rarely used. The side effects of these drugs are similar to those listed for lignocaine. In addition, gastrointestinal symptoms, especially nausea, are a common complaint.

1C DRUGS: FLECAINIDE, ENCAINIDE, LORCAINIDE, PROPAFENONE

These drugs, of which only flecainide is freely available in Australia, are discussed briefly. There are a number of studies indicating that all three are very effective in suppressing both supraventricular and ventricular arrhythmias. It should be noted, however, that they also have considerable negative inotropic properties and tend to prolong intracardiac conduction times, even in therapeutic concentrations. Arrhythmogenesis has been reported for encainide and flecainide, and led to their withdrawal from the CAST study, a large American study of antiarrhythmic drug therapy in 1991.

Class II agents

Beta-blocking agents are often effective both in reversion of, and in prophylaxis against, supraventricular tachycardia, where they probably act largely by prolonging refractoriness and slowing conduction in the AV node. Their role in this arrhythmia (particularly for acute therapy) has, however, been largely overshadowed by verapamil. In atrial fibrillation and flutter (especially if due to thyrotoxicosis), beta-blocking agents can be useful in slowing the ventricular response by their effect on the AV node, but they are generally of little use in restoring sinus rhythm. An exception to this is sotalol, which is discussed with Class III drugs.

Beta-blocking agents also have value in the therapy of ventricular tachyarrhythmias though they have not generally been used as first-line drugs for this indication in the past. They are of particular use in arrhythmias caused by increased circulating catecholamines (anxiety, exercise, phaeochromocytoma), and arrhythmias of the congenital long QT interval syndrome. Some recent studies have also shown a reduction in ventricular arrhythmias in acute myocardial infarction after the early intravenous administration of beta-blocking drugs.

Class III agents

The best-known drug of this class is amiodarone. It was first used in France in 1962 as a vascular smooth-muscle relaxant and has been widely used in Europe and South America as an antiarrhythmic agent for well over a decade. It did not, however, come into use in the United States and Australia until the 1980s. Apart from its marked ability to prolong the duration of the cardiac action potential (Class III activity), amiodarone is also a smooth-muscle relaxant, a non-competitive antiadrenergic agent, and demonstrates some degree of Class I and IV activity, at least *in vitro*.

Whatever its basic mechanism (or mechanisms) of action, it is a very useful antiarrhythmic agent with demonstrated effectiveness in the therapy and prophylaxis of most types of arrhythmia. It is particularly effective in the treatment of atrial fibrillation, supraventricular arrhythmias associated with Wolff–Parkinson–White Syndrome, ventricular arrhythmias complicating hypertrophic cardiomyopathy (which responds poorly to beta-blocking agents or calcium antagonists) and refractory, recurrent ventricular tachycardia and fibrillation. In the latter life-threatening situation, amiodarone has proved effective in large numbers of patients whose condition had failed to respond to a series of other established and experimental drugs.

As often happens in medicine, such benefits come at a price. Amiodarone's clinical use is complicated by its very unusual pharmacokinetics and unwanted side effects.

Administration of amiodarone (normally by mouth) is complicated by a variable bioavailability (20%–80%), a huge volume of distribution (5000 litres) and a terminal half-life of elimination which is usually 35–40 days, but may exceed 100 days. The major metabolite accumulates in high concentration in plasma and tissues, and possesses very similar electrophysiological properties to amiodarone. Dosage regimens vary from clinician to clinician, but most recommend a loading dose of 600–2000 mg/day for 1–8 weeks, followed by reduction to a maintenance dose, usually of the order of 200–400 mg/day. Many of the side effects are dose-dependent and each patient should receive the minimum effective dose.

Cardiovascular side effects can include hypotension (usually a problem only with intravenous use), bradycardia (which may be aggravated by concomitant therapy with beta-blocking drugs or verapamil), and QT interval prolongation (normally therapeutic, but occasionally excessive and rarely associated with ventricular tachycardias). Non-cardiac effects include photosensitivity, disturbances of sleep, resting tremor, thyrotoxicosis and hypothyroidism, and pulmonary alveolitis (sometimes fatal). The interaction between amiodarone and the thyroid is complex and has been well described. While thyroid function should be assessed before the start of amiodarone therapy, overt thyroid disease develops in less than 2% of patients. One of the best known, but least important, side effects of amiodarone therapy is the development of corneal microdeposits, which can be seen in 98% of patients receiving long-term treatment. These deposits rarely produce symptoms; blurred and halo vision occurs in 1%–2% of cases and diminishes after reduction of the dose. Amiodarone may interact with other drugs. Its additive effects with beta-blocking agents and verapamil, and its ability to elevate serum digoxin levels have already been noted. In addition, potentiation of the effects of warfarin may occur, which usually necessitates reduction of the warfarin dose by about half.

Sotalol is a non-cardioselective beta-blocking agent with marked Class III activity. Unlike other beta-blocking agents the prolongation of the duration of the action potential is apparent at once (within minutes, if administered intravenously), and this drug is showing promise in clinical trials in the treatment of supraventricular and ventricular arrhythmias. The oral bioavailability of sotalol is about 60%, and there is no significant hepatic first-pass metabolism. Sotalol can produce any of the characteristic side effects associated with beta-blockers, and in addition has been reported to cause polymorphic ventricular tachycardia ('torsade de pointes') associated with lengthening of the QT interval. This side effect, which may be fatal, is probably more common in the presence of high sotalol concentrations, potassium depletion or the co-administration of other drugs known to prolong the QT interval.

Class IV agents

Verapamil is the prototype for this class of drug. It has been in clinical use since 1966, and has become the drug of first choice for short-term therapy of supraventricular tachycardia, in which it acts by blocking the slow conducting (AV nodal) limb of the re-entrant circuit. The usual dosage is 5–10 mg administered intravenously over 5–10 minutes, with careful monitoring of the ECG and blood pressure. In atrial fibrillation or flutter, verapamil usually slows the ventricular response, but is unlikely to induce reversion to sinus rhythm. Long-term oral therapy with verapamil can be useful in prophylaxis against recurrent supraventricular tachycardias, but can be complicated by the pharmacokinetics of the drug. Verapamil is not generally employed for treatment of recurrent ventricular tachyarrhythmias. Some studies have demonstrated a good response to verapamil in a small subgroup of patients with recurrent ventricular tachycardia.

Cardiac depression is the most serious side effect of verapamil. It is rarely a problem in patients with normal left ventricular function but can be quite severe in already diseased or beta-blocked hearts, especially when verapamil is administered intravenously. Non-cardiac side effects are occasionally a problem. These include tiredness, constipation, pruritus, headache and vertigo. Constipation in particular can be very troublesome, especially to elderly patients.

Because of their additive effects on the AV node and on myocardial contractility, the combination of verapamil and beta-blocking agents is potentially dangerous. Recent experience suggests that they can be safely administered together in many patients, but the initiation of such therapy is best carried out under careful supervision. Similarly, the combined administration of digoxin and verapamil can be very useful, especially in atrial fibrillation, but caution must be exercised both because of their additive effects on AV conduction and because verapamil tends to elevate serum levels of digoxin.

ANTIPLATELET AGENTS

These drugs are discussed in Chapter 23.

ANTITHROMBOTIC AGENTS

Heparin

Heparin was first isolated from the canine liver by a medical student in 1916 and has been in regular clinical use for over 50 years. Structurally it is a mixture of sulphated glycosaminoglycans, ranging in molecular weight from less than 5,000 to more than 30,000 daltons with an average of 12,000–15,000 daltons, depending on the source. Only about one third of this heparin mixture has significant anticoagulant effect.

Heparin exerts most of its anticoagulant effect by binding to and greatly increasing the activity of an alpha2-globulin called antithrombin III. Antithrombin-III normally complexes with and inactivates a number of activated clotting factors, particularly thrombin and Factor Xa. When heparin binds to antithrombin III it produces a conformational change that dramatically increases the affinity of antithrombin III for thrombin, factor Xa and other protease enzymes of the coagulation cascade. This eventually leads to a dose-dependent prolongation of blood clotting which can be monitored with assays such as the activated partial thromboplastin time (APTT) and the thrombin time (TT). Heparin has other effects including some inhibition of platelet function, increased permeability of vessel walls and inhibition of proliferation of vascular smooth muscle, but this presentation concentrates on the antithrombotic actions of this agent.

While thrombin is more sensitive to inhibition by the heparin-antithrombin-III complex than is factor Xa, it has recently become recognised that the low molecular weight components of the heparin mixture (those with fewer saccharide residues), are unable to bind to thrombin and antithrombin-III simultaneously, and thus selectively inhibit factor Xa activity. This has led to the marketing and promotion of specific low molecular weight fractions of heparin for antithrombotic prophylaxis, the aim being to inhibit factor Xa and hence intravascular coagulation, without inhibiting thrombin activation and seriously impairing normal haemostasis. In this way it may prove possible to separate the beneficial actions and the bleeding complications of heparin, and further enhance the clinical value of this compound.

Heparin is poorly absorbed orally, and must be administered by intravenous or subcutaneous injection. Since there is no satisfactory assay for circulating heparin, the dosage is normally adjusted according to the APPT or TT as noted above. The dose response curve for heparin is not linear; the anticoagulant response increases disproportionately in intensity and duration as the dose increases. The apparent biological half-life of intravenous heparin is of the order of 30–60 minutes, increasing somewhat with dosage. Heparin binds initially to saturable sites on endothelial cells. Heparin is eliminated by mechanisms which are still unclear, but there are reports of reduced heparin requirements in patients with renal failure.

It has been confirmed that fibrin binds to thrombin and protects it from inactivation by the heparin-antithrombin-III complex. The result of this is that about twenty times more heparin is needed to inactivate fibrin-bound thrombin than to inactivate prothrombin. This does not apply to a number of more recently introduced thrombin inhibitors such as bivalirudin (or hirudin—see below). This effect explains the observation that preventing extension of established venous thrombosis requires higher concentrations of heparin than does preventing its formation, as well as the relative inefficacy of heparin in inhibiting thrombin activity after successful coronary thrombolysis.

The most common and feared side effect of heparin is bleeding. With well-monitored administration intravenously or subcutaneously the incidence of major bleeding appears to range from about 4% to 6%. This can be increased by concomitant use of aspirin, co-existent alcoholic liver disease or other major hepatic dysfunction and possibly renal failure. Thrombocytopenia is also a well-recognised and usually asymptomatic complication of heparin therapy, with an incidence ranging from 2% or less, up to over 20%. In a much smaller number of patients (probably well under 1% of those given heparin), thrombocytopenia is associated with arterial or venous thrombosis (this combination is sometimes known as 'HITT': Heparin Induced Thrombocytopenia and Thrombosis). Venous thrombosis in particular may also result from heparin resistance caused by the neutralising effect of heparin-induced release of platelet factor 4. In patients with persistent heparin-induced thrombocytopenia and who require continuing antithrombotic therapy, low molecular weight heparin may have cross-reactivity with standard heparin, and use of heparinoid appears to be a more successful alternative. Less common side effects of heparin in long-term use include various allergic reactions, alopecia and osteoporosis.

Low molecular weight heparins

There are several low molecular weight versions of heparin available of which enoxaparin is by far the most widely used in Australia (dalteparin much less commonly). These have more predictable and longer half-lives and are usually given by once or twice-daily subcutaneous injections. They are largely anti-factor Xa drugs. Advantages include ease of administration and much less likelihood of HITT, as well as usually having no need to monitor effect continuously as with heparin. Disadvantages include high renal excretion necessitating care in patients with renal impairment (acute or chronic).

Bivalirudin

Bivalirudin (once known as hirudin) is a parenteral direct thrombin inhibitor. On the basis of some clinical trial data comparing it to intravenous heparin, it has become popular as an alternative to heparin in cardiac catheterisation laboratories in some countries, particularly in North America.

Warfarin (coumadin)

Dishydroxycoumarin (dicumarol) was identified in 1939 as the causative agent for the haemorrhagic disorder described in cattle that ingested spoiled sweet clover. A few years later a synthetic congener named warfarin was developed. In the 1950s, warfarin and related compounds became widespread therapy for the prevention and treatment of thromboembolic disease. The chemistry and pharmacology of these agents is well described in the literature and are only outlined here. In the remainder of this section the term warfarin is used, but most of what is presented applies equally to the other coumadin derivatives.

Warfarin is an antagonist of vitamin K. The coagulation factors II, VII, IX and X and the anticoagulant proteins C and S require vitamin C as a co-factor for their activation. All of these factors, except possibly protein S, are synthesised mainly in the liver. Therapeutic doses of warfarin decrease both the amount and activity of each of the vitamin K dependent coagulation factors. Warfarin has no direct effect on the activity of any fully activated coagulation factors already present in the blood, and hence the time required for the effects of warfarin to manifest depends on individual rates of clearance of each of the factors. Factor VII and protein C have half-lives of approximately 6–8 hours. The half-lives of factors IV, X and II are approximately 24, 36 and 54 hours respectively, and the half-life of protein S is approximately 30 hours. Thus the effects of the reduction in factor VII and protein C are manifested long before effects on other coagulation factors. Because factor VII is of limited relevance to intravascular coagulation, patients in the first 24 hours or so after the introduction of warfarin therapy may manifest a 'hypercoaguable' state secondary to the reduction in protein C. For this reason, and also because of the long half-lives of the other vitamin K dependent clotting factors which are more important than factor VII in intravascular coagulation, concomitant heparin therapy should be continued for several days after the introduction of warfarin.

Warfarin is well absorbed orally, although food can reduce this to some extent. It freely crosses the placenta. Warfarin is transformed into inactive metabolites by the liver and kidneys and eliminated with a half-life ranging from 20 to 60 hours. There are large numbers of potentially important interactions between warfarin and other ingested substances including many drugs. These are well covered in standard textbooks. The major toxic complication of warfarin is of course bleeding. If necessary, the effects of warfarin can be reversed with vitamin K, or by replacing clotting factors exogenously using fresh frozen plasma or transfusions of fresh whole blood. Warfarin should not be used during pregnancy because of its teratogenic effects on the foetus and risk of maternal bleeding. Other occasional reactions to warfarin include rashes, itching, fever and gastrointestinal upsets.

Regular monitoring is an important part of therapy with warfarin. Originally this was done using the prothrombin time or its inverse the pro-thombin index. Prolongation of prothrombin time relative to a controlled sample of plasma occurs when any of factors V, II, VII or X are decreased significantly. All countries have introduced the International Normalised Ratio (INR) for report-ing and standardising warfarin effect. This is based on the ratio of the patient prothrombin time to a controlled prothrombin time that would have been obtained using a standard World Health Organisation technique.

Recommendations for the ideal therapeutic level of the prothrombin time or INR vary accord-ing to indication but a target range of 2–3 is usual. Efficacy falls off quickly at INR's less than 1 and bleeding risk starts to rise significantly as INR goes above 4.

NOVEL ORAL ANTICOAGULANTS

The last 5 years or so have seen the rapid emer-gence of a new group of orally active anticoagu-lants (novel or direct oral anticoagulants, NOAC or DOAC). These include dabigatran, apixaban and rivaroxaban, all available for various indications in Australia, and edoxaban, which is used in some countries as well.

Dabigatran differs from apixaban and riva-roxaban in that it is a direct thrombin inhibi-tor whereas the other two agents are direct factor Xa inhibitors. All share similar half-lives of 8–12 hours or so although rivaroxaban is usually administered once-daily and the other two twice daily. They do not normally require monitor-ing and their effects are much more predictable, and these properties make them very attractive as replacements for warfarin. They do however require care in the presence of renal impairment and details for each are available in their product information.

Clinically their greatest advantage over war-farin is that they reduce by 50%–75% the risk of intracerebral haemorrhage (by far the most feared complication of anticoagulation) compared to warfarin even when monitored and dosed ideally. The reason for this is not yet clear. It is important to know that these drugs have been shown to be ineffective compared to warfarin in patients with mechanical heart valves and so must not be used in this setting.

THROMBOLYTIC (FIBRINOLYTIC) AGENTS

Widespread use of thrombolytic agents has revolu-tionised the management of acute myocardial infarc-tion in the past decade. The following is only a very brief outline of the biochemistry and pharmacology of some of the more important of these new agents.

Thrombolytics convert plasminogen into plasmin, a serine protease (790 amino acids) that breaks the arginine-lysine bonds found in many clotting-cascade proteins including fibrin. 'Specificity' for fibrin is only due to the facts that plasminogen binds selectively to partially lysed fibrin, and plasminogen is more readily converted to plasmin when already bound to fibrin. Inactive plasminogen is converted to plasmin by a number of activators including tissue plasminogen activator (tPA), urokinase and streptokinase-plasminogen complex. There are a number of endogenous plasmin inhibitors: Alpha2-antiplasmin, alpha2-macroglobulin, alpha1-antitrypsin, C1-esterase inhibitor and antithrombin III. Extensive activation of circulating plasminogen to plasmin (e.g. by streptokinase), results in its mopping up of all available alpha2-antiplasmin, the most important of the endogenous inhibitors. Since there is more plasminogen than alpha2-antiplasmin, this eventually produces a systemic lytic state. This is seen with streptokinase and urokinase and high doses of tPA, and produces depletion of plasminogen and fibrinogen. Generally fibrinogen and fibrin degradation products are indistinguishable, but the 'D-D dimer' fragment is relatively specific for fibrin degradation, and has been used to monitor successful lysis of fibrin.

tPA is a 527 amino acid glycoprotein made by many cell types including endothelial cells, liver and myocardium. It binds to fibrin as well as plas-minogen (hence 'clot-selectivity'). When given pharmacologically, any tPA that does not quickly bind to fibrin tends to bind to an inactivator (PAI-1) and circulates in blood in this inactive form. tPA has a redistribution half-life of 3–6 minutes and a beta half-life of 20–40 minutes. It was the agent used in many early trials of reperfusion therapy for acute myocardial infarction and these were very successful. Thrombolysis can clearly lead to satis-factory outcomes in acute infarction and should be administered in settings where percutaneous intervention with angioplasty and stenting is not available. However percutaneous coronary stenting has become the standard of care for hospitals with facilities to perform this procedure.

A number of molecules were developed that contain modest improvements on tPA, and the commonest of these currently in use in Australia is tenectoplase.

FURTHER READING

Brunton LL, Knollmann BC, Hilal-Dandan R. *Goodman & Gilman's the Pharmacological Basis of Therapeutics*. 13th ed. New York: McGraw-Hill; 2018. p. 1419.

23

Drug therapy in the cardiac catheterisation laboratory: A guide to commonly used drugs

JOHN EDWARD BOLAND, FUYUE JIANG AND ANDREW FENNING

INTRODUCTION

Drugs used in cardiology may be categorised in various ways, either alphabetically, by mode of action, frequency of use, or pharmacological activity. In this presentation, the most commonly used drugs in the cardiac catheterisation laboratory (CCL) are grouped according to their major clinical effects and are discussed under the following major headings: (1) **Pain Relief**, (2) **Antiplatelet and Anticoagulation Therapy** (including antithrombin and thrombolytic agents), (3) **Control** of **Blood Pressure**, (4) **Treatment of Arrhythmia** (including inotropes, chronotropes, alpha blockers and beta blockers), (5) **Premedication and Sedation**, (6) **Treatment of Nausea**, and (7) **Other Conditions**. Alternatively, these pharmacological interventions can also be classified under two different headings: (1) as adjuvants to primary care (pain relief, premedication and sedation, treatment of nausea, and other conditions) and (2) for direct treatment of a cardiovascular pathophysiology (antiplatelet and anticoagulant therapy, control of blood pressure, and treatment of arrhythmia).

Traditionally, drugs are named according to their effect (stimulatory or inhibitory) on nerve fibres (sympathetic or parasympathetic), or according to the type of neurotransmitter or cell receptor involved (acetylcholine or norepinephrine [noradrenaline]) (see Table 23.1). Thus, **Parasympathomimetic**

Table 23.1 Pharmacological classification model of major drugs

Drug type	Action
Sympathomimetic agents	Increase force and/or rate of cardiac contraction (Adrenaline, noradrenaline, dopamine, dobutamine)
Sympatholytic agents	Decrease force and/or rate of cardiac contraction (Include beta blockers)
Centrally-acting antihypertensive agents	Control blood pressure (Include alpha-methyldopa, clonidine)
Peripherally-acting antihypertensive agents	Control blood pressure (Include sympatholytic agents, alpha blockers, calcium antagonists, nitrovasodilators, ACE inhibitors)
Antiarrhythmic agents	Class I (Ia, Ib, Ic) Class II (beta blockers, sympathomimetics) Class III (amiodarone, sotalol) Class IV (calcium antagonists)
Antiplatelet agents	Aspirin, clopidogrel, ticlopidine, glycoprotein IIb/IIIa antagonists
Antigoagulant agents	Heparin (unfractionated and low molecular weight), warfarin, direct thrombin inhibitors
Thrombolytic agents	Tissue plasminogen activator, urokinase, streptokinase, reteplase
Hypertensive agents (Pressors)	Metaraminol (adrenergic agent used to raise blood pressure)
Anticholinergic (or vagolytic) agents	Atropine

agents stimulate parasympathetic nerves; **Parasympatholytic** agents block or inhibit parasympathetic nerves; **Sympathomimetic** agents stimulate sympathetic nerves; and **Sympatholytic** agents block or inhibit sympathetic nerves. **Cholinergic** drugs stimulate receptor sites mediated by the neurotransmitter acetylcholine; and **Anticholinergic** drugs block acetylcholine receptors. **Adrenergic** drugs stimulate sympathetic neuroeffector sites for epinephrine (adrenaline) or norepinephrine (noradrenaline); and **Antiadrenergic** drugs block epinephrine (adrenaline) or norepinephrine (noradrenaline) receptors (note acetylcholine is not exclusively a neurotransmitter for parasympathetic sites). Most drugs are designed to mimic the activity or chemical structure of endogenous ligands and are typically classified as agonists, partial agonists, antagonists or enzyme inhibitors targeting traditional protein receptors, voltage gated ion channels, or key cellular enzymes. Table 23.1 lists the major categories of cardiac drugs according to their pharmacological modes of action. This provides a reference from which to identify and compare the individual drugs discussed herein. A common feature of cardiovascular pharmacotherapy is the notion that one class of agents is often effective for the management of multiple conditions. Important examples are medication classes such as the β-adrenoceptor antagonists and calcium channel antagonists, with drugs from both being effective treatments for hypertension, arrhythmia, angina and heart failure. The following text presents the medications in the cardiovascular pharmacology classes most relevant to the CCL.

PAIN RELIEF (SEE TABLE 23.2)

Pain killers (analgesics) operate by blocking transmission of nerve impulses from pain receptors, or by altering the brain's perception of pain. However, if the acute myocardial hypoxia is also relieved either through surgical intervention or nitrovasodilator therapy pain relief is also achieved. The most commonly used opiate analgesics for relieving angina are fentanyl, morphine and historically, pethidine. All opiates are narcotics and operate on the central nervous system.

Fentanyl is a narcotic and a relative of morphine. It is available in 100 mcg vials, is administered intravenously and is short acting, with a half-life

Table 23.2 Pain relief

	Dose	Action	Side effects
Fentanyl	25 mcg iv	Immediate, short-acting (20 minutes)	Nausea, drowsiness hypoventilation
Morphine	2.5 mcg iv (can be oral rectal, sc, im)	Immediate, Long-acting (4 hours)	As for fentanyl

of 20 minutes. The standard dose is 25 mcg, with additional dosages given in aliquots of 25 mcg as required. Possible side effects are nausea, drowsiness and hypoventilation. Patients are therefore usually given oxygen with fentanyl and are also monitored with a digital pulse oximeter. Fentanyl is often administered with an anti-emetic agent to alleviate opioid-induced dysphoria and nausea (see below).

Morphine is an opiate, meaning it operates on cerebral opiate receptors, thereby altering a patient's perception of pain. It is available in 5 mg vials and can be administered orally, rectally, intravenously, subcutaneously or by intramuscular injection. In the CCL it is given intravenously at a dosage of 2.5 mg. It is a long-lasting agent, its effects often persisting long after the case is finished. Side effects are similar to those of fentanyl.

Pethidine, although not used in the CCL, is also an opiate and is generally administered subcutaneously or intramuscularly. It has a slightly shorter half-life than morphine (3 hours instead of 4). Dosage is usually 25 mg, which is equivalent to 2.5 mg of morphine, or to 25 mcg of fentanyl.

Anginine and other vasodilators such as glyceryl trinitrate (**GTN** or **Tridil**) and Isosorbide dinitrate (**Isordil**) are not considered pain killers per se. Nitrates and nitrites cause peripheral venous dilatation, with a corresponding drop in blood pressure. This results in a reduction of stroke volume and cardiac workload, which in turn relieves acute myocardial hypoxia. Pain relief is thus achieved primarily by reducing preload, as GTN is a relatively weak arterial vasodilator. The nitrovasodilators are further discussed below for their use in managing hypertension during cardiac catheterisation procedures.

ANTIPLATELET AND ANTICOAGULATION THERAPY

Antiplatelet, anticoagulation and thrombolytic pharmacology is a mainstay of both primary and secondary prevention of acute coronary syndromes. The coagulation process begins with activation of platelets and ends with formation of a stable fibrin clot following a complex series of interactions involving vascular endothelium, platelets and circulating plasma proteins (see Chapter 4). The dominant role of platelets, thrombin and positive feedback agents such as adenosine diphosphate (ADP) provide excellent opportunities for new and improved drugs to focus on two main strategies: To reduce thrombin production and to inhibit platelet activity. Platelet aggregation is essential to coagulation, while thrombin plays a central role in platelet activation and fibrin production.

The commonly used antiplatelet and anticoagulant agents are aspirin, clopidogrel, ticagrelor, prasugrel, dypiridamole, abciximab, tirofiban, enoxaparin, heparin, warfarin and the thrombolytic agents tissue plasminogen activator (tPA), reteplase and streptokinase.

It is useful to differentiate between specific antiplatelet agents such as aspirin, clopidogrel, abciximab and tirofiban, which directly inhibit platelet activity, and the anticoagulants such as heparin and its derivatives that interfere with some aspect of the coagulation process, usually by blocking plasma protein interactions.

Thrombolytics act by dissolving a clot after it is formed, while the antithrombin agents inhibit thrombin formation by targeting thrombin activity either directly (hirudin and bivalirudin) or indirectly (heparin and its derivatives again, and warfarin).

Antiplatelet agents

Antiplatelet agents are a diverse group of pharmacological medications targeting enzymes, cell surface receptors, inflammatory mediators and calcium homeostasis within the platelet (Table 23.3).

ASPIRIN

Aspirin is a potent, though limited, platelet inhibitor and is extensively used as a first line of treatment

Table 23.3 Antiplatelet agents

	Dose	Action	Side effects
Aspirin	600 mg loading 75–300 mg pd oral	Long-lasting (days)	Bleeding, gastro-intestinal ulcers, bruising
Dipyridamole	100 mg × 4 pd oral	Long-lasting	Increased heart rate, bleeding, bruising
Clopidogrel	600 mg loading 75 mg pd oral	Long-lasting	Bleeding, bruising
Prasugrel	60 mg loading 10 mg pd oral	Rapid onset	Bleeding, bruising
Ticagrelor	180 mg loading + 90 mg 2 × pd oral	Fast-acting	Bleeding, dyspnea, hepatic impairment, bradycardia
Abciximab	0.25 mg/kg bolus + 0.125 mcg/kg 12-h infusion	Fast-acting, long-lasting	Bleeding, allergic reaction, antibody reaction
Tirofiban	0.4 mcg/kg/min 30-min infusion +0.1 mcg/kg/min Maintenance for 48–108 h	Fast-acting, long-lasting	Bleeding

in a variety of conditions where platelet inhibition is desired. Numerous trials have substantiated the benefits of aspirin as standard treatment for acute myocardial infarction and unstable angina, and to a lesser extent, as long-term prophylactic use for the prevention of primary and secondary ischemic or thrombotic events.[1] Aspirin affects arachidonic acid metabolism by reducing production of thromboxane A2 (TXA2) via inhibition of the cyclooxygenase (COX-1) enzyme, a platelet derivative that promotes platelet activation. The effects of aspirin on platelets are irreversible and last for the life of the platelet, which is typically eight to ten days. It has no effect on other platelet activators such as thrombin and is often prescribed in combination with other drugs. It is usually taken orally at a dose of 75–300 mg daily; 600 mg is usually given before coronary intervention, followed by 300 mg daily for 3 months, then 100 mg daily for life. Potential side effects are excessive bleeding and formation of gastro-intestinal ulcers from chronic COX-1 inhibition.

DIPYRIDAMOLE

Dipyridamole is an antiplatelet agent similar to aspirin, but unlike aspirin does not inhibit platelet production of cyclo-oxygenase. It acts by preventing adenosine re-uptake by red blood cells, and blocks AMP phosphodiesterase and cGMP phosphodiesterase. Although no longer used by interventional cardiologists it was originally used mainly in combination with aspirin postoperatively for secondary prevention of stroke at a dose of 100 mg tablets 4 times daily. In large doses it causes an increase in heart rate and was used to emulate stress for sestamibi studies.

THIENOPYRIDINES (CLOPIDOGREL, PRASUGREL, TICAGRELOR)

The thienopyridines are similar to aspirin, but with a different mode of action. They do not interfere with TXA2 production, but inhibit binding of ADP to platelet surface receptors (specifically by blocking the P2Y12 platelet surface receptor) thereby inhibiting ADP-induced platelet aggregation. Clopidogrel is available as 75 mg tablets and has replaced ticlopidine, which caused neutropenia as a side effect. A loading dose of four tablets (600 mg) is usually given prior to angioplasty or stenting, and in combination with 300 mg aspirin is the preferred loading dose preceding percutaneous coronary intervention (PCI).[2] Its optimum effect is reached after 3–4 hours. Side effects are bleeding, rash and a low platelet count. Suppression of platelet activity is very effectively achieved by a combination of aspirin and clopidogrel,[3] and is of particular benefit in preventing in-stent thrombosis following drug-eluting stent deployment. Long-term dual antiplatelet therapy with 300 mg clopidogrel and low-dose aspirin is now a Class IA recommendation.[4]

Prasugrel is a relatively new, third-generation thienopyridine that targets the platelet ADP receptor, much like clopidogrel. For planned PCI, it reportedly achieves more rapid onset and substantially greater and more consistent inhibition of platelet aggregation with a loading dose of 60 mg followed by 10 mg per day, and has less patient variability compared with a 600 mg loading dose of clopidogrel followed by 150 mg per day.[5] In patients presenting with acute coronary syndrome (ACS),[6] prasugrel-treated patients showed lower rates of myocardial infarction, urgent target-vessel revascularisation and stent thrombosis than clopidogrel-treated patients. Major bleeding rates tended to be higher with the prasugrel group and there was no difference in mortality between the two groups. The TRITON-TIMI 38 Trial reported that prasugrel reduced cardiovascular events compared with clopidogrel in patients with acute coronary syndromes.[7]

Ticagrelor, another of the newer ADP P2Y12 platelet receptor inhibitors, was found to have more pronounced platelet inhibition than clopidogrel in patients presenting with ACS. The PLATO study[8] compared ticagrelor with aspirin versus clopidogrel with aspirin and found that ticagrelor reduced the primary composite endpoint (cardiovascular death, myocardial infarction, stroke) by 12% at 30 days, and by 16% at 12 months for cardiovascular death and myocardial infarction but not stroke, with no significant difference in total major bleeding. There was also a lower rate of in-stent thrombosis with ticagrelor. Initial loading dose was 180 mg with a maintenance dose of 90 mg twice daily.

GLYCOPROTEIN IIb/IIIa INHIBITORS

Abciximab

Abciximab is a monoclonal antiplatelet antibody that targets the platelet GP IIb/IIIa surface receptor. The other GP IIb/IIIa antagonists are the peptide **eptifibatide** (a derivative of rattlesnake venom) and a group of smaller peptides (**tirofiban**, **lamifiban** and **xemilofiban**). Abciximab was widely used in association with stent deployment, or as required to prevent or treat acute clotting scenarios. It is delivered intravenously according to a weight-adjusted chart. Initial administration is as an intravenous bolus in solution (0.25 mg/kg) followed by a 12-hours infusion at 0.125 mcg/kg/min (to a maximum of 10 ug/min). Again, side effects are bleeding complications and possible

allergic reactions that drop the platelet count. The latter may be associated with formation of human anti chimeric antibodies. Abciximab is fast-acting, achieving receptor blockade greater than 80% after the first bolus. Its effects are irreversible and last for 24–36 hours. A platelet transfusion is necessary to effect reversibility. Abciximab also reduced the incidence of death and myocardial infarction in patients presenting with ACS,[9,10] but demonstrated no added benefit to stable patients pre-treated with aspirin and clopidogrel prior to elective coronary intervention.[11] Use of abciximab has declined considerably in recent years and is now used almost exclusively in association with thrombus formation during coronary intervention.

Tirofiban

Tirofiban is manufactured synthetically and belongs to the same group of antiplatelet agents as abciximab, yet different dosing regimens resulted in mixed results when originally compared in clinical trials. A meta-analysis of randomised clinical trials comparing tirofiban versus placebo or versus abciximab suggested that the safety profile favoured tirofiban over abciximab, and other studies have supported its efficacy as adjunctive therapy for ST-elevation myocardial infarction patients undergoing PCI.[12] Like abciximab, however, tirofiban is not generally used during PCI and is currently favoured for patients in emergency transit from remote or country areas to the catheterisation unit. In this setting it is given as a weight-adjusted infusion, with a loading infusion rate 0.4 mcg/kg/min for 30 minutes and a maintenance infusion rate of 0.1 mcg/kg/min over 48–108 hours. In patients undergoing PCI for non-ST elevation myocardial infarction, tirofiban was found to be non-inferior to abciximab. Like abciximab, however, routine use of tirofiban during PCI has been largely discontinued.

Anticoagulants (see Table 23.4)

HEPARIN

Heparin is a naturally occurring, biologically active compound with a variety of functions. Heparin alone is not an anticoagulant. It acts primarily by enhancing the anticoagulant and antithrombotic

Table 23.4 Anticoagulation, thrombolytic and antithrombin agents

	Dose	Action	Side effects
Anticoagulants			
Heparin	70–100 IU/kg iv	Immediate, long-lasting (1 hour)	Bleeding, HITTS
LMWH Enoxaparin	sc	Activity dose-dependent	Bleeding, HITTS, can induce heparin resistance
Thrombolytics			
tPA	Weight-related protocol	3–6 minutes, 80% complete reperfusion in <90 minutes	Allergic reaction, bleeding, reperfusion arrhythmia, can promote antibodies
Urokinase	Weight-related protocol		Bleeding
Streptokinase	Weight-related protocol		
Reteplase	Weight-related protocol		
Direct Antithrombins			
Bivalirudin	0.25 mg/kg bolus iv + 0.175 mcg/kg/12 hours Infusion up to 4 hours	Acts within minutes, short-acting, reversible	Irritation, bleeding, nausea

Abbreviations: HITTS, heparin-induced thrombotic thrombocytopenia; tPA, tissue plasminogen activator.

effects of antithrombin III (another naturally occurring plasma protein) that inhibits thrombin and other coagulation factors, thus preventing thrombus formation. Its effects are limited, however, as it is ineffective against thrombin already bound to fibrin and is itself inhibited by other circulating factors such as heparinase and platelet factor 4.

Heparin is poorly absorbed by the gut so is usually given intravenously, intra-arterially or subcutaneously. Standard dosage preceding catheterisation is 2500 IU, with additional doses for coronary angioplasty. Recommended doses for this vary, but are generally between 70 and 100 IU per kg. As with most drugs, it is inactivated by the liver and excreted in urine, with a half-life of about 1 hour and, as with many other anticoagulants, bleeding can be a serious side effect. Heparin dosage is routinely monitored by the Activated Partial Thromboplastin Time (APTT) test and by the benchside Activated Clotting Time (ACT) test (see Chapter 6).

Recent studies have shown that low-dose heparin provides comparable protection against thromboembolic episodes following angioplasty as does high-dose heparin, but with fewer complications.[13] Different dosages provide different levels of anticoagulation and wear off at different rates. During

coronary intervention, the coagulation status of whole blood (as measured by the ACT test) is an appropriate means of determining heparin dosage and helpful in reducing bleeding complications. Target ACT levels are 250–300 seconds, or 200–250 seconds when used in combination with abciximab. For routine diagnostic angiography, some operators prefer to flush catheters with heparinised saline prior to use and forgo systemic heparin administration altogether. ACT levels are also useful for guiding use of percutaneous closure devices following intervention.

Protamine is not an anticoagulant but is mentioned here because it reverses the effects of heparin and is given intravenously. Injection of 25 mg protamine reverses the effects of 2500 IU heparin. It was at one time administered to permit prompt sheath removal following diagnostic angiography, but its use for this purpose has been largely discontinued.

LOW MOLECULAR WEIGHT HEPARIN

Heparin is available as unfractionated heparin or as low molecular weight heparin (LMWH), e.g. enoxaparin. LMWH is manufactured by modifying the unfractionated heparin chain (average molecular weight 15000 daltons) and has a molecular weight of less than 6000 daltons. LMWH has a longer half-life (24 hours), allowing subcutaneous administration once or twice daily. Despite certain advantages, there are a number of problems associated with LMWH. Its effects are not fully reversed by protamine, it stays in the body much longer than unfractionated heparin, and the assay for quantifying its activity (anti-factor Xa level) is not routinely performed. If a diagnostic procedure proceeds to a coronary intervention, it can be difficult to determine how much additional heparin to give the patient. This results in a clinical advantage by not requiring an intravenous drip for administration, and a haemostatic closure device can still be applied at the end of the procedure. Generally, LMWH is considered a more effective anticoagulant than heparin but is also more problematic. Nevertheless, LMWH is useful in preventing deep venous thrombosis following surgery,[14] and remains the anticoagulant of choice during cardiopulmonary bypass surgery.[15] The SYNERGY trial showed that enoxaparin may be better than heparin in ACS, albeit with higher bleeding complications. As yet, enoxaparin is not favoured during coronary intervention.

NEW ORAL ANTICOAGULANTS (NOACs)

Other, relatively new orally active drugs called NOACs (e.g. apixaban, rivaroxaban, dabigatran) that target specific coagulation factors are available as possible alternatives to heparin and warfarin. The NOAC class provides significant clinical advantages, particularly compared to warfarin, such as reliable pharmacokinetics, standardised dosing without the requirement of frequent monitoring, a wider therapeutic window and fewer non-specific drug interactions. NOACs are useful in the management of clotting disorders associated with venous thromboembolic disease and atrial fibrillation. NOACs fall into two specific categories based on their mechanism of action. **Rivaroxaban** and **apixaban** inhibit factor Xa of the coagulation cascade, whereas **dabigatran** directly inhibits thrombin (factor IIa), which consequently inactivates soluble and fibrin-bound thrombin, thus inhibiting thrombus formation.

THROMBOLYTICS (SEE TABLE 23.4)

The function of thrombolytics is to dissolve a formed clot. They are used for treating acute myocardial infarction, particularly when cardiac catheterisation is not immediately available, and are effective in 50% of cases.[16] Dosages vary. A large dose or infusion is usually indicated according to a weight-adjusted protocol. Thrombolytics are delivered intravenously. Direct intracoronary injections during cardiac catheterisation are only rarely attempted, as the efficacy of this delivery is questionable. Bleeding is a possible side effect, along with arrhythmia resulting from a reperfusion effect. It is also possible to suffer a distal arterial insult from the flushing effect of atheromatous debris once the clot starts to dissolve.

Thrombolytics act by converting circulating plasminogen into plasmin, a serine protease that breaks down fibrin. tPA and urokinase, (both are enzymes and endogenous plasminogen activators) and streptokinase (a derivative of Streptococcus), are the most common thrombolytic agents. A bolus of tPA, with a recirculation half-life of 3–6 minutes, in combination with intravenous heparin is favoured over streptokinase. Urokinase is more expensive, and repeated use of streptokinase can lead to allergic reactions and formation of streptokinase antibodies. A more recent product, reteplase, is a modification of tPA, and has some advantages.[17] The TIMI-14 and GUSTO trials demonstrated more effective thrombolysis when the newer fibrinolytic agents reteplase and alteplase respectively were administered in conjunction with the antiplatelet agent abciximab: 80% of patients achieved complete reperfusion within 90 minutes of treatment, a result comparable with primary angioplasty.[18] The PAMI and other trials, however, subsequently established the overall superiority of primary intervention over thrombolysis for patients presenting with ST-elevation ACS.[19]

ANTITHROMBINS (SEE TABLE 23.4)

Thrombin, a powerful platelet activator, stabilises a clot by converting fibrinogen to fibrin and is generated by the final pathway of the coagulation cascade, which is itself a crucial and complicated component of thrombosis.

Indirect thrombin inhibitors such as heparin act via antithrombin. Antithrombin neutralises enzymes in the clotting cascade (especially thrombin, factor Xa, and factor IXa) by forming irreversible, non-functioning complexes with thrombin. Inhibition of thrombin and factor Xa by antithrombin alone is relatively slow (minutes) but binding of heparin to antithrombin accelerates the inactivating process by 1000- to 4000-fold. In addition, heparin-induced inactivation of thrombin requires formation of a ternary complex in which heparin binds to both antithrombin and thrombin. This binding occurs with unfractionated heparin and not LMWH because the LMWH molecule is not long enough to bind both antithrombin and thrombin. Thus, LMWHs act mainly via inactivation of Xa. Fibrin-bound thrombin is relatively protected from inactivation by indirect thrombin inhibitors because the binding sites are protected within the clot.

Unfractionated heparin has various limitations, e.g. it binds non-specifically to plasma proteins and endothelial cells, resulting in a variable and unpredictable anticoagulant effect, it cannot inactivate thrombin already bound within clot which continues to activate platelets and the clotting cascade and can paradoxically induce platelet activation, it has a dose-dependent half-life, and patients can develop heparin resistance and form anti-heparin antibodies leading to heparin-induced thrombotic thrombocytopaenia syndrome (HITTS). The direct thrombin inhibitors bind directly to thrombin, do not have the above limitations and may prove more useful, particularly in dealing with ACS, where inactivation of clot-bound thrombin is critical.

The direct thrombin inhibitor bivalirudin is a bivalent, synthetic analog of hirudin (the prototypic direct thrombin inhibitor). It does not activate platelets and has reversible binding to thrombin, whether circulating or clot-bound. It has linear pharmacokinetics intravenously with a half-life of 25 minutes and coagulation times return to normal within 2 hours of cessation of administration. It is degraded by peptidases then cleared by the kidneys and so requires dose adjustment in severe renal impairment. Its activity can be measured by the activated clotting time (ACT).

The REPLACE 2 trial[20] confirmed bivalirudin as an acceptable alternative to heparin in patients with stable coronary artery disease or low-risk ACS undergoing percutaneous coronary intervention (PCI). It found a lower risk of bleeding complications and was as effective as heparin plus a Gp IIb/IIIa inhibitor. Patients in high-risk subgroups showed a trend towards lower mortality at 1 year follow-up.

The ACUITY trial evaluated different regimens of antithrombotic therapy, including bivalirudin alone or plus a GP IIb/IIIa inhibitor vs. heparin plus GP IIb/IIIa inhibition following intervention and treatment for ACS.[21] The conclusions from ACUITY are that bivalirudin is as effective as UFH or enoxaparin plus a GP IIb/IIIa inhibitor in

patients with moderate to high risk ACS undergoing PCI and is associated with a lower risk of bleeding (3% vs. 5.7%, $p < 0.0001$) but did not improve overall clinical outcomes. These results extended to a 1-year follow-up.[22] ACUITY also demonstrated that major bleeding was associated with increased mortality, increased ischaemic events and increased stent thrombosis.[23]

Initial dosage of bivalirudin is 0.75 mg/kg intravenous bolus followed by a 1.75 mg/kg/h infusion up to 4 hours after intervention.

Use of direct thrombin inhibitors was also assessed for ST-Elevation Myocardial Infarction patients in the HORIZONS trial.[24] This study found that bivalirudin therapy is associated with improved net clinical outcomes when compared to heparin plus GP IIb/IIIa inhibition, and this net benefit is explained entirely by a reduction in risk of bleeding complications.

In REPLACE, ACUITY and HORIZONS, GP IIb/IIIa inhibitors were used in 7%–10% of the bivalirudin group if thrombus was seen at PCI or if flow was impaired post-PCI. Current opinion is that bivalirudin does not offer any clinical advantage over heparin.[25]

CONTROL OF BLOOD PRESSURE

Treatment of hypertension (see Table 23.5)

The main pharmacological strategies in the treatment of hypertension involve inhibition of components of the renin-angiotensin-aldosterone system, inhibition of the sympathetic nervous system, inhibition of cardiac and vascular calcium release, enhancement of vasodilation and a decrease in blood volume. Primary hypertension is a chronic condition caused by a generalised increase in peripheral vascular resistance, and it is not uncommon for patients to present for cardiac catheterisation under treatment with a variety of antihypertensive drugs. Secondary hypertension results as a secondary response to a specific condition (e.g. pregnancy, renal disease). Although treatment for hypertension depends on its severity, most antihypertensive drugs act by relaxing arteriolar smooth muscle, by reducing the effect of the sympathetic nervous system on arteriolar smooth muscle (that constricts arterioles), inhibiting humoral pressor hormones and

Table 23.5 Treatment of hypertension (and tachy-arrhythmias)

	Dose	Action	Side effects
ACE Inhibitors (approx 12 on market)			
Captopril	Up to 50 mg pd × 3 for patients within 10 d of AMI	Block ACE in lungs	Cough, can impair renal function
Enalopril	5–20 mg × 1		
Lisinopril	5–20 mg × 1		
Ramipril	5–20 mg × 1		
Angiotensin Receptor Blockers (approx 12 on market)			
Losartan	50 mg pd oral	Rarely used	Angio-oedema, can lower blood pressure
Valsartan	160 mg pd	Blocks angiotensin	
Nitrates			
Isosorbide mononitrate	30–120 g pd oral, or 600 mg iv, or transdermal, or 5 mg sublingual, or 50–100 mcg bolus iv, or 50 mg in 500 mL 5% glucose as variable iv infusion	Vasodilators	Headache Tolerance
Alpha Blockers			
Hydralazine	25–50 bd	Vasodilators	Lupus &1A dose effect
Prazosin	25–50 bd		
Beta Blockers			
Metoprolol (for VT, AF)	40–160 mg bd oral	Cardiac and peripheral action (vasoconstriction)	Asthma
Atenolol (for VT, AF)	25–100 mg pd oral		
Propranolol (for VT, AF)	10–160 mg bd oral		

Abbreviations: AMI, acute myocardial infarction; ACE, angiotensin converting enzyme; BP, blood pressure; VT, ventricular tachycardia; AF, atrial fibrillation.

inflammatory mediators or by acting directly on the brain. Diuretics are also useful as a first-line or adjunctive treatment for hypertension. Although a diverse groups of drugs, antihypertensives act primarily by promoting vasodilation, reducing blood volume, and reducing stroke volume and vascular resistance. This meets the clinical target of primary prevention of the haemodynamic sequela, and also prevents the secondary humoral effects damaging heart muscle, blood vessels, kidney and brain.

The most commonly used drug for treating hypertension during catheterisation is the nitro-vasodilator GTN. GTN is absorbed via mucous membranes so can be administered sublingually in tablet form (anginine) at either 300 mg or 600 mg, or in solution as an intracoronary injection or intravenous infusion, or transdermally as a skin patch. Tridil acts more quickly than anginine and is given as an intra-coronary bolus of 50–100 mcg. In dilating arteries it also reduces blood pressure and can cause headaches. An intracoronary bolus is also useful for evaluating vessel patency immediately post-stenting to eliminate localised spasm that often accompanies coronary artery cannulation and stent deployment. Some centres prefer sodium nitroprusside (nipride), a short-acting calcium channel blocker (see later). In this setting, calcium channel blockers cause arterial dilatation.

Isordil can be given as a substitute if patients cannot tolerate anginine. It is given as a 5 mg tablet sub-lingually. In wards, GTN is generally given as a venous infusion of Tridil in 5% dextrose (10 mL ampoule containing 50 mg GTN in 500 mL glucose 5%). Plastic absorbs GTN, thereby reducing the dosage delivered, so it is packaged with special resistant tubing for direct delivery. Dose rate is variable, the patient is monitored and tubing is changed every 24 hours.

The sedative lorazepam and contrast media also lower blood pressure as a side effect. Blood pressure can also drop during coronary angiography as a result of a catheter blocking blood supply during positioning. Metaraminol (see below) is a useful, short-acting agent that may be used to ameliorate hypertension if severe or symptomatic.

Inhibition of angiotensin II – angiotensin receptor (ACE) inhibitors and angiotensin receptor blockers (ARB)

Many patients routinely present for cardiac catheterisation taking daily doses of ACE inhibitors or ARB, although these drugs are not given during the case. ACE inhibitors and ARBs (AT1 receptor antagonists) are in widespread use for treatment of hypertension and heart failure, following an acute myocardial infarction and for diabetic patients.[26,27] These medications are characterised by protecting the heart, blood vessels and kidney from cardiometabolic damage. As their name suggests, ACE inhibitors and ARBs work via different pathways by blocking the effects of angiotensin, a hormone that causes vascular constriction. The renin-angiotensin-aldosterone system (by which increased renin secretion elevates arterial blood pressure) operates on a number of local systems within individual organs or tissues, including the heart. Simply put, a drop in renal arterial pressure, or a low serum sodium level (hyponatremia), or an increase in sympathetic tone causes release of renin from the renal juxtaglomerular apparatus. Renin splits circulating angiotensinogen to form inactive angiotensin-I, which is converted by angiotensin converting enzyme (ACE) into its active form, angiotensin-II.

Angiotensin-II then binds to the AT1 receptor exerting its cellular effects. Angiotensin-II regulates a number of complex physiological effects, including constriction of vascular smooth muscle and increased myocardial contractility. It also maintains vasoconstriction of the afferent arteriole of the glomerulus, essential in maintaining glomerular filtration pressure.

A major meta-analysis reported that ACE inhibitors and ARBs had similar blood-pressure-dependent effects for risks of stroke, coronary disease and heart failure, while for ACE inhibitors but not ARBs, there was evidence of blood pressure-independent effects on risk of major coronary events.[28] It is possible, however, that ARBs may increase the risk of myocardial infarction[29,30] but their proven benefits override this small risk and both ACE inhibitors and ARBs are commonly used in patients with ischaemic heart disease. Clinically, both drug types lower blood pressure, improve congestive heart failure, inhibit diabetic renal disease and reduce stroke rates. Side effects of ACE inhibitors are angio-oedema, hypotension, coughing and deterioration in renal function (in patients with renal artery stenosis).

Aldosterone secretion by the adrenal cortex is the second major factor in regulating arterial blood pressure. As well as stimulating renin secretion, a marked fall in arterial pressure also causes increased aldosterone secretion, which reduces excretion of salt and water in urine, in turn increasing blood volume and thus returning blood pressure to normal levels.

A raised creatinine level (above 0.12 mmol/L) requires contrast injection to be kept to a minimum. Iodinated contrast media can be nephrotoxic and are recognised as a leading cause of hospital-acquired renal failure.[31]

Treatment of hypotension (see Table 23.6)

The preferred drugs for hypotension in the CCL are the sympathomimetic agents metaraminol and adrenaline (epinephrine). Norpinephrine (noradrenaline) is a neurotransmitter released from the adrenal medulla as a result of sympathetic activation. Adrenergic drugs such as adrenaline thus stimulate sympathetic neuroeffector sites. There are two types of sympathetic adrenergic receptors;

Table 23.6 Treatment of hypotension

	Dose	Action	Side effects
Metaraminol	0.5 mg bolus iv (10 mg lethal)	5–10 minutes Agonist	Arrhythmia (VF)
Adrenaline	0.1 mg bolus iv (never ia), or 0.3 mg sc, or 1 mg in 20 mL N/saline endotracheal, or 1 mg/10 mL Normal saline bolus iv	≤5 minute Agonist, rate-accelerator	Relieves bronchospasm, arterial constriction

Abbreviation: VF, ventricular fibrillation.

alpha and beta, and adrenergic drugs affect both types of receptors. When stimulated, alpha receptors cause excitation, except for the intestinal and central nervous systems, which are relaxed or inhibited by alpha receptor activity. Conversely, beta receptors cause relaxation or inhibition, except for the heart, which is stimulated by beta receptor activity. As alpha sympathetic receptors occur in peripheral vasculature, stimulation leads to peripheral vasoconstriction. Beta receptors occur in smooth muscle cells of the respiratory passage and in cardiac muscle cells. Stimulation of these receptors results in increased heart rate and contractility and dilatation of respiratory airways.

Acetylcholine is the neurotransmitter for motor (somatic) neurones, as well as for parasympathetic and sympathetic responses, but not for those sites stimulated by norepinephrine.

Metaraminol is an alpha-adrenergic agonist, meaning it stimulates alpha receptors, causing widespread vasoconstriction and a corresponding increase in blood pressure. As cerebral and coronary arteries have few alpha receptors, blood pressure is elevated without compromising cardiac or cerebral blood flow. It is packaged as 10 mg ampoules and is routinely given as 0.5 mg intravenous boluses and has a half-life of 5–10 minutes. Excessive doses can lead to ventricular fibrillation. A dose of 10 mg is lethal.

Adrenaline stimulates both alpha and beta receptors (see below), causing an increase primarily in systolic rather than diastolic blood pressure. It can be administered either as a bolus or an intravenous infusion depending on the desired effect, which can be complex. It is generally

administered in dosages of 0.1 mg intravenously, or 0.3 mg subcutaneously for hypotension. It is packaged in pre-loaded syringes for use in cardiac arrest, when it is given as a bolus dose of 1 mg/10 mL. Administration via an endotracheal tube is possible if intravenous access cannot be obtained (1 mg adrenaline in 20 mL Normal saline). Its predominant effect is to increase heart rate and contractility of the heart, resulting in an increase in blood pressure. It also acts on beta receptors in the lungs, meaning it can relieve bronchospasm and is therefore used to treat anaphylactic shock. It should never be given intra-arterially, as it causes arterial constriction and can result in limb ischaemia and subsequent amputation. It has a half-life of 5 minutes or less.

Calcium channel blockers and β- and α-adrenoceptor antagonists (see below) are also widely used for both hypertension and arrhythmia.

TREATMENT OF ARRHYTHMIA

Bradycardia and tachycardia are potential arrhythmic presentations in the CCL. Specific treatment depends on the individual presentation and cause of the arrhythmia. For bradycardias, which have the dual undesired effect of lowered blood pressure along with reduced heart rate, the force-increasing (inotropic) and/or rate-increasing (chronotropic) catecholamines and other sympathomimetic agents such as adrenaline or metaraminol are used to enhance rapid recovery of cardiac performance. Treatment of tachycardias is equally complex depending on their underlying pathology and causative factors and may include defibrillation. Associated with the effects of many of these drug types are secondary effects on either lowering or increasing blood pressure, which can be desirable or undesirable depending on circumstances. Hence, many drugs used to treat blood pressure are also used to regulate arrhythmias and are often used in combination.

Historically, antiarrhythmic drugs were classified into four main categories according to their mode of action (the Vaughan and Williams system) and are called Class I, Class II, Class III and Class IV and Class V, depending on their effects on different phases of the action potential (see Table 23.7). Class I drugs can be toxic and act by blocking the fast sodium current during phase 0, and are further classified into three sub-categories called IA (quinidine, procainamide, disopyramide), IB (lignocaine, mexiletine, tocainide), and IC (flecainide, encainide). Class II drugs generally refer to beta-blockers and include the generally safe sympathomimetic agents; they inhibit cardiac adrenergic stimulation. Class III drugs (amiodarone and sotalol) lengthen duration of phase 3 of the action potential. Class IV drugs are the calcium antagonists verapamil and ditiazem that inhibit the slow calcium channel during phase 2. Not all of these drugs are used in the CCL, and not all antiarrhythmics fit this classification system (e.g. digoxin, atropine, noradrenaline). Hence the need for a fifth class, Class V, that includes antiarrhythmics with an unknown mechanism of action. Atropine and adrenaline are discussed above and can be selectively given with other drugs to regulate heart rhythm along with rate (Table 23.8).

Digoxin is a cardiac glycoside used to treat rapid atrial fibrillation. The first dose given is 500 mcg orally or intravenously, then 250 mcg 4 hours later. Digoxin reduces heart rate by targeting the atrioventricular pacemaker, the AV node. It is considered a dangerous drug, particularly with heart failure patients, and amiodarone, flecainide or sotalol are usually preferred as frontline therapy for atrial fibrillation.

Lignocaine has been used routinely for ventricular tachycardia but is now being supplanted by sotalol and amiodarone. Standard dose is 100 mg intravenously and can be given as a continuous infusion. Side effects are confusion, seizures or coma, usually from infusion rather than a single dose.

Sotalol is a Class III agent as well as a beta blocker. It is used primarily for ventricular tachycardia or atrial fibrillation and can be given intravenously or per os. Standard dose is 80–160 mg. It causes a drop in blood pressure and reduces heart rate, hence is useful as a prophylactic agent for patients at risk of ventricular tachycardia.

Amiodarone is the most-used Class III agent and is a very useful antiarrhythmic, particularly for ventricular tachycardia. During catheterisation it is given for ventricular arrhythmias or atrial fibrillation. Intravenous dosage is 150–300 mg over one minute. It is also available as a 200 mg tablet for oral administration. Amiodarone is

Table 23.7 Classification of antiarrhythmic drugs

	Drugs	Action
Class I	IA: Quinidine, procainamide disopyramide	Block fast sodium current, lengthen action potential duration
	IB: Lignocaine, tocainide, mexiletine	Block fast sodium current, shorten action potential duration
	IC: Flecainide, encainide	Block fast sodium current, no effect on action potential duration
Class II	Beta blockers (metoprolol, atenolol)	Block effects of catecholamines
Class III	Potassium channel blockers (amiodarone, sotalol)	Lengthen action potential duration
Class IV	Verapamil, diltiazem	Calcium antagonists
Class V	Adenosine, digoxin	Mechanism unknown

Table 23.8 Treatment of tachy-arrhythmias

Atrial fibrillation		
Initial dose	**Action**	**Side effects**
Digoxin 500 g oral, iv + 250 mcg 4 hours later	AV nodal blockade	Cardiac and cerebral toxicity, GI effects
Sotalol 80–160 mg iv, oral	For AF, VT	Hypotension
Flecainide 1 mg/kg/min iv		Avoid in LV dysfunction or BBB
Amiodarone 150–300 mg/min Iv; oral 200 for 2/52	Rate reducing, reversal of atrial flutter, AF/VT	Hypotension, Bradycardia. If iv: Phlebitis, thyroid/lung/skin/liver problems
Maintenance Dose		
Sotalol 40–160 bd		
Flecainide 25–100 bd	Slows conduction (class IA)	May slow atrial rate and organise to 1:1 flutter; should not be used in LV systolic dysfunction
Amiodarone 200 mg pd		
Atrial Flutter		
Digoxin 500 g oral, iv + 500 mcg 4 hours later	AV nodal blockade	
Amiodarone 150–300 mg/min iv, oral	AV nodal blockade	Hypotension, bradycardia
Ventricular tachycardia (in setting of AMI +/− DC cardioversion)		
Lignocaine 100 mg iv mg/kg	Class IA. For ischaemic VT	Confusion, coma, seizures, bradycardia
Sotalol 80–160 mg iv, oral	Class III. For acute reversal of AF/VT	Hypotension
Amiodarone 150–300 mg/min iv, oral	Mixed Class III & β-blocker, rate reduction, reversal of AF/VT	Hypotension, bradycardia
Adenosine 6–24 mg iv stat	AV node blocker, reversal of SVT	Sense of 'impending death', Ventricular arrhythmia

Abbreviations: AV, atrioventricular; AF, atrial fibrillation, VT, ventricular tachycardia; GI, gastro-intestinal; BBB, bundle branch block; SVT, supraventricular tachycardia.

now preferred over lignocaine. Cardiovascular side effects are hypotension and bradycardia with known additional toxicities, and initial dose is only administered under hospital supervision.

Cardiovascular tissues contain alpha-1 receptors and two types of beta receptors, called beta 1 (β1) and beta 2 (β2). Alpha and beta receptors are found mainly in myocardium and vascular smooth muscle cells. Alpha receptor activation causes a small increase in myocardial contraction, and vasoconstriction in vascular walls. Beta receptor activation induces increased myocardial contractility and vasodilatation (with a decrease in blood pressure) in vessel walls. β1 receptors are found mainly in the lungs, heart and blood vessels. β2 receptors are found in the lungs. Activation of β2 lung receptors by drugs such as salbutamol (Ventolin) dilates pulmonary airways. Beta blockers, as implied by name, do the opposite, causing airway constriction by inhibiting beta receptor activity (Table 23.9).

Table 23.9 Treatment of other arrhythmias

	Dose	Action	Side effects
Beta Blockers			
Sotalol (for VT, AF)	40–160 mg bd oral	Negative inotropy	Hypotension
Metoprolol (for VT, AF)	25–100 mg bd oral		
Atenolol (for VT, AF)	25–50 mg pd oral		
Ca Channel Blockers			
Verapamil	5–10 mg iv, or oral for long-term treatment	AV node slowing, reversal of SVT	Decreases AV-node conduction; dangerous with beta-blockers and LV dysfunction
Diltiazem	Oral, no iv	For long-term use	
Anti-brady-arrhythmics			
Atropine	600 mcg bolus iv, ia	For brady-arrhythmias only	Mouth dryness
Noradrenaline	Weight-dependent iv	Sympatho-mimetic	Mouth dryness

Abbreviations: VT, ventricular tachycardia; AF, atrial fibrillation; AV, atrioventricular; LV, left ventricle.

Alpha blockers: These are alpha-adrenergic antagonists (e.g. Prazosin, used for hypertension), and have limited application in cardiology. Most of these drug types affect the sympathetic system to cause vasodilatation with a drop in blood pressure, but this is counteracted by baroreceptor reflexes that result in increased heart rate and cardiac output. They also have been found to increase the risk of heart attack in some situations, when used unopposed.

Phentolamine is a calcium channel blocker that causes arterial dilatation with an associated drop in blood pressure but is now rarely used.

Beta blockers: All beta-adrenergic blocking agents are structurally similar to catecholamines and inhibit beta receptors, resulting in a decrease in heart rate and myocardial contractility, hence reducing stroke volume, oxygen demand and relieving myocardial ischaemia. Stimulating beta receptors causes an increase in heart rate, blood pressure and cardiac output. Beta blockers are useful for treating angina, arrhythmia and hypertension, but should be prescribed with caution to people with diabetes, asthma and chronic obstructive lung disease. Beta blockers

are indicated in patients with systolic heart failure in patients who do not have a contraindication (systolic hypertension, advanced heart block or bradycardia, cardiogenic shock, fluid overload, bronchospasm). **Carvedilol**, **sotalol** and **metoprolol** are the most well-known beta blockers currently in use.

Carvedilol acts as a non-selective vasodilating beta blocker, an alpha1 blocker and has antioxidant properties. This combination is considered beneficial in assisting the failing heart, so carvedilol is gaining increasing favour for long-term treatment of heart failure, although it is not generally used in the catheterisation setting. **Sotalol** is a non-selective beta-blocker that antagonises both β1 and β2 beta-adrenergic effects.

Cardioselective β1 blockers (e.g. **metoprolol, atenolol**) that act specifically on β1 receptors are available. Metoprolol is a selective beta blocker that stimulates cardiac contraction and reduces heart rate and blood pressure. Hence it is useful as a rate control agent in patients with atrial fibrillation and heart disease. A potential unwanted side effect is hypotension.

Calcium channel blockers: Calcium channel blockers have been in use for treating hypertension for several decades. These drugs work by blocking the effects of calcium in initiating myocardial activation and reducing vascular tone. **Verapamil** is a calcium channel blocker that reduces heart rate by slowing atrio-ventricular node conduction and reduces blood pressure by arterial dilatation. It is thus used for hypertension and to treat fast rhythms such as supraventricular tachycardia or atrial fibrillation, or to relieve spasm of the brachial or radial artery (nitrates are not as effective at dilating peripheral arteries). It is also used as an infusion in combination with heparin and nitrates to prevent spasm during coronary rotational atherectomy.

Usual dose is 5–10 mg intravenously over 5–10 minutes and can be given orally for long-term therapy. Combination therapy with beta-blockers can be potentially dangerous as the combination can induce profound bradycardia and heart block. **Diltiazem** has similar rate controlling effects. Dihydropyridine calcium channel blockers such as **amlodipine** and **felodipine** do not slow ventricular rate and can be used in combination with beta blockers, but should not be used unopposed in patients with ischaemic heart disease, as they may induce ischaemia due to tachycardia.

Atropine is the main agent used to treat bradycardia. Atropine is an anticholinergic, meaning it blocks the acetylcholine receptor site, preventing acetylcholine from transmitting parasympathetic nerve impulses across the postganglionic nerve terminal to the effector organ. It is usually given for bradycardia rather than just hypotension, although it does have some effect on increasing blood pressure. Atropine is also a sympatholytic agent and acts by blocking the vagus nerve response that slows the sinus and atrioventricular nodes, thus causing an increase in both heart rate and the speed of conduction along the atrioventricular

pathway. It is available in 600 μg ampoules and can be administered at this dose intravenously or intra-arterially. A side effect can be dryness of the mouth.

PREMEDICATION AND SEDATION (SEE TABLE 23.10)

Routine premedication prior to transfer to the CCL includes administration of antihistamines such as **loratadine** and a sedative such as **lorazepam**. If necessary, this can be supplemented by additional sedation with **midazolam**, which is a short-acting and shorter-lasting sedative.

Loratadine can be given to patients orally before angiography as a 10 mg tablet to reduce risk of contrast allergy. **Lorazepam** is given sublingually as a 1 mg tablet. It induces drowsiness and reduces heart rate and blood pressure. **Diazepam**, a different sedative, is available as 10 mg ampoules and can be given as an injection. **Midazolam**, also a sedative and similar to diazepam, can be given as a 1 mg intravenous injection prior to angiography. It is relatively short-acting, usually lasting less than 1 hour, and can be continued for up to 4 hours. It causes anterograde amnesia and keeps patients sleepy and contented, a boon to any invasive cardiologist. Side effects are hypotension and hypoventilation, so oxygen saturation should be monitored.

OTHER CONDITIONS (SEE TABLE 23.11)

Treatment of nausea

Metoclopramide (Maxolon) is an antiemetic and is the drug of choice for treating nausea during catheterisation. This compound is an antagonist

Table 23.10 Premedication and sedation (benzodiazepines)

	Dose	Action	Side effects
Loratadine	10 mg oral	Antihistamine	Drowsiness, headache
Lorazepam	1 mg sublingual	Sedative Intermediate-acting	Drowsiness, bradycardia, hypotension
Diazepam (valium)	10 mg iv, oral	Sedative Long-acting	Drowsiness, dizziness
Midazolam	1 mg iv	Sedative Short-acting	Hypotension, hypoventilation

Table 23.11 Treatment of other conditions

	Dose	Action	Side effects
Nausea			
Metoclopramide	10 mg iv or oral	Anti-emetic	Nil
Antibiotics			
Cephazolin	1 g iv	Antibiotic	Cross-reaction
Cephalexin	500 mg oral 4× daily		with penicillin, allergy
Contrast Reaction			
Hydrocortisone	10 mg iv	Fast-acting, short-lasting	Nil
Prednisone	Oral, weight adjusted dose	Pre-conditioning	Nil
Drug Challenge			
Ergotamine	500 mcg/5 mL Normal saline for 100 mcg/mL solution; 50 mcg+100 mcg at 1 minute interval up to 500 mcg		Headache, numbness, brady- or tachycardia
Adenosine	20–30 mcg in RCA, 30–40 mcg in LCA, or 5 mcg in 500 mL Normal saline for 5000 mcg in 500 mL solution (i.e. 10 mg/mL)	Vasodilator, immediate and short-acting	Harmless angina-like symptoms, bronchoconstriction, hypotension, dyspnoea, headache
Isoprenaline	1–3 mcg iv in 1 mcg/mL	Chronotrope	

Abbreviations: RCA, right coronary artery; LCA, left coronary artery.

of brain dopamine (D2) receptors and serotonin (5-HT) receptors at higher doses. Nausea, sweatiness and vomiting are generally caused by a vaso-vagal reaction. Dosage is normally 10 mg, administered either by intravenous or intramuscular injection. The drug takes effect within minutes and lasts 1–2 hours.

Antibiotics

Cephazolin and **cephalexin, both cephalosporins** (broad spectrum bactericidal agents that inhibit bacterial cell wall synthesis), are currently the preferred antibiotic for prophylactic treatment following potential contamination of the groin puncture site, or after insertion of a transcutaneous closure device such as Angioseal™ or Perclose™, or after implantation of septal occluder devices. Usual dosage is 1 mg intravenously. It should be noted that cephalosporins have a known cross-reactivity with penicillin allergy. **Ampicillin**, **flucoxicillin** and penicillin are only rarely used. **Gentamicin** (240 mg intravenously) in combination with **cephazolin** (1 g

intravenously) can also be used for Gram negative organisms, but because of its potential renal toxicity and more rare ototoxicity (causing deafness) it is used only rarely.

Contrast media and acetylcysteine

Contrast media can be toxic to a patient, mainly due to the effects of direct chemical toxicity, and to hyperosmolality.[31] The water-soluble, non-ionic (and hence uncharged), low-osmolar agents currently in use are generally safe and enjoy widespread application. All contrast media can impair kidney function, but contrast-media induced nephrotoxicity is usually reversible. Patients presenting with renal failure or a raised creatinine level are routinely assessed for their suitability for coronary angiography. Diabetic patients are usually prehydrated, contrast is used in diluted form and injections are minimised. It has also been reported that hydration with sodium bicarbonate before contrast exposure is more effective than hydration with sodium chloride for prophylaxis of contrast-induced renal failure.[32]

Hydrocortisone

True hypersensitivity to modern contrast agents is rare. Reactions can vary from an itch or rash to anaphylactic shock. If a patient has a history of contrast allergy, a common pretreatment regimen includes hydrocortisone, promethazine, loratidine, or ranitidine. In patients with a history of severe allergy, corticosteroid administration should commence 24–48 hours pre-procedure. Adrenaline should be ready for use if required during the procedure.

Ergometrine is a vasoconstrictor previously used during coronary angiography to diagnose coronary artery spasm and confirm the absence of coronary artery disease in angiographically normal patients. It was used particularly in symptomatic young patients to exclude coronary disease. A 500 mcg vial is diluted in 5 mL normal saline to give a 100 mcg/mL solution. Increasing doses commencing with 50 mcg (0.5 mL) are given as a first dose followed by 100 mcg doses at 1 minute intervals, up to 500 mcg, noting ST segment inversions and/or haemodynamic changes until either a positive or negative response is confirmed. A negative response indicates absence of disease. A positive response induces localised spasm with corresponding angina. Ergometrine challenge is no longer practiced.

Adenosine is a vasodilator and atrio-ventricular node blocker. The effect is immediate and short-acting. It is used to improve distal coronary circulation in the event of poor reflow following intervention. A dose of 24 mcg is appropriate in this situation, although 20–30 mcg in the right coronary and 30–40 mcg in the left coronary is safely tolerated in most patients. One ampoule contains 2 mL (6 mg) of drug. From this, 1.7 mL (5 mg) is added to 500 mL saline to give a solution of 5000 mcg in 500 mL, i.e. 10 mcg/mL. It is also used during a pressure wire study to quantify fractional flow reserve in diseased coronary arteries, where it is preferable to administer by intravenous infusion at a dose of 140 mcg/kg/min via a femoral line. Adenosine is supplied as 6 mg/2 mL vials and is diluted to a total of 50 mL saline. Infusion rate is set at 750 mL/h via minimal volume tubing. Intracoronary nitrate should be administered before commencing infusion to prevent vasospasm. Major side effects include bronchoconstriction and should be avoided in asthmatics. Other side effects include chest tightness, dyspnoea, headache and hypotension. It is often associated with angina-like symptom, but this is harmless if patients are warned, and does not indicate ischaemia.

Dopamine (the metabolic precursor of noradrenaline and adrenaline) has a complex dose-related effect on the cardiovascular, renal, mesenteric and nervous systems, and is not commonly used in the CCL. **Dobutamine,** structurally similar to dopamine, is used to induce pharmacological stress exercise in patients during myocardial stress imaging. It acts on both alpha and beta adrenergic receptors, causing a sinus tachycardia and increasing myocardial oxygen demand.

Isoprenaline is a chronotrope used for diagnosis of hypertrophic obstructive cardiomyopathy (HOCM). HOCM is a disease that causes ventricular hypertrophy, particularly the interventricular septum, resulting in a left ventricular cavity of reduced volume and compliance. The thickened septum may obstruct the outflow tract during systole, causing a drop in aortic pressure and a corresponding rise in ventricular pressure. The hypertrophy may cause obstruction with a pressure gradient even at rest and is especially pronounced after an ectopic beat with a longer filling time. It is important to distinguish between obstructive and non-obstructive disease. Isoprenaline increases heart rate and may increase the amount of obstruction. The drug is diluted to a 1 mcg/mL solution and is usually given as 1–3 mcg injections until a positive or negative result is determined from intracardiac pressure recordings.

SUMMARY

The preceding is in essence a summary of cardiac drugs that are or have been in common use in the CCL, and a summary of these is effectively contained in the introduction. A working knowledge of the many categories and sub-categories of these drugs, together with their application and dosage is invaluable for all staff in the CCL.

REFERENCES

1. Campbell C, Steinhubl S. The irony of chronic aspirin therapy: Fewer events, worse outcomes? *Acute Cor Syndromes.* 2002;5(1):2–9.
2. Gurbel PA, Bliden KP, Zaman KA, Yoho JA, Hayes KM, Tantry US. Clopidogrel loading with eptifibatide to arrest the reactivity

of platelets: Results of the Clopidogrel Loading With Eptifibatide to Arrest the Reactivity of Platelets (CLEAR PLATELETS) study. *Circulation*. 2005;111(9):1153–1159.

3. Investigators CiUAtPRET. Effects of clopidogrel in addition to aspirin in patients with acute coronary syndromes without ST-segment elevation. *N Engl J Med*. 2001;345(7):494–502.

4. Mauri L, Kereiakes DJ, Yeh RW, Driscoll-Shempp P, Cutlip DE, Steg PG, et al. Twelve or 30 months of dual antiplatelet therapy after drug-eluting stents. *N Engl J Med*. 2014;371(23):2155–2166.

5. Wiviott SD, Trenk D, Frelinger AL, O'Donoghue M, Neumann F-J, Michelson AD, et al. Prasugrel compared with high loading-and maintenance-dose clopidogrel in patients with planned percutaneous coronary intervention: The prasugrel in comparison to clopidogrel for inhibition of platelet activation and aggregation–Thrombolysis In Myocardial Infarction 44 trial. *Circulation*. 2007;116(25):2923–2932.

6. Wiviott SD, Braunwald E, McCabe CH, Montalescot G, Ruzyllo W, Gottlieb S, et al. Prasugrel versus clopidogrel in patients with acute coronary syndromes. *N Engl J Med*. 2007;357(20):2001–2015.

7. Murphy SA, Antman EM, Wiviott SD, Weerakkody G, Morocutti G, Huber K, et al. Reduction in recurrent cardiovascular events with prasugrel compared with clopidogrel in patients with acute coronary syndromes from the TRITON-TIMI 38 trial. *Eur Heart J*. 2008;29(20):2473–2479.

8. Wallentin L, Becker RC, Budaj A, Cannon CP, Emanuelsson H, Held C, et al. Ticagrelor versus clopidogrel in patients with acute coronary syndromes. *N Engl J Med*. 2009;361(11):1045–1057.

9. Boersma E, Harrington RA, Moliterno DJ, White H, Théroux P, Van de Werf F, et al. Platelet glycoprotein IIb/IIIa inhibitors in acute coronary syndromes: A meta-analysis of all major randomised clinical trials. *Lancet*. 2002;359(9302):189–198.

10. Kastrati A, Mehilli J, Schühlen H, Dirschinger J, Dotzer F, ten Berg JM, et al. A clinical trial of abciximab in elective percutaneous coronary intervention after pretreatment with clopidogrel. *N Engl J Med*. 2004;350(3):232–238.

11. Valgimigli M, Percoco G, Barbieri D, Ferrari F, Guardigli G, Parrinello G, et al. The additive value of tirofiban administered with the high-dose bolus in the prevention of ischemic complications during high-risk coronary angioplasty: The ADVANCE Trial. *J Am Coll Cardiol*. 2004;44(1):14–19.

12. Shen J, Zhang Q, Zhang RY, Zhang JS, Hu J, Yang Z-k, et al. Clinical benefits of adjunctive tirofiban therapy in patients with acute ST-segment elevation myocardial infarction undergoing primary percutaneous coronary intervention. *Coron Artery Dis*. 2008;19(4):271–277.

13. Vainer J, Fleisch M, Gunnes P, Ramamurthy S, Garachemani A, Kaufmann UP, et al. Low-dose heparin for routine coronary angioplasty and stenting. *Am J Cardiol*. 996;78(8):964–966.

14. Boneu B. Low molecular weight heparins: Are they superior to unfractionated heparins to prevent and to treat deep vein thrombosis? *Thromb Res*. 2000;100(2):113–120.

15. Hirsh J, O'Donnell M, Eikelboom JW. Beyond unfractionated heparin and warfarin: Current and future advances. *Circulation*. 2007;116(5):552–560.

16. Goldman LE, Eisenberg MJ. Identification and management of patients with failed thrombolysis after acute myocardial infarction. *Ann Intern Med*. 2000;132(7):556–565.

17. Topol EJ, Ohman EM, Armstrong PW, Wilcox R, Skene AM, Aylward P, et al. Survival outcomes 1 year after reperfusion therapy with either alteplase or reteplase for acute myocardial infarction: Results from the Global Utilization of Streptokinase and t-PA for Occluded Coronary Arteries (GUSTO) III Trial. *Circulation*. 2000;102(15):1761–1765.

18. Investigators GV. Reperfusion therapy for acute myocardial infarction with fibrinolytic therapy or combination reduced fibrinolytic therapy and platelet glycoprotein IIb/IIIa inhibition: The GUSTO V randomised trial. *Lancet*. 2001;357(9272):1905–1914.

19. Aversano T, Aversano LT, Passamani E, Knatterud GL, Terrin ML, Williams DO, et al. Thrombolytic therapy vs primary percutaneous coronary intervention for myocardial infarction in patients presenting to hospitals without on-site cardiac surgery: A randomized controlled trial. *JAMA*. 2002;287(15):1943–1951.

20. Lincoff AM, Bittl JA, Harrington RA, Feit F, Kleiman NS, Jackman JD, et al. Bivalirudin and provisional glycoprotein IIb/IIIa blockade compared with heparin and planned glycoprotein IIb/IIIa blockade during percutaneous coronary intervention: REPLACE-2 randomized trial. *JAMA*. 2003;289(7):853–863.

21. Stone GW, McLaurin BT, Cox DA, Bertrand ME, Lincoff AM, Moses JW, et al. Bivalirudin for patients with acute coronary syndromes. *N Engl J Med*. 2006;355(21):2203–2216.

22. White HD, Ohman EM, Lincoff AM, Bertrand ME, Colombo A, McLaurin BT, et al. Safety and efficacy of bivalirudin with and without glycoprotein IIb/IIIa inhibitors in patients with acute coronary syndromes undergoing percutaneous coronary intervention: 1-year results from the ACUITY (Acute Catheterization and Urgent Intervention Triage strategY) trial. *J Am Coll Cardiol*. 2008;52(10):807–814.

23. Manoukian SV, Feit F, Mehran R, Voeltz MD, Ebrahimi R, Hamon M, et al. Impact of major bleeding on 30-day mortality and clinical outcomes in patients with acute coronary syndromes: An analysis from the ACUITY Trial. *J Am Coll Cardiol*. 2007;49(12):1362–1368.

24. Mehran R, Lansky AJ, Witzenbichler B, Guagliumi G, Peruga JZ, Brodie BR, et al. Bivalirudin in patients undergoing primary angioplasty for acute myocardial infarction (HORIZONS-AMI): 1-year results of a randomised controlled trial. *Lancet*. 2009;374(9696):1149–1159.

25. Constantinos A, Maniotis C, Koutouzis M The rise and fall of anticoagulation with bivalirudin during percutaneous coronary intervention: A review article. *Cardiol Ther*. 2017. doi: 10.1007/s40119-017-0082-x.

26. McMurray J, Cohen-Solal A, Dietz R, Eichhorn E, Erhardt L, Hobbs F, et al. Practical recommendations for the use of ACE inhibitors, beta-blockers, aldosterone antagonists and angiotensin receptor blockers in heart failure: Putting guidelines into practice. *Eur J Heart Fail*. 2005;7(5):710–721.

27. Lowy AJ, Howes LG. ACE inhibitors and angiotensin receptor blockers in type 2 diabetes. *Curr Ther*. 2002;43(5):47.

28. Turnbull F, Neal B, Pfeffer M, Kostis J, Algert C, Woodward M. Blood Pressure Lowering Treatment Trialists' Collaboration. Blood pressure dependent and independent effects of agents that inhibit the renin-angiotensin system. *J Hypertens*. 2007;25(5):951–958.

29. Strauss MH, Hall A. Do angiotensin receptor blockers increase the risk of myocardial infarction?: Angiotensin Receptor Blockers May increase risk of Myocardial Infarction: Unraveling the ARB-MI Paradox. *Circulation*. 2006;114:838–854.

30. Graber MA, Dachs R, Darby-Stewart A. The "ARB-MI paradox": Real or a fluke? *Am Fam Physician*. 2012;86(2):136–141.

31. Bartorelli AL, Marenzi G. Contrast-induced nephropathy. *J Interv Cardiol*. 2008;21(1):74–85.

32. Vasheghani-Farahani A, Sadigh G, Kassaian SE, Khatami SM, Fotouhi A, Razavi SA, et al. Sodium bicarbonate plus isotonic saline versus saline for prevention of contrast-induced nephropathy in patients undergoing coronary angiography: A randomized controlled trial. *Am J Kidney Dis*. 2009;54(4):610–618.

24

Antiplatelet therapy in interventional cardiology

CHRISTOPHER YU AND HARRY C. LOWE

'The patient is given aspirin (1.0 g per day) for three days, starting the day before the procedure. Heparin and low molecular weight dextran are administered during dilatation; warfarin is started after the procedure and is continued until the follow-up study six to nine months later.'

Andreas R Gruntzig, 12th July, 1979.[1]

INTRODUCTION

Ischaemic heart disease is the leading cause of death in Australia, accounting for 12% of all deaths in Australia in 2016.[2] The use of therapeutic coronary intervention is the gold standard in treating culprit lesions in acute coronary syndrome, as per American (American College of Cardiology, AAC, and American Heart Association, AHA, and European (European Society of Cardiology, ESC) guidelines.[3-6] Despite improvements in coronary stent technology, antiplatelet therapy continues to have an important role in reducing post-interventional thrombosis.

RATIONALE FOR DRUG USE IN CORONARY INTERVENTION

Coronary balloon angioplasty, by its very nature, causes atherosclerotic plaque rupture, exposure of the subendothelium to flowing blood, platelet adherence and aggregation, thrombin formation and the generation of fibrin. The coronary stent adds a potent thrombogenic stimulus to this already prothrombotic environment.[7] For this reason, despite recent advances in coronary stenting, antiplatelet therapy is important to mitigate this inherent tendency to thrombosis.

Cyclo-oxygenase (COX) inhibitors (Aspirin)

Aspirin was first tested clinically for a variety of rheumatic conditions in 1899, and its use in cardiovascular disease was first described over 40 years ago, demonstrating a protective effect in acute myocardial infarction (MI)[8] that was later found to be due to an inhibitory effect on platelets.[9] Aspirin inhibits platelet thromboxane A2 and prostaglandin I2 synthesis by the irreversible acetylation of COX-1.[10] This occurs rapidly, within approximately 30 minutes, and lasts for the lifetime of the platelet, around 10 days. The effect is dose-dependent from 5 mg to 100 mg, with 100 mg causing almost complete inhibition of thromboxane A2.[10] Aspirin has a number of disadvantages, however. It is a relatively weak antiplatelet agent; it has no effect on thromboxane A2 independent pathways; it does not alter platelet adhesion or secretion and its effects are variable between individuals. Aspirin causes a dose-dependent risk of major upper gastrointestinal tract bleeding of up to three-fold in doses up to 325 mg.[11] The risk is not eliminated by doses less than 100 mg or by coated formulations, and is increased further in doses greater than 325 mg.[10,11] Aspirin also causes dose-dependent increases in nausea, epigastric pain and intracranial haemorrhage, and a non dose-dependent increase in constipation.[10]

ADP receptor/P2Y12 inhibitors

THIENOPYRIDINE DERIVATIVES (CLOPIDOGREL, PRASUGREL AND TICLOPIDINE)

This class of antiplatelet agents target adenosine diphosphate (ADP) 2 receptors on the surface of platelets. Ticlopidine was the first drug in this class; however, significant side effects, albeit at low rates (neutropenia and thrombotic thrombocytopenic purpura) compared to clopidogrel, contributed to cessation of its widespread use.[12]

These drugs are inactive in vitro, but active orally following hepatic metabolism via cytochrome P450 (CYP) isoforms to one or more metabolically active forms, making them indirectly-acting platelet inhibitors. The active metabolites covalently and irreversibly bind to the P2Y12 receptor for the remaining lifespan of the platelet.[13] Excretion is principally renal.[14,15] Like aspirin, these drugs provide irreversible platelet inhibition that persists after ceasing therapy. The effect is present for 7–10 days, equivalent to the lifespan of the platelet.[16]

Inhibition is dose-dependent; 20%–30% platelet inhibition is achieved in 2–3 days of treatment with 500 mg/day ticlopidine or 75 mg/day clopidogrel.[17,18] The reason for this delay in effect is not known. Furthermore, studies have shown up to nearly a third of patients are non-responders to clopidogrel, giving rise to the term clopidogrel resistance.[19] This is due to the reduced-function allele of CYP 2C19.[20] Prasugrel has demonstrated a more rapid onset of action in preclinical studies and greater platelet inhibition in phase 1 studies when compared to clopidogrel.[21–23] In addition, there is evidence that thienopyridine resistance may be less frequent post-loading doses of prasugrel compared with clopidogrel.[19] Subsequently, these attributes stimulated the Trial to Assess Improvement in Therapeutic Outcomes by Optimizing Platelet Inhibition with Prasugrel–Thrombolysis in Myocardial Infarction (TRITON–TIMI) 38 study.[24]

Clopidogrel and prasugrel share a number of side effects. In general, however, side effects occur less frequently with clopidogrel therapy, such that its side effect profile is similar to that of aspirin.[17] Neutropenia is uncommon with clopidogrel. In a trial of 19,185 patients given either clopidogrel or aspirin chronically, severe neutropenia occurred in 0.1%, which did not differ significantly from aspirin (0.17%).[25] Other side effects shared by the two agents are gastrointestinal (diarrhoea, nausea and dyspepsia) and dermatologic (rash, urticaria).[26]

The main concern with prasugrel is increased bleeding. In the TRITON-TIMI 38 trial, TIMI-major haemorrhage (not related to coronary artery bypass) occurred in 2.4% (prasugrel group) vs. 1.8% (clopidogrel group) with a hazard ratio, 1.32; 95% CI, 1.03 to 1.68; $P = 0.03$.[24] The bleeding risk of prasugrel was also increased when bleeds were categorised into fatal and non-fatal.[24] Data from TRITON-TIMI 38 has led to the American Geriatric Society (AGS) including prasugrel in the 2015, Beers Criteria, a list of potentially inappropriate medications to be avoided in older adults.[27] The AGS have advised caution in using prasugrel in adults ≥75 years old given the smaller relative reduction in primary efficacy events, coupled with higher absolute TIMI major bleeding rates.[24, 27] Additional patients with a known history of stroke or transient ischemic attack before enrolment in TRITON–TIMI 38 had an increase in stroke and higher rate of bleeding, in particular intracranial haemorrhage.[24] Patients with low body weight (<60 kg) also have higher rates of bleeding.[24] The most frequent side effects of prasugrel include: hypertension (7.5%), hyperlipidaemia (7%), headache (5.5%), back pain (5%), dyspnea (4.9%) and nausea (4.6%). Post-marking there have been reports of thrombotic thrombocytopenic purpura and hypersensitivity reactions including anaphylaxis.

NON-THIENOPYRIDINE P2Y12 RECEPTOR ANTAGONISTS (TICAGRELOR, CANGRELOR)

This class of anti-platelet drugs consists of the direct-acting and reversible antagonists of the adenosine diphosphate receptor P2Y12. The ability to work without metabolic activation allows faster platelet inhibition, and this is one of the advantages of these antiplatelet drugs.

Ticagrelor, an oral agent, provides faster and greater P2Y12 inhibition than clopidogrel.[28,29] Furthermore, ticagrelor can overcome the issues related to clopidogrel resistance.[30] Concentrations of ticagrelor increase in plasma in a dose-dependent manner.[29] Despite ticagrelor not requiring activation, it undergoes hepatic metabolism via CYP3A4 and CYP3A5 forming an active metabolite AR-C124910XX.[31] Maximum plasma concentrations and maximum platelet inhibition are reached 1–3 hours after treatment. The plasma half-life is 6–13 hours and, accordingly, the treatment requires twice daily administration.[13] Subsequently, ticagrelor can be ceased three days prior to non-acute surgery.[31]

Cangrelor is an intravenous agent that reaches steady-state concentrations in plasma within 30 minutes from start of infusion.[13] Cangrelor is rapidly cleared from plasma and has a very short half-life (<6 minutes) with platelet function restored within 1 hour post cessation of the infusion.[32–34] Cangrelor is metabolised in the circulation by dephosphorylation and this is independent of hepatic function. It is 58% renally-excreted, and the remainder via the biliary system.

Bleeding is the most common adverse reaction with this drug class. Bleeding is increased with ticagrelor and cangrelor compared to clopidogrel.

In the Platelet Inhibition and Patient Outcomes (PLATO) trial there was a higher rate of non-coronary bypass-related major bleeding (4.5% vs. 3.8%, $P = 0.03$) and the TIMI criteria (2.8% vs. 2.2%, $P = 0.03$).[35] In addition, there were increased episodes of intracranial bleeding with ticagrelor (0.3% vs. 0.2%, $P = 0.06$), including fatal intracranial bleeding (0.1% vs. 0.01%, $P = 0.02$).[35]

Both agents can cause dyspnoea, though cangrelor-induced dyspnoea occurs less than with ticagrelor. Ticagrelor-induced dyspnoea is dose-dependent.[36] The mechanism is unclear; however, the dyspnoea can be transient and in the PLATO trial, despite a 13.8% experience of dyspnoea, only 0.9% ceased therapy due to dyspnoea.[35] Other common side effects in PLATO include dizziness (4.5%), diarrhoea (4.3%) and ventricular pauses (6% vs. 3.5% clopidogrel group).[35] The cangrelor side-effect profile is currently limited to trial data. It achieved Food and Drug Administration approval in 2015. From the CHAMPION PHOENIX trial, participants in the cangrelor arm experienced increased hypersensitivity (0.05% vs. 0.02%) and decreased renal function (3.2% vs. 1.4%), particularly in patients with creatinine clearance <30 mL/min.[37] Table 24.1 presents a summary of current antiplatelet drugs in use.

Glycoprotein IIb/IIIa (GP IIb/IIIa) inhibitors

GP IIb/IIIa inhibitors prevent fibrinogen binding to activated GP IIb/IIIa receptor and the final common pathway of platelet aggregation, which is the formation of fibrinogen bridges between platelets.[38] Abciximab, an intravenous IIb/IIIa receptor antagonist, is a chimeric humanised Fab fragment of a monoclonal antibody to the IIb/IIIa (αIIbβ3) receptor. It also binds with equal affinity to the vitronectin (αvβ3) receptor, which is present on vascular endothelial and smooth muscle cells as well as the platelet, and shares the same β3 subunit as the GP IIb/IIIa receptor.[39]

There are two other principal groups of IIb/IIIa antagonists. The first, the peptide eptifibatide, is a synthetic analogue of barbourin, a naturally occurring disintegrin from the venom of the rattlesnake Sistrurus barbouri.[40] The second is a group of smaller peptides having the Arg-Gly-Asp (RGD) sequence in common. These include

Table 24.1 Summary table of the current antiplatelet drugs in use

	Aspirin	Clopidogrel	Prasugrel	Ticagrelor	Cangrelor
Drug class	Nonsteroidal anti-inflammatory	Second-generation Thienopyridine	Third-generation Thienopyridine	Cyclo-pentyl-triazolo-pyrimidine	Stabilised ATP analogue
Administration	Oral	Oral	Oral	Oral	Intravenous
Prodrug	Yes	Yes	Yes	No	No
Dosing	Loading dose: 300 mg Standard dose: 100 mg daily	Loading dose: 300–600 mg Standard dose: 75 mg daily	Loading dose: 60 mg Standard dose: 10 mg daily	Loading dose: 180 mg Standard dose: 90 mg daily	IV Bolus: 30 µg/kg Immediately followed by IV infusion 4 µg/kg/min
Reversibility	No	No	No	Yes	Yes
Onset of action	1–3 hours	2–6 hours	30 minutes	30 minutes	2 minutes
Duration of effect	10 days	3–10 days	7–10 days	3–5 days	1–2 hours
CYP metabolism	No	CYP2C19	CYP3A4, CYP2B6	CYP3A4 CYP3A%	No
Withhold prior to surgery	7 days	At least 5 days	At least 7 days	At least 3 days	1 hour

Abbreviation: IV, intravenous.

tirofiban, lamifiban and xemilofiban. Despite the diverse structure and methods of synthesis, these agents all bind resting and activated platelets.

Oral GP IIb/IIIa inhibitors (xemilofiban, orbo-fiban, sibrafiban and lotrafiban) have been investigated in phase III clinical trial but demonstrated increased mortality with nil clinical benefit, so development has been abandoned.[41–43]

The role of GP IIb/IIIa inhibitors in intervention has reduced over the last decade with the rise of dual antiplatelet therapy (DAPT) with aspirin and P2Y12 receptor blockers. Current guidelines suggest use of GP IIb/IIIa inhibitors in combination with heparin at the time of PCI among patients with high-risk clinical and angiographic characteristics, or for treating thrombotic complications among patients with acute coronary syndrome (ACS).[44]

Abciximab is given as a bolus (0.25 mg/kg) followed by a 12 hours infusion (0.125 µg/kg/min).[45] Abciximab has a high affinity for the GP IIb/IIIa receptor, a rapid onset of action and provides greater than 80% receptor blockade after bolus administration.[46] Platelet function as assessed by standard means returns to normal within 24–36 hours of treatment with a bolus and 12 hours infusion.[47,48] However, flow cytometric analyses have shown that at 8 and 15 days after treatment, abciximab still provides 29% and 13% receptor blockade.[49] This suggests a longer term effect on platelets not detected by standard means.

Eptifibatide is a non-immunogenic cyclic heptapeptide that reversibly inhibits the platelet IIb/IIIa receptor as a competitive inhibitor of the fibrinogen-binding site. It is rapid but short acting (2–4 hours) with a half-life of 2.5 hours. It should be used with caution in patients with renal impairment as it is renally excreted. The PURSUIT study examined the role of eptifibatide in acute coronary syndromes.[50] The dose used was a 180 µg/kg bolus followed by a 2.0 µg/kg/min infusion. There was a small but significant reduction in death or non-fatal MI (14.2% vs. 15.7% $p = 0.004$).[50]

Tirofiban is a competitive inhibitor of the fibrinogen-binding site. It is short acting (2–4 hours) with a half-life of 2 hours. Tirofiban was trialled in 2139 patients with acute coronary syndromes undergoing percutaneous revascularisation.[51] Over 90% were treated with angioplasty alone. Patients received either placebo or tirofiban (10 µg/kg bolus followed by a 36 hours infusion

of 0.15 µg/kg/min). At 30 days, the combined endpoint of death, MI, revascularisation or need for non-elective stenting during the procedure was not significantly different in the tirofiban and placebo groups (10% vs. 12.2% $p = 0.16$), although there was a difference at 7 days (7.6% vs. 10.4% $p = 0.022$).

Thrombocytopenia occurs with the IIb/IIIa antagonists. In some cases, this appears clinically similar to, and is difficult to distinguish from, heparin-induced thrombocytopenia.[52] In some cases it appears to be a particular effect of abciximab, with an acute (<24 hours after drug initiation) and marked (to <20 × 10 × 9 platelets/mL) fall in platelet count. This occurs in between 0.3% and 0.79% of patients and responds to cessation of all antiplatelet and anticoagulant therapy and platelet infusion, without major complication.[53,54] The pathogenesis is unclear, although it may be related to the generation of human antichimeric antibodies, which occurs in up to 6% of abciximab treated patients.[45]

Phosphodiesterase (PDE) inhibitors

Cilostazol is a PDE inhibitor with vasodilator and anti-platelet effects and exerts it antiplatelet effect through inhibition of phosphodiesterase III inhibitor, which subsequently increases cyclic adenosine monophosphate within platelets.[55] Cilostazol (100 mg twice daily) added to a standard combination of aspirin plus clopidogrel has been found to increase platelet aggregation inhibition when compared with aspirin and clopidogrel in high-risk patients.[56,57]

Dipyridamole exerts its effect through selectively inhibiting the cGMP phosphodiesterase type V enzyme, resulting in antiplatelet effects of the nitric oxide – cGMP signalling pathway.[58]

PAR-1 antagonists

Vorapaxar and atopaxar are PAR-1 inhibitors that have been investigated in secondary prevention of ischaemic events with mixed results.[59,60] They work by blocking the binding of thrombin to PAR-1, thus inhibiting thrombin-induced platelet activation and aggregation.

In non-ST-elevation (NSTE) ACS, a Phase III clinical trial investigating the role of vorapaxer was ceased early due to a significant increase in the risk of major bleeding without a significant reduction in the primary composite end point.[61] A meta-analysis has highlighted the higher risk of major bleeding, including intracranial haemorrhage, with PAR-1 inhibitors.[62]

Other antiplatelet agents

Thromboxane receptors, which mediate thromboxane A2-induced platelet activation, have been an area of interest, as despite aspirin blockade of COX-1, platelets continue to be exposed to thromboxane A2.[63] Various thromboxane receptor antagonists (picotamide, ridogrel, terutroban) have been trialled with overall disappointing results. [64–66]

An antibody to von Willebrand Factor (ARC1779) has previously been investigated but the trial was terminated due to the mode of administration of drug being unfeasible.[67]

Treatment following coronary angioplasty

Aspirin was used with heparin, dextran and warfarin in the very first cases of angioplasty in the late 1970s.[1] Ticlopidine in combination with aspirin in the 1980s reduced ischemic complications related to angioplasty.[68]

Unfractionated heparin remains the standard of care for peri-procedural anticoagulation. It has not, however, been the subject of randomised trials for this indication, but experimental animal data and its efficacy in reducing thrombotic complications in the setting of unstable angina suggest these trials will not be undertaken.[69] Since the introduction of IIb/IIIa receptor antagonists in combination with heparin, the EPILOG trial demonstrated equal efficacy, and reduced bleeding complications with a weight-adjusted heparin dose of 70 μg/kg, aiming for an activated clotting time (ACT) of >200 seconds, compared to a standard heparin dose of 100 μg/kg.[45]

The thrombin inhibitors bivalirudin and hirudin have both been used as alternatives to heparin in coronary angioplasty. However, in recent times clinical trials have demonstrated no reduction in major cardiovascular event involving bivalirudin in acute coronary syndrome undergoing invasive treatment versus unfractionated heparin.[70,71]

Overall, the role of isolated coronary angioplasty has reduced over the last decade with the increasing role of coronary stenting using drug eluting stents (DES). However, guidelines using data from trials investigating patients who have drug-coated balloon therapy for in-stent restenosis have recommended an antiplatelet treatment duration of between 3 and 12 months.[72–75]

Treatment following coronary stenting

The early experience of coronary stenting has been well documented and well-reviewed[76] and was associated with high rates of stent thrombosis—up to 6%–20% despite heavy antithrombotic regimens including aspirin, dipyridamole, dextran, heparin and warfarin. These early studies also reported excessive bleeding.[76,77] Intravascular ultrasound was pivotal in demonstrating that many stents with satisfactory angiographic appearance were under-deployed.[78] This provided a reason for the initially high rates of stent thrombosis, and a rationale for proceeding to high-pressure balloon inflation to ensure optimal stent deployment, following this with a simplified antiplatelet regimen without anticoagulation. A number of the initial registries used only aspirin and ticlopidine, with or without heparin, and reported stent thrombosis rates 0%–1.4% and bleeding rates of 0%–2.2%.[78,79] Two subsequent randomised but not blinded trials, ISAR and STARS, confirmed the registry findings.[80,81] In the ISAR trial, the aspirin and ticlopidine group had a 1.6% combined cardiac endpoint compared to 6.2% ($P < 0.01$) for the phenprocoumon group, and no incidence of stent thrombosis compared to 5.0% ($P < 0.01$).[81] The STARS trial demonstrated a similar improvement of 0.5% vs. 2.7% ($p = 0.07$) in a combined cardiac endpoint for aspirin and ticlopidine versus warfarin.[80] The STARS study included a group randomised to aspirin alone. This group had a combined endpoint of 3.6%, higher than the warfarin group.[80] This field has evolved with the newer generation P2Y12 receptor antagonists and DES.

ANTIPLATELET THERAPY IN ACUTE PERCUTANEOUS CORONARY INTERVENTION (PCI) FOR ACS

In patients with NSTE ACS, undergoing PCI, ticagrelor (180 mg loading and 90 mg twice daily maintenance dose) is recommended regardless of the initial treatment strategy, including patients pre-treated with clopidogre.[72] Alternatively, if there is a contraindication to ticagrelor, clopidogrel (600 mg loading and 150 mg/day maintenance dose) may be used. Prasugrel is not recommended for NSTE ACS for patients in whom the coronary anatomy is not known.[72,82]

In patients with STEMI, prasugrel (60 mg loading and 10 mg/day maintenance dose), or ticagrelor (180 mg loading and 90 mg twice daily maintenance dose) is the first line P2Y12 inhibitor.[72] Clopidogrel (600 mg loading and 150 mg/day maintenance dose) is an alternative should there be a contraindication to the newer P2Y12 inhibitor.

Current guidelines recommend 12 months of DAPT unless there is a contraindication such as excessive bleeding risk.[24,35,72,83] The role of DAPT beyond 12 months has been investigated in the PEGASUS trial with ticagrelor.[84] PEGASUS recruited 21,162 patients with a history of MI 1–3 years previously. The participants were randomly assigned to ticagrelor 90 mg BD, ticagrelor 60 mg BD or placebo in addition to aspirin. The primary efficacy endpoint was the composite of cardiovascular death, MI, or stroke at 3 years and was 7.85% ($P = 0.008$) in the 90 mg group, 7.77% ($P = 0.004$) in the 60 mg group, and 9.04% in the placebo group.[84] There was a trend for a reduction in cardiovascular mortality, and all-cause mortality was neutral. The primary safety endpoint of TIMI major bleeding was observed more frequently with ticagrelor (2.60%; $P < 0.001$ with 90 mg and 2.30%; $P < 0.001$ with 60 mg) than with placebo (1.06%).[84] The small risk–benefit ratio from prolonged DAPT with ticagrelor beyond 12 months should be used with caution, given the risk of harm from bleeding.

Furthermore, non-prespecified analysis from the DAPT trial assessed the benefit and risk of extended versus standard duration of DAPT among patients with or without MI.[85] Prasugrel was used in one-third of the patients with MI and clopidogrel in the remainder. Within the MI cohort, extended DAPT as compared with aspirin alone significantly reduced stent thrombosis (0.5% vs. 1.9%; $P < 0.001$) and major adverse cardiac events (MACE: 3.9% vs. 6.8%; $P < 0.001$). However, extended DAPT significantly increased GUSTO moderate or severe bleeding (1.9% vs. 0.8%, $P = 0.005$). Interestingly, compared to the main study findings there was no difference in all-cause mortality.

A meta-analysis by Udell et al. assessed the role of extended DAPT in secondary prevention using predominantly the subgroup of large trials,

which included PEGASUS, DAPT, CHARISMA, PRODIGY and DES-LATE.[86] The PEGASUS study was the only study used in its entirety and its data contributed >60% to the pooled endpoint estimates, as well as being the only appropriately powered study for post-MI patients, thus it does expose the results to bias. Extended DAPT decreased the risk of MACE compared with aspirin alone (6.4% vs. 7.5%; $P = 0.001$). However, there was significantly increased major bleeding (1.85% vs. 1.09%; $P = 0.004$). Thus, one may consider the role of switching P2Y12 inhibitor to clopidogrel after being stable 12 months post MI in patients, given its low bleeding risk.

Regarding the interruption of P2Y12 inhibitor treatment, PEGASUS-TIMI 54 involving ticagrelor investigated stable patient with a median 1.7 year post MI.[87] It concluded that patients who continued ticagrelor without a >30-day interruption derived a larger benefit from extended ticagrelor intake than patients who interrupted treatment for >30 days.[87]

Reduced DAPT duration to three months comes at increased ischaemic risk.[88] However, shortened DAPT duration may be necessary in patients with a high bleeding risk. This is a 'grey area' as most of the DAPT studies excluded high bleeding-risk patients. There is no dedicated trial assessing optimal DAPT duration. As a result, the latest guidelines recommend considering discontinuation of P2Y12 inhibitor therapy after 6 months, in patients with high bleeding risk.[72] The ESC 2017 DAPT guidelines on duration of DATP post-PCI in ACS are summarised in Figure 24.1.

ANTIPLATELET THERAPY IN ELECTIVE PCI

In PCI for stable CAD, 600 mg clopidogrel loading dose followed by 75 mg/day should be administered.[72] Pre-treatment is recommended for elective PCI if coronary anatomy has been pre-established.[72] There is evidence that systematic clopidogrel preloading before diagnostic coronary angiography lowers risk of major coronary events but does not affect mortality, with comparable bleeding rates.[89] The role of GP IIb/IIIa inhibitor is often limited to high-risk patients or 'bailout" situations in the elective PCI setting as there is no additive benefit of GP IIb/IIIa inhibitor in addition to loading dose clopidogrel in low-risk elective PCI.[90–92]

DAPT is the gold standard of care post PCI. As mentioned earlier, the ISAR trial established the utility of DAPT post stenting.[81] Subsequently,

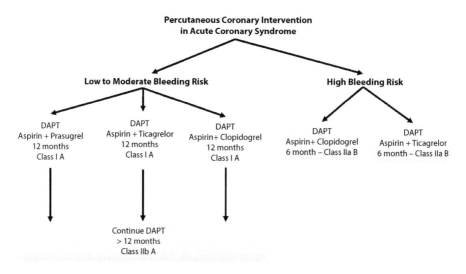

Figure 24.1 Duration of dual antiplatelet therapy (DAPT) post-percutaneous coronary intervention in acute coronary syndrome. (Adapted from the ESC 2017 Antiplatelet Guidelines.)

12-months or more of DAPT duration has been recommended by guidelines.[72] There is no study to date that specifically assesses different DAPT durations on stable CAD patients undergoing PCI. Thus, recommendations in this group are based on subgroup analyses from larger studies.[85,93] It is important to note that there are no trial data involving use of ticagrelor or prasugrel in stable CAD patients undergoing PCI.

Various trials have studied DAPT duration from three months to 24 months. One of the largest studies to date is Intracoronary Stenting and Antithrombotic Regimen: Safety and Efficacy of 6 Months Dual Antiplatelet Therapy After Drug-Eluting Stenting (ISAR-SAFE).[94] ISAR-SAFE was ceased early due to the low event rate and slow recruitment. In this multicentre, randomised, double-blind, placebo-controlled trial, 4005 patients (2394 with stable CAD) were recruited. Patients at 6 months post-DES implantation were randomly assigned to either a 6-month period of placebo or an additional 6-month period of clopidogrel. The event rate was low (1.5% 6 months of clopidogrel vs. 1.6% 12 months of clopidogrel) with no significant difference in 12 months of DATP over 6 months of DATP. In addition, the ITALIC (6 months DATP vs. 24 months DATP) and SECURITY (6 months DATP vs. 12 months DATP) trials demonstrated consistent results.[95,96]

Three-month DAPT (aspirin and clopidogrel) duration has been studied in The Real Safety and Efficacy of 3-Month Dual Antiplatelet Therapy Following Endeavor Zotarolimus-Eluting Stent Implantation (RESET) and in the Optimised Duration of Clopidogrel Therapy Following Treatment With the Zotarolimus-Eluting Stent in Real-World Clinical Practice (OPTIMIZE) trials.[97,98] Both studies did not show significant harm with 3 months DATP vs. 12 months DATP, 0.8% vs. 1.3%; $P = 0.48$ (composite endpoint included any death, MI, or stent thrombosis) in RESET and 1-year incidence of MACE was 8.3% in the 3 months DATP group and 7.4% in the 12 months DATP group (HR 1.12, 95% CI 0.87–1.45) in OPTIMIZE. Both studies used Endeavor Zotarolimus-Eluting Stents, which are no longer available, so it is unclear how transferable the results are to other DES.

The pivotal DAPT study was an international, multicentre, randomised, placebo-controlled trial that was designed to determine the benefits and risks of continuing dual antiplatelet therapy beyond 1 year after the placement of a coronary stent.[99] Patients who were still on DAPT and had not experienced any bleeding or ischaemic events were recruited at 12 months post-DES placement. For another 18 months, 9961 patients were subsequently randomly allocated to thienopyridine or placebo. Thirty months DAPT vs. 12 months DAPT reduced the rates of stent thrombosis (0.4% vs. 1.4%; $P < 0.001$), major adverse cardiovascular and cerebrovascular events (4.3% vs. 5.9%; $P < 0.001$) and there were lower rates of MI (2.1% vs. 4.1%; $P < 0.001$). However, the rate of moderate or severe bleeding was increased with continued DAPT treatment (2.5% vs. 1.6%, $P = 0.001$). In addition, a meta-analysis for the AHA 2016 DAPT guidelines assessing of 11 randomised, controlled trials involving 33,051 patients showed weak evidence of increased mortality rate with prolonged DAPT usage.[100]

Consequently, it is clear that prolonged DAPT therapy post-DES placement has benefits of reduced stent thrombosis and cardiac events. However, this is at the expense of increased risk of bleeding and a possible signal for increased mortality. The guidelines acknowledge this, and thus DAPT duration is guided according to the patient's bleeding risk, with some consideration to the type of stent used, and with the largest benefit being in patients with a paclitaxel-eluting stent compared to the smallest benefit with an everolimus-eluting stent.[72,101]

The evidence for bioresorbable stents remains limited, with no dedicated study assessing the optimal duration of DAPT. The current recommendation for 12 months of DAPT is from the largest bioresorable stent clinical trial.[102] Two-year outcome data was assessed in a meta-analysis demonstrating that the cumulative 2-year incidence of device thrombosis was significantly higher with bioresorbable stents than with DES (RR 3.35 [95% CI 1.96–5.72], $P < 0.0001$).[103] This area remains a rapidly evolving field, and although there is a clear rational for more potent P2Y12 inhibitors and possibly longer DATP, improvements in bioresorbable stents are needed. The ESC 2017 DAPT guidelines on duration of DATP post-PCI in stable coronary artery disease are summarised in Figure 24.2.

Switching antiplatelet agents

The last decade has brought an increase in the number of P2Y12 inhibitors, and a consequent requirement to change agents on occasions. However, only the transition between clopidogrel to ticagrelor has been formally investigated.[35] As a consequence of PLATO, guidelines recommend switching from clopidogrel to ticagrelor in ACS patients who have previously had clopidogrel exposure.[72] Patients should be loaded with 180 mg of ticagrelor regardless of their last clopidogrel dose.[72] This data contrasts with TRITON-TIMI 38, which excluded

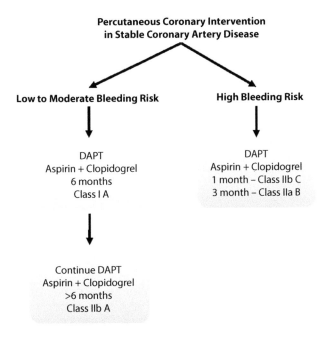

Figure 24.2 Duration of dual antiplatelet therapy (DATP) post-percutaneous coronary intervention in stable coronary artery disease. (Adapted from the ESC 2017 Antiplatelet Guidelines.)

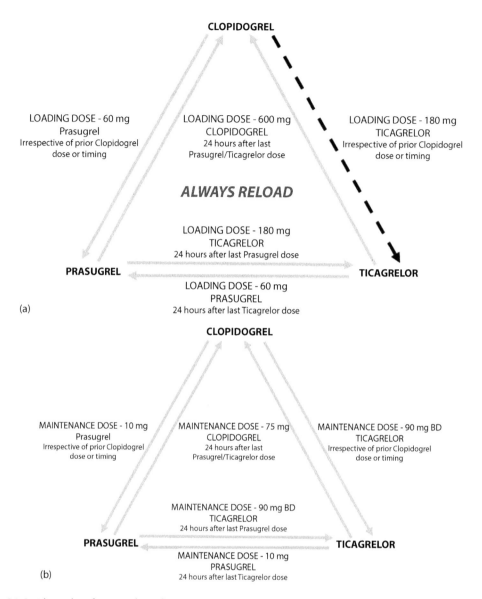

Figure 24.3 Algorithm for switching between oral P2Y12 inhibitors in the acute (a) and chronic (b) setting. Dashed arrow = Class I; solid arrow = Class IIb. (Adapted from the ESC 2017 Antiplatelet Guidelines.)

participants who had exposure of patients to a P2Y12 receptor.[24] Thus, registry data provides limited information with regards to switching from clopidogrel to prasugrel.[104] In addition, there is no outcome data on switching between ticagrelor and prasugrel, as well as ticagrelor/prasugrel to clopidogrel. As a result, the latest ESC guidelines discourage switching P2Y12 inhibitors due to a lack of safety/efficacy data.[72] However the guidelines do recognise that agents may need to be switched for clinical reason and thus offer the guidance summarised in Figure 24.3.

Antiplatelets in structural heart disease intervention

Advances in cardiac care have led to increases in the role of cardiac intervention. The role of antiplatelet agents is important in reducing the increased thromboembolic risk these procedures cause.

PATENT FORAMEN OVALE (PFO) AND ATRIAL SEPTAL DEFECT (ASD) CLOSURE

There is variability in the use of antiplatelet therapy post PFO/ASD closure. If there is no indication for antiplatelet therapy prior to PFO/ASD closure, patients generally commence aspirin 100 mg 3–5 days before. If there are contraindications to aspirin, clopidogrel 75 mg daily is an alternative. Post-procedure antiplatelet therapy is generally continued for 6 months to allow device endothelialisation. Antiplatelet therapy is often ceased at 6 months, contingent on other co-morbidities.

TRANSCATHETER AORTIC VALVE IMPLANTATION (TAVI)

Given the often-present co-morbidities in this population, patients are often on antiplatelet therapy prior to TAVI. Current guidelines also suggest post procedural antiplatelet therapy. Currently, aspirin and clopidogrel for 3–6 months, followed by life-long aspirin.[105,106] Concern has been raised about subclinical valvular thrombosis, and that DAPT compared to single antiplatelet therapy increases the incidence of haemorrhagic events, with no benefits in terms of thrombotic events and cardiovascular mortality.[107,108] The optimal antiplatelet regimen following TAVI is thus an evolving field of investigation.

MITRACLIP

There are no guidelines on antiplatelet therapy following Mitraclip use for mitral regurgitation. In EVEREST II, the first study of mitraclip use, aspirin 325 mg was administered for 6–12 months, along with clopidogrel 75 mg daily for one month.[109] Given the concern surrounding thrombotic events, Alsidawi and Effat published a suggested regimen of aspirin 325 mg and clopidogrel 75 mg immediately after the procedure for 6 to 12 months,[110] but similarly to other structural interventions, this is a field of active investigation.

FUTURE PROSPECTS

The pace of change in antiplatelet and anticoagulant therapies in the last decade has been rapid, with several factors influencing future improvements. Significantly, the endpoints of stent thrombosis and cardiovascular morbidity have become low. Thus, any new drug therapy is likely to need randomised trials involving large numbers of patients to demonstrate an improvement in efficacy over standard therapy.[111] However, there are multiple agents currently under development: PZ-128, targeting intracellular signalling on PAR-1; BMS-986141, a PAR-4 antagonist; MRS2179 a P2Y1 antagonist as well as a combined P2Y1 and P2 Y12 antagonist.[112–115] In addition, numerous questions remain unanswered about the optimal type, use and duration of antiplatelet therapy during and after PCI. Although unlikely to occur a randomised, multicentre direct comparison between prasugrel, ticagrelor and clopidogrel to evaluate their relative efficacy and safety is desirable, as this evolving field aims to continue to discover the best treatment for patients.

REFERENCES

1. Grüntzig AR, Senning Å and Siegenthaler WE. Nonoperative Dilatation of Coronary-Artery Stenosis. *N Engl J Med.* 1979;301:61–68.
2. Causes of Death, Australia, 2016. 2017.
3. O'gara PT, Kushner FG, Ascheim DD, Casey DE, Chung MK, De Lemos JA, et al. 2013 ACCF/AHA guideline for the management of ST-elevation myocardial infarction: Executive summary: A report of the American College of Cardiology Foundation/American Heart Association Task Force on Practice Guidelines. *J Am Coll Cardiol.* 2013;61(4):485–510.
4. Ibanez B, James S, Agewall S, Antunes MJ, Bucciarelli-Ducci C, Bueno H, et al. 2017 ESC guidelines for the management of acute myocardial infarction in patients presenting with ST-segment elevation: The Task Force for the management of acute myocardial infarction in patients presenting with ST-segment elevation of the European Society of Cardiology (ESC). *Eur Heart J.* 2017;39(2):119–177.
5. Roffi M, Patrono C, Collet J-P, Mueller C, Valgimigli M, Andreotti F, et al. 2015 ESC Guidelines for the management of acute coronary syndromes in patients presenting without persistent ST-segment elevation: Task Force for the management of acute

coronary syndromes in patients presenting without persistent ST-segment elevation of the European Society of Cardiology (ESC). *Eur Heart J*. 2016;37(3):267–315.

6. Amsterdam EA, Wenger NK, Brindis RG, Casey DE, Ganiats TG, Holmes DR, et al. 2014 AHA/ACC guideline for the management of patients with non–ST-elevation acute coronary syndromes: A report of the American College of Cardiology/American Heart Association Task Force on Practice Guidelines. *J Am Coll Cardiol*. 2014;64(24):e139–e228.

7. Serruys PW, Strauss BH, Beatt KJ, Bertrand ME, Puel J, Rickards AF, et al. Angiographic follow-up after placement of a self-expanding coronary-artery stent. *N Engl J Med*. 1991;324:13–17.

8. Craven LL. Experiences with aspirin (Acetylsalicylic acid) in the nonspecific prophylaxis of coronary thrombosis. *Miss Valley Med J*. 1953;75:38–44.

9. Weiss HJ and Aledort LM. Impaired platelet-connective-tissue reaction in man after aspirin ingestion. *Lancet*. 1967;2:495–497.

10. Patrono C. Aspirin as an antiplatelet drug. *N Engl J Med*. 1994;330:1287–1294.

11. Kelly JP, Kaufman DW, Jurgelon JM, Sheehan J, Koff RS, Shapiro S. Risk of aspirin-associated major upper-gastrointestinal bleeding with enteric-coated or buffered product. *Lancet*. 1996;348:1413–1416.

12. Kastrati A, Schomig A, Schomig E. Are we making efficient use of clopidogrel? *Eur Heart J*. 2004;25:454–456.

13. Wallentin L. P2Y12 inhibitors: Differences in properties and mechanisms of action and potential consequences for clinical use. *Eur Heart J*. 2009;30:1964–1977.

14. Verstraete M and Zoldhelyi P. Novel antithrombotic drugs in development. *Drugs*. 1995;49:856–884.

15. Dobesh PP. Pharmacokinetics and pharmacodynamics of prasugrel, a thienopyridine P2Y12 inhibitor. *Pharmacotherapy*. 2009;29:1089–1102.

16. Ford I. Coming safely to a stop: A review of platelet activity after cessation of antiplatelet drugs. *Ther Adv Drug Saf*. 2015;6:141–150.

17. Herbert JM, Frehel D, Vallee E, Kieffer G, Gouy D, Berger Y, et al. Clopidogrel, A novel antiplatelet and antithrombotic agent. *Cardiovasc Drug Rev*. 1993;11:180–198.

18. Coukell AJ and Markham A. Clopidogrel. *Drugs*. 1997;54:745–750; discussion 751.

19. Jernberg T, Payne CD, Winters KJ, Darstein C, Brandt JT, Jakubowski JA, et al. Prasugrel achieves greater inhibition of platelet aggregation and a lower rate of non-responders compared with clopidogrel in aspirin-treated patients with stable coronary artery disease. *Eur Heart J*. 2006;27:1166–1173.

20. Simon T, Verstuyft C, Mary-Krause M, Quteineh L, Drouet E, Méneveau N, Steg PG, Ferrières J, Danchin N, Becquemont L. Genetic determinants of response to clopidogrel and cardiovascular events. *N Engl J Med*. 2009;360:363–375.

21. Sugidachi A, Asai F, Ogawa T, Inoue T, Koike H. The in vivo pharmacological profile of CS-747, a novel antiplatelet agent with platelet ADP receptor antagonist properties. *Br J Pharmacol*. 2000;129:1439–1446.

22. Wiviott SD, Antman EM, Winters KJ, Weerakkody G, Murphy SA, Behounek BD, et al. Randomized comparison of prasugrel (CS-747, LY640315), a novel thienopyridine P2Y12 antagonist, with clopidogrel in percutaneous coronary intervention: Results of the Joint Utilization of Medications to Block Platelets Optimally (JUMBO)-TIMI 26 trial. *Circulation*. 2005;111:3366–3373.

23. Brandt JT, Payne CD, Wiviott SD, Weerakkody G, Farid NA, Small DS, et al. A comparison of prasugrel and clopidogrel loading doses on platelet function: Magnitude of platelet inhibition is related to active metabolite formation. *Am Heart J*. 2007;153:66.e9–16.

24. Wiviott SD, Braunwald E, McCabe CH, Montalescot G, Ruzyllo W, Gottlieb S, et al. Prasugrel versus clopidogrel in patients with acute coronary syndromes. *N Engl J Med*. 2007;357:2001–2015.

25. Committee CS. A randomised, blinded, trial of clopidogrel versus aspirin in patients at risk of ischaemic events (CAPRIE). CAPRIE Steering Committee. *Lancet*. 1996;348:1329–1339.

26. Hass WK, Easton JD, Adams HP, Jr., Pryse-Phillips W, Molony BA, Anderson S, Kamm B. A randomized trial comparing ticlopidine hydrochloride with aspirin for the prevention of stroke in high-risk patients. Ticlopidine Aspirin Stroke Study Group. *N Engl J Med.* 1989;321:501–507.

27. By the American Geriatrics Society Beers Criteria Update Expert P. American Geriatrics Society 2015 updated beers criteria for potentially inappropriate medication use in older adults. *J Am Geriatr Soc.* 2015;63:2227–2246.

28. Storey RF, Husted S, Harrington RA, Heptinstall S, Wilcox RG, Peters G, et al. Inhibition of platelet aggregation by AZD6140, a reversible oral P2Y12 receptor antagonist, compared with clopidogrel in patients with acute coronary syndromes. *J Am Coll Cardiol.* 2007;50:1852–1856.

29. Husted S, Emanuelsson H, Heptinstall S, Sandset PM, Wickens M, Peters G. Pharmacodynamics, pharmacokinetics, and safety of the oral reversible P2Y12 antagonist AZD6140 with aspirin in patients with atherosclerosis: A double-blind comparison to clopidogrel with aspirin. *Eur Heart J.* 2006;27:1038–1047.

30. Gurbel PA, Bliden KP, Butler K, Antonino MJ, Wei C, Teng R, et al. Response to ticagrelor in clopidogrel non-responders and responders and effect of switching therapies: The RESPOND study. *Circulation.* 2010;121:1188–1199.

31. Patrono C, Morais J, Baigent C, Collet JP, Fitzgerald D, Halvorsen S, et al. Antiplatelet agents for the treatment and prevention of coronary atherothrombosis. *J Am Coll Cardiol.* 2017;70:1760–1776.

32. Jacobsson F, Swahn E, Wallentin L, Ellborg M. Safety profile and tolerability of intravenous AR-C69931MX, a new anti-platelet drug, in unstable angina pectoris and non-Q-wave myocardial infarction. *Clin Ther.* 2002;24:752–765.

33. Storey RF, Oldroyd KG, Wilcox RG. Open multicentre study of the P2T receptor antagonist AR-C69931MX assessing safety, tolerability and activity in patients with acute coronary syndromes. *Thromb Haemost.* 2001;85:401–407.

34. Angiolillo DJ, Schneider DJ, Bhatt DL, French WJ, Price MJ, Saucedo JF, et al. Pharmacodynamic effects of cangrelor and clopidogrel: The platelet function substudy from the cangrelor versus standard therapy to achieve optimal management of platelet inhibition (CHAMPION) trials. *J Thromb Thrombolysis.* 2012;34:44–55.

35. Wallentin L, Becker RC, Budaj A, Cannon CP, Emanuelsson H, Held C, et al. Ticagrelor versus Clopidogrel in Patients with Acute Coronary Syndromes. *N Engl J Med.* 2009;361:1045–1057.

36. Cannon CP, Husted S, Harrington RA, Scirica BM, Emanuelsson H, Peters G, Storey RF. Safety, tolerability, and initial efficacy of AZD6140, the first reversible oral adenosine diphosphate receptor antagonist, compared with clopidogrel, in patients with non-ST-segment elevation acute coronary syndrome: Primary results of the DISPERSE-2 trial. *J Am Coll Cardiol.* 2007;50:1844–1851.

37. Bhatt DL, Stone GW, Mahaffey KW, Gibson CM, Steg PG, Hamm CW, et al. Effect of platelet inhibition with cangrelor during PCI on ischemic events. *N Engl J Med.* 2013;368:1303–1313.

38. Coller BS. alphaIIbbeta3: Structure and function. *J Thromb Haemost.* 2015;13 Suppl 1:S17–25.

39. Nakada MT JR, Knight DM. Abciximab (ReoPro, chimeric 7E3 Fab) cross-specificity with [alpha]V [beta]3 integrin receptors: A potential mechanism for the prevention of restenosis. *J Am Coll Cardiol.* 1997;29:A243.

40. Scarborough RM. Development of eptifibatide. *Am Heart J.* 1999;138:1093–1104.

41. O'Neill WW, Serruys P, Knudtson M, van Es G-A, Timmis GC, van der Zwaan C, et al. Long-term treatment with a platelet glycoprotein-receptor antagonist after percutaneous coronary revascularization. *N Engl J Med.* 2000;342:1316–1324.

42. Cannon CP, McCabe CH, Wilcox RG, Langer A, Caspi A, Berink P, et al. Oralg glycoprotein IIb/IIIa inhibition with orbofiban in patients with unstable coronary syndromes (OPUS-TIMI 16) trial. *Circulation.* 2000;102:149–156.

43. Chew DP, Bhatt DL, Sapp S, Topol EJ. Increased mortality with oral platelet glyco-protein IIb/IIIa antagonists: A meta-analysis of phase III multicenter randomized trials. *Circulation*. 2001;103:201–206.

44. Chew DP, Scott IA, Cullen L, French JK, Briffa TG, Tideman PA, et al. National Heart Foundation of Australia & Cardiac Society of Australia and New Zealand: Australian clinical guidelines for the man-agement of acute coronary syndromes 2016. *Heart Lung Circ*. 2016;25:895–951.

45. Investigators TE. Platelet glycopro-tein IIb/IIIa receptor blockade and low-dose heparin during percutaneous coronary revascularization. *N Engl J Med*. 1997;336:1689–1697.

46. Coller BS, Scudder LE, Beer J, Gold HK, Folts JD, Cavagnaro J, et al. Monoclonal antibodies to platelet glycoprotein IIb/IIIa as antithrombotic agents. *Ann N Y Acad Sci*. 1991;614:193–213.

47. Mascelli MA, Worley S, Veriabo NJ, Lance ET, Mack S, Schaible T, et al. Rapid assessment of platelet function with a modified whole-blood aggregometer in percutaneous transluminal coronary angio-plasty patients receiving anti-GP IIb/IIIa therapy. *Circulation*. 1997;96:3860–3866.

48. Tcheng JE, Ellis SG, George BS, Kereiakes DJ, Kleiman NS, Talley JD, et al. Pharmacodynamics of chimeric glycopro-tein IIb/IIIa integrin antiplatelet antibody Fab 7E3 in high-risk coronary angioplasty. *Circulation*. 1994;90:1757–1764.

49. Mascelli MA, Lance ET, Damaraju L, Wagner CL, Weisman HF, Jordan RE. Pharmacodynamic profile of short-term abciximab treatment demonstrates pro-longed platelet inhibition with gradual recovery from GP IIb/IIIa receptor blockade. *Circulation*. 1998;97:1680–1688.

50. Investigators TPT. Inhibition of platelet glycoprotein IIb/IIIa with eptifibatide in patients with acute coronary syndromes. *N Engl J Med*. 1998;339:436–443.

51. Gibson CM, Goel M, Cohen DJ, Piana RN, Deckelbaum LI, Harris KE, King SB, 3rd. Six-month angiographic and clinical follow-up of patients prospectively random-ized to receive either tirofiban or placebo during angioplasty in the RESTORE trial. Randomized Efficacy Study of Tirofiban for Outcomes and Restenosis. *J Am Coll Cardiol*. 1998;32:28–34.

52. Madan M, Berkowitz SD, Tcheng JE. Glycoprotein IIb/IIIa integrin blockade. *Circulation*. 1998;98:2629–2635.

53. Berkowitz SD, Harrington RA, Rund MM, Tcheng JE. Acute profound thrombo-cytopenia after c7E3 Fab (abciximab) therapy. *Circulation*. 1997;95:809–813.

54. Investigators TC. Randomised placebo-controlled trial of abciximab before and during coronary intervention in refrac-tory unstable angina: The CAPTURE study. *Lancet*. 349:1429–1435.

55. Schror K. The pharmacology of cilo-stazol. *Diabetes Obes Metab*. 2002;4 Suppl 2:S14–9.

56. Park KW, Kang S-H, Park JJ, Yang H-M, Kang H-J, Koo B-K, et al. Adjunctive cilo-stazol versus double-dose clopidogrel after drug-eluting stent implantation: The host-assure randomized trial (harmonizing optimal strategy for treatment of coronary artery stenosis–safety & effectiveness of drug-eluting stents & anti-platelet regimen). *JACC: Cardiovasc Interv*. 2013;6:932–942.

57. Jeong YH, Lee SW, Choi BR, Kim IS, Seo MK, Kwak CH, et al. Randomized com-parison of adjunctive cilostazol versus high maintenance dose clopidogrel in patients with high post-treatment platelet reactiv-ity: Results of the ACCEL-RESISTANCE (Adjunctive Cilostazol Versus High Maintenance Dose Clopidogrel in Patients With Clopidogrel Resistance) randomized study. *J Am Coll Cardiol*. 2009;53(13):1101–1109.

58. Aktas B, Utz A, Hoenig-Liedl P, Walter U, Geiger J. Dipyridamole enhances NO/cGMP-mediated vasodilator-stimulated phosphoprotein phosphorylation and signaling in human platelets: In vitro and in vivo/ex vivo studies. *Stroke*. 2003;34:764–769.

59. Morrow DA, Braunwald E, Bonaca MP, Ameriso SF, Dalby AJ, Fish MP, et al. Vorapaxar in the secondary prevention of atherothrombotic events. *N Engl J Med*. 2012;366:1404–1413.

60. Wiviott SD, Flather MD, O'Donoghue ML, Goto S, Fitzgerald DJ, Cura F, et al. Randomized trial of atopaxar in the treatment of patients with coronary artery disease: The lessons from antagonizing the cellular effect of Thrombin-Coronary Artery Disease Trial. *Circulation*. 2011;123:1854–1863.

61. Tricoci P, Huang Z, Held C, Moliterno DJ, Armstrong PW, Van de Werf F, et al. Thrombin-receptor antagonist vorapaxar in acute coronary syndromes. *New Engl J Med*. 2012;366(1):20–33.

62. Capodanno D, Bhatt DL, Goto S, O'Donoghue ML, Moliterno DJ, Tamburino C, Angiolillo DJ. Safety and efficacy of protease-activated receptor-1 antagonists in patients with coronary artery disease: A meta-analysis of randomized clinical trials. *J Thromb Haemost: JTH*. 2012;10:2006–2015.

63. Chamorro A. TP receptor antagonism: A new concept in atherothrombosis and stroke prevention. *Cerebrovasc Dis*. 2009;27 Suppl 3:20–27.

64. Neri Serneri GG, Coccheri S, Marubini E, Violi F. Picotamide, a combined inhibitor of thromboxane A2 synthase and receptor, reduces 2-year mortality in diabetics with peripheral arterial disease: The DAVID study. *Eur Heart J*. 2004;25:1845–1852.

65. van der Wieken LR, Simoons ML, Laarman GJ, Van den Brand M, Nijssen KM, Dellborg M, et al. Ridogrel as an adjunct to thrombolysis in acute myocardial infarction. *Int J Cardiol*. 1995;52:125–134.

66. Bousser M-G, Amarenco P, Chamorro A, Fisher M, Ford I, Fox KM, et al. Terutroban versus aspirin in patients with cerebral ischaemic events (PERFORM): A randomised, double-blind, parallel-group trial. *Lancet*. 2011;377:2013–2022.

67. Gibson M. Study of ARC1779 in patients with acute myocardial infarction undergoing percutaneous coronary intervention (PCI) (vITAL-1). 2008. - https://clinicaltrials.gov/ct2/show/NCT00507338

68. White CW, Chaitman B, Lassar TA, Marcus ML, Chisholm RJ, Knudson M, et al. Antiplatelet agents are effective in reducing the immediate complications of PTCA: Results from the ticlopidine multicenter trial. *Circulation*. 1987;76(Suppl).

69. Heras M, Chesebro JH, Penny WJ, Bailey KR, Lam JY, Holmes DR, et al. Importance of adequate heparin dosage in arterial angioplasty in a porcine model. *Circulation*. 1988;78:654–660.

70. Leonardi S, Frigoli E, Rothenbühler M, Navarese E, Calabró P, Bellotti P, et al. Bivalirudin or unfractionated heparin in patients with acute coronary syndromes managed invasively with and without ST elevation (MATRIX): Randomised controlled trial. *BMJ*. 2016;354:i4935.

71. Valgimigli M, Frigoli E, Leonardi S, Rothenbühler M, Gagnor A, Calabrò P, et al. Bivalirudin or unfractionated heparin in acute coronary syndromes. *N Engl J Med*. 2015;373:997–1009.

72. Valgimigli M, Bueno H, Byrne RA, Collet J-P, Costa F, Jeppsson A, et al. 2017 ESC focused update on dual antiplatelet therapy in coronary artery disease developed in collaboration with EACTSThe Task Force for dual antiplatelet therapy in coronary artery disease of the European Society of Cardiology (ESC) and of the European Association for Cardio-Thoracic Surgery (EACTS). *Eur Heart J*. 2017:ehx419–ehx419.

73. Xu B, Gao R, Wang J, Yang Y, Chen S, Liu B, et al. A prospective, multicenter, randomized trial of paclitaxel-coated balloon versus paclitaxel-eluting stent for the treatment of drug-eluting stent in-stent restenosis: Results from the PEPCAD China ISR trial. *JACC Cardiovasc interv*. 2014;7:204–211.

74. Byrne RA, Neumann FJ, Mehilli J, Pinieck S, Wolff B, Tiroch K, et al. Paclitaxel-eluting balloons, paclitaxel-eluting stents, and balloon angioplasty in patients with restenosis after implantation of a drug-eluting stent (ISAR-DESIRE 3): A randomised, open-label trial. *Lancet*. 2013;381:461–467.

75. Alfonso F, Perez-Vizcayno MJ, Cardenas A, Garcia del Blanco B, Garcia-Touchard A, Lopez-Minguez JR, et al. A prospective randomized trial of drug-eluting balloons versus everolimus-eluting stents in patients with in-stent restenosis of drug-eluting stents: The RIBS IV randomized clinical trial. *J Am Coll Cardiol*. 2015;66:23–33.

76. Eeckhout E, Kappenberger L, Goy J-J. Stents for intracoronary placement: Current status and future directions. *J Am Coll Cardiol*. 1996;27:757–765.

77. Mak KH, Belli G, Ellis SG, Moliterno DJ. Subacute stent thrombosis: Evolving issues and current concepts. *J Am Coll Cardiol*. 1996;27:494–503.

78. Colombo A, Hall P, Nakamura S, Almagor Y, Maiello L, Martini G, et al. Intracoronary stenting without antico-agulation accomplished with intravas-cular ultrasound guidance. *Circulation*. 1995;91:1676–1688.

79. Karrillon GJ, Morice MC, Benveniste E, Bunouf P, Aubry P, Cattan S, et al. Intracoronary stent implantation without ultrasound guidance and with replacement of conventional anticoagulation by anti-platelet therapy. 30-day clinical outcome of the French Multicenter Registry. *Circulation*. 1996;94:1519–1527.

80. Leon MB, Baim DS, Popma JJ, Gordon PC, Cutlip DE, Ho KKL, et al. A clinical trial comparing three antithrombotic-drug regimens after coronary-artery stenting. *N Engl J Med*. 1998;339:1665–1671.

81. Schömig A, Neumann F-J, Kastrati A, Schühlen H, Blasini R, Hadamitzky M, et al. A randomized comparison of anti-platelet and anticoagulant therapy after the placement of coronary-artery stents. *N Engl J Med*. 1996;334:1084–1089.

82. Montalescot G, Bolognese L, Dudek D, Goldstein P, Hamm C, Tanguay JF, et al. Pretreatment with prasugrel in non-ST-segment elevation acute coronary syndromes. *N Engl J Med*. 2013;369:999–1010.

83. Yusuf S, Zhao F, Mehta SR, Chrolavicius S, Tognoni G, Fox KK. Effects of clopido-grel in addition to aspirin in patients with acute coronary syndromes without ST-segment elevation. *N Engl J Med*. 2001;345:494–502.

84. Bonaca MP, Bhatt DL, Cohen M, Steg PG, Storey RF, Jensen EC, et al. Long-term use of ticagrelor in patients with prior myocardial infarction. *N Engl J Med*. 2015;372:1791–1800.

85. Yeh RW, Kereiakes DJ, Steg PG, Windecker S, Rinaldi MJ, Gershlick AH, et al. Benefits and risks of extended duration dual antiplatelet therapy after PCI in patients with and without acute myocardial infarc-tion. *J Am Coll Cardiol*. 2015;65:2211–2221.

86. Udell JA, Bonaca MP, Collet JP, Lincoff AM, Kereiakes DJ, Costa F, et al. Long-term dual antiplatelet therapy for secondary preven-tion of cardiovascular events in the sub-group of patients with previous myocardial infarction: A collaborative meta-analysis of randomized trials. *Eur Heart J*. 2016;37:390–399.

87. Bonaca MP, Bhatt DL, Steg PG, Storey RF, Cohen M, Im K, et al. Ischaemic risk and efficacy of ticagrelor in relation to time from P2Y12 inhibitor withdrawal in patients with prior myocardial infarction: Insights from PEGASUS-TIMI 54. *Eur Heart J*. 2016;37:1133–1142.

88. Palmerini T, Della Riva D, Benedetto U, Bacchi Reggiani L, Feres F, Abizaid A, et al. Three, six, or twelve months of dual antiplatelet therapy after DES implantation in patients with or without acute coronary syndromes: An individual patient data pairwise and network meta-analysis of six randomized trials and 11 473 patients. *Eur Hear J*. 2017;38:1034–1043.

89. Bellemain-Appaix A, O'Connor SA, Silvain J, Cucherat M, Beygui F, Barthelemy O, et al. Association of clopidogrel pretreatment with mortality, cardiovascular events, and major bleeding among patients undergoing percutaneous coronary intervention: A sys-tematic review and meta-analysis. *JAMA*. 2012;308:2507–2516.

90. Members ATF, Kolh P, Windecker S, Alfonso F, Collet J-P, Cremer J, et al. 2014 ESC/EACTS guidelines on myocardial revas-cularization: The Task Force on myocardial revascularization of the European Society of Cardiology (ESC) and the European Association for Cardio-Thoracic Surgery (EACTS) developed with the special con-tribution of the European Association of Percutaneous Cardiovascular Interventions (EAPCI). *Eur J Cardiothorac Surg*. 2014;46(4):517–592.

91. Kastrati A, Mehilli J, Schuhlen H, Dirschinger J, Dotzer F, ten Berg JM, et al. A clinical trial of abciximab in elective percutaneous coronary intervention after pretreatment with clopidogrel. *N Engl J Med.* 2004;350:232–238.

92. Valgimigli M, Percoco G, Barbieri D, Ferrari F, Guardigli G, Parrinello G, et al. The additive value of tirofiban administered with the high-dose bolus in the prevention of ischemic complications during high-risk coronary angioplasty: The ADVANCE Trial. *J Am Coll Cardiol.* 2004;44:14–19.

93. Costa F, Vranckx P, Leonardi S, Moscarella E, Ando G, Calabro P, et al. Impact of clinical presentation on ischaemic and bleeding outcomes in patients receiving 6- or 24-month duration of dual-antiplatelet therapy after stent implantation: A pre-specified analysis from the PRODIGY (Prolonging Dual-Antiplatelet Treatment After Grading Stent-Induced Intimal Hyperplasia) trial. *Eur Hear J.* 2015;36:1242–1251.

94. Schulz-Schupke S, Byrne RA, Ten Berg JM, Neumann FJ, Han Y, Adriaenssens T, Tolg R, et al. ISAR-SAFE: A randomized, double-blind, placebo-controlled trial of 6 vs. 12 months of clopidogrel therapy after drug-eluting stenting. *Eur Hear J.* 2015;36:1252–1263.

95. Gilard M, Barragan P, Noryani AAL, Noor HA, Majwal T, Hovasse T, et al. 6- versus 24-month dual antiplatelet therapy after implantation of drug-eluting stents in patients nonresistant to aspirin: The randomized, multicenter ITALIC trial. *J Am Coll Cardiol.* 2015;65:777–786.

96. Colombo A, Chieffo A, Frasheri A, Garbo R, Masotti-Centol M, Salvatella N, et al. Second-generation drug-eluting stent implantation followed by 6- versus 12-month dual antiplatelet therapy: The SECURITY randomized clinical trial. *J Am Coll Cardiol.* 2014;64:2086–2097.

97. Feres F, Costa RA, Abizaid A, Leon MB, Marin-Neto JA, Botelho RV, et al. Three vs twelve months of dual antiplatelet therapy after zotarolimus-eluting stents: The OPTIMIZE randomized trial. *JAMA.* 2013;310:2510–2522.

98. Kim BK, Hong MK, Shin DH, Nam CM, Kim JS, Ko YG, et al. A new strategy for discontinuation of dual antiplatelet therapy: The RESET Trial (REal Safety and Efficacy of 3-month dual antiplatelet Therapy following Endeavor zotarolimus-eluting stent implantation). *J Am Coll Cardiol.* 2012;60:1340–1348.

99. Mauri L, Kereiakes DJ, Yeh RW, Driscoll-Shempp P, Cutlip DE, Steg PG, et al. Twelve or 30 months of dual antiplatelet therapy after drug-eluting stents. *N Engl J Med.* 2014;371:2155–2166.

100. Bittl JA, Baber U, Bradley SM, Wijeysundera DN. Duration of dual antiplatelet therapy: A systematic review for the 2016 ACC/AHA Guideline Focused Update on Duration of Dual Antiplatelet Therapy in Patients With Coronary Artery Disease: A report of the American College of Cardiology/American Heart Association Task Force on Clinical Practice Guidelines. *J Am Coll Cardiol.* 2016;68:1116–1139.

101. Hermiller JB, Krucoff MW, Kereiakes DJ, Windecker S, Steg PG, Yeh RW, et al. Benefits and risks of extended dual antiplatelet therapy after everolimus-eluting stents. *JACC Cardiovasc Interv.* 2016;9:138–147.

102. Ellis SG, Kereiakes DJ, Metzger DC, Caputo RP, Rizik DG, Teirstein PS, et al. Everolimus-eluting bioresorbable scaffolds for coronary artery disease. *N Engl J Med.* 2015;373:1905–1915.

103. Ali ZA, Serruys PW, Kimura T, Gao R, Ellis SG, Kereiakes DJ, et al. 2-year outcomes with the Absorb bioresorbable scaffold for treatment of coronary artery disease: A systematic review and meta-analysis of seven randomised trials with an individual patient data substudy. Lancet. 2017;390:760–772.

104. Bagai A, Peterson ED, Honeycutt E, Effron MB, Cohen DJ, Goodman SG, et al. In-hospital switching between adenosine diphosphate receptor inhibitors in patients with acute myocardial infarction treated with percutaneous coronary intervention: Insights into contemporary practice from the TRANSLATE-ACS study. *Eur Heart J: Acute Cardiovasc Care.* 2015;4(6):499–508.

105. Baumgartner H, Falk V, Bax JJ, De Bonis M, Hamm C, Holm PJ, et al. 2017 ESC/EACTS guidelines for the management of valvular heart disease. *Eur Hear J.* 2017;38:2739–2791.

106. Holmes DR, Jr., Mack MJ, Kaul S, Agnihotri A, Alexander KP, Bailey SR, et al. 2012 ACCF/AATS/SCAI/STS expert consensus document on transcatheter aortic valve replacement. *J Am Coll Cardiol.* 2012;59:1200–1254.

107. Hansson NC, Grove EL, Andersen HR, Leipsic J, Mathiassen ON, Jensen JM, et al. Transcatheter aortic valve thrombosis: Incidence, predisposing factors, and clinical implications. *J Am Coll Cardiol.* 2016;68(19):2059–2069.

108. Vavuranakis M, Siasos G, Zografos T, Oikonomou E, Vrachatis D, Kalogeras K, et al. Dual or single antiplatelet therapy after transcatheter aortic valve implantation? A systematic review and meta-analysis. *Curr Pharm Des.* 2016;22(29):4596–4603.

109. Feldman T, Foster E, Glower DD, Kar S, Rinaldi MJ, Fail PS, et al. Percutaneous repair or surgery for mitral regurgitation. *N Engl J Med.* 2011;364:1395–1406.

110. Alsidawi S, Effat M. Peri-procedural management of anti-platelets and anticoagulation in patients undergoing MitraClip procedure. *J Thromb Thrombolysis.* 2014;38:416–419.

111. Califf RM. A perspective on the regulation of the evaluation of new antithrombotic drugs. *Am J Cardiol.* 1998;82:25–35.

112. Dunne H, Cowman, Kenny D. MRS2179: A novel inhibitor of platelet function. *BMC Proceedings.* 2015;9:A2–A2.

113. Wong PC, Watson CA, Bostwick J, Banville J, Wexler RR, Priestley ES, et al. Abstract 13794: An orally-active small-molecule antagonist of the platelet protease-activated receptor-4, BMS-986141, prevents aeterial thrombosis with low bleeding liability in cynomolgus monkeys. *Circulation.* 2017;136:A13794–A13794.

114. Yanachkov IB, Chang H, Yanachkova MI, Dix EJ, Berny-Lang MA, Gremmel T, et al. New highly active antiplatelet agents with dual specificity for platelet P2Y1 and P2Y12 adenosine diphosphate receptors. *Eur J Med Chem.* 2016;107:204–218.

115. Gurbel PA, Bliden KP, Turner SE, Tantry US, Gesheff MG, Barr TP, Covic L, Kuliopulos A. Cell-penetrating pepducin therapy targeting par1 in subjects with coronary artery disease. *Arterioscler Thromb Vasc Biol.* 2016;36:189–197.

PART 4

Diagnostic procedures

25

Coronary angiography:
Techniques and tools of the trade

ROBERTO SPINA AND TOM GAVAGHAN

INTRODUCTION

Cardiac catheterisation consists of the invasive assessment of the left and right heart, and has evolved over the last few decades into a sophisticated, highly specialised and low-risk diagnostic procedure that requires considerable skills, intensive training and dedicated support staff. As an invasive imaging modality, coronary angiography is currently considered the gold standard in the diagnosis of the coronary tree. It may be performed concomitantly with left ventriculography and/or right heart catheterisation, and the findings direct percutaneous coronary intervention. The diversity of catheters from various companies and improvements in imaging equipment through digital cardiac technology have made this a predictably safe, reliable and accurate test in the investigation of the cardiac patient. This chapter discusses the indications, equipment and various technical aspects in the performance of cardiac catheterisation and coronary angiography.

INDICATIONS FOR CORONARY ANGIOGRAPHY

Coronary angiography is performed to investigate coronary artery disease in the setting of acute coronary syndrome, stable angina, or in response to adverse or inconclusive results on non-invasive testing such as stress echocardiography or myocardial perfusion testing. Cardiac catheterisation is valuable in the investigation of valvular and congenital cardiac abnormalities and to assess the patient with cardiomyopathy, pulmonary hypertension, cardiac shunting, pericardial disease and arrhythmias.

Cardiac catheterisation, due to its invasive nature, carries risk of serious complications. Therefore, determining the appropriate use of diagnostic coronary angiography is of utmost importance. According to the ACCF/SCAI/AATS/AHA/ASE/ASNC/HFSA/HRS/SCCM/SCCT/SCMR/STS 2012 Appropriate Use Criteria for Diagnostic Catheterisation, 'an appropriate diagnostic cardiac catheterisation (left heart, right heart, ventriculography, and/or coronary angiography) is one in which the expected incremental information combined with clinical judgment exceeds the negative consequences by a sufficiently wide margin for a specific indication that the procedure is generally considered acceptable care and a reasonable approach for the indication'.[1] The above-mentioned document contains a detailed list of appropriate uses of cardiac catheterisation.

Diagnostic coronary angiography is now frequently followed by additional procedures, including adjunctive pharmacological treatments (nitroglycerine, verapamil and thrombolytic drugs); intracoronary ultrasound (IVUS) to accurately quantify coronary atherosclerosis and the effects of coronary interventions; and insertion of a coronary pressure wire to study the haemodynamic significance of a coronary stenosis and for evaluation of interventional techniques (angioplasty, stenting, and /or rotational atherectomy).

Vascular access

Historically, the arterial and venous circulation were accessed by direct surgical approach (femoral or brachial). This approach has been largely abandoned with the advent of percutaneous techniques of cannulating the femoral and radial vessels.

Initially the femoral approach was the predominant access route for diagnostic cardiac catherisation, but in the last decade, transradial access has gained wide popularity and acceptance because of a lower vascular complication rate and better patient acceptance and has become the predominant access modality worldwide.

The importance of a thorough and meticulous approach to insertion of angiography catheters into the vascular system cannot be overemphasised. This one step, completed successfully, enables the operator to perform the insertion and manipulation of diagnostic catheters with remarkable efficiency and accuracy and to minimise the potential complications of a prolonged procedure.

Percutaneous technique. Sites for arterial puncture include femoral, radial, brachial and axillary arteries, as shown in Figure 25.1.

Prior to formal draping of the patient, laboratory personnel should accurately assess the patient's peripheral vascular status for later comparison after removal of the arterial sheath. Depending on the arm or leg approach, proper positioning of the

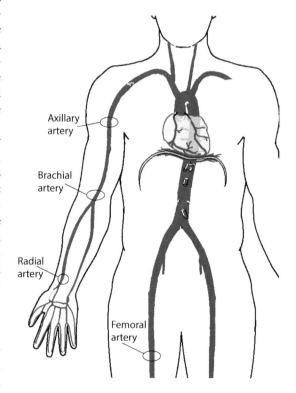

Figure 25.1 Illustration of arterial pathway and puncture sites for radial, brachial, axillary and femoral arteries.

patient toward the head of the catheter table and a stable, comfortable position of the patient's arms allows smooth progress throughout the procedure.

FEMORAL ARTERY

Historically, arterial access in the cardiac catheterisation laboratory has been obtained using anatomic landmarks, along with pulsation and/or fluoroscopic guidance for femoral access. Despite wide acceptance outside the cardiac catheterisation laboratory for vascular access with guideline recommendations endorsing its use, use of ultrasound in the cardiac catheterisation laboratory remains infrequent. Rather than relying on a single approach, contemporary femoral access should ideally be obtained combining all four available techniques: (1) Fluoroscopy; (2) ultrasound; (3) micropuncture access; (4) femoral angiography.

Contemporary techniques for obtaining femoral vascular access include the following steps (Figure 25.2).[2] After appropriate skin sterilisation and draping of the right or left groin with sterile, disposable angiographic setup packages, the artery is palpated immediately beneath the inguinal skin crease using the middle and index fingers of the left hand. Local anaesthetic (1% or 2% xylocaine) is infiltrated into the skin 1 or 2 cm distal to the point of anticipated arterial puncture. Further infiltration is performed down to the arterial surface, taking care, with frequent aspiration, to avoid injecting directly into the artery. Up to 15 mL is used to adequately anaesthetise this area and assist in the possible deployment of a percutaneous vascular closure device at the end of the procedure. A small 3 mm incision is made using a scalpel blade and a subcutaneous tunnel is opened with blunt dissection from curved arterial forceps. A haemostat is used to identify the lower edge of the femoral head (Figure 25.2a), and position is confirmed with fluoroscopy, as in Figure 25.2b. Ultrasound may be used to visualise the bifurcation of the common femoral artery into superficial femoral and profunda femoris (Figure 25.2c–f). A sharp 18-gauge needle is held between thumb and index finger of the right hand, and firm palpation is made with the left hand to stabilise the femoral artery above and below the skin incision. With the needle tip bevel directed upwards, the needle is slowly advanced at an angle of 40°–45° with the horizontal plane and, usually, a firm pulsatile resistance is felt as the needle abuts the wall of the vessel. Further gentle

advancement is required, and then a strong pulsatile jet of blood indicates that the needle has entered the true lumen of the artery. As indicated in Figure 25.3, while stabilising the needle with the left hand, a soft J-tipped guidewire is passed through the needle under fluoroscopic guidance about 15–20 cm into the proximal vessel without resistance. Needle entry position (arrow) is assessed using fluoroscopy (Figure 25.2g). The introducing needle is then withdrawn while pressure is maintained over the puncture site with the left hand. An appropriately sized sheath and dilator are passed along the clean guidewire with a forward, twisting motion into the femoral artery. In the patient with significant tortuosity of the iliac artery, it may be advantageous to use a 23–30 cm long sheath in order to facilitate subsequent catheter exchanges and to improve torque control of the distal end of the diagnostic catheter. Once the sheath has been inserted into the femoral artery, an iliofemoral angiogram should be performed to confirm satisfactory entry position (Figure 25.2h). A 20°–30° ipsilateral angulation of the detector will identify the entry point of the sheath, as well as the femoral bifurcation.

It is important to achieve femoral arterial puncture at the level of the common femoral artery, in a space delimited superiorly by the inguinal ligament and inferiorly by the bifurcation of the common femoral artery into the superficial femoral artery and the profunda femoris artery (Figure 25.4). Arteriotomy sites at this level are compressible. Punctures that are above the inguinal ligament lie in a non-compressible space, and risk injuring the inferior epigastric artery. These high punctures increase the risk of serious and occasionally life-threatening retroperitoneal haemorrhage.[3] Punctures below the bifurcation of the common femoral artery may be difficult to compress because of the soft tissue overlying it. These low punctures are associated with an increased risk of arterial pseudoaneurysm and arteriovenous fistula formation.[3]

RADIAL ARTERY

This approach is possible if the patient has an easily-palpable radial pulse and a negative Allen test (intact ipsilateral ulnar circulation). However, many operators do not routinely test the patency of the ulnar circulation based on the findings of two randomised trials that demonstrated no clinical or

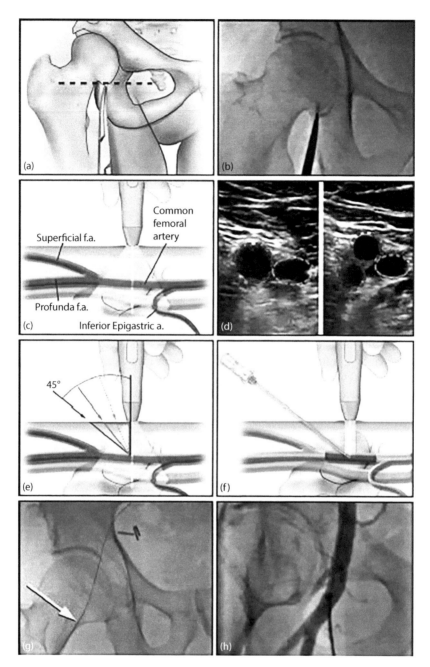

Figure 25.2 A haemostat is used to identify lower edge of femoral head (a), and position is confirmed with fluoroscopy (b). Ultrasound may be used to visualise the bifurcation of the common femoral artery bifurcation into superficial femoral and profunda femoris. (c–f). Needle is advanced until pulsatile flow is observed, and guidewire is advanced into the artery. Needle entry position (arrow) assessed using fluoroscopy (g). Once the sheath has been inserted into the femoral artery, an ilio-femoral angiogram should be performed to confirm satisfactory entry position (h). (Reproduced with permission from Sandoval, Y., et al., *JACC Cardiovasc. Interv.*, 10, 2233–2241, 2017.)

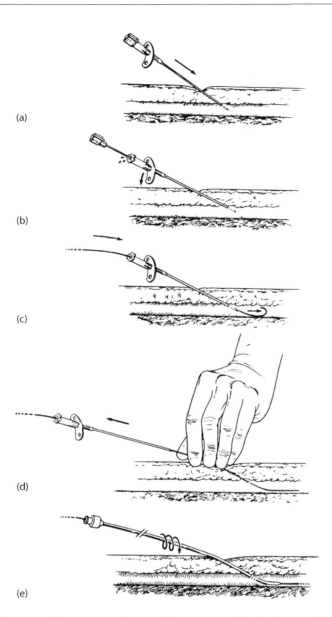

(a)

(b)

(c)

(d)

(e)

Figure 25.3 The Seldinger technique. (a) The vessel is punctured with the needle at a 30° to 40° angle. (b) The stylet is removed and free blood flow is observed; the angle of the needle is then reduced. (c) The flexible tip of the guidewire is passed through the needle into the vessel. (d) The needle is removed over the wire while firm pressure is applied at the site. (e) The tip of the catheter is passed over the wire and advanced into the vessel with a rotating motion. (Reprinted from *Cardiovascular Procedures: Diagnostic Techniques and Therapeutic Procedures*, Tilkian, A.G. and Daly, E.K., Copyright (1986), with permission from Elsevier.)

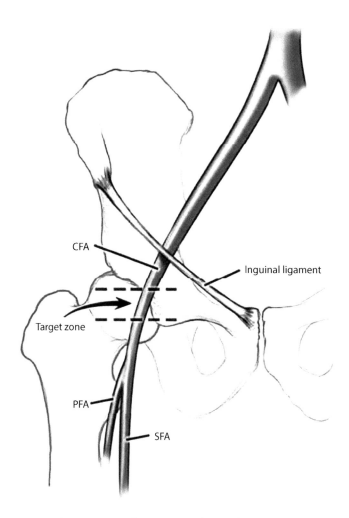

Figure 25.4 The target zone for access to the common femoral artery is delimited superiorly by the inguinal ligament, and inferiorly by the bifurcation of the common femoral into the superficial femoral artery and profunda femoris artery. CFA, common femoral artery; PFA, profunda femoris artery; SFA, superficial femoral artery. (Reproduced from Bhatty, S., et al., *Interv. Cardiol.*, 3, 503–514, 2011. With permission.)

subclinical signs of hand ischemia and no major ischemic complications in patients with abnormal Allen or Barbeau tests.[4,5] The radial artery is a small-calibre vessel and has a tendency to spasm upon instrumentation. Using the Seldinger technique, the 18-gauge needle is very carefully advanced at 45° into the radial artery and upon bleed-back a very soft 0.018-inch guidewire is advanced into the vessel, then a 5 Fr or 6 Fr sheath is passed smoothly into the artery up to the full length of the sheath. Following sheath insertion, intra-arterial nitro or verapamil are injected to prevent radial artery spasm, and heparin (2000–5000 U) is administered to reduce risk of radial artery occlusion.

In the event of radial artery spasm not responding to intra-arterial administration of spasmolytics, additional analgesia and sedation might be of benefit. Sheath and catheter downsizing (i.e. 6 Fr to 5 Fr or 5 Fr to 4 Fr) and minimisation of wire and catheter movement and exchanges might also help. Occasionally radial artery spasm may be so severe that catheter entrapment occurs, requiring deep sedation with general anaesthesia to retrieve the equipment.

BRACHIAL AND AXILLARY ARTERIES

These approaches are less commonly used because of difficulty in securing adequate haemostasis after removal of the sheath. Both sites are nonetheless valuable in the patient with inaccessible femoral vessels and with inadequate collateral perfusion of the hand. Venous access for right heart catheterisation is possible via the major central veins (subclavian and internal jugular), as well as femoral and antecubital veins. The percutaneous approach is similar to that for arterial access but aspiration on the venous needle for brisk drawback of blood is necessary to confirm that the tip of the needle is intravascular, before proceeding to insert the guidewire and sheath.

SELECTION OF DIAGNOSTIC CATHETERS

Once there is stable arterial and/or venous access it is necessary to choose appropriate size, length and shape of diagnostic catheters. Ideally, one would choose a catheter with good torque control to allow accurate transmission of manipulative movement from the hub of the catheter to the distal tip, and a catheter with moderate stiffness, sufficient radio-opacity, good memory and an adequate internal lumen to facilitate injection of contrast. Diagnostic catheters vary in size from 4 Fr to 9 Fr and most diagnostic studies are performed with 5 Fr or 6 Fr catheters. There is lower risk of femoral haematoma with 5 Fr catheters. This has implications for outpatient angiography in the current cost-conscious healthcare environment.

There is great variety in subtle characteristics (stiffness, radio-opacity, torque control and memory) among catheters of various companies and it is only possible to find the best individual feel by comparing different products.

The guidewire provides the safest means by which an open-ended catheter can be passed from a distal insertion point along the circulatory tree to the vessel to be examined. There is a large selection available and the most commonly used wires include the 0.035- or 0.038-inch J-tipped standard wire, the 0.035-inch movable core wire (with variable length distal flexible tip), and the 0.038-inch teflon-coated Glidewire for patients with marked tortuosity or atherosclerotic disease of the iliac system. These wires are usually curved and soft in the tip and stiffer in the shaft to avoid any trauma to the vessel wall and yet allow smooth passage of the catheter to the region of interest. The straight-tipped Glidewire is often used inside a pigtail,

Judkins right or Amplatz (AL1) diagnostic catheter as a means of crossing the aortic valve in significant aortic stenosis.

CORONARY ANGIOGRAPHIC CATHETERS

Femoral approach

Judkins left and right coronary catheters have preformed curves that allow relatively easy positioning of catheters in the ostium of the relevant coronary artery. Judkins catheters are available in different-sized curves according to the size of the aortic root and, to a lesser degree, the take-off of the coronary artery.

Amplatz left and right coronary catheters are also preshaped catheters that are used for angiography of both native coronary vessels and difficult graft studies. These catheters can be used for angiography via the radial and brachial approach. In all cases, however, there is a higher incidence of coronary dissection due to the rather aggressive hook shape of the distal end of the catheter.

The Multipurpose catheter is designed such that it is capable of selectively catheterising both left and right coronary arteries and can then be used to perform ventriculography without the need to exchange to other diagnostic catheters. This inherently requires greater manipulative skills and involves longer fluoroscopy times, hence making the multipurpose catheter a second choice for most operators. Coronary vein graft catheters (left and right) are specifically designed to cater for the high, anterior origin of the left grafts and the vertically oriented take-off of right grafts. In difficult cases, it is often possible to selectively cannulate the grafts using Amplatz and/or Multipurpose catheters.

The internal mammary artery graft catheter is designed to fit the acute inferior take-off of either mammary artery and may be useful in the catheterisation of left coronary grafts.

Brachial approach

The brachial artery was the original access site via surgical cutdown for percutaneous entry, but is now rarely used. The Sones catheter is a straight catheter with a tapered tip that is advanced carefully over a guidewire around the tortuous brachiocephalic vessels to the proximal aorta and then manipulated into both left and right coronary arteries. This requires considerable training before adequate competency is achieved.

Judkins, Amplatz and Multipurpose catheters are acceptable alternatives for coronary angiography from the right brachial approach and, due to their preformed shape, these catheters usually sit securely in the ostium of the coronary artery once intubated. Amplatz catheters are well suited to cannulate a superiorly-directed high-takeoff left main coronary artery and to engage the origin of both left and right bypass grafts (venous or free-pedicle arterial grafts).

Radial approach

The transradial approach to coronary angiography may be significantly more challenging compared to the femoral approach, due to smaller vessel size and greater vessel tortuosity. Figure 25.5a demonstrates the different catheter course in transfemoral versus transradial coronary angiography: Whereas one area of resistance is encountered transfemorally, two areas of resistance are found in transradial angiography. Commonly used catheter shapes used in transradial angiography are also illustrated in Figure 25.5b.

The Judkins catheters are the frontline shapes used to perform coronary angiography from the radial artery. For the engagement of the left main coronary ostium from the right radial artery, a Judkins left 3.50 is usually the most appropriate catheter choice. When approaching the left main trunk from the left radial artery, a catheter with a longer distance between primary and secondary curves, such as the Judkins left 4.0 coronary catheter, is necessary. Engagement of the right coronary ostium is usually performed with a Judkins right 4.0 diagnostic catheter. If engagement is difficult with these catheters, the Amplatz left curves are usually successful in reaching both left and right coronary ostia. In the presence of significant brachiocephalic tortuosity, the following manoeuvres and additional steps might allow for easier intubation: (1) Deep inspiration will stretch the subclavian and innominate arteries and the aorta vertically, making coronary incubation easier; (2) using the stiff end of the standard J-wire to deploy the catheter tip near the coronary ostia; (3) using a stiff wire such as an Amplatz extra-stiff or super-stiff guidewire (taking care not to allow the stiff wire to exit the catheter distally, to prevent aortic trauma) to deploy

the catheter tip near the coronary ostia; (4) upgrading the French size of the catheter; (5) using a guide catheter with or without guidewire support. If all these measures are unsuccessful, conversion to the femoral approach might be necessary.

Additional diagnostic catheters have been developed to meet specific challenges of transradial angiography. These shapes are illustrated in Figure 25.5c. The Tiger diagnostic catheter is designed to allow intubation of both left and right coronary ostia without exchanging catheter. However, successful intubation of both coronary ostia is not always possible, and intubation of the left coronary ostium via the left radial approach may prove challenging with the Tiger catheter.

VENTRICULOGRAPHY CATHETERS

Femoral approach

Typically, the multiple side-hole Pigtail catheter is passed retrogradely through the aortic valve into the body of the left ventricle.

Brachial and radial approach

The multipurpose, NIH, pigtail or Sones catheters can be used for left ventriculography from these approaches. Catheters with a single endhole should not be used for ventriculography because of the risk of myocardial perforation.

TECHNIQUES OF ANGIOGRAPHY

General principles

MANIFOLD MANAGEMENT

A two- or three-port, plastic, disposable manifold is commonly used for diagnostic and/or interventional coronary procedures. The manifold acts as an airtight closed junction between the catheter, pressure manometer, radio-opaque dye line, infusion port and injecting port. Rigid attention throughout the procedure to ensure that the line and manifold are free of air minimises the chance of significant air embolism to the coronary bed or aorta. The injection syringe should be held constantly in a downward sloping direction to prevent inadvertent injection of air bubbles during image acquisition. Accurate arterial waveform recognition is necessary during angiography in order to

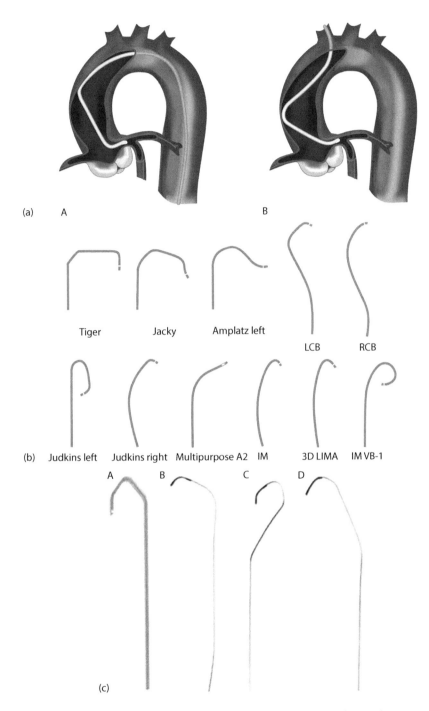

Figure 25.5 **(a)** This figure illustrates the different catheter course in transfemoral versus transradial coronary angiography. Whereas one point of contact/area of resistance is encountered transfemorally (A), two points of contact/areas of resistance are found in transradial angiography (B); **(b)** commonly used diagnostic catheters in transradial coronary angiography; **(c)** specialty catheters designed specifically for use via the radial approach. A: Kimny; B: Tiger; C: Ikari left; D: Ikari right. ([a] Courtesy of Medtronic Australasia; [b] Courtesy of Terumo; [c] Courtesy of Cardiac Interventions Today.)

detect damping of the pressure trace. This may indicate air in the system or possible catheter tip impaction against the arterial intima or an ostial obstruction. Further injection of dye under force may precipitate intimal dissection. Usually, gentle withdrawal of the catheter resolves this problem without injury to the vessel wall.

CONTRAST INJECTION

All angiographic contrast media currently in use are derivatives of tri-iodinated benzene. In recent years, improved patient tolerance and a lower incidence of adverse effects have favoured an increased preference for non-ionic hydrophylic agents with low viscosity and low osmolarity and osmolality, particularly for patients with renal impairment. In most angiography suites ionic agents are no longer used. The incidence of renal failure requiring dialysis after contrast administration is greatly increased in diabetics and patients with a history of renal failure. Contrast-induced acute renal failure following angiography can occur in as many as 8% of in-patients with healthy kidneys, and contrast administration still accounts for 11% of hospital-acquired cases of renal failure.[6] Concern over potential toxicity and osmotic load stress restricts dosages given to a conservative level. True anaphylactoid responses are not dose-dependent.

Contrast media (often called dye) can be injected either manually through a refillable syringe or via a power automated injector. Contrast is usually injected at 2–4 mL/sec with volumes of 3–6 mL for the right coronary and 6–10 mL for the left coronary artery. During faster heart rates, a higher rate of injection is required.

Catheter manipulation

After the syringe and manifold have been correctly set up and the pressure trace is clear and pulsatile, the operator must concentrate on placement of the diagnostic catheter into the relevant artery under fluoroscopic control in a specified X-ray viewing plane. Manipulation of the catheter is usually done by one of two methods:

Method 1: First, the doctor may elect to have the scrub nurse stabilise the manifold/syringe with manual support while using the right hand to rotate the hub of the catheter and the left hand to provide forward or backward motion to the

catheter after it enters the femoral, brachial or radial sheath.

Method 2: The doctor may prefer to support the manifold and catheter hub assembly in the right hand and use the left hand for forward/backward motion on the catheter shaft as it enters the sheath. With this approach, the manifold is stabilised between the third, fourth and fifth fingers of the right hand and right palm, leaving the thumb and index finger to provide rotation of the hub as desired. Although greater dexterity is required with this approach, it allows for smoother, more subtle movement of the diagnostic catheter during a difficult cannulation. It is essential to recognise that one-to-one torque transmission from the hub to the distal catheter tip is greatly facilitated by gentle back-and-forth movement on the catheter with the left hand while rotating the hub with the right hand. This tends to avoid the sudden whip-like rotation of the catheter tip that results from excess build-up of non-transmitted torque.

Panning

Most operators acquire coronary images using the five- to six-inch (17 cm) field size to enable sufficient magnification of the coronary arteriogram and reduce image distortion from overlying lung and diaphragm. In order to account for the reduced field of view it is necessary for the operator to move (or pan) the X-ray table during the latter third of each imaging sequence to follow the flow of dye from the proximal to the more distal segments of each coronary artery. This requires practice in the various viewing planes and is essential for accurate assessment of late-filling collateral vessels and unsuspected anatomical variants. Generally, in the right anterior oblique (RAO) view, the table is moved slowly towards the operator and slightly cranially. In the left anterior oblique (LAO) view the table is panned in a cranial direction. Figure 25.6 illustrates the viewing planes formed by positioning the X-ray source and detector at various angles around the patient.

Cardiologists refer to the orientation of the U-arm according to the position of the detector (above the table) in relation to the patient's left side as the LAO projection, with the generator (below the table) on the patient's right side. Radiologists

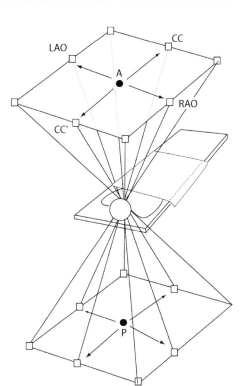

Figure 25.6 Positioning of X-ray camera around the patient, illustrating the various viewing planes and angiographic projections (*Abbreviations:* RAO, right anterior oblique; LAO, left anterior oblique; A, anterior; P, posterior; CC, caudo-cranial; CC', cranio-caudal). The cardiologist's preference for determining C-arm orientation in relation to position of the detector rather than the generator is followed.

refer to the position of the generator in relation to the patient's left (with the detector on the patient's right) as the LAO projection. Hence, the terms RAO and LAO to a cardiologist mean the opposite to a radiologist; similarly, with the terms caudo-cranial and cranio-caudal. The terminology used in this text refers to the cardiologist's viewpoint.

Angiographic views

In most modern cardiac catheterisation laboratories, the X-ray source (the generator) is beneath the table and the camera (detector) is above the patient. In the LAO projection, the detector is rotated in the transverse plane to the left of the patient. On the resulting angiogram, the spine is usually seen on the right side of the image. The RAO projection is the opposite and entails rotation of the detector

to the patient's right, the spine being seen on the left side of the subsequent images. In specific cases, the detector is rotated toward the patient's head (cranial) or feet (caudal) in order to accurately outline otherwise overlapping vessels.

As a general rule, cranial views are helpful for assessment of the left anterior descending coronary artery (LAD) and caudal views for the left circumflex artery (LCx). For graft angiography the standard views are important, with emphasis on the left lateral view for distal LAD anastomoses, LAO cranial for distal right coronary artery anastomoses and RAO/LAO caudal for left circumflex anastomoses.

Left ventriculography provides essential information on ventricular contractility, particularly in cases of myocardial infarction and cardiomyopathy, along with aortic and mitral valve function. When left ventriculography is performed, the standard view is 30° RAO for single-plane assessment and calculation of the ejection fraction. For additional information on regional left ventricular function or shunting, an additional 30°–60° LAO view provides complete biplane ventriculography.

At times it is necessary to perform aortography to complete the cardiac catheter investigation. The proximal and arch aortogram is set up in the LAO using digital subtraction angiography as the preferred mode of acquisition and with the lowest X-ray magnification (largest field size). Usually 40–50 mL of dye at 20–25 mL/sec is sufficient with a power injector. The aortogram provides essential data for complete assessment of aortic valve disease, aortic dissection, aortic aneurysm, coarctation of the aorta and patent ductus arteriosus.

Coronary anatomy

The key to identifying coronary artery anatomy lies in mentally forming a three-dimensional (3D) image of the heart from the 2D pictures presented on screen. The heart may be considered in 3D as an oval football shape, with two imaginary planes of reference transsecting the football longitudinally (Figure 25.7a, top panels) across two orthogonal planes of cross-section equivalent to the echocardiographic parasternal long and short axis views. The LAD courses along the longitudinal plane, running along the seam of the football before curving anteriorly, while the LCx courses clockwise around the circumference of the football in the short axis

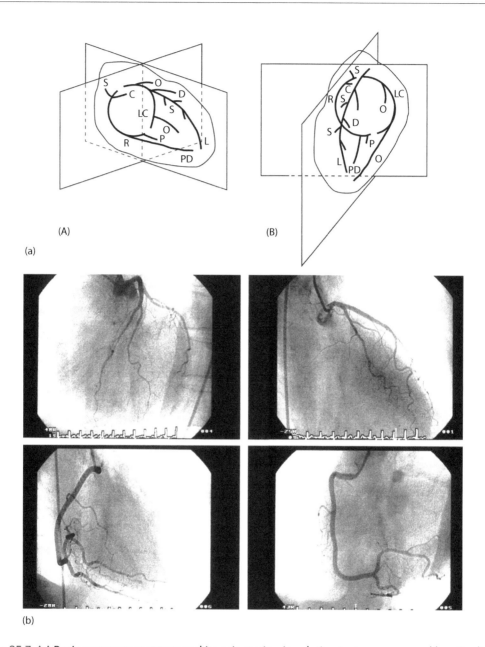

(a)

(A)　　　　　　　　　　　(B)

(b)

Figure 25.7 **(a)** Basic coronary anatomy and its orientation in relation to transverse and longitudinal planes of cross-section. (A): Right anterior oblique view (RAO), (B): Left anterior oblique view (LAO). (R, right coronary artery; LC, left circumflex coronary artery; L, left anterior descending coronary artery; D, diagonal branch; L, lateral branch; S, septal branch). **(b)** Set of angiographs showing the typical angiographic presentation of left and right coronary arteries. Clockwise from top left: Left coronary artery in LAO projection; left coronary artery in RAO projection; right coronary artery in LAO projection; right coronary artery in RAO projection with cranial tilt. Exact angulation is shown by numbers at bottom corners of each frame.

plane, tracking along the atrio-ventricular groove. The proximal right coronary artery (RCA) runs counter-clockwise along the same plane as the LCx, branching distally to form the posterior descending and posterolateral branches.

The LAD can be identified in the RAO view by the septal perforators tracking downwards at right angles from its main trunk, with the diagonal branches extending to the right. In the LAO views, septal vessels project towards the left of the LAD, the diagonals to the right. The LCx gives rise to the obtuse marginal and lateral ventricular branches.

The RCA is anatomically less complex and can be readily identified in any view. The conus and right atrial branches arise proximally from the RCA. Distally, the point at which the RCA bifurcates into the posterior descending and posterolateral branches is called the crux. The main trunk of the posterior descending branch of the RCA lies in the same longitudinal plane as the LAD. The main trunks of the LCx and RCA lie along the same plane.

Standard viewing planes for left and right coronary arteries are summarised in Table 25.1. The angiographic anatomy of normal left and right coronary arteries is shown in Figure 25.7b (bottom four panels).

SELECTIVE CORONARY ANGIOGRAPHY

Femoral technique

After successful insertion of the femoral artery sheath, a preshaped left and right catheter (usually Judkins or Amplatz design) or a Multipurpose catheter can be used for selective angiography of the coronary vessels. The appropriate catheter with preloaded 0.035-inch guidewire is inserted through the femoral sheath, and under fluoroscopic guidance the wire is gently advanced ahead of the catheter along the abdominal aorta, around the aortic arch and to the mid-ascending aorta. The diagnostic catheter is positioned just above the sinuses of Valsalva and the wire is withdrawn carefully. After

Table 25.1 Standard viewing planes for angiographic examination of left and right coronary arteries

Coronary segment	Standard views	Other views
Left main	RAO caudal	AP
	LAO cranial	
	LAO caudal	
Proximal LAD	LAO cranial	AP caudal
	RAO cranial	
Mid LAD	LAO cranial	AP cranial
Distal LAD	RAO cranial	Lateral
Diagonal	LAO cranial	LAO caudal
	RAO cranial	
Proximal LCx	RAO caudal	AP caudal
Intermediate,	LAO caudal	
Obtuse marginal		
Left posterolateral	LAO cranial	LAO caudal
Posterior descending artery	RAO cranial	
Proximal RCA	LAO	Lateral
Mid RCA	LAO	Lateral
Distal RCA	LAO cranial	Lateral
	AP cranial	
PDA, Posterolateral	LAO cranial	RAO cranial
	AP cranial	

Abbreviations: LAD, Left anterior descending; LCx, left circumflex; RCA, right coronary artery; LAO, left anterior oblique; RAO, right anterior oblique; AP, anterio-posterior.

meticulous aspiration and flushing technique to ensure that no air bubbles or thrombus lie within the system, the catheter assembly is now ready for manipulation into the relevant coronary artery.

The Judkins catheters

Selection of appropriate left Judkins catheter (JL3.5, JL4.0, JL5.0, JL6.0) depends primarily on the operator's assessment of the size of the aortic root. A small female often requires a JL3.5 catheter whereas for severe aortic stenosis, Marfan's syndrome or prominent aortic unfolding, the JL5 or JL6 is appropriate. The Judkins left catheter requires slow advancement and minimal manipulation to cannulate the left coronary artery. Usually inserted in the LAO view, it is important to ensure that the tip of this end-hole catheter is not deeply engaged against the roof of the left main coronary artery, with the risk of inducing dissection in this area. Alteration or damping of the pressure wave may indicate such occurrence and hence gentle withdrawal and test injection is required to confirm a safer, more axial orientation with the left main orifice. The Judkins left catheter is then exchanged for the right and is best advanced towards the right coronary in the LAO projection. Initially the catheter is directed toward the left coronary sinus. Gentle clockwise torque on the hub, coupled with a smooth push/pull movement on the catheter shaft causes the tube to migrate anteriorly and then either into or just below the origin of the right coronary artery. Excessive rotation usually results in the catheter flicking out of the ostium during inspiration and then the same manoeuvre must be repeated. Preformed catheters that do not require rotation are available and are particularly useful in patients with severe peripheral vascular disease or dilated aortas.

The Amplatz catheters

These preshaped catheters have a rounded distal curve leading to a sharply angulated terminal hook for the left coronary and a less sharp hook for the right coronary artery. The most commonly used left coronary Amplatz catheter (AL2) is advanced in the LAO view towards the left sinus and then gently moved forward to make the tip climb up towards the left main ostium. This is a more aggressive catheter shape, and care is needed when disengaging the left Amplatz by pushing slightly forward to move the catheter tip above the left main coronary for safe removal. The right (modified) Amplatz catheter is inserted in the LAO view by the same approach as the right Judkins, starting with clockwise rotation from the left coronary sinus.

The multipurpose catheter

This catheter makes for a faster and more efficient diagnostic angiogram but does require greater manipulative skills on the part of the operator. The technique is similar to the Sones technique and requires formation of a terminal loop on the catheter either in the LAO or RAO projection. In the LAO view, for cannulation of the left coronary artery the loop is enlarged by forward motion and slight counter-clockwise rotation until the catheter tip is near the left main ostium. At this point, slight clockwise rotation moves the tip to the left main and, if desired, the tip may enter the ostium farther during inspiration by slight withdrawal of the catheter. To approach the right coronary, a less pronounced loop is used in the LAO projection. The catheter tip is directed towards the left sinus and then rotated clockwise from the left cusp until the tip is pointing toward the right sinus and slightly cranially. This usually engages the ostium of the right coronary artery. During inspiration, care must be taken to avoid deep cannulation of vertical, downward take-off right coronary vessels.

Brachial and radial techniques

The brachial artery is entered by either open cutdown or percutaneous puncture; the radial artery is entered only by percutaneous puncture. Most commonly, the Sones catheter (5–6 Fr) is used with this approach and is a multipurpose catheter for coronary angiography and ventriculography. The catheter is usually inserted with a guidewire through the subclavian artery (often acutely angulated and tortuous) into the ascending aorta. The more flexible tip may be preshaped by the operator before insertion, thus allowing easier formation of a loop in the left coronary sinus after withdrawal of the guidewire. In the LAO view, this loop can be enlarged by forward/backward motion and counter-clockwise rotation of the catheter until the tip reaches the left main ostium. During inspiration, the tip can be 'lifted' into the left ostium by gentle withdrawal and clockwise rotation. After completion of the left coronary runs, the Sones catheter tip is withdrawn and a less pronounced loop is formed in the left coronary sinus. A smooth clockwise rotation and gentle push/pull movement of the catheter shaft rotates the tip and loop towards the right coronary sinus and the tip enters the right coronary ostium. The catheter tends to deeply intubate the right coronary artery and may need gentle withdrawal during respiratory movements.

The preshaped Amplatz catheters can be used from both brachial and radial approaches but must be inserted over a guidewire. They tend to sit snugly in the ostia of the coronary arteries once engaged.

SELECTIVE CORONARY BYPASS GRAFT ANGIOGRAPHY

From the femoral approach, graft angiography (either vein grafts or free mammary or radial grafts) can often be performed using the same right Judkins or modified right Amplatz catheters used for the native right coronary injections. These catheters should be placed in the mid-ascending aorta in the LAO view, and clockwise rotation usually causes the catheter to seat in the graft ostium. If the grafts are placed in a more anterior position on the aorta, then a left coronary bypass graft catheter or Amplatz AL2 catheter can be used to find the graft ostium. Right coronary grafts (vertically downward takeoff) can usually be found by the right Judkins, right modified Amplatz or Multipurpose catheter rotated clockwise from a slightly more proximal aortic position.

Mammary artery grafts are most often approached from the femoral artery using an acutely angulated preshaped mammary artery catheter. After passage of this catheter to the proximal aortic arch over the preferred guidewire, a reliable method of accessing the left subclavian artery is described. The guidewire is withdrawn approximately 8–10 cm into the catheter and then gentle withdrawal of the catheter with mild counter-clockwise rotation causes the catheter to access sequentially the right innominate, then the left common carotid and then the left subclavian artery. Once at the origin of the left subclavian, the guidewire is passed forward into the axillary artery and the mammary catheter is moved forward along the wire just beyond the origin of the left internal mammary artery. After withdrawing the wire and flushing the system, the catheter is

carefully withdrawn with slight counter-clockwise (anterior) rotation. This frequently causes the catheter tip to subtly drop into the ostium of the mammary artery. Small test injections and occasional minor forward or backward adjustment of the catheter facilitate proper selective injections.

For patients with severe peripheral vascular disease, the right and/or left radial or brachial approach is needed to find the mammary arteries, using the same diagnostic catheters. Great care is needed when intubating the mammary ostium to avoid dissection or spasm at this delicate area. An over-forceful graft injection may cause intense chest wall burning to the patient.

Accessory imaging modalities

Selective coronary angiography remains the standard for assessment of coronary artery anatomy. Ancillary imaging modalities such as IVUS and optical coherence tomography provide more detailed anatomical information on specific intravascular characteristics (dissection, stent apposition, extent of vessel calcification, virtual histology). These modalities, however, do not provide assessment of the functional significance of a coronary stenosis. Fractional flow reserve (FFR) and the instantaneous wave-free ratio (iFR) provide direct physiological assessment of the extent to which a coronary stenosis restricts epicardial myocardial blood flow and cause ischemia (see Chapter 26). FFR must be measured during maximal hyperemia, which is typically induced with administration of a potent intravenous or intracoronary vasodilator, such as adenosine. iFR is a pressure-derived index of stenosis severity that does not require administration of a vasodilator, thus making assessment of the functional significance of a stenosis faster, safer, and more cost-efficient. In two large, recent, multicentre, randomised, controlled, open-label clinical trials enrolling patients with stable angina or an acute coronary syndrome, an iFR-guided revascularisation strategy was non-inferior to an FFR-guided revascularisation strategy with respect to the rate of major adverse cardiac events at 12 months.[7-8]

FUTURE DIRECTIONS

Modern-day diagnostic cardiac catheterisation is a safe invasive procedure providing useful anatomical and physiological assessment of the coronary tree and the state of myocardial perfusion. Future directions at further minimising risk of adverse events to patients and operators alike include: (1) Reducing the radiation dose absorbed by operators and patients by using low-dose fluoroscopy only instead of high-dose acquisition or by using remotely-controlled robotic coronary angiography; (2) use of IVUS instead of contrast angiography and the development of less nephrotoxic iodinated contrast media in patients with renal dysfunction; (3) wider adoption of transradial angiography; (4) improvement of closure devices for femoral access angiography. With continued advances in angiographic imaging technology, it may even be possible to acquire a single continuous acquisition of each coronary artery with 270° rotational view (the 'spin' technique) currently in use for transcatheter aortic valve implantation procedures. Ultimately, it may even be possible to enhance ultrasound technology (echocardiography) to permit transthoracic coronary artery imaging. As the technology, both physical and virtual (algorithms) improves, axial modalities such as magnetic resonance imaging (MRI) and computed tomography (CT) will become more specific, more spatially accurate, and less limited in terms of physical limitations (calcium/beam hardening artefact and voxel resolution in CT, or time resolution/movement artefact and availability for MRI). For now, however, traditional methods endure.

REFERENCES

1. Patel MR, Bailey SR, Bonow RO, Chambers CE, Chan PS, Dehmer GJ, et al. ACCF/SCAI/AATS/AHA/ASE/ASNC/HFSA/HRS/SCCM/SCCT/SCMR/STS 2012 appropriate use criteria for diagnostic catheterization: A report of the American College of Cardiology Foundation Appropriate Use Criteria Task Force, Society for Cardiovascular Angiography and Interventions, American Association for Thoracic Surgery, American Heart Association, American Society of Echocardiography, American Society of Nuclear Cardiology, Heart Failure Society of America, Heart Rhythm Society, Society of Critical Care Medicine, Society of Cardiovascular Computed Tomography, Society for Cardiovascular Magnetic Resonance, and Society of Thoracic Surgeons. J Am Coll Cardiol. 2012;59:1995–2027.
2. Sandoval Y, Burke MN, Lobo AS, Lips DL, Seto AH, Chavez I, et al. Contemporary arterial access in the cardiac catheterization laboratory. JACC Cardiovasc Interv. 2017;10:2233–2241.
3. Bhatty S, Cooke R, Shetty R, Jovin IS. Femoral vascular access-site complications in the cardiac catheterization laboratory: Diagnosis and management. Interv Cardiol. 2011;3:503–514.
4. Valgimigli M, Gagnor A, Calabró P, Frigoli E, Leonardi S, Zaro T, et al. Radial versus femoral access in patients with acute coronary syndromes undergoing invasive management: A randomised multicenter trial. Lancet. 2015;385:2465–2476.
5. Valgimigli M, Campo G, Penzo C, Tebaldi M, Biscaglia S, Ferrari R, for the RADAR investigators. Transradial coronary catheterization and intervention across the whole spectrum of Allen test results. J Am Coll Cardiol. 2014;63:1833–1841.
6. Bartorelli AL, Marenzi G. Contrast-induced nephropathy. J Interv Cardiol. 2008;21(1):74–85.
7. Götberg M, Christiansen EH, Gudmundsdottir IJ, Sandhall L, Danielewicz M, Jakobsen L. Instantaneous wave-free ratio versus fractional flow reserve to guide PCI. N Engl J Med. 2017;376:1813–1823.
8. Davies JE, Sen S, Dehbi HM, Al-Lamee R, Petraco R, Nijjer SS. Use of the instantaneous wave-free ratio or fractional flow reserve in PCI. N Engl J Med. 2017;11:376:1824–1834.
9. Tilkian, A.G., Daly, E.K. Cardiovascular Procedures: Diagnostic Techniques and Therapeutic Procedures, St. Louis, MO, 1986.

HISTORICAL REFERENCES

1. Judkins MP. Selective coronary angiography: 1. A percutaneous transfemoral technic. Radiology. 1967;89:815–824.
2. Judkins MP, Gander M. Prevention of complications of coronary angiography (editorial). Circulation. 1974;49:599–602.

3. Kiemeneij F, Laarman GJ. Percutaneous tran-sradial artery approach for coronary Palmaz-Schatz stent implantation. *Am Heart J.* 1994;128:167–174.

FURTHER READING

Fihn SD, Blankenship JC, Alexander KP, Bittl JA, Byrne JG, Fletcher BJ, et al. 2014 ACC/AHA/ AATS/PCNA/SCAI/STS focused update of the guideline for the diagnosis and management of patients with stable ischemic heart disease: A report of the American College of Cardiology/American Heart Association Task Force on Practice Guidelines, and the American Association for Thoracic Surgery, Preventive Cardiovascular Nurses Association, Society for Cardiovascular Angiography and Interventions, and Society of Thoracic Surgeons. *J Thorac Cardiovasc Surg.* 2015;149(3):e5–e23.

Kern MJ, Sorajja P, Lim MJ. *The Cardiac Catheterization Handbook.* 6th ed. Philadelphia, PA: Elsevier; 2016. 416 p.

Moscucci M, editor. *Grossman & Baim's Cardiac Catheterization, Angiography, and Intervention.* 8th ed. Philadelphia, PA: Wolters Kluwer/ Lippincott Williams & Wilkins; 2014. 1141 p.

Vasheghani-Farahani A, Sadigh G, Kassaian SE, Khatami SM, Fotouhi A, Razavi SA, et al. Sodium bicarbonate plus isotonic saline versus saline for prevention of contrast-induced nephropathy in patients undergoing coronary angiography: A randomized controlled trial. *Am J Kidney Dis.* 2009;54(4):610–618.

26

Physiological assessment of coronary lesion severity

USAID ALLAHWALA AND RAVINAY BHINDI

INTRODUCTION

Coronary artery disease (CAD) is the commonest cause of morbidity and mortality in Australia and much of the world.[1] The decision to institute interventions for CAD, including percutaneous coronary intervention (PCI) has traditionally relied on diagnostic coronary angiography alone. This had traditionally been instituted when an epicardial coronary lesion was considered 'significant' – conventionally determined by a stenosis ≥50% in the left main coronary artery, or ≥70% stenosis in other major epicardial vessels. However, over the past few decades it has become increasingly apparent that angiography alone cannot determine whether a lesion produces ischaemia, and that adjunctive use of coronary physiology results in improved clinical outcomes and cost-effectivenes.[2] The most commonly adopted invasive physiologic indices are fractional flow reserve (FFR) and instantaneous wave-free ratio (iFR). While use of coronary physiology has been well established in those with stable CAD, it is widely expanding its role to include assessment during acute coronary syndromes (ACS), and following PCI to assess reduction in ischaemia burden as well as use in those with co-existing conditions affecting haemodynamics such as valvular heart disease.

Similarly, intracoronary imaging has provided additional benefit in the diagnosis and performance of PCI. The commonly used imaging modalities of intravascular ultrasound (IVUS) and optical coherence tomography (OCT) has allowed near-histological level of detail of coronary vessels with implications for providing more informed interventions.

A comprehensive understanding of the rationale, performance and interpretation of coronary physiology is paramount to sound clinical work for all clinical staff involved in interventional cardiology. Similarly, intravascular imaging will continue to be more readily adopted routinely, and its performance will be a pre-requisite for those wanting to work within the ever-adapting field of interventional cardiology.

CORONARY PHYSIOLOGY

Fractional flow reserve

RATIONALE FOR FRACTIONAL FLOW RESERVE (FFR)

FFR is the ratio of the mean coronary pressure distal to a stenosis (P_d) to the mean aortic pressure (Pa) at maximal hyperaemia, i.e. when myocardial resistance is at its presumed absolute minimum. This condition allows pressure and flow to be linearly related, and hence FFR represents the fraction of normal coronary blood flow across a stenosis, with a normal value being 1.0, meaning flow proximal and distal is equivalent at any time. FFR requires the induction of maximal hyperaemia, which most commonly is achieved with administration of adenosine, either via an intravenous (IV) infusion or as an intracoronary bolus (Figure 26.1). Adenosine results in vasodilation of the microcirculation, counteracting autoregulation, and ensures maximal hyperaemia.

PERFORMING FFR

FFR is measured with use of ultra-thin 0.015-inch angioplasty pressure monitoring guidewires. After diagnostic angiography is performed, lesions determined to be 'intermediate' in severity are

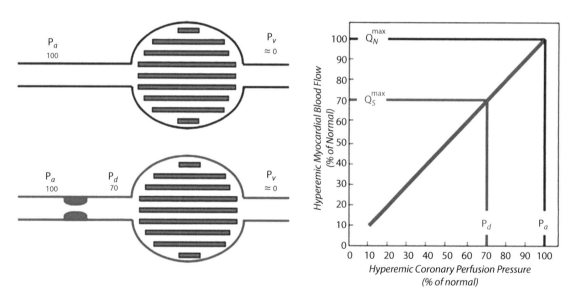

Figure 26.1 Concept of fractional flow reserve measurements: When no epicardial stenosis is present (top blue lines), the driving pressure P_a determines a normal (100%) maximal myocardial blood flow. In the case of stenosis responsible for a hyperaemic pressure gradient of 30 mmHg (bottom red lines), the driving pressure will no longer be 1000 mmHg but instead will be 70 mmHg (P_d). Because the relationship between driving pressure and myocardial blood flow is linear during maximal hyperaemia, myocardial blood flow will only reach 70% of its normal value. This numerical example shows how a ratio of 2 pressure (P_d/P_a) corresponds to a ratio of 2 flows (Q_s^{max}/Q_N^{max}). It also demonstrates how important it is to induce maximal hyperemisa. P_v = central venous pressure. (Adapted from Pijls, N.H. and Sels, J.W., J. Am. Coll. Cardiol., 9, 1045–1057, 2012.)

identified by interrogation with FFR. The pressure guidewire is introduced into the vessel, with the pressure monitor and the aortic guiding catheter transducer both being calibrated, or 'zeroed', as for any diagnostic angiogram, to atmospheric pressure as the reference point. Once the pressure wire sensor is within the vessel (but proximal to the stenosis) it should be 'equalised' or 'normalised' to ensure the $P_d/P_a = 1$, as pressure (and hence flow) should be equal in the aorta and coronary artery, in the absence of any epicardial stenosis. This ensures there are no confounders to results once the wire is distal to the stenosis. The sensor (which is located just proximal to the radio-opaque distal component of the pressure-wire) is then advanced distal to the lesion.

Administration of adenosine can be performed via intracoronary bolus administration of between 100–480 µg, but IV administration is preferable and should be performed for at least 90 seconds at a dose of 140 µg/kg/minute. Side effects with adenosine are common and patients should be warned of these. The commonest side effects are of dyspnoea and chest heaviness, reported by 20% and 7.2% of patients respectively.[3] Less common side effects include heart rhythm disturbances (~5%), hypotension, nausea and vomiting, ventricular arrhythmia and bronchospasm. Given the very short half-life of adenosine these adverse effects are transient, but should be recognised, with appropriate provisions for emergent management available. In the case of intracoronary boluses, repeat procedures may be performed to ensure reproducibility. Following acquisition of an FFR value, the sensor should be withdrawn to a location proximal to the lesion to ensure the P_d/P_a is 1 and ensure there has been 'no drift'. If a significant change in the P_d/P_a is noticed – repeat equalisation and subsequent repeat FFR measurements may be necessary (Figure 26.2, top panel).

INTERPRETATION OF FFR

In 1996, Pijls and colleagues published their landmark paper,[4] in which they compared the validity of FFR to accurately detect haemodynamically significant lesions that appeared only moderate in severity on diagnostic angiography, against established noninvasive measures of myocardial ischaemia. Three important studies have followed,

DEFER,[5] FAME[6] and FAME II,[7] that firmly established FFR as an integral tool in the assessment of coronary artery disease severity, illustrating both safety in deferral of PCI for lesions with a non-significant FFR, as well as improvement in major adverse cardiac events in the treatment of those with a significant FFR. While initial studies suggest a threshold of 0.75, the threshold has been raised to 0.80 to improve the sensitivity of FFR, and it is the threshold endorsed by the American College of Cardiology (ACC), American Heart Association (AHA), Society for Cardiovascular Angiography and Interventions (SCAI), and European Society of Cardiology (ESC) in their guidelines for PCI.

IMPACT OF RIGHT ATRIAL PRESSURE ON FFR

The FFR equation used above (where FFR = P_d/P_a), is an abbreviated version of the equation for myocardial fractional flow reserve (where $FFR_{myo} = [P_d - RAP]/[P_a - RAP]$, and RAP = right atrial pressure). The abbreviated version applies when RAP is minimal, or near-zero. If RAP is low, there is little or no resistance to venous return, or on myocardial perfusion and flow, but if RAP is elevated (say above 10 mmHg), there is increased resistance to venous drainage. This increased resistance may compromise the baseline requirement for maximal hyperaemia. Removing RAP from both numerator and denominator in the FFR equation, particularly when RAP is low, compensates for this effect. It has been demonstrated, however, that actual differences between FFR_{myo} and FFR are minimal, and the impact of RAP is negligible, even in patients with markedly increased RAP.[8]

FFR IN ACUTE CORONARY SYNDROMES

The utility of FFR in acute coronary syndromes (ACS), and in particular during ST elevation myocardial infarction (STEMI), has been controversial, predominantly due to concerns in the ability to reliably achieve maximal hyperaemia in a dysfunctional microcirculation. Consequently, a sub-hyperemic response to adenosine would result in an underestimation of stenosis severity so that an FFR >0.80 at the time of a STEMI may increase several days later as the injured myocardial bed recovers and flow increases to the area. However, studies have shown FFR has excellent accuracy in predicting perfusion defects on cardiac magnetic resonance imaging in patients with ACS.[9] Similarly, in the DANAMI3-PRIMULTI trial,[10] FFR-guided complete revascularisation during the index admission for non-infarct related arteries following a STEMI was associated with a significant reduction in the primary endpoint, primarily driven by a reduction in ischaemia-driven revascularisation. In the COMPARE-ACUTE trial,[11] FFR-guided complete revascularisation was done during the index procedure following a STEMI, a time when the microcirculation is believed to be dysfunctional. FFR-guided complete revascularisation was associated with lower mortality, AMI and need for revascularisation, while approximately 50% of those lesions that were angiographically significant were not physiologically significant.

The ideal threshold for FFR in the ACS population has been debated, with studies finding that a threshold of 0.8 in those with a ACS was associated with a three-fold increase in the risk of subsequent AMI and target vessel failure compared with those with stable CAD, and perhaps a cut off of 0.85 should be applied to those presenting with ACS.[12]

FFR following PCI

FFR post PCI has not been studied in large randomised trials, with meta-analysis of smaller studies suggesting a higher FFR value associated with significant reduction in MACE, and an FFR of ≥ 0.90 associated with a 55% relative risk reduction in need for repeat PCI and a 30% reduction in MACE.[13] However, the paucity of randomised evidence showing the clinical utility of routine post PCI FFR measurements suggests it should only be performed in specific situations.

Instantaneous wave-free ratio

The *instantaneous wave-free ratio* (iFR) is a resting index used to assess severity of an intracoronary stenosis. It measures the ratio of P_d to the P_a during an isolated period of diastole (the 'wave-free period'). A cut-off value of 0.89 has been identified as a marker of ischaemia. It is an attractive

alternative to FFR because it does not require hyperemia, and therefore has a lower incidence of patient discomfort, side effects, and shorter procedural time. In the DEFINE-FLAIR[3] and iFR-SWEDEHEART[14] trials, iFR was found to be non-inferior to FFR for guiding revascularisation with respect to MACE.

While FFR and iFR generally have a high rate of concordance, in 20% of cases there is discordance, raising clinical decision-making dilemmas. Which, if either, index is superior remains uncertain and is an area of ongoing research.

Tandem lesions

In the setting of serial (tandem) stenosis within a vessel, FFR values of a proximal lesion can be underestimated, most commonly as a result of an inability to induce maximal hyperaemia with adenosine. Thus, while the FFR value gives a summative FFR for the entire vessel in the setting of tandem lesions, it does not distinguish which lesion would be contributing most, and hence cannot be used in isolation to determine which lesion would benefit from PCI. As such, FFR values may often need to be repeated following PCI to a distal lesion. While equations to compute FFR for each lesion, correcting for the presence of the other, have been validated,[15] these require measuring pressure during balloon occlusion of the vessel (highly impractical) (Figure 26.2, bottom panel). One alternative is to perform a pressure wire pullback. After obtaining an FFR of the vessel, if it is <0.80 then perform a pullback FFR during an IV adenosine infusion and measure the change in pressure (ΔP) across each lesion. Once the pullback is completed, the lesion with the greatest pressure gradient (ΔP, rather than absolute change), should be treated with PCI first. A repeat FFR should subsequently be performed, and if the value remains <0.80, further PCI should be performed.

While this process is time-intensive and cumbersome, iFR has the advantage of independently assessing each lesion to determine the ischaemic potential of each lesion, without needing to attain maximal hyperemia. Newer co-registration technologies allow iFR lesions to be seen on the fluoroscopic image of the vessel in real time, allowing the operator to determine the optimal location for PCI.

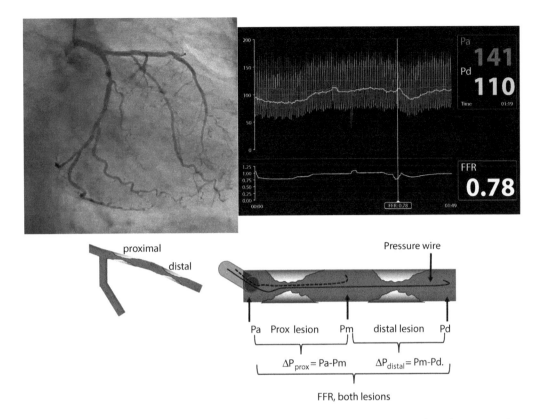

Figure 26.2 (Top panel) Fractional flow reserve (FFR) assessment in an intermediate lesion: A 68 year old male presenting with Canadian Class 3 angina. Fluoroscopic image showing an intermediate mid left circumflex lesion, which was determined to be 65% stenosis by quantitative coronary angiography. FFR value of 0.78 was recorded and subsequent revascularisation was performed; (Bottom panel): FFR in Tandem lesions. Diagram of pressures and pressure gradients across lesions in series (Pa, aortic pressure; Pm, mid pressure between lesions; Pd, distal pressure; ΔP, pressure gradients produced be each lesion.) (Adapted from Kern, M., *Cath. Lab. Digest.*, 20, 2012.)

INTRAVASCULAR IMAGING

Optical coherence tomography

BACKGROUND

Optical coherence tomography (OCT) is an imaging modality whereby an image of the lumen and deep structures up to 3 mm is created by directing an optical beam of infrared light onto the tissue, and measuring the reflected intensity of light.[16] OCT allows exquisite assessment of the luminal wall and structure to a near-histological tissue assessment level. This can add value to angiography as a diagnostic and/or interventional tool for PCI guidance. It has multiple uses in diagnosing,

procedural planning and early identification of complications. It is important that appropriate performance and interpretation of OCT is established for clinical staff working within the cardiac catheterisation laboratory.

PERFORMANCE

The OCT catheter is inserted into the vessel along a guidewire, ensuring the imaging component is distal to the lesion. As erythrocytes can degrade image quality, the vessel must be 'flushed' clear of blood with either iodinated contrast or crystalloid solution while the imaging catheter is simultaneously and automatically pulled back to create a cross-sectional image of the vessel of interest.

CLINICAL UTILITY OF OCT

One of the primary benefits of OCT is that of determining aetiology of lesions identified on angiography, particularly during an ACS.[17] OCT has 100% sensitivity of identifying intracoronary thrombus, compared with 33% for IVUS,[18] which is particularly useful in cases of ambiguity between calcium and thrombus, as it drastically alters management. Similarly, OCT is the gold standard for identifying acute plaque rupture[18] and is twice as sensitive as IVUS.

OCT allows operators to accurately identify features of the lesion to be stented, including identifying degree and depth of calcification, which results in superior lesion preparation and which may dictate need for rotational athrectomy or scoring balloons. Furthermore, adequate sizing and appropriate over-sized stent selection (and hence aggressive post dilatation to ensure adequate stent expansion) can be more accurately determined with OCT. Intravascular OCT-derived minimal lumen area (MLA) has a tendency to be smaller than IVUS calculations,[19] which may result in under-sizing of a stent, and hence measuring the diameter from the external elastic lamina has been advocated.[20] OCT is not generally able to accurately estimate the MLA of the left main stem as it is difficult to clear blood from contrast, and hence physiological interrogation with IVUS or a combination of both is typically recommended in such situations.

OCT post PCI can also be performed allowing immediate identification of complications with a very high degree of sensitivity, including edge dissection,[21] tissue prolapse, stent malapposition[16] and stent under-expansion,[22] the latter of which is most closely correlated with clinical sequelae of stent failure (Figure 26.3).

There is an important distinction to be re-iterated, that while OCT allows very accurate and detailed cross-sectional and longitudinal luminal analysis, it cannot predict the

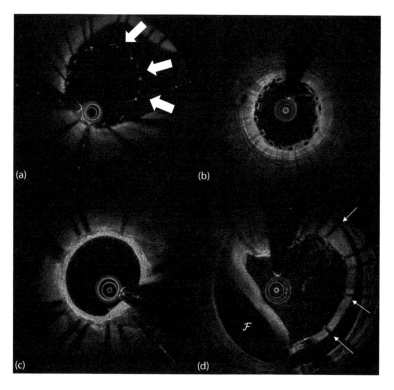

Figure 26.3 Optical coherence tomography (OCT) images. **(a)** OCT image of a metallic stent which is significantly underexpanded, with stent struts not apposed to the vessel intima (thick arrows); **(b)** OCT images of bioresorbable scaffold, identifiable by its thicker, box shaped struts; **(c)** neoatherosclerosis seen within a previously well-expanded metallic stent; **(d)** spiral coronary artery dissection complicating coronary intervention with metallic stents. The false lumen (labelled *F*) is seen well with OCT imaging, with underexpanded metallic stents seen in the true lumen.

physiological implication of the lesion, and hence cannot be used to determine whether ischaemia is present, and should ideally be used in conjunction with haemodynamic assessment of the vessel.

INTRAVASCULAR ULTRASOUND

Intravascular ultrasound (IVUS) is a modality that, similarly to OCT, allows use of sound waves to create a cross sectional image of a vessel, allowing a more informed performance of PCI. Most commercially available IVUS catheters contain a rotating transducer within a short, monorail imaging sheath to create cross-sectional IVUS images. Unlike OCT, blood does not need to be flushed from the vessel of interest during image acquisition, and a manual pullback of the catheter is performed.

While we have covered the evidence for use of haemodynamic assessment to determine the ischaemic potential of a lesion, studies have shown a modest correlation between IVUS-derived MLA and ischaemia. With a cut-off of 3 mm^2 advocated in some studies, IVUS-derived MLA appears to have a high negative predictive value (75%–90%) but a relatively poor positive predictive value (40%–70%), suggesting that while it may be acceptable to defer PCI based on IVUS, it should not be solely relied upon to determine suitability of PCI.[23] Conversely, interrogation of an intermediate left main stenosis has relative equipoise between IVUS and haemodynamic assessment. An MLA of <6 mm^2 has been shown to be a predictor of poor outcomes, similar to an FFR of <0.80,[24] although care should be taken in patients of differing ethnicities, sex and body surface area.[25,26]

IVUS is similar to OCT in regard to identification of lesion characteristics, with the exception of not being able to image calcium depth, although allowing more overall penetration of the vessel wall and imaging of larger vessels. Numerous studies have shown that use of IVUS as an adjunct to angiography reduces early and intermediate rates of MACE, including mortality.[27,28] Similarly, IVUS has been shown to reduce MACE following percutaneous chronic total occlusion PCI,[29] as well as significantly reduce contrast load[30] and can actually be cost-saving[31] when compared to angiography alone.

OCT vs. IVUS

While there are certain situations where OCT may be superior to IVUS (e.g. identifying thrombus) and vice versa (e.g. imaging left main coronary artery stenosis), there has been a paucity of data directly comparing IVUS with OCT in clinical outcomes. The ILLUMIEN III trial[20] was a crossover study comparing OCT-directed, IVUS-directed and angiography-alone PCI. The primary endpoint of OCT-derived minimum stent area showed OCT was non-inferior to IVUS, although OCT was not superior to angiography alone. While there are inherent dangers in extrapolating surrogate measures for clinical benefit, further research is needed to determine in which situations one imaging modality is preferable to the other.

CONCLUSION

Interventional cardiology has progressed substantially over the last 60 years since the first recorded selective coronary angiogram. The modern coronary catheterisation laboratory is equipped not only for diagnostic coronary angiography, but for interrogation of the haemodynamics of pressure and flow within the coronary vasculature, as well as providing exquisite detail of vascular structures and disease processes. Use of physiological assessment has improved detection of lesions capable of ischaemia, as well as improved clinical outcomes when used to guide revascularisation. Intracoronary imaging, namely OCT and IVUS, has revealed the underlying pathobiological process of CAD, allowing detailed and informed sizing for stents as well as identifying complications following PCI. Whether this translates to meaningful improvements in clinical outcomes is currently being investigated, but initial studies certainly suggest an inherent benefit in their use in selected situations.

REFERENCES

1. ABS3303. Causes of Death. Australian Bureau of Statistics, 2013. 2013.
2. Fearon WF, Yeung AC, Lee DP, Yock PG, Heidenreich PA. Cost-effectiveness of measuring fractional flow reserve to guide coronary interventions. *Am Heart J.* 2003;145(5):882–887.

3. Davies JE, Sen S, Dehbi HM, Al-Lamee R, Petraco R, Nijjer SS, et al. Use of the instantaneous wave-free ratio or fractional flow reserve in PCI. *N Engl J Med.* 2017;376(19):1824–1834.

4. Pijls NH, De Bruyne B, Peels K, Van Der Voort PH, Bonnier HJ, Bartunek JKJJ, et al. Measurement of fractional flow reserve to assess the functional severity of coronary-artery stenoses. *N Engl J Med.* 1996;334(26):1703–1708.

5. Bech GJ, De Bruyne B, Pijls NH, de Muinck ED, Hoorntje JC, Escaned J, et al. Fractional flow reserve to determine the appropriateness of angioplasty in moderate coronary stenosis: A randomized trial. *Circulation.* 2001;103(24):2928–2934.

6. Tonino PA, De Bruyne B, Pijls NH, Siebert U, Ikeno F, van' t Veer M, et al. Fractional flow reserve versus angiography for guiding percutaneous coronary intervention. *N Engl J Med.* 2009;360(3):213–324.

7. De Bruyne B, Pijls NH, Kalesan B, Barbato E, Tonino PA, Piroth Z, et al. Fractional flow reserve-guided PCI versus medical therapy in stable coronary disease. *N Engl J Med.* 2012;367(11):991–1001.

8. Toth GG, De Bruyne B, Rusinaru D, Di Gioia G, Bartunek J, Pellicano M, et al. Impact of right atrial pressure on fractional flow reserve measurements: Comparison of fractional flow reserve and myocardial Fractional flow reserve in 1,600 coronary stenoses. *JACC Cardiovasc Interv.* 2016;9(5):453–459.

9. Layland J, Rauhalammi S, Watkins S, Ahmed N, McClure J, Lee MM, et al. Assessment of fractional flow reserve in patients with recent non-ST-segment-elevation myocardial infarction: Comparative study with 3-T stress perfusion cardiac magnetic resonance imaging. *Circ Cardiovasc Interv.* 2015;8(8):e002207.

10. Engstrom T, Kelbaek H, Helqvist S, Hofsten DE, Klovgaard L, Holmvang L, et al. Complete revascularisation versus treatment of the culprit lesion only in patients with ST-segment elevation myocardial infarction and multivessel disease (DANAMI-3-PRIMULTI): An open-label, randomised controlled trial. *Lancet.* 2015;386(9994):665–671.

11. Smits PC, Abdel-Wahab M, Neumann FJ, Boxma-de Klerk BM, Lunde K, Schotborgh CE, et al. Fractional flow reserve-guided multivessel angioplasty in myocardial infarction. *N Engl J Med.* 2017;376(13):1234–1244.

12. Hakeem A, Edupuganti MM, Almomani A, Pothineni NV, Payne J, Abualsuod AM, et al. Long-term prognosis of deferred acute coronary syndrome lesions based on non-ischemic fractional flow reserve. *J Am Coll Cardiol.* 2016;68(11):1181–1191.

13. Rimac G, Fearon WF, De Bruyne B, Ikeno F, Matsuo H, Piroth Z, et al. Clinical value of post-percutaneous coronary intervention fractional flow reserve value: A systematic review and meta-analysis. *Am Heart J.* 2017;183:1–9.

14. Gotberg M, Christiansen EH, Gudmundsdottir IJ, Sandhall L, Danielewicz M, Jakobsen L, et al. Instantaneous wave-free ratio versus fractional flow reserve to guide PCI. *N Engl J Med.* 2017;376(19):1813–1823.

15. Pijls NH, De Bruyne B, Bech GJ, Liistro F, Heyndrickx GR, Bonnier HJ, et al. Coronary pressure measurement to assess the hemodynamic significance of serial stenoses within one coronary artery: Validation in humans. *Circulation.* 2000;102(19):2371–2377.

16. Bezerra HG, Costa MA, Guagliumi G, Rollins AM, Simon DI. Intracoronary optical coherence tomography: A comprehensive review clinical and research applications. *JACC Cardiovasc Interv.* 2009;2(11):1035–1046.

17. Guagliumi G, Capodanno D, Saia F, Musumeci G, Tarantini G, Garbo R, et al. Mechanisms of atherothrombosis and vascular response to primary percutaneous coronary intervention in women versus men with acute myocardial infarction: Results of the OCTAVIA study. *JACC Cardiovasc Interv.* 2014;7(9):958–968.

18. Kubo T, Imanishi T, Takarada S, Kuroi A, Ueno S, Yamano T, et al. Assessment of culprit lesion morphology in acute myocardial infarction: Ability of optical coherence tomography compared with intravascular ultrasound and coronary angioscopy. *J Am Coll Cardiol.* 2007;50(10):933–939.

19. Bezerra HG, Attizzani GF, Sirbu V, Musumeci G, Lortkipanidze N, Fujino Y, et al. Optical coherence tomography versus intravascular ultrasound to evaluate coronary artery disease and percutaneous coronary intervention. *JACC Cardiovasc Interv.* 2013;6(3):228–236.

20. Ali ZA, Maehara A, Genereux P, Shlofmitz RA, Fabbiocchi F, Nazif TM, et al. Optical coherence tomography compared with intravascular ultrasound and with angiography to guide coronary stent implantation (ILUMIEN III: OPTIMIZE PCI): A randomised controlled trial. *Lancet.* 2016;388(10060):2618–2628.

21. Chamie D, Bezerra HG, Attizzani GF, Yamamoto H, Kanaya T, Stefano GT, et al. Incidence, predictors, morphological characteristics, and clinical outcomes of stent edge dissections detected by optical coherence tomography. *JACC Cardiovasc Interv.* 2013;6(8):800–813.

22. Liu X, Doi H, Maehara A, Mintz GS, Costa Jde R, Jr., Sano K, et al. A volumetric intravascular ultrasound comparison of early drug-eluting stent thrombosis versus restenosis. *JACC Cardiovasc Interv.* 2009;2(5):428–434.

23. Mintz GS. IVUS in PCI guidance. *JACC.* 2016;Expert Analysis.

24. Kang SJ, Ahn JM, Kim WJ, Lee JY, Park DW, Lee SW, et al. Functional and morphological assessment of side branch after left main coronary artery bifurcation stenting with cross-over technique. *Catheter Cardiovasc Interv.* 2014;83(4):545–552.

25. de la Torre Hernandez JM, Hernandez Hernandez F, Alfonso F, Rumoroso JR, Lopez-Palop R, Sadaba M, et al. Prospective application of pre-defined intravascular ultrasound criteria for assessment of intermediate left main coronary artery lesions results from the multicenter LITRO study. *J Am Coll Cardiol.* 2011;58(4):351–358.

26. Park SJ, Ahn JM, Kang SJ, Yoon SH, Koo BK, Lee JY, et al. Intravascular ultrasound-derived minimal lumen area criteria for functionally significant left main coronary artery stenosis. *JACC Cardiovasc Interv.* 2014;7(8):868–874.

27. Elgendy IY, Mahmoud AN, Elgendy AY, Bavry AA. Outcomes with intravascular ultrasound-guided stentImplantation: A meta-analysis of randomized trials in the era of drug-eluting stents. *Circ Cardiovasc Interv.* 2016;9(4):e003700.

28. Hong SJ, Kim BK, Shin DH, Nam CM, Kim JS, Ko YG, et al. Effect of intravascular ultrasound-guided vs angiography-guidede everolimus-eluting stent implantation: The IVUS-XPL Randomized Clinical Trial. *JAMA.* 2015;314(20):2155–2163.

29. Kim BK, Shin DH, Hong MK, Park HS, Rha SW, Mintz GS, et al. Clinical impact of intravascular ultrasound-guided chronic total occlusion intervention with zotarolimus-eluting versus biolimus-eluting stent implantation: Randomized study. *Circ Cardiovasc Interv.* 2015;8(7):e002592.

30. Mariani J, Jr., Guedes C, Soares P, Zalc S, Campos CM, Lopes AC, et al. Intravascular ultrasound guidance to minimize the use of iodine contrast in percutaneous coronary intervention: The MOZART (Minimizing cOntrast utiliZation With IVUS Guidance in coRonary angioplasTy) randomized controlled trial. *JACC Cardiovasc Interv.* 2014;7(11):1287–1293.

31. Alberti A, Giudice P, Gelera A, Stefanini L, Priest V, Simmonds M, et al. Understanding the economic impact of intravascular ultrasound (IVUS). *Eur J Health Econ.* 2016;17(2):185–193.

32. Pijls NH, Sels JW. Functional measurement of coronary stenosis. *J Am Coll Cardiol.* 2012;59(12):1045–1057.

33. Kern M. Serial lesion FFR made simple. *Cath Lab Digest.* 2012;20(9).

27

Non-invasive assessment of ischaemic heart disease

JAMES OTTON, PATRICK PENDER AND NEVILLE SAMMEL

INTRODUCTION

While invasive assessment of the coronary arteries is excellent at detecting coronary atherosclerosis and guiding treatment, non-invasive assessment of ischaemic heart disease (IHD) is often the preferred initial strategy for diagnosis and, in the modern era, provides an invaluable guide to medical, surgical and percutaneous treatment of coronary artery disease. Non-invasive techniques can be broadly classified into tests for ischemia, viability and anatomy. Each method has its own role in the management of ischemic heart disease.

ISCHAEMIC TESTING

In the past, treatment of coronary artery disease was frequently based upon anatomical appearance alone, such as the degree of luminal artery stenosis as seen by invasive coronary angiography. Current views from multiple sources of evidence, however, now point to the functional significance of coronary disease as the prime prognostic indicator and determinant of therapeutic benefit. Several studies including the FAME trial[1] have demonstrated the superiority of functional testing with invasive Fractional Flow Reserve (FFR) over anatomical assessment of coronary disease. Likewise, the long-term follow-up of the DEFER trial[2] indicates that percutaneous intervention and stenting in situations where the FFR indicates little or no functional significance (i.e. FFR > 0.80) is most likely detrimental to the patient over the long term. Consequently, FFR has become the de facto gold standard for the assessment of coronary stenosis, although it is sometimes forgotten that FFR validation and the chosen FFR threshold was based upon non-invasive imaging techniques.[3] Although robust, randomised trial evidence for non-invasive ischemia testing to guide PCI awaits the NIH sponsored ISCHEMIA trial,[4] a wealth of evidence suggests that ischemia is both a good prognostic indicator, and also a marker of treatment benefit for both medical and invasive treatments.[5] These data and the high concordance of non-invasive ischemic imaging techniques with invasive methods such as FFR have underscored the critical role of non-invasive assessment of ischemia in cardiology and cardiac catheterisation.

Non-invasive assessment of ischemia is used to guide coronary intervention before the procedure, or it may be used after diagnostic invasive coronary angiography where invasive functional measurement with FFR is not feasible or unavailable.

Exercise stress testing (EST)

EST is a non-invasive investigation using a treadmill, electrocardiogram (ECG) and blood pressure cuff. Patients are attached to a traditional 12-lead ECG and non-invasive blood pressure cuff and then exercised at increments to monitor heart rate, blood pressure response, and ECG patterns at varying levels of exertion. The test is widely available, inexpensive, has minimal technical demand and no burden of radiation, but has poor sensitivity and specificity in terms of diagnosing IHD.

Relative to other testing modalities, the stress ECG has lower sensitivity and specificity for detecting coronary disease and is dependent on its pre-test probability for coronary artery disease (Range Sensitivity 66%–80%, Range Specificity 65%–75% to detect coronary artery disease).[6] In those with intermediate pre-test risk, EST has been shown to have only 66% sensitivity and 75% specificity in a recent systematic review and meta-analysis.[6] In those with even lower pre-test probability, the specificity is poorer still, while those with a high pre-test probability have a low sensitivity, and EST is often unhelpful, as a negative result does not rule out coronary artery disease with any degree of certainty. As such, EST is not recommended for diagnosis of obstructive coronary disease where other modalities are available.

Screening EST in asymptomatic individuals has not been shown to be beneficial; however, EST may be useful to objectively quantify exercise capacity and the haemodynamic response in heart rate and blood pressure to exercise; assess for exercise-induced arrhythmias; as well as overall prognosis.

Stress echocardiography

Stress echocardiography combines a stress ECG with an echocardiogram performed immediately before and after stress. This can be achieved either through exercise (treadmill or bicycle) or a pharmacologic stress agent such as dobutamine.

Protocol guidelines from the American Society of Echocardiography[7] (ASE) recommend symptom-limited exercise according to standard protocols using either a treadmill or bicycle. With exercise regimens, the patient is required to transfer from treadmill to the sonographer's table into a recumbent position within a few seconds so that a complete set of images can be obtained as rapidly as possible (usually within 60 seconds following cessation of exercise).

In pharmacological stress testing, graded infusion of dobutamine is given in five stages, beginning at 5 µg/kg/min and incrementing to 10, 20, 30, and 40 µg/kg/min at 3-minute intervals. Images are acquired at rest, and then following completion of each stage and during recovery phase. This allows echocardiographic assessment prior to, during and after stress.

Use of digitised images permits side-by-side comparison of rest and post-exercise images in order to maximise accuracy of interpretation. If a cycle ergometer is used, then the stress echocardiogram can be performed during the end of exercise. Where there is insufficient perfusion to a myocardial area due to a coronary obstruction, the corresponding myocardium will be unable to contract normally due to demand ischemia (stress-induced segmental wall motion abnormalities). Stress echocardiography therefore shows areas of the heart that are ischemic or poorly supplied.

Furthermore, by combining Doppler evaluation alongside two-dimensional (2D) imaging, stress echocardiogram can also evaluate valvular function, pulmonary artery pressure, left ventricular outflow gradients, and diastolic function.

Contraindications to stress echocardiogram are the same as those for standard EST including active chest pain. Additional contraindications to pharmaceutical dobutamine stress test include tachyarrhythmias and uncontrolled systemic hypertension.[8] Poor imaging echocardiographic windows may hamper accurate testing. In this situation, an injection of soluble micro-bubble echo contrast agent may be of assistance, as these agents greatly enhance delineation between the blood pool and endocardium.

Radionuclide myocardial perfusion imaging

SINGLE PHOTON EMISSION COMPUTED TOMOGRAPHY (SPECT)

Nuclear perfusion imaging is generally performed with an intravenous injection of a radiopharmaceutical tracer, most typically technetium 99 m sestamibi. Most outpatient protocols take 2 to 3 hours. The test compares myocardial perfusion at rest with myocardial perfusion with 'stress'. Stress imaging can be achieved with either exercise or adenosine. Adenosine dilates normal coronary arteries but is unable to dilate stenosed arteries, thereby causing differential myocardial perfusion.

The tracer is taken up by intact viable myocardial cells. Areas of the heart that are relatively under-perfused receive less tracer, which is visible on computationally reconstructed scans (Figure 27.1). The rest and stress images are compared side by side. Comparison of these images determines whether regional perfusion is normal, with normal perfusion at both rest and stress, or due to ischemia with reduced perfusion at stress only, or due to infarction with reduced perfusion both at rest and stress.

The accuracy of nuclear perfusion is similar to that of stress echocardiography in most situations, with a large meta-analysis[9] reporting that myocardial perfusion imaging has 80% sensitivity and 73% specificity for detecting significant coronary disease. The main downside to nuclear perfusion imaging is radiation exposure and it is generally avoided in younger patients. A false negative test may occur in patients with balanced ischemia, e.g. left main coronary disease. The test is most beneficial for older patients with renal failure, arrhythmias or obesity, who would not be suitable for computed tomography (CT) coronary angiography or stress echocardiography.

CARDIAC POSITRON EMISSION TOMOGRAPHY (PET)

PET is a nuclear medicine technique used to image tissues and is based on the distinct ways normal and abnormal tissue metabolise positron-emitting radionuclides. Various PET imaging compounds, most typically ammonia, rubidium chloride, and fluoro-2-deoxy-d-glucose (FDG), include an isotopic label that emit a positron, the antimatter counterpart of an electron. On emission the positron meets and annihilates a corresponding electron, releasing two high-energy photons (gamma rays) with opposite momentum. These gamma rays are detected by an external array of elements in the PET scaffold and are digitally reconstructed into images.

PET imaging is most commonly used for viability testing,[10,11] although ammonia and rubidium PET tracers can also be used for ischemia quantification,

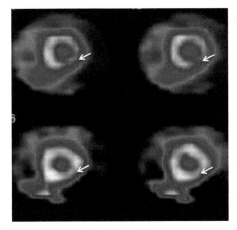
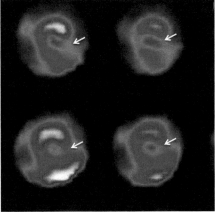

Figure 27.1 Myocardial perfusion: Technetium sestamibi single photon emission computed tomography (SPECT). The left panel shows a mild reversible perfusion deficit in the inferolateral wall. The deficit is present at stress (upper image) but normalises at rest. By contrast, on the right panel the deficit is severe and does not change with stress (upper image) or rest (lower image).

and appears highly accurate for diagnosing myocardial perfusion abnormalities[12]. PET tracers, however, tend to be more costly and have shorter half-lives than their SPECT counterparts.

Magnetic resonance imaging (MRI)

MRI imaging uses a strong magnetic field, proton nuclear spin and radiofrequency stimulation of proton spin in water molecules to generate an image. Unique among imaging modalities, the MRI image may be 'tuned' to exacerbate certain tissue qualities, such as oedema or fibrosis. T1, T2 ('Time to relaxation', weighted scans that describe the interaction of protons with nearby material) and proton density vary according to tissue type.

Cardiac MRI can provide very high-quality images of heart motion (cine imaging) and is frequently used to assess cardiac function. It can also assess for myocarditis using sequences where T2 (associated with oedema) is exacerbated. Tissue properties in cardiac tumours or unusual hypertrophy can be measured, and fat 'saturated' or removed from the image.

For assessment of ischemic heart disease function, perfusion imaging and direct imaging of the coronary arteries by MRI may be used. In perfusion testing, adenosine is administered while the patient is in the MRI scanner receiving an infusion of intravenous adenosine. A bolus of gadolinium-based contrast is then injected. The adenosine causes coronary vascular and microvascular dilatation, but where a fixed stenosis is present, there is relative hypoperfusion of downstream tissue. This is seen on the MRI perfusion scan as an area of reduced and delayed contrast wash in. A rest perfusion scan is usually performed to aid diagnosis. An advantage of MRI is that supplemental scanning to measure '*late gadolinium enhancement*' which can be used to assess areas of scar. This enables differentiation of hypoperfusion due to coronary stenosis compared to hypoperfusion due to prior infarction, as shown in Figure 27.2. Stress myocardial perfusion has been shown to be superior to nuclear perfusion in some studies,[13] and to correspond well to invasive haemodynamic assessments in detecting reversible ischemia.

Coronary imaging with cardiac MRI is also possible, although this is not as accurate as CT based coronary imaging.[14] It is mostly used to assess coronary anomalies in younger patients in whom exposure to ionising radiation is to be avoided.

A major contraindication of MRI scanning is that many older model implantable defibrillators and pacemakers are not certified for use within an MRI environment. Additional limitations of MRI include patient claustrophobia from the small image scanner, time-consuming acquisition, and metal foreign bodies (including intra-coronary stents) which produce metal artefact image distortion and potentially mask adjacent lesions.

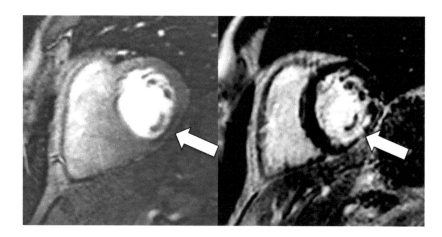

Figure 27.2 Still images of cardiac perfusion imaging (left) and late gadolinium enhancement (right). On perfusion assessment there is an area of subendocardial hypoperfusion in the inferolateral wall (arrow). The corresponding late gadolinium enhancement image, however, shows extensive late enhancement (myocardial scar) in the corresponding area.

VIABILITY TESTING

Myocardial revascularisation (coronary bypass surgery, angioplasty or stenting) is usually undertaken to relieve angina or to abolish myocardial ischemia. In some patients with impaired left ventricular contractility, revascularisation may be indicated to improve left ventricular function. In these patients it is necessary to identify '*hibernating myocardium*', i.e. myocardium that is not contracting but is still viable and can be expected to contract when perfusion is restored. Where no viability exists, intervention or surgery is generally futile. Viability testing is used to differentiate between ischemic and infarcted tissues. Such testing can also be used to evaluate '*stunned myocardium*', i.e. myocardium, usually recently vascularised, that is perfused but is temporarily poorly contractile, and has the ability to improve in function over time.

Dobutamine stress echocardiography

Ischemic, hibernating and stunned myocardium may be differentiated with the pattern of response to dobutamine, as detected by echocardiography. Hibernation is usually caused by chronically low myocardial blood flow. At low levels of dobutamine infusion, hibernating myocardium, stimulated by the adrenergic response, increases in contractility. At higher levels of dobutamine increased oxygen demand may provoke ischemia and a reduction in myocardial contractility. This biphasic response to increased rates of dobutamine infusion is suggestive of myocardial viability with hibernation. Infarcted tissues will not increase contractility at any rate of infusion, while stunned myocardium may remain hypokinetic until near-maximum dobutamine infusion rates are administered.

Cardiac positron emission tomography

Cardiac PET viability assessment may occur in two parts, by combining perfusion assessment using radionuclides Nitrogen-13 labelled ammonia ($^{13}NH_3$) or rhubidium-82, and by metabolic assessment using Fluorodeoxyglucose-18 (FDG-18). In some centres, perfusion assessment may take place using SPECT techniques where FDG is taken up by metabolically active tissue. This generally indicates preserved myocardial viability, but the specific pattern of perfusion and metabolic function provided by PET may indicate various pathophysiologies:

1. Perfusion-metabolism mismatch with reduced myocardial perfusion and contractile function in the setting of preserved FDG uptake indicating viable 'hibernating' myocardium.
2. Regions of normal perfusion and normal metabolism in dysfunctional segments (may represent myocardial stunning, or remodelling).
3. Reduction in both perfusion and metabolism (myocardial scar).
4. Reversed-mismatch whereby there is normal perfusion but reduced FDG-18 uptake. This can occur in diabetes mellitus, but also following revascularisation early after myocardial infarction and in left bundle branch block.[15]

Magnetic resonance imaging

For detection of scar and viability, a cardiac MRI technique of *inversion recovery,* otherwise known as tissue-nulling, is used. After administration of contrast, a period of time from 3 to 10 minutes is given to allow contrast redistribution into the extracellular space. In the normal myocardium, within many cells with intact cellular membranes the extracellular space is small. Where areas of fibrosis or scar exist the extracellular space is high, resulting in higher concentrations of gadolinium contrast. The inversion recovery sequence results in little to no signal coming from normal tissue. Abnormal tissue reflecting myocardial scar is very bright, and the images generally have excellent signal-to-noise ratios.

The extent and thickness of myocardial fibrosis and scar can be measured, and this directly corresponds with the likelihood of functional recovery after revascularisation.[16]

NON-INVASIVE ANATOMICAL TESTING

Coronary calcium score

The coronary calcium score is a CT-based measurement of calcified plaques within the coronary arteries. The calcium score is a prognostic test, not a diagnostic test, i.e. the calcium score is insufficient for the assessment of symptoms of chest pain or dyspnea. The test is most appropriate for risk stratification in asymptomatic individuals with intermediate cardiovascular risk. The test indicates short-term and medium-term risk by the absolute calcium score while long-term and lifetime risk is indicated by the calcium score centile, which measures the degree of calcification relative to other individuals of the same age.

Computed tomography coronary angiography (CTCA) and cardiac CT

CTCA uses an ECG-gated CT scan to capture the heart and coronary arteries in a three-dimensional image of high resolution. Procurement of the CT image is the same as for all CT scanners: The X-ray tube of the CT scanner rotates rapidly around the patient and the image is created via computer-assisted tomography. In CT coronary angiography, however, the image is acquired or reconstructed only from those portions of the cardiac cycle where coronary motion is relatively quiescent, typically mid-diastole. Frequently, 150 ms or less is required for complete image cardiac acquisition. Radiation dose associated with the technique was once high but is now in the order of 1 or 2 years background radiation.[17]

CTCA enables direct visualisation of the coronary artery and vessel wall. It is frequently used to assess the coronary anatomy, for example in the setting of coronary anomalies as seen in Figure 27.3, or to assess for coronary stenosis. Although predominantly useful for imaging the coronary arteries, ECG-gated cardiac CT may also be used to image the myocardium, pericardium and great vessels. In addition, CTCA has a unique benefit of assessing early development of coronary atherosclerosis within the vessel wall,[18] which is sometimes invisible by invasive angiography. Certain features of the atheroma may be useful in assessing future cardiovascular risk, including high volume non-calcified plaque, low attenuation plaque, unstable plaque, micro-calcification and positive remodelling.

When used to assess for obstructive or occlusive coronary artery disease, the negative predictive value of CT coronary angiography is excellent; where a CT coronary angiogram is normal or demonstrates only non-obstructive disease, it is very unlikely that significant coronary disease is present. A meta-analysis comparing CTCA to invasive coronary angiography demonstrated 99% sensitivity, 83% specificity, 93% positive predictive value and 100% negative predictive value.[19]

Conditions that reduce the utility of CTCA include significant calcification, as seen in

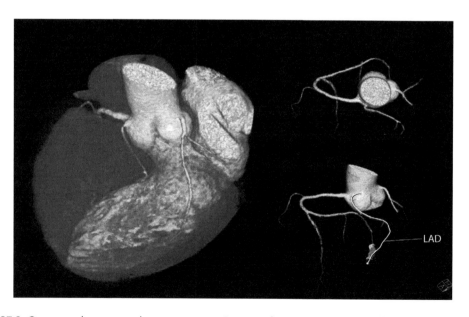

Figure 27.3 Computed tomography coronary angiogram demonstrating a small anomalous left anterior descending coronary artery arising from the right coronary artery. The left circumflex artery has a separate origin.

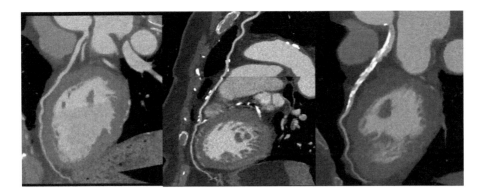

Figure 27.4 Examples of computed tomography (CT) coronary angiogram images. CT has excellent negative predictive value and a normal coronary artery (left panel) reliably indicates the absence of significant disease. CT is also excellent at evaluating grafts (centre panel). In the setting of high calcium levels, the accuracy of the technique is poorer, as significant artefact can occur (right panel).

Figure 27.4, and coronary artery stents (which cause image distortion through artefact production), high heart rates (which contribute to motion artefact), inability to breath-hold for five seconds, and narrow or small coronary arteries (Diameter < 1.5 mm), which are difficult to visualise.

CT fractional flow reserve

While anatomic techniques are excellent in terms of detecting coronary disease and guiding medical therapy, percutaneous intervention and surgery are generally best guided by the functional significance of the coronary stenosis, with invasive FFR serving as the reference standard.

Recent advancements in imaging and computational flow dynamics have enabled estimation of FFR measurement through CT anatomical imaging alone. The process of CT FFR involves extraction of geometric models of the coronary anatomy and application of computational flow dynamics to the imaged vessels. The process of CT FFR computation is complex and is dependent not only on coronary anatomy but also on myocardial volume and multiple physiological assumptions. Nevertheless, initial data indicate that CT FFR significantly augments the diagnostic utility of CT coronary angiography, in many cases by causing a significant reduction in false positives without compromising test sensitivity.[20] An example image of a CT FFR analysis is shown in Figure 27.5.

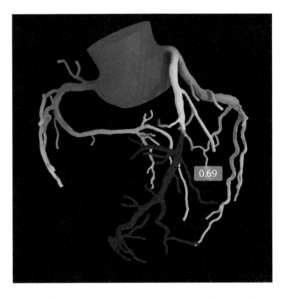

Figure 27.5 Computed tomography-fractional flow reserve (CT-FFR). A processed CT image shows a significant stenosis at the mid-left anterior descending coronary artery with an estimated FFR of 0.69 in the distal vessel. (Courtesy of HeartFlow.)

SUMMARY

- Cardiac investigations for assessment of coronary artery disease have advanced rapidly. Non-invasive techniques can be broadly classified into tests for ischemia, viability and anatomy.

- Non-invasive assessment modalities are generally the preferred initial strategy for diagnosis except where there is a high likelihood of obstructive coronary disease that may require intervention. In this case, the patient should be referred directly for invasive coronary angiography.
- Ischemic testing includes stress schocardiography, radionuclide myocardial perfusion imaging and cardiac MRI.
- Viability studies include dobutamine stress echocardiography, MRI and cardiac PET.
- The Coronary Calcium score calculated during a non-contrast CT scan is used as a prognostic test to assess an asymptomatic individual's absolute and relative cardiovascular risk.
- When assessing low-to-intermediate risk populations with chest pain, anatomical non-invasive imaging techniques such as CT coronary angiography can be used.
- CT coronary angiography helps assess future cardiovascular risk (using factors such as non-calcified plaque, positive remodelling and micro-calcification) and the degree of anatomical stenosis.

REFERENCES

1. Tonino PA, Fearon WF, De Bruyne B, et al. Angiographic versus functional severity of coronary artery stenosis in the FAME study fractional flow reserve versus angiography in multivessel evaluation. *J Am Coll Cardiol.* 2010;55:2816–2821.
2. Zimmermann FN, Ferrara A, Johnson NP, et al. Deferral vs. performance of percutaneous coronary intervention of functionally non – significant coronary stenosis: 15-year follow- up of the, DEFER trial. *Eur Heart J.* 2010;36:36182–36188.
3. De Bruyne B, Bartunek J, Sys SU, Heyndrickx GR. Relation between myocardial fractional flow reserve calculated from coronary pressure measurements and exercise-induced myocardial ischemia. *Circulation.* 1995;92:39–46.
4. Hochman JS, Maron DJ. International Study of Comparative Health Effectiveness With Medical and Invasive Approaches (ISCHEMIA) clinical trials.gov Identifier: NCT01471522. Available at: https://clinicaltrials.gov/ct2/show/NCT01471522
5. Hachamovitch R, Berman DS, Shaw LJ, et al. Incremental prognostic value of myocardial perfusion single photon emission computed tomography for the prediction of cardiac death: Differential stratification for risk of cardiac death and myocardial infarction. *Circulation* 1998;97:535.
6. Yin X, Wang J, Zheng W, Ma J, Hao P, Chen Y. Diagnostic performance of coronary computed tomography angiography versus exercise electrocardiography for coronary artery disease: A systematic review and meta-analysis. *J Thorac Dis.* 2016;8(7):1688–1696.
7. Pellikka PA, Nagueh SF, Elhendy AA, et al. American Society of Echocardiography recommendations for performance, interpretation, and application of stress echocardiography. *J Am Soc Echocardiogr.* 2007;20:1021.
8. Sicari R, Nihoyannopoulos P, Evangelista A, et al. Stress echocardiography expert consensus statement: European Association of Echocardiography (EAE) (a registered branch of the ESC). *Eur J Echocardiogr.* 2008;9:415.
9. Klocke FJ, Baird MG, Lorell BH, et al. ACC/AHA/ASNC guidelines for the clinical use of cardiac radionuclide imaging – executive summary: A report of the American College of Cardiology/American Heart Association Task Force on Practice Guidelines (ACC/AHA/ASNC Committee to Revise the 1995 Guidelines for the Clinical Use of Cardiac Radionuclide Imaging). *Circulation.* 2003;8:1404–1418.
10. Lim SP, Mc Ardle BA, Beanlands RS, Hessian RC. Myocardial viability: It is still alive. *Semin Nucl Med.* 2014;44:358–374.
11. Camici PG, Prasad SK, Rimoldi OE. Stunning, hibernation and assessment of myocardial viability. *Circulation.* 2008;117:103–114.
12. McArdle BA, Dowsley TF, deKemp RA, Wells GA, Beanlands RS. Does Rubidium-82 PET have superior accuracy to SPECT perfusion imaging for the diagnosis of obstructive coronary disease? A systematic review and meta-analysis. *J Am Coll Cardiol.* 2012;60:1828–1837.

13. Greenwood JP, Maredia N, Younger JF, Brown JM, Nixon J, Everett CC, Bijsterveld P, Ridgway JP, Radjenovic A, Dickinson CJ, et al. Cardiovascular magnetic resonance and single-photon emission computed tomography for diagnosis of coronary heart disease (CE-MARC): A prospective trial. *Lancet* 2012;379:453–460.

14. Schuijf JD, Bax JJ, Shaw LJ, et al. Meta-analysis of comparative diagnostic performance of magnetic resonance imaging and multislice computed tomography for noninvasive coronary angiography. *Am Heart J.* 2006;151:404.

15. Gould KL, Hamilton GW, Lipscomb K, Ritchie JL, Kennedy JW. Method for assessing stress-induced regional malperfusion during coronary arteri-ography. Experimental validation and clinical application. *J Am Coll Cardiol.* 1974;34:557–564.

16. Kim RJ, Wu E, Rafael A, Chen EL, Parker MA, Simonetti O, Klocke FJ, Bonow RO, Judd RM. The use of contrast-enhanced magnetic resonance imaging to identify reversible myocardial dysfunction. *N Engl J Med.* 2000;343(20):1445–1453.

17. Deseivre S, Chen MY Korosoglou G, Hausleiter J. Prospective randomized trial on radiation dose estimates of CT angiography applying iterative image reconstruction: The PROTECTION V study. *JACC: Cardiovasc Imaging.* 2015;8(8):888–896.

18. Eckert J, Schmidt M, Magedanz A, Voigtländer T, Schmermund A. Coronary CT angiography in managing atherosclerosis. *Int J of Mol Sci.* 2015;16(2):3740–3756.

19. Budoff MJ, Dowe D, Jollis JG, Gitter M, Sutherland J, Halamert E, et al. Diagnostic performance of 64-multidetector row coronary computed tomographic angiography for evaluation of coronary artery stenosis in individuals without known coronary artery disease: Results from the prospective multicenter ACCURACY trial. *J Am Coll Cardiol.* 2008;55:1724–1732.

20. Min JK, Koo BK, Erglis A, et al. Effect of image quality on diagnostic accuracy of noninvasive fractional flow reserve: Results from the prospective multicenter international DISCOVER- FLOW study. *J Cardiovasc Comput Tomogr.* 2012;6:191–199.

28

Right heart catheterisation and evaluation of the pulmonary hypertension patient

EUGENE KOTLYAR AND ANNE KEOGH

INTRODUCTION

Right heart catheterisation dates to 1929, when a surgical student in Germany, Werner Forsmann, who later became a urologist, inserted a Foley's catheter into the cubital vein of his own forearm, advanced it to the right atrium (RA) and took an X-ray.[1] This represented the first right heart catheterisation (RHC) in man.

Further development occurred in the 1940s. Drs André Cournand and Dickinson Richards developed catheters that could be advanced to the pulmonary artery (PA) and used them to study congenital and acquired heart disease. In 1956, in recognition of their efforts, Cournand, Richards, and Forsmann received the Nobel Prize for Physiology and Medicine. In 1967, a balloon-tipped, flow-guided catheter was refined by Drs Swan and Ganz and in the 1970s and this was also used for immediate bedside monitoring.[2] Balloon flotation catheters, known as 'Swan-Ganz' catheters, were further developed for measuring cardiac output (CO) by the thermodilution technique, for right atrial and right ventricular pacing, and for measuring right-sided pressures, including pulmonary arterial wedge pressure (PAWP).[3,4] Infusion pores were incorporated to facilitate administration of drugs with the same catheter.

In the 1970s and 80s, RHC was performed at the same time as left heart catheterisation to assess suitability for valvular surgery. With the advent, improvement and widespread use of echocardiography, RHC was not considered to provide additional relevant information by some cardiologists. Developments in the cardiac catheterisation laboratory resulted in percutaneous procedures such as angioplasty and stenting. As a result, new cardiology trainees from the 1990s and onward were not sufficiently trained in RHC technique and pulmonary haemodynamics, but RHC was still important in cardiac transplantation centres to assess suitability for orthotopic heart transplantation (see Chapter 29). Since 2004, when oral pulmonary arterial hypertension (PAH) specific therapies became available in Australia, RHC has made somewhat of a comeback in its importance to general cardiology, yet it is still underused and suboptimally performed in modern cardiology practice.

WHY IS RHC IMPORTANT?

RHC is the gold standard for diagnosis of pulmonary hypertension (PH) and PAH. RHC is also required to assess the severity of haemodynamic impairment, and to undertake vasoreactivity testing of the pulmonary circulation in selected patients[5] (Tables 28.1 through 28.4). There are five clinical groups of PH: group 1 – PAH; group 2 – PH due to left heart disease (LHD); group 3 – PH due to lung diseases and/or hypoxia; group 4 – chronic thromboembolic PH; group 5 – PH with unclear and multifactorial mechanisms.[6] RHC allows further subdivision of these groups according to various combinations of mean pulmonary artery pressure (mPAP), PAWP, CO, diastolic pressure gradient (DPG) and pulmonary vascular resistance (PVR), into pre-capillary PH (groups 1, 3, 4 and 5) and post-capillary (groups 2 and 5), with PH depending on a PAWP reading of > or $\leq$15 mmHg[7] (Table 28.5). Post-capillary PH can be further divided into isolated post-capillary PH (Ipc-PH), and combined pre-capillary and post-capillary PH (Cpc-PH) (Table 28.5).

PH is a life-threatening condition that was defined by a mPAP $\geq$ 25 mmHg measured by RHC in the supine position at rest since the 1st World Symposium of Pulmonary hypertension (WSPH) in 1973, Geneva, Switzerland. Accumulating data in healthy individuals, however, suggest that a normal mPAP at rest is 14 $\pm$ 3.3 mmHg.[8] At the recent 6th World Symposium of Pulmonary hypertension, Nice, France (6th WSPH 2018), the upper limit of

Table 28.1 Right heart catheterisation in pulmonary hypertension[5]

Recommendations	Class	Level
RHC is recommended to confirm the diagnosis of pulmonary artery hypertension (group 1) and to support treatment decisions.	I	C
In patients with pulmonary hypertension, it is recommended to perform RHC in expert centres as it is technically demanding and may be associated with serious complications.	I	B
RHC should be considered in pulmonary artery hypertension (Group 1) to assess the treatment effect of drugs.	IIa	C
RHC is recommended in patients with congenital cardiac shunts to support decisions on correction.	I	C
RHC is recommended in patients with pulmonary hypertension due to left heart disease (Group 2) or lung disease (Group 3) if organ transplantation is considered.	I	C
When measurement of pulmonary artery wedge pressure is unreliable, left heart catheterisation should be considered to measure left ventricular EDP.	IIa	C
RHC may be considered in patients with suspected pulmonary hypertension and left heart disease (Group 2) or lung disease (Group 3) to assist in the differential diagnosis and support treatment decisions.	IIb	C
RHC is indicated in patients with chronic thromboembolic pulmonary hypertension (Group 4) to confirm the diagnosis and support treatment decisions.	I	C

Source: Galie, N. et al., Eur. Respir. J., 46, 903, 2015.

Table 28.2 Risk assessment of pulmonary artery hypertension

Determinants of prognosis (estimated 1-year mortality)	Low risk <5%	Intermediate risk 5%–10%	High risk >10%
Clinical signs of RHF	Absent	Absent	Present
Progression of symptoms	No	Slow	Rapid
Syncope	No	Occasional	Repeated
WHO functional class	I, II	III	IV
6MWD	>440 m	165–440 m	<165 m
CPET	Peak $VO_2 > 15$ mL/kg/min (65% pred.) VE/VCO$_2$ slope <36	Peak VO_2 11–15 mL/kg/min (35%–65% pred.) VE/VCO$_2$ slope 36–44.9	Peak $VO_2 < 11$ mL/kg/min (<35% pred.) VE/VCO$_2$ slope $\geq$45
NT-pro-BNP/BNP plasma levels	BNP < 50 ng/L NT-proBNP < 300 ng/L	BNP 50–300 ng/L NT-proBNP 300–1400 ng/L	BNP > 300 ng/L NT-proBNP > 1400 ng/L
Imaging (Echo, cMR)	RA area < 18 cm^2 No pericardial effusion	RA area 18–26 cm^2 No or minimal pericardial effusion	RA area > 26 cm^2 Pericardial effusion
Haemodynamics	RA < 8 mmHg CI $\geq$ 2.5 L/min/m^2 SvO$_2$ > 65%	RA 8–14 mmHg CI 2.0–2.5 L/min/m^2 SvO$_2$ 60%–65%	RA > 14 mmHg CI < 2.0 L/min/m^2 SvO$_2$ < 60%

Source: From European Society of Cardiology/European respiratory Society, *Eur. Respir. J.*, 46, 903–975, 2015; Simonneau, G., *J. Am. Coll. Cardiol.*, 62, D34–D41, 2013.

Abbreviations: RHF, right heart failure; WHO, World Health Organization; 6MWD, six minute walking distance; CPET, cardiopulmonary exercise test; VO_2, oxygen consumption; VE/VCO$_2$, ventilatory equivalents for carbon dioxide; NT-proBNP, N-terminal probrain type natriuretic peptide; CI, cardiac index; RA, right atrium.

Table 28.3 Simplified Risk Stratification in pulmonary artery hypertension (WSPH 2018, Nice)

	Prognostic criteria	Low risk variables	Intermediate risk variables	High risk variables
A.	WHO functional class	I, II	III	IV
B.	6MWD	>440 m	165–440 m	<165 m
C.	NT-pro-BNP/BNP plasma levels OR RA pressure	BNP < 50 ng/L NT-proBNP < 300 ng/L RA < 8 mmHg	BNP 50–300 ng/L NT-proBNP 300–1400 ng/L RA 8–14 mmHg	BNP < 50 ng/L NT-proBNP > 1400 ng/L RA > 14 mmHg
D.	CI or SvO$_2$	CI $\geq$ 2.5 L/min/m^2 SvO$_2$ > 65%	CI 2.0–2.5 L/min/m^2 SvO$_2$ 60%–65%	CI < 2.0 L/min/m^2 SvO$_2$ < 60%

Abbreviations: WHO, World Health Organization; 6MWD, six-minute walking distance; RA, right atrium; CI, cardiac index; CO, cardiac output; SvO$_2$, mixed venous oxygen saturation.

Table 28.4 Simplified Risk Stratification in pulmonary artery hypertension (WSPH 2018, Nice)

Low risk	Intermediate risk	High risk
At least 3 low risk variables and no high risk variables	Definitions of low and high risk not fulfilled	At least 2 high risk variables including CI or SvO$_2$

Abbreviations: CI, cardiac index; SvO$_2$, mixed venous oxygen saturation.

Table 28.5 Haemodynamic classification of pulmonary hypertension

Definition	Characteristics	Clinical group (s)
PH	mPAP ≥ 25 mmHg	All
Pre-capillary PH	mPAP ≥ 25 mmHg PAWP ≤ 15 mmHg	1. PAH 2. PH due to ling diseases 3. CTEPH 4. PH with unclear and/or multifactorial mechanisms
Post-capillary PH	mPAP ≥ 25 mmHg PAWP ≥ 15 mmHg	1. PH due to LHD 2. PH with unclear and/or multifactorial mechanisms
Isolated post-capillary PH (Ipc-PH)	DPG < 7 mmHg and/or PVR ≤ 3 WU	
Combined post-capillary and pre-capillary PH (Cpc-PH)	DPG < 7 mmHg and/or PVR ≤ 3 WU	

Source: Simonneau, G. et al., J. Am. Coll. Cardiol. 62, D34–D41, 2013.
Abbreviations: mPAP, mean pulmonary artery pressure; PAH, pulmonary artery hypertension; PH, pulmonary hypertension; CTEPH, chronic thromboembolic pulmonary hypertension; LHD, left heart disease; DPG, diastolic pulmonary gradient; WU, Wood units; Ipc, Isolated post-capillary; Cpc, Combined post-capillary and pre-capillary.

normal value was altered to be 20 mmHg, calculated as the mean normal value of 14 mmHg plus 2 standard deviations.[9] This was based on recognition that in a number of conditions, mPAP > 20 mmHg was associated with increased mortality.[10–13] As the increase in mPAP can be due to many conditions, such as increase in the CO, elevation in PAWP, left to right shunt, and pre-capillary PH with pulmonary vascular disease (PVD), it was considered important to *redefine pre-capillary PH as mPAP > 20 mmHg, PAWP < 15 mmHg and PVR > 3 Wood Units* (WU).[9] This is because in this setting, some therapies in certain conditions have been shown to improve outcome. In particular, in PH group 1 (PAH), medications targeting the endothelin, nitric oxide and prostacyclin pathways and PH group 4, chronic thromboembolic pulmonary hypertension (CTEPH), pulmonary endarterectomy,[14] balloon pulmonary angioplasty[15] and riociguat.[16]

The PVR >3 WU has been arbitrarily chosen in the definition of PAH since the WSPH, 2013, Venice,[17] was used for inclusion in most randomised controlled trials, in the definition of Cpc-PH and to characterise patients for whom correction of congenital systemic to pulmonary shunting becomes questionable. There are emerging data that in pre-capillary PH with mPAP 21–24 mmHg, PVR is usually >3WU.[13,14,18,19]

RHC is therefore central to the new definition of PAH, which is characterised by the presence of precapillary PH (PAWP ≤ 15 mmHg), mPAP > 20 mmHg and PVR >3 WU at rest.[9] The impact of the new definition on the number of precapillary PH patients identified is estimated to be low, with preliminary data suggesting a less than 10% increase.[9] It is hoped that the new definition may allow earlier identification of PVD, with potential for early treatment and improved outcomes.

RHC in PAH also provides the clinician with an indication of disease severity, including the effects of PAH on right heart function, establishes prognosis[6] (Tables 28.2 through 28.4), guides choice, and determines response to therapy. Pulmonary vasodilation reserve can also be assessed during acute vasodilator challenge and if positive, the patient can now be classified in the new PAH subgroup of 1.2, PAH with vasoreactivity.[9]

DIAGNOSTIC ALGORITHM FOR PAH

The 2015 European Society of Cardiology (ESC)/ European Respiratory Society (ERS) guidelines, as well as the most recent proceedings of the WSPH 2018, stress the importance of RHC in the definitive diagnosis of PAH (Figure 28.1a and b). These documents initially recommend that patients with unexplained exertional symptoms of dyspnoea, syncope and signs of right heart dysfunction should be assessed for suspected PH/PAH with transthoracic echocardiography (Tables 28.6 and 28.7) and RHC would then be used to confirm the diagnosis.[5,20]

RHC TECHNIQUE

RHC should be performed in a clinically stable patient who is resting quietly with legs positioned flat on the X-ray table. The procedure can be performed via a number of venous access sites depending on the experience of the operator, availability of the equipment and the possible requirement of other concurrent procedures. For example, if an endomyocardial biopsy is required, right internal jugular venous access would be the best option. If a supine bicycle ergometer exercise study is required,

then internal jugular or antecubital venous access would be most appropriate. If a left heart catheter is also required, then femoral vein and artery access would be convenient, or an antecubital vein and radial arterial combination could be employed.

In our institution, RHC is usually performed via the right internal jugular vein. It commonly takes 15–20 minutes and can be performed in an outpatient setting. As no fasting is required, this gives the most accurate physiological determination of cardiopulmonary haemodynamics. In order to avoid thromboembolic complications, anticoagulation does not need to be interrupted with an International Normalised Ratio (INR) kept between 2 and 3 if on warfarin. Direct oral anticoagulant therapy can also be continued but omitted on the morning of the procedure, providing there is no concern about recent deterioration of renal function.

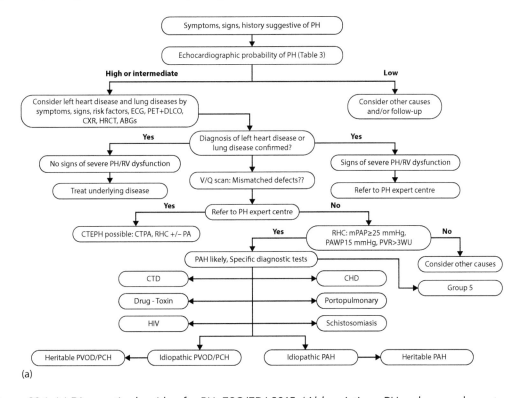

(a)

Figure 28.1 (a) Diagnostic algorithm for PH, ESC/ERJ 2015. (*Abbreviations:* PH, pulmonary hypertension; PFT, pulmonary functions testing, DLCO, diffusing capacity of carbon monoxide; CXR, chest X-ray; HRCT, high resolution CT; ABGs, arterial blood gases; RV, right ventricle; V/Q, nuclear ventilation perfusion scan; CTEPH, chronic thromboembolic pulmonary hypertension; CTPA, CT pulmonary angiography; RHC, right heart catheterisation; PA, pulmonary angiography; PAWP, pulmonary arterial wedge pressure; PVR, pulmonary vascular resistance; PAH, pulmonary arterial hypertension; CTD, connective tissue disease; CHD, congenital heart disease; HIV, human immunodeficiency virus; PVOD pulmonary venooc-clusive disease, pulmonary capillary haemangiomatosis, pulmonary capillary haemangiomatosis);

(*Continued*)

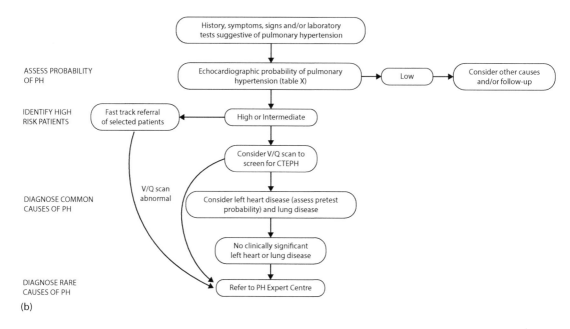

Figure 28.1 (Continued) **(b)** New diagnostic algorithm for PH, WSPH 2018, Nice (*Abbreviations: CTEPH,* chronic thromboembolic pulmonary hypertension; PAH, pulmonary arterial hypertension; PH, pulmonary hypertension; V/Q, nuclear ventilation perfusion scan). ([a] Reproduced with permission of the © 2018 European Society of Cardiology & European Respiratory Society. *Eur. Respir. J.*, 46, 903–975, 2015; [b] Gibbs, S. et al., *JACC*, 2018, in press.)

Table 28.6 Echocardiographic (Echo) probability of pulmonary hypertension in symptomatic patients with a suspicion of pulmonary hypertension (PH)

Peak tricuspid regurgitation velocity (m/s)	Presence of other Echo 'PH signs'[a]	Echo probability of PH
<2.8 or not measurable	No	Low
<2.8 or not measurable	Yes	Intermediate
2.9–3.4	No	Intermediate
2.9–3.4	Yes	High
>3.4	Not required	High

Source: Galie, N. et al., *Eur. Heart J.*, 37, 67, 2016.
[a] See Table 28.7.

The patient is positioned supine, preferably without a pillow on a fluoroscopy table, breathing room air, with head turned to the left and neck slightly extended. The operator can then identify anatomical landmarks, such as the triangle formed by the sternal and clavicular heads of the right sternocleidomastoid muscle and the clavicle. Anatomical landmarks can be made more prominent by asking the patient to lift the head slightly off the bed or turn the head left against resistance. A prominent jugular venous pulsation can be seen in the presence of significant tricuspid regurgitation.

Local anaesthetic (4 mL of 1% lignocaine buffered with 1 mL sodium bicarbonate) is injected at a point approximately two fingerbreadths above the clavicle in the apex of the triangle. A 22-gauge (G) needle is used to locate the internal jugular vein, advancing approximately 40° from vertical and 20° to the right. The vein is usually situated at a depth of 1–2.5 cm below the skin. If the vein is not located, the same approach is repeated with more lateral angulation,

Table 28.7 Echocardiographic signs suggesting pulmonary hypertension used to assess the probability of pulmonary hypertension in addition to tricuspid regurgitation velocity measurement in Table 28.6

A: The ventricles[a]	B: Pulmonary artery[a]	C: Inferior vena cava and right atrium[a]
Right ventricle/left ventricle basal diameter ratio >1.0	Right ventricular outflow Doppler acceleration time <105 ms and/or midsystolic notching	Inferior vena cava >21 mm with decreased inspiratory collapse (<50% with a sniff or <20% with quite inspiration)
Flattening of the interventricular septum (left ventricular eccentricity index >1.1 in systole and/or diastole)	Early diastolic pulmonary regurgitation velocity >2.2 m/s	Right atrial area (end-systole) >18 cm^2
	Pulmonary artery diameter >25 mm	

Source: Galie, N. et al., Eur. Heart J., 37, 67, 2016.
[a] Echocardiographic signs from at least two different categories (A/B/C) from the list should be present to alter the level of echocardiographic probability of pulmonary hypertension.

and if unsuccessful, a medial approach can be used. Medial angulation must be approached with caution, as the carotid artery lies deep and medial to the internal jugular vein. If venous pressure is low, a head-down tilt by 15°–30° (Trendelenburg position), elevation of legs and Valsalva manoeuvre may help increase the venous return and make internal jugular venous cannulation easier.

More recently, localisation of the internal jugular vein has become considerably easier by the availability of a portable ultrasound probe (SonoSite, US) and, if available, should be used routinely during the procedure.

Once the right internal jugular vein is located and, under ultrasound guidance if possible, a puncture with a larger (18G) needle can be made following the same angle, through which the J guide-wire is advanced into the RA. A small nick is then made in the skin at the entry point with a scalpel blade. The needle is then removed and an 8F sheath is inserted over the guidewire. A Swan-Ganz thermodilution catheter, the lumen of which has been prefilled with normal saline, can then be inserted via the sheath. Catheter passage is made easier with fluoroscopic guidance, especially in patients with right ventricular enlargement and significant tricuspid regurgitation. The J-shaped curvature of the Swan-Ganz catheter, as well as balloon flotation, facilitates passage from the superior vena cava to the pulmonary artery (PA). When the catheter tip reaches the RA, the balloon at the distal end is inflated with 2 mL of air and then floated through the tricuspid valve into

the right ventricle (RV) by gently rotating the proximal end of the catheter counter-clockwise, aided by the fluoroscopic guidance. When the tip reaches the PA, continuing to advance the balloon-inflated tip will result in the catheter becoming wedged in one of the segmental pulmonary arteries (usually in the right inferior or right middle lobar region). As the catheter is progressively advanced from a suitable vein to the superior vena cava and to the contiguous right heart chambers, the pressures are recorded at each location: RA, RV, PA and PAWP. Occasionally, pressures may need to be measured in reverse order, i.e. PAWP, PA, PAWP and RV to prevent the catheter losing its 'tongue'. This is especially useful when the RV is very large and the catheter tends to hold and loop within the RV.

If there is some difficulty in passage of the catheter, deep inspiration, cough or elevating the right shoulder can help. In the presence of pacing or defibrillator device wires or in a congenital heart study, the Emerald guidewire (Cordis, FL, USA) with a J-tip may be required to increase the stiffness of the catheter and allow passage of the tip to the required location in the pulmonary arterial tree in order to 'wedge' the tip in the PAWP position. At this point, it may be helpful to draw blood from the distal tip to ascertain that the catheter tip is fully wedged as evidenced by the bright red appearance of oxygenated blood, which can be confirmed by blood gas analysis. The arterial oxygen saturation obtained can also be used in the Fick calculation of CO (see Chapter 16).

After recording the PAWP, the balloon is deflated and the pulmonary arterial pressure (PAP) is again recorded. Two blood samples from the distal tip of the catheter are then obtained for mixed venous oxygen saturation.

PRESSURE MEASUREMENT SYSTEMS

Accurate recording of pressure waveforms and correct interpretation of physiological data derived from these waveforms is the main goal of RHC. A pressure wave from a cardiac chamber is a cyclical force, and its amplitude and duration are influenced by various mechanical and physiological parameters, such as the force of the contracting chamber and its surrounding structures, the contiguous heart chambers, pericardium, lungs and the vasculature. The heart rate and the respiratory cycle also influence pressure waveforms (see Chapters 14 and 15).[21,22]

PRESSURE TRANSDUCER AND ZEROING

Intravascular pressures are recorded using a fluid-filled catheter connected to a pressure transducer. The lack of standardisation regarding the exact position of the transducer may lead to differences up to 8 mmHg.[23] The ideal zero reference should not only be independent of the chest diameter but also be insensitive to changes in body position, and represent a 'hydrostatic indifference point'.[24] Current international standardisation of zero level is at the mid-thoracic line with a suggested reference point defined by the intersection of the frontal plane at the mid-thoracic level, the transverse plane at the fourth intercostal space and the midsagittal plane.[25] If the patient is in the supine position, this corresponds to a halfway point between the anterior sternum and the bed surface. This zero-reference point represents the level of the left atrium (LA). Once levelling to the mid-thoracic level is completed, zeroing the transducer to atmospheric pressure should then be performed.

HAEMODYNAMIC MEASUREMENTS

The following measurements are recorded during RHC at end-expiration: RA pressure (RAP), RV pressure (RVP) (systole, diastole, end-diastole), PAWP, and PA pressures (systole, diastole and mean). CO is most commonly measured using the thermodilution method, although the direct Fick method can be more accurate in the settings of severe tricuspid regurgitation, congenital heart disease or low cardiac output (see Chapters 16 and 17 for more details). It is our practice to measure intracardiac pressures twice, 10 minutes apart or until two consecutive values differ by less than 10%. It is important to note that it is the cardiac index (CI), i.e. the CO corrected for body surface area, that has the prognostic importance.

Blood is subsequently taken from the distal port for determination of mixed venous oxygen saturation. Comparison of oxygen saturations in the superior vena cava, inferior vena cava, RA, RV and PA permits assessment of the presence of shunting at the atrial, ventricular, or pulmonary arterial level, manifested as an increase ('step-up') in the oxygen saturation of blood as it traverses these vessels and chambers (see Chapter 16).

Systemic blood pressure (systole, diastole and mean) and heart rate (HR) can be measured non-invasively.

RHC-derived haemodynamic parameters are shown in Table 28.8.[26] Table 28.9 illustrates the expected range of cardiovascular pressures measured during RHC for the disease-free and the PAH patient at rest.[8,26–28] It has been demonstrated, however, that normal haemodynamics vary with age (Table 28.10), having a normal range of 15–150 dynes·sec·cm^{-5} (0.2–2.0 WU), with doubling of PVR over the first five decades of life.[8,29–33] Modelling indicates that a PVR > 2 WU with a CO of 5 L/min identifies 25% of pulmonary vascular loss.[28]

Furthermore, PVR is linearly related to the viscosity of blood, and viscosity and hematocrit are exponentially related, but more evidence is required to define clinical relevance of hematocrit-corrected PVR.[34]

CORRECT PRESSURE WAVEFORMS

Each heart chamber pressure waveform is unique, specific to that chamber, and reflects the physiology or pathophysiology in that chamber.

The right atrial pressure trace and electrocardiogram (ECG) timing

The atrial trace has three positive deflections, the *a*, *c* and *v* waves (see Chapter 14). The *a* wave results from atrial systole and occurs after the P waveduring

Table 28.8 Calculated parameters at time of right heart catheterisation

Transpulmonary gradient (TPG) = (mPAP – PAWP)
Pulmonary vascular resistance (PVR) = (mPAP – PAWP)/CO)
Total pulmonary resistance (TPG) = mPAP/CO
Cardiac Index (CI) = CO/BSA*
Stroke volume (SV) = CO/HR
Stroke volume = SV/BSA*

Source: Arnold, R. et al., *Cardiology and Cardiac Catheterisation: The Essential Guide*, Harwood Academic Publishers, Amsterdam, the Netherlands, 2001.
Note: Cardiac index (CI) is calculated to adjust for the body surface area (BSA) to compare individuals of different body weight and sizes; *BSA = 0.007184 × (weight $^{0.425}$ × height$^{0.725}$) – Dubois formula.
Abbreviations: mPAP, mean pulmonary artery pressure; PAWP, pulmonary artery wedge pressure; PCWP, pulmonary capillary wedge pressure; CO, cardiac output; BSA, body surface area.

Table 28.9 The expected range of the cardiovascular pressures measured by the pulmonary artery catheter for disease-free and pulmonary artery hypertension patient at rest

	Normal subject	PAH patient
Right atrium (mmHg)	0–7	normal or elevated
Right ventricle (mmHg)		
Systolic:	15–25	>30
Diastolic:	1–8	Normal or elevated
PAP (mmHg)		
Systolic:	13–30	96
Diastolic:	6–15	38
Mean	8–20	61
PAWP (mmHg)	5–12	≤15
PPC (mmHg)	8–12	8–12
TPG (mmHg)	2–12	>12
DPG (mmHg)	0–5	>3
Cardiac output (L/min)	4–8	2.5
Cardiac index (L/min/m²)	2.5–4.5	1.7
PVR (WU)	0.2–1.2	>3
SVR (WU)	8.8–20	PVR/SVR: <0.75

Source: Galie, N. et al., *Eur. Heart J.*, 37, 67, 2016; Arnold, R. et al., *Cardiology and Cardiac Catheterisation: The Essential Guide*, Harwood Academic Publishers, Amsterdam, the Netherlands, 2001; Rosenkranz, S., Preston, I.R., *Eur. Respir. Rev.*, 24, 642, 2015; Naeije, R., *Pulmonary Circulation Diseases and their Treatment*, CRC Press, Boca Raton, FL, 2016.
Abbreviations: PAP, pulmonary artery pressure; PAWP, pulmonary artery wedge pressure; PPC, pulmonary capillary pressure; TPG, Transpulmonary gradient; DPG, diastolic pulmonary gradient; PVR, pulmonary vascular resistance; SVR, systemic vascular resistance.

the PR interval of the ECG (Figure 28.2a and b). The height of the a wave depends on atrial contractility and the resistance to RV filling.[21] The c wave corresponds to right ventricular contraction causing the tricuspid valve to bulge toward the RA.[21] It occurs with closure of the tricuspid valve and the initiation of atrial filling, and when present it is seen at the end of the QRS complex (RST junction).

The x descent follows the a wave and occurs as a result of the RV pulling the tricuspid valve downward during ventricular systole. The x descent corresponds to atrial relaxation and rapid atrial filling

Table 28.10 The influence of age on pulmonary haemodynamics

Age	16–28	61–83
n	22	16
Cardiac output L/min	7.6 ± 1.2	5.6 ± 1.0
mPAP, mmHg	13 ± 3	16 ± 2
PAWP, mmHg	8 ± 2	9 ± 2
PVR (dynes.s.cm^{-5})	54 ± 29	96 ± 25

Source: Galie, N. et al., *Eur. Heart J.*, 37, 67, 2016; Holmgren, A. et al., *Acta Physiol. Scand.*, 49, 343–63, 1960; Granath, A. et al., *Acta Med. Scand.*, 176, 425–46, 1964; Granath, A., Strandell T., *Acta Med. Scand.*, 176, 447–66, 1964; Bevegard, S. et al., *Acta Physiol. Scand.*, 49, 279–98, 1960; Kovacs, G. et al., *Eur. Respir. J.*, 39(2), 319–28, 2012.

Abbreviations: mPAP, mean artery pressure; PAWP, pulmonary artery wedge pressure; PVR, pulmonary vascular resistance.

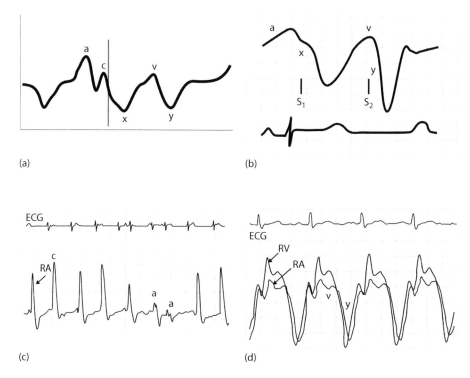

Figure 28.2 The right atrial pressure trace. **(a)** Components of the right atrial pressure trace (a, c, and v waves, x and y descents); **(b)** ECG timing of the right atrial pressure trace (S1 and S2 represent timing of first and second heart sounds); **(c)** Cannon a waves occurring during atrio-ventricular dysynchrony – atrial contraction is occurring against a closed tricuspid valve; **(d)** Large atrial v waves that occur with severe tricuspid regurgitation. (Adapted from Davidson, C.J. et al., *Heart Disease: A Textbook of Cardiovascular Medicine.* 1, W. S. Saunders Company, Philadelphia, PA, 1997.)

due to the low pressure in the RA. Pressure in the RA then rises after the x descent and peaks as the v wave. The v wave occurs with passive venous blood filling of the RA while the tricuspid valve is closed during RV systole. It appears after the T wave of the ECG. The height of the v wave is related to atrial compliance and the amount of blood returning to the atrium.[21] The y descent corresponds to rapid emptying of the RA into the RV following opening of the tricuspid valve. During normal breathing, RA pressure falls during inspiration as intrathoracic pressures decreases, and increases during expiration as intrathoracic pressure increase. The opposite effect occurs during mechanical ventilation.[21]

RA haemodynamic pathology

Elevated *a* wave occurs in tricuspid stenosis and when there is decrease in RV compliance, such as in PH and pulmonary stenosis.

Cannon *a* waves can be seen during atrio-ventricular asynchrony when the atrium contracts against a closed tricuspid valve (Figure 28.2c). This is seen in complete heart block or during ventricular tachycardia.

Absent *a* wave occurs in atrial fibrillation or standstill, and in atrial flutter.

Elevated or prominent *v* wave occurs with tricuspid regurgitation (Figure 28.2c), right ventricular failure and in conditions of reduced atrial compliance, e.g. in restrictive cardiomyopathy.

The PAWP tracing

The PAWP tracing is similar to the RA waveform but is higher, reflecting a higher left pressure system. It is also slightly damped and delayed as a result of transmission through the lungs (Figure 28.3a–d). In addition, the *v* wave is higher than the *a* wave due to LA constraint by the pulmonary veins posteriorly, whereas the RA can decompress via the superior and inferior venae cavae. The *a* wave represents LA contraction, and the *c* wave represents closure of the mitral valve. The *v* wave represents filling of the LA while the mitral valve is closed during left ventricular systole. The *x* and *y* descents are visible but the *c* wave is often not well seen.[21]

CURRENT ISSUES WITH PAWP

The PAWP is an approximation of LA pressure (LAP) and LV end-diastolic pressure (LVEDP) (see Chapter 14). The PAWP may over-estimate LAP in acute respiratory failure, chronic obstructive pulmonary disease in PH, pulmonary venoconstriction, and if the catheter size is small for the given PA, with the balloon tip being too small. The LAP is greater than the LVEDP in the setting of significant mitral regurgitation or stenosis. The LVEDP is greater than LAP in acute aortic regurgitation and in a non-compliant left ventricle.

The technical quality of PAWP, or 'wedge' tracing should be perfects; however, in 31% of some cases, it has been found technically inadequate.[35] Correct interpretation of PAWP is essential, but in some studies, it was found that 50% of the tracings are misinterpreted.[36,37]

It is important to obtain a good wedge waveform and to be aware of the over- and under-damped tracing. In some instances, the PAWP quality can be improved by partially deflating the balloon and gentle forward advancement of the catheter in order to better seat the catheter against the walls of the PA branch. The abnormally or unexpectedly elevated PAWP measurements can be validated by gently withdrawing a blood sample from the distal port of the RHC during balloon inflation and PAWP recording, to ensure that the saturation of the sample is consistent with arterial oxygen saturation.

Reading PAWP tracing within the respiratory cycle

A systematic review by Kovacs et al.[24] was performed to provide practical recommendations on how to interpret respiratory swings. Their key conclusions were that the effect of elastic recoil was minimal at functional residual capacity (end-expiration). Larger effects of intrathoracic pressure changes, however, occur in patients with lung disease. In these situations, the inspiratory and expiratory pressure swings may cancel each other out, so the authors proposed that instead of relying on the readings at end-expiration, the pulmonary vascular pressures should be *averaged* throughout three respiratory swings.[24] In another study by LeVarge,[38] elevated end-expiratory PAWP (>15 mmHg) occurred in 29% of subjects with pre-capillary PH. In this study, the end-expiratory PAWP measurements led to misclassification of patients with a pre-capillary phenotype as post-capillary PH in 29% of the patients in this series. The authors thus argued that PAWP averaged throughout the respiratory cycle *may be* a more accurate measurement, especially in patients in whom spontaneous positive end-expiratory intrathoracic pressure may contribute to high end-expiratory PAWP, such as in the setting of obesity and chronic obstructive pulmonary disease (COPD).[38] Forty-four percent of this cohort, however, had post-capillary phenotype but had a respiratory mean PAWP ≤15 mmHg and would

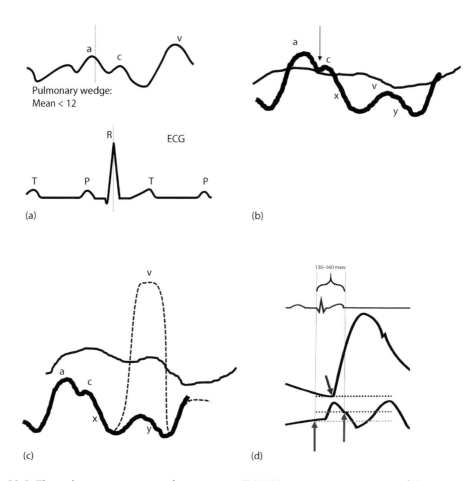

Figure 28.3 The pulmonary artery wedge pressure (PAWP) trace. **(a)** ECG timing of the PAWP wave; **(b)** Close correlation between mean PAWP (pale thin line) and end-diastolic PAWP (the pre-*c* wave pressure, arrow); **(c)** Exaggeration of mean PAWP with large *v* wave; **(d)** PAWP is phase delayed by 130–160 ms from the ECG. Thus, end-diastolic PAWP (pre *c*-wave pressure; right arrow) occurs later than the QRS-gated PAWP used (left arrow). By subtracting the diastolic pulmonary artery pressure (middle arrow and top dotted line) from the QRS-gated value (bottom dotted line), it is possible that one overestimates the true diastolic pulmonary gradient (difference between top dotted line and middle dotted line). ([b,c] Adapted from Tedford, R. et al., *JACC*, 2018 in press; [d] Houston, B.A., Tedford, R.J., *Circ Heart Fail*, 10, 2017.)

also have been misclassified. The end-expiratory method is supported by an earlier study, which showed that use of the digitised mean PAWP can under-estimate LVEDP by 4.4 mmHg and lead to misclassification of PH in 30% of the cohort reported by Ryan et al.[39]

Hence, PAWP is affected by respiratory swings and, at the Sixth World Symposium on PH, it was recommended that it should, in most situations, continue to be measured at end-expiration, when the effects of intrathoracic pressure swings are minimal and when the end-expiratory PAWP is approximately equal to LVEDP.

Reading PAWP tracing within the cardiac cycle

The purpose of measuring the PAWP is to record the reflected LAP and LVEDP, hence the end-diastolic PAWP should be measured. This is delayed by 130–200 ms from the QRS.[40] The PAWP that is averaged throughout the cardiac cycle overestimates the PAWP and underestimates the DPG, if the *v*-wave is incorporated. End-diastolic or QRS-gated PAWP better approximates LVEDP and better defines the pre-capillary component.

The measured PAWP in atrial fibrillation overestimated the LVEDP by 4.76 mmHg and underestimated the LVEDP in sinus rhythm by 2.96 mmHg.[41] This confirmed the earlier study by Halpern et al., who found that PAWP underestimated LVEDP by 2.9 mmHg.[42]

At the Sixth World Symposium of PH, it was acknowledged that earlier studies that considered a normal PAWP to be ≤12 mmHg was due to use of the respiratory mean rather than PAWP measured at end-expiration.

Current recommendations for PAWP/LVEDP measurement

At the Fifth World Symposium of PH in 2013, it was decided that the term Pulmonary *Capillary* Wedge Pressure was misleading, and it was recommended that PAWP or Pulmonary Arterial Occlusion Pressure should be used. It was also deemed that the cut-off for pre-capillary PH should remain ≤15 mmHg as this has been used in almost all randomised controlled trials. It was considered that the sponsors of future trials may decide to use PAWP ≤12 mmHg. There have been limited new data since that time and as this also concurs with the ESC guidelines, at the sixth WSPH in 2018 there was no recommendation to change this definition.

With respect to the cardiac cycle, it was recommended to measure PAWP at end-diastole as this more closely reflects the LVEDP. In sinus rhythm, the *a*-wave should be averaged to obtain the end-diastolic measurement. In atrial fibrillation, the PAWP should be measured 130–160 ms after the onset of the QRS and before the *v*-wave (Figure 28.3d).[40,43,44]

Again, with respect to the respiratory cycle, assessment of PAWP at end-expiration was still recommended, as measuring the mean of the respiratory cycle would reclassify many post-capillary PH patients to pre-capillary disease. It was acknowledged, however, that some data supports averaging over several respiratory cycles, instead of only at expiration, particularly in patients with COPD and in the obese. Inspection of the tracing is essential for final determination of the pulmonary vascular pressure reading.

The PAWP is sufficient in such right heart studies when recordings are reliable and patient history (e.g. metabolic syndrome) and non-invasive testing, including echocardiography, yield no evidence of LHD.

Furthermore, invasive haemodynamics and especially the PAWP measurement, need to be placed in the context of the clinical, echocardiographic and/or cardiac magnetic resonance imaging data with regard to the probability of presence of LHD[7,27,45-48] (Tables 28.11 and 28.12; Figure 28.4a and b).

The PAP trace and ECG timing

As the catheter advances from the RV outflow track to the PA, there is a systolic notch indicating ventricular contraction followed by closure of the pulmonary valve, and then a gradual decline in pressure until the next systolic phase. Closure of the pulmonary valve is indicated by the dicrotic notch. Peak systole correlates with the T wave, whereas end-diastole correlates with the QRS complex on ECG.

PAP haemodynamic pathology

Elevated PA systolic pressure occurs in idiopathic PAH, mitral stenosis or regurgitation, restrictive myopathies, significant left to right shunting, and pulmonary disease, and PH secondary to LV systolic and diastolic function or left-sided valvular disease and pulmonary vein stenosis (i.e. after pulmonary venous isolation for atrial fibrillation).

Reduced PA systolic pressure is seen in PA stenosis, Ebstein's anomaly, Tricuspid stenosis and atresia.

Reduced pulse pressure can be seen in RV ischaemia, acute pulmonary embolism and pericardial tamponade.

Bifid PA waveform is seen when a large left atrial *v* wave is transmitted backward, as occurs in severe mitral regurgitation.

PADP greater than PAWP can occur in pulmonary disease, pulmonary embolus and tachycardia.

RISKS ASSOCIATED WITH RHC

The risks of RHC are those associated with central vein line placement and include haematoma (1 in 200) and pneumothorax (1 in 500). These risks have been considerably decreased by use of ultrasound

Table 28.11 Clinical phenotype commonly found in PH LHD Recommendations for PH due to left heart disease

Clinical presentation	Echocardiography	Other features
Age > 60	Structural left heart abnormality:	Electrocardiogram:
Symptoms of left heart failure	LV systolic dysfunction	LVH and/or LAE
	Left heart valve disease	Atrial fibrillation
(most useful: orthopnoea, PND)	LA enlargement (>42 mm, LAVI > 34 mL/m²)	Left bundle branch block
		Q waves
Obesity, hgypertension, dyslipidaemia, glucose intolerance, diabetes	Concentric LVH	CXR/HRCT:
	LV mass index ≥ 115 g/m² (M), ≥95 g/m² (F)	Pulmonary oedema
		Kerley B lines
Metabolic syndrome	Doppler indices of increased filling pressures:	Pleural effusion
History of cardiac disease (past or current)	Increased mean/lateral E/e' ≥ 13	CPET:
		Exercise oscillatory ventilation
Atrial fibrillation	Grade 2–3 mitral inflow abnormality	Elevated VE/VCO₂ slope (i.e. >36)
RF ablation		
CAD/valvular disease		Cardiac MR:
Cardiac intervention		LA/RA > 1
		LA area > 20 cm²
		LA strain

Source: Galie, N. et al., *Eur. Heart J.*, 37, 67–119, 2016; Simonneau, G. et al. *J. Am. Coll. Cardiol.*, 62, D34–D41, 2013; Rosenkranz, S., Preston, I.R., *Eur. Respir. Rev.*, 24, 642–652, 2015; Wright, S.P. et al., *Circ. Heart Fail.*, 10, 2017; Tedford, R. et al., *JACC*, 2018; Caravita, S. et al., *J. Heart Lung Transplant.*, 36, 754–62, 2017; Jacobs, W. et al., *Eur. Respir. J.*, 46, 422–430, 2015.

Abbreviations: LV, left ventricle; LA, left atrium: LAVI, left atrial volume index; LVH, left ventricular hypertrophy; LAE, left atrial enlargement; M, male gender; F, female gender; CXR, chest X-ray; HRCT, high resolution computerised tomography scan; PND, paroxysmal nocturnal dyspnoea; VE/VCO₂, ventilatory equivalent for carbon dioxide; RF, radiofrequency; CAD, coronary artery disease; RA, right atrium.

guidance. Temporary hoarseness can occur if the local anaesthetic is injected around the recurrent laryngeal nerve.

Other risks are associated with PA catheter insertion and include serious arrhythmia (1 in 1000), as atrial or ventricular arrhythmias, which can be transient or sustained. Sustained atrial arrhythmia can be overdriven during the procedure by introducing a pacing wire into the RA via the sheath. Other risks of PA catheter insertion are infection, pulmonary infarction, PA or RV perforation. The latter can be minimised by floating the balloon-tipped catheter into the PA to the wedge position rather than attempting to wedge once the deflated tip is in the artery. One large study examined the complication rate in 7218 patients undergoing RHC in 15 experienced centres in Europe and the United States. Among the proceduralists, 57% were pulmonologists and 43% were cardiologists. Almost 72.7% of procedures were via the internal jugular vein. The outcomes of 5,727 patients were collected retrospectively over a 5-year period and 1,491 patient data were collected prospectively over six months. Serious adverse events occurred in 76 (1.1%, 0.08%–1.3%) and there were four fatal events (0.055%, 0.01%–0.099%): (1) PA rupture resulting in massive haemoptysis and asphyxiation; (2) arrest 15 minutes following pulmonary angiography due to intrapulmonary haemorrhage; (3) sudden cardiac death during preparation of the patient for the procedure due to massive acute pulmonary embolism with warfarin stopped 5 days pre-procedure; and (4) sudden cardiac death occurring the day after the RHC procedure in a patient with an underlying

Table 28.12 Pretest probability to differentiate between pulmonary artery hypertension and pulmonary hypertension due to heart failure with preserved ejection fraction (HFpEF)

Feature	High probability of LHD	Intermediate probability of LHD	Low probability of LHD
Age	>70	60–70	<60
Obesity, hypertension, dyslipidaemia, glucose intolerance, DM	>2	1–2	None
Previous cardiac intervention	Yes	No	No
Atrial fibrillation	Current	Previous	No
Structural LHD	Present	No	No
Electrocardiogram	LBBB or LVH	Mild LVH	Normal or RV strain
Echocardiography	LA dilatation Mitral inflow grade >2	No LA dilatation Mitral inflow grade <2	No E/e′ < 13
CPET	Mildly elevated VE/VCO^2 Exercise oscillatory ventilation	Elevated VE/VCO^2 Exercise oscillatory ventilation	High VE/VCO^2 slope No exercise oscillatory ventilation
cMR	LA strain or LA/RA >1		No left heart abnormalities

Source: Simonneau, G., J. Am. Coll. Cardiol., 62, D34–D41, 2013.
Abbreviations: LHD, left heart disease; DM, diabetes mellitus; LBBB, left bundle branch block; LVH, left ventricular hypertrophy; RV, right ventricle; LA, left atrium; VE/VCO^2, ventilatory equivalent for carbon dioxide; CPET, cardiopulmonary exercise testing; cMR, cardiac magnetic resonance imaging.

dilated cardiomyopathy. Most frequent complications ($n = 72$), however, were of mild to moderate intensity and included 0.3% access-related complications such as haematoma, pneumothorax, arrhythmia and hypotension. Hypotension was the result of a vagal reaction during acute vasodilator challenge.[49] Contraindications to RHC are listed in Table 28.13.[50–52]

LIMITATIONS IN RHC MEASUREMENTS

Measurements are generally obtained only under resting conditions in the supine position. These may not be representative of haemodynamic responses in the upright posture, during activity, or sleep, and even under these static circumstances, measurements may vary.

Prolonged measurement of pulmonary haemodynamics in a group of 12 patients with PAH found wide intra-individual spontaneous variability, with PAP varying by >20 mmHg in some patients; the mean coefficient of variability was 8%.[53]

ACUTE VASODILATOR TESTING

In a healthy situation, the pulmonary circulation is a low-pressure, low-resistance and highly distensible system. Acute vasoreactivity testing during RHC helps identify those likely to benefit from treatment with calcium channel blockers (CCB). Only a minority of patients with PAH subsequently respond to oral long-term administration of CCB. Patients with no evidence of an acute haemodynamic response to vasodilator testing are unlikely to benefit from chronic

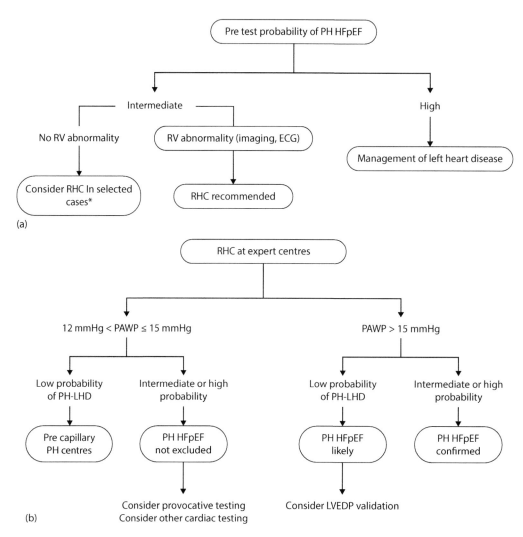

Figure 28.4 (a, b) **(a)** Flow chart to determine who requires haemodynamic assessment in pulmonary artery hypertension vs. pulmonary hypertensive left heart disease for patients with high/intermediate probability of pulmonary hypertension by echocardiography (Tables 28.6 and 28.7). Patients with low probability of LHD follow the general pulmonary hypertension diagnostic algorithm; **(b)** Flow chart to interpret the haemodynamic assessment in pulmonary artery hypertension vs. pulmonary hypertensive LHD. ([a] Adapted from Galie, N., *Eur. Heart J.*, 37, 67–119, 2016; Rosenkranz, S., Preston, I.R., *Eur. Respir. Rev.*, 24, 642–52, 2015; Caravita, S. et al., *J. Heart Lung Transplant.*, 36, 754–62, 2017; Jacobs, W. et al., *Eur. Respir. J.*, 46, 422–30, 2015; Opotowsky, A.R. et al., *Circ. Cardiovasc. Imaging*, 5, 765–75, 2012; Berthelot, E. et al., *J. Card. Fail.*, 23, 29–35, 2017; [b] Galie, N., *Eur. Heart J.*, 37, 67–119, 2016.)

therapy. The agents for testing vasoreactivity are listed in Table 28.14. Inhaled nitric oxide at 10–20 parts per million is the recommended agent for pulmonary vasoreactivity testing. Intravenous epoprostenol (2–12 ng/kg/min), intravenous adenosine (50–350 µg/min), and inhaled iloprost (5 µg) can be used as alternatives. Use of oxygen, phosphodiesterase 5 inhibitors, or other vasodilators for acute pulmonary vasoreactivity testing is not recommended.[7] Acute testing with CCB is not recommended due to a high incidence of severe deleterious effects, especially in non-responders.[54–57]

Acute vasodilator response is defined as a decrease in mPAP >10 mmHg, to reach mPAP of <40 mmHg, with a normal or a high CO. Long-term treatment with CCB must be started *only* in patients displaying acute vasoreactivity. Acute responders

Table 28.13 Complications and contraindications to right heart catheterisation

Contraindications	Absolute	Mechanical tricuspid and pulmonary valve
		Right heart masses (thrombus, tumour)
		Right sided endocarditis
	Relative	Coagulopathy
		Pacemaker
		Bioprosthetic mechanical tricuspid and pulmonary valve
		LBBB
		Arrhythmias
		Skin site infections
Complications		Haematoma
		Pneumothorax
		Arrhythmias
		Vasovagal episodes
		Hypotension
		Pulmonary haemorrhage

Source: Opotowsky, A.R. et al., *Circ. Cardiovasc. Imaging*, 5, 765–775, 2012; Berthelot, E. et al. *J. Card. Fail.*, 23, 29–35, 2017; Hoeper, M.M. et al., *J. Am. Coll. Cardiol.*, 48, 2546–2552, 2006; Gupta, D. et al., *Cardiology: An Illustrated Textbook*, Jaypee Brothers Medical Publishers, New Delhi, India, 2012.

Table 28.14 Acute vasoreactivity agents

	Route	t1/2	Dose range[a]	Increments[b]	Duration[c]
Nitric Oxide	inh	15–30 sec	10–20 ppm	–	5 min[d]
Epoprostenol	IV	3 min	2–12 ng/kg/min	2 ng/kg/min	10 min
Adenosine	IV	5–10 sec	50–350 mcg/kg/min	50 mcg/kg/min	2 min
Iloprost	inh	30 min	5–20 mcg		15 min

Source: Coughlan, G.F. et al., *Eur. Respir. J.*, 51, 2018; Galie, N. et al., *Eur. Respir. J.*, 46, 903–975, 2015.
[a] Initial dose and maximal dose suggested.
[b] Increments of dose by each step.
[c] Duration of administration on each step.
[d] For NO a single step within the dose range is suggested.

should be monitored for long-term clinical and haemodynamic effects at about 3–4 months of therapy. Of 557 consecutive patients with idiopathic PAH (iPAH) from the French registry, only 70 (12.6%) were acute responders who were commenced on high dose CCB. Subsequently, only 38 (6.8%) were long-term responders at 1 year with World Health Organisation functional class I or II that did not require the introduction of PAH-specific therapy.[58]

In a further study, patients with PAH associated with heritable (HPAH), anorexigens, connective tissue disease, portopulmonary, HIV, congenital heart disease and pulmonary vaso-oclusive disease and pulmonary capillary haemangiomatosis, conditions were assessed for acute and long-term vasodilator responsiveness. Of all the subsets, only PAH

associated with anorexigen use was found to have sustained long-term response in 9.4% of cases.[59]

The guidelines therefore recommend that acute vasodilator testing should only be performed in iPAH, HPAH and drug- and toxin-induced PAH. As there appears to be an early diagnostic tool providing specific management with high doses of CCB and carrying better prognosis, in the most recent WSPH 2018, these patients have been reclassified into subgroup 1.2, PAH with vasoreactivity.

ROLE OF EXERCISE DURING RHC

In healthy subjects, stroke volume increases by 20%–50% with exercise, due to the increase in venous return and cardiac inotropy before reaching a plateau at about 50% of maximum oxygen consumption (VO_2 max).[60] HR increases linearly in a progressive effort. The increased CO results in minimal increase in PAP due to recruitment and distension of pulmonary arteriolar resistive units.[8]

Measuring PVR is essential in the current diagnosis of PH and PVD. The formula PVR = mPAP − PAWP/CO assumes that the pressure-flow relationship is linear and crosses the origin, so that the PVR is flow and pressure independent. Kovacs et al. found that PVR in young adults decreases with increasing CO, and by 15%–20% when CO >10 L/min, but does not significantly change after 70 years of age.[33] PVR in PAH decreases with increasing CO, and this is not explained by pulmonary vascular distension but by recruitment of pulmonary vasculature. The increase in CO with exercise is then reflected as a disproportionate increase in PAP. Due to the increase in RV afterload, PAH patients have a decrease in stroke volume that remains unchanged during exercise.[61] The increase in CO with exercise is thus dependent on the chronotropic response and explains the low tolerance of PAH patients taking negative chronotropic agents such as beta-blockers.[62]

In addition, PA distensibility predicts cardiovascular mortality.[63] Refined multipoint pressure-flow derived PVR by exercise or dobutamine challenge may detect early PVD and better define therapeutic responses.[64,65]

Pulmonary hypertensive response to exercise can be seen in a number of settings. This could be a normal variant as it occurs in elite athletes.[66] Late pulmonary vasoconstriction during incremental exercise occurs as in other well-described 'thresholds' noted during incremental exercise, including those of arterial blood lactate concentration, ventilation, carbon dioxide output and humoral catecholamines.

There is some evidence that exercise haemodynamics may be a more accurate predictor of long-term outcomes in PAH than are haemodynamic parameters at rest.[67,68]

The promise of exercise testing is to correlate patients' symptoms on exertion to their haemodynamics in order to detect early PVD or pulmonary venous hypertension in heart failure with preserved ejection fraction, which may lead to research into earlier introduction of therapies and better outcomes.

Exercise testing during RHC

This is performed in the supine position on a cycle ergometer secured to the catheter table. The haemodynamic values are initially measured at rest with the patient's legs positioned on the bed. Measurements are then repeated with patient's legs positioned in the pedals. The patient is then instructed to pedal at a rate of 60 revolutions per minute. The workload is increased stepwise by 10 W every 3 minutes up to 40 W or more depending on functional tolerance. The haemodynamic parameters are measured during the last minute of each exercise level, at a steady state (when mPAP and heart rate values are stable).[61]

WHY WAS EXERCISE mPAP >30 mmHg EXCLUDED FROM THE DEFINITION OF PH?

Before the 4th WSPH in 2008, PH had been defined by a mPAP of >30 mmHg at exercise.[17] This was removed from the definition because the degree of exercise has not been clearly defined and standardised, and the normal response of mPAP to exercise varies with age and degree of exercise[69] and almost 50% of healthy subjects older than 50 meet this definition on light exercise[8] (Table 28.15), making it difficult to have an upper limit of normal value for exercise-induced PH. Furthermore, elite athletes can reach mPAP of >30 mmHg with normal lung function due to their ability to achieve very high CO.[70] There was also lack of clear data supporting its clinical relevance: Natural history of exercise PH, treatment effect and mechanism were not well known.[71]

Some patients with PVD are not symptomatic at rest but have symptoms with exertion. Hence, there is potential for exercise or volume challenge during RHC to better diagnose early PVD. Patients at high risk for PH with mPAP on exercise >30 mmHg and normal mPAP at rest might be considered as an early manifestation of pulmonary vasculopathy.[72] In a UK study by Condcliffe et al.,

Table 28.15 Upper limit of normal mean pulmonary artery pressure (mmHg) according to age and during exercise

Age	<30	30–50	>50
Rest (mmHg)	19	19	22.7[a]
Mild exercise (mmHg)	29	29	46.2[a]
Submaximal exercise (mmHg)	33	36	47[a]

Source: Kovacs, G. et al., Eur. Respir. J., 34, 888–894, 2009.

[a] $p < 0.001$ compared with <30 yo

of 42 patients with mPAP on exercise >30 mmHg and normal mPAP at rest, 5 patients died: 4 of PH or right heart failure and 8 (19%) showed evidence of disease progression with development of PAH at rest, and mean time to PAH at rest was 838 ± 477 days from diagnosis.[73] Furthermore, exercise RHC may help explain exertional dyspnea in some patients. Recent studies have provided additional knowledge of the relationship of mPAP and CO in health and disease.[74,75]

The ERS 2017 statement and WSPH 2018 proposed the following criteria for exercise PH: mPAP >30 mmHg with total pulmonary resistance of >3 mmHg per litre of CO at maximum exercise. This could occur due to unmasking early PVD, exercise-induced rise in LAP and PAWP or both. The latter requires careful assessment of exercise PAWP, using a clinical score for LHD (Table 28.12) and possibly the use of exercise echocardiography or cardiac magnetic resonance imaging.

It is important to stress, however, that without further data on the natural history of exercise PH, mechanistic information on pathophysiology and trials of treatment efficacy, these proposed criteria are not ready for identification of treatable PAH patients and hence not yet part of the definition of PH.

FLUID CHALLENGE DURING RHC

A number of studies have addressed the utility of the fluid challenge. In patients with heart failure with preserved ejection (HFpEF), who have been adequately diuresed and in those with occult pulmonary venous hypertension, a normal PAWP could lead to the incorrect diagnosis of PAH.[76,77] Fluid challenge could be useful in these situations.

In a retrospective study of 207 patients meeting resting haemodynamic criteria of PAH, pulmonary venous hypertension, defined as PAWP >15 mmHg, was found in 22.2% of patients after a 500 mL bolus of intravenous normal saline over 5–10 minutes.[77] In another study, occult LHD in scleroderma patients with PH was also uncovered with a similar fluid challenge protocol.[78] The study by Fujimoto et al.[79] found that in healthy subjects, PAWP increased from 10 ± 2 mmHg to 16 + 3 mmHg after 1 litre of saline.[79] Older women had steeper increase in PAWP compared to younger men and women and older men. Patients with HFpEF displayed a steeper increase in PAWP relative to the infused volume compared to healthy young and older subjects (Figure 28.5a), and no healthy subject would have increased the PAWP >18 mmHg with 500 mL of saline.[79] Exercise challenge in this group may have provided a clearer distinction between HFpEF and PVD.[80] As mentioned earlier, exercise has the advantage of patient symptom assessment, but requires a specific complex setting and expertise in conducting the test. There are also difficulties in pressure reading during the exercise test, and the range of normal response is still uncertain. The fluid loading, on the other hand, is easy to perform with standardised protocol, requires no special equipment, and there is minimal risk of misinterpretation of pressure reading. There is also a more established cut-off, defining an abnormal increase in PAWP, but age-dependency of response has been observed.

At the WSPH 2018, it was suggested that PAWP of 15 mmHg should still be the upper limit of normal for pre-capillary PH at rest. In patients with PAWP between 13 and 15 mmHg and intermediate to high probability of PH HFpEF (Table 28.8), a fluid-loading challenge should be considered with 500 mL of normal saline over 5 minutes. A PAWP of >18 mmHg after fluid administration is considered abnormal, but how that should impact patient management is currently uncertain.

DIASTOLIC PULMONARY GRADIENT (DPG)

This controversial parameter was first suggested in 2013 by Naeije et al. due to the fact that the traditional markers such as transpulmonary gradient and PVR used to describe PVD 'out of proportion' to LHD were affected by flow state and the impact of left heart failure on pulmonary vascular compliance.[81]

By assessing diastolic pressure, the DPG examines the pulmonary vessels in late diastole at cardiac diastasis, when the pressure gradient or the difference between the diastolic PAP and LAP should be minimal, with no contribution of flow or effect of PA Windkessel function.[81]

A 2013 study by Gerges et al. suggested that a DPG >7 mmHg predicted worse median survival in patients with post-capillary PH and a TPG >12 mmHg[82] (Figure 28.5b and c). Subsequent studies, however, found that DPG does not predict survival in patients with PH due to LHD and have no

impact on post-transplant survival in patients with PH and an elevated TPG and PVR[83,84] (Figure 28.5d). Recently, it has been suggested that variations in the reporting and measurement of PAWP is responsible for these differences.[85] In the calculation of the DPG, represented by a small number, small variations in measurement technique will result in a potentially small margin for error.[40]

During the Fifth World Symposium on Pulmonary Hypertension it was proposed that a DPG ≥7 mmHg alone should define combined post- and pre-capillary PH (CpcPH).[86] Since then, due to the abovementioned studies exploring the prognostic value of DPG that have yielded mixed results, the more recent guidelines have included PVR into the CpcPH definition.[5]

CpcPH, defined by DPG, transpulmonary gradient and PVR is not only common in group 2 PH,[5] but numerous studies have shown it confers increased risk of mortality in the LHD population beyond isolated post-capillary PH (IpcPH).[83,87] The question of whether DPG can or should predict clinical outcome in PH-LHD remains controversial, and it may be that the alternative parameters of pre-capillary PH may be better suited to identify PVD in left heart dysfunction incorporating measurements of RV and pulmonary vascular function.[88]

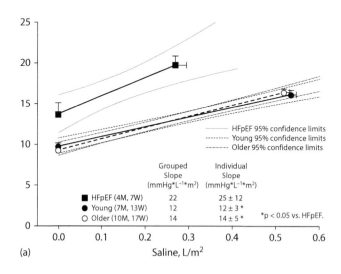

Figure 28.5 **(a)** Pulmonary wedge pressure (PCWP) relative to saline in patients with heart failure with preserved ejection fraction (HFpEF), young subjects, and older subjects after the first set of saline infusions. Dashed line indicates 95% confidence limits. *(Continued)*

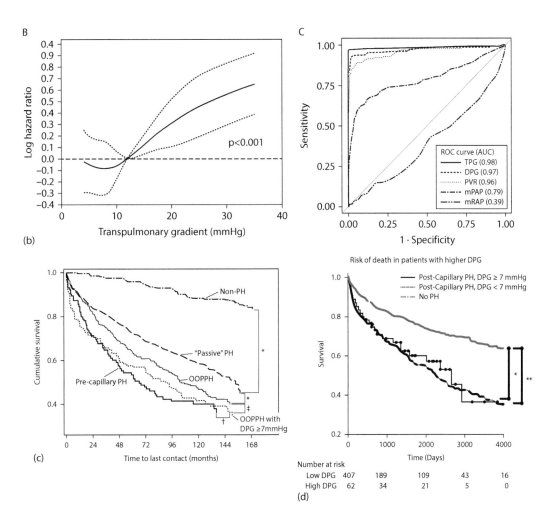

Figure 28.5 (Continued) **(b)** Transpulmonary gradient as a predictor of death in patients with pre- and postcapillary pulmonary hypertension. The vertical line marks a change in the slope of the regression line at 12 mmHg. Dashed lines marks confidence intervals of the hazard function. C. ROC curves of transpulmonary gradient (TPG), diastolic pulmonary gradient (DPG), pulmonary vascular resistance (PVR), mean pulmonary arterial pressure (mPAP) and mean right atrial pressure (mRAP) for the discrimination between precapillary and postcapillary 'passive' pulmonary hypertension. **(c)** Survival curves illustrating a population of 'non-pulmonary hypertension' group (non-PH) (dashed-dotted line) patients with precapillary PH (closed line), 'passive' PH (dashed line), out of proportion pulmonary hypertension (OOPPH) (thin closed line), and OOPPH with diastolic pulmonary gradient (DPG) ≥7 mmHg (dotted line), all adjusted for age, sex, stable ischaemic heart disease, and creatinine clearance <60 mL/min. (Symbols indicate significance levels: † $P = 0.908$, *$P < 0.001$; ‡$P = 0.01$. **(d)** The diastolic pulmonary gradient (DPG), DPG (≥7 mmHg), did not predict survival in patients with pulmonary hypertension due to left heart disease (PH-LHD) (mPAP ≥ 25 and PCWP ≥ 15 mmHg; *$P < 0.05$, **$P < 0.001$). ([a] Reproduced from Fujimoto, N. et al., *Circulation*, 127, 55–62, 2013. With permission; [b,c] Reproduced from Gerges, C. et al., *Chest*, 143, 758–766, 2013. With permission; [d] Reproduced with permission from Tampakakis, E. et al., *JACC Heart Fail.*, 3, 9–16, 2015.)

CONCLUSION

RHC is the gold standard investigation to reliably and definitively diagnose PAH. It is associated with low risk of serious complications. It is paramount that attention to detail is employed during RHC in order to derive the correct pulmonary haemodynamic values at rest, during exercise and fluid challenges. Haemodynamic parameters measured during RHC guide response to therapy and provide information on prognosis to guide clinical decisions on therapy. Furthermore, there is a need to apply standardised protocols to further improve standardisation in achieving optimal application of RHC, with resulting positive implications for diagnosis and earlier intervention for patients with PAH in routine clinical practice.

REFERENCES

1. Chatterjee K. The Swan-Ganz catheters: Past, present, and future. A viewpoint. *Circulation*. 2009;119(1):147–152.
2. Nossaman BD, Scruggs BA, Nossaman VE, Murthy SN, Kadowitz PJ. History of right heart catheterization: 100 years of experimentation and methodology development. *Cardiol Rev*. 2010;18(2):94–101.
3. Forrester JS, Ganz W, Diamond G, McHugh T, Chonette DW, Swan HJ. Thermodilution cardiac output determination with a single flow-directed catheter. *Am Heart J*. 1972;83(3):306–311.
4. Chatterjee K, Swan HJ, Ganz W, Gray R, Loebel H, Forrester JS, et al. Use of a balloon-tipped flotation electrode catheter for cardiac mounting. *Am J Cardiol*. 1975;36(1):56–61.
5. Galie N, Humbert M, Vachiery JL, Gibbs S, Lang I, Torbicki A, et al. 2015 ESC/ERS Guidelines for the diagnosis and treatment of pulmonary hypertension: The Joint Task Force for the Diagnosis and Treatment of Pulmonary Hypertension of the European Society of Cardiology (ESC) and the European Respiratory Society (ERS): Endorsed by: Association for European Paediatric and Congenital Cardiology (AEPC), International Society for Heart and Lung Transplantation (ISHLT). *Eur Respir J*. 2015;46(4):903–975.
6. Simonneau G, Gatzoulis MA, Adatia I, Celermajer D, Denton C, Ghofrani A, et al. Updated clinical classification of pulmonary hypertension. *J Am Coll Cardiol*. 2013;62(25 Suppl):D34–D41.
7. Galie N, Humbert M, Vachiery JL, Gibbs S, Lang I, Torbicki A, et al. 2015 ESC/ERS Guidelines for the diagnosis and treatment of pulmonary hypertension: The Joint Task Force for the Diagnosis and Treatment of Pulmonary Hypertension of the European Society of Cardiology (ESC) and the European Respiratory Society (ERS): Endorsed by: Association for European Paediatric and Congenital Cardiology (AEPC), International Society for Heart and Lung Transplantation (ISHLT). *Eur Heart J*. 2016;37(1):67–119.
8. Kovacs G, Berghold A, Scheidl S, Olschewski H. Pulmonary arterial pressure during rest and exercise in healthy subjects: A systematic review. *Eur Respir J*. 2009;34(4):888–894.
9. Simonneau G, Souza R, Celermajer D, Denton C, Gatzoulis M, Krowka M, et al. PH haemodynamic definitions and clinical classifications and characteristics of specific PAH Subgroups. *J Am Coll Cardiol*. 2018.
10. Bishop JM, Cross KW. Physiological variables and mortality in patients with various categories of chronic respiratory disease. *Bull Eur Physiopathol Respir*. 1984;20(6):495–500.
11. Maron BA, Hess E, Maddox TM, Opotowsky AR, Tedford RJ, Lahm T, et al. Association of borderline pulmonary hypertension with mortality and hospitalization in a large patient cohort: Insights from the veterans affairs clinical assessment, reporting, and tracking program. *Circulation*. 2016;133(13):1240–1248.
12. Assad TR, Maron BA, Robbins IM, Xu M, Huang S, Harrell FE, et al. Prognostic effect and longitudinal hemodynamic assessment of borderline pulmonary hypertension. *JAMA Cardiol*. 2017;2(12):1361–1368.
13. Douschan P, Kovacs G, Avian A, Foris V, Gruber F, Olschewski A, et al. Mild elevation of pulmonary arterial pressure as a predictor of mortality. *Am J Respir Crit Care Med*. 2018;197(4):509–516.

14. Taboada D, Pepke-Zaba J, Jenkins DP, Berman M, Treacy CM, Cannon JE, et al. Outcome of pulmonary endarterectomy in symptomatic chronic thromboembolic disease. *Eur Respir J*. 2014;44(6):1635–1645.

15. Ogawa A, Satoh T, Fukuda T, Sugimura K, Fukumoto Y, Emoto N, et al. Balloon pulmonary angioplasty for chronic thromboembolic pulmonary hypertension: Results of a multicenter registry. *Circ Cardiovasc Qual Outcomes*. 2017;10(11):e004029.

16. Ghofrani HA, D'Armini AM, Grimminger F, Hoeper MM, Jansa P, Kim NH, et al. Riociguat for the treatment of chronic thromboembolic pulmonary hypertension. *N Engl J Med*. 2013;369(4):319–329.

17. Barst RJ, McGoon M, Torbicki A, Sitbon O, Krowka MJ, Olschewski H, et al. Diagnosis and differential assessment of pulmonary arterial hypertension. *J Am Coll Cardiol*. 2004;43(12 Suppl S):40S–47S.

18. Valerio CJ, Schreiber BE, Handler CE, Denton CP, Coghlan JG. Borderline mean pulmonary artery pressure in patients with systemic sclerosis: Transpulmonary gradient predicts risk of developing pulmonary hypertension. *Arthritis Rheum*. 2013;65(4):1074–1084.

19. Coughlan GF, Wolf M, Distler O, Denton CP, Doelberg M, Harutyunova S, et al. Incidence of pulmonary hypertension and determining factors in patients with systemic sclerosis. *Eur Respir J*. 2018;51(4):1701197.

20. Gibbs S, Frost AE, Torbicki A, Gopalan D, Khanna D, Manes A, et al. Diagnosis of pulmonary hypertension. *JACC*. 2018 (in press).

21. Davidson CJ, Fishman RF, Bonow RO. Cardiac Catheterisation. In: Braunwald E, editor. *Heart Disease: A Textbook of Cardiovascular Medicine*. 1. Philadelphia, PA: W. S. Saunders Company; 1997. p. 188.

22. Moscucci M, Grossman W. Pressure measurement. In: Moscucci M, editor. *Cardiac Catheterization, Angiography, and Intervention*. 8th ed. Philadelphia, PA: Lea and Febiger; 2014. p. 223–244.

23. Kovacs G, Avian A, Olschewski A, Olschewski H. Zero reference level for right heart catheterisation. *Eur Respir J*. 2013;42(6):1586–1594.

24. Kovacs G, Avian A, Pienn M, Naeije R, Olschewski H. Reading pulmonary vascular pressure tracings. How to handle the problems of zero leveling and respiratory swings. *Am J Respir Crit Care Med*. 2014;190(3):252–257.

25. Hoeper MM, Bogaard HJ, Condliffe R, Frantz R, Khanna D, Kurzyna M, et al. Definitions and diagnosis of pulmonary hypertension. *J Am Coll Cardiol*. 2013;62(25 Suppl):D42–D50.

26. Arnold R, Keogh A, Macdonald P. Right heart catheterisation and haemodynamic evaluation of the heart transplant patient. In: Boland J, Muller DWM, editors. *Cardiology and Cardiac Catheterisation: The Essential Guide*. Amsterdam, the Netherlands: Harwood Academic Publishers; 2001. p. 297–304.

27. Rosenkranz S, Preston IR. Right heart catheterisation: Best practice and pitfalls in pulmonary hypertension. *Eur Respir Rev*. 2015;24(138):642–652.

28. Naeije R. Pulmonary vascular function. In: Peacock AJ, Naeije R, Rubin LJ, editors. *Pulmonary Circulation Diseases and their Treatment*. 4th ed. Boca Raton, FL: CRC Press; 2016. p. 11–24.

29. Holmgren A, Jonsson B, Sjostrand T. Circulatory data in normal subjects at rest and during exercise in recumbent position, with special reference to the stroke volume at different work intensities. *Acta Physiol Scand*. 1960;49:343–363.

30. Granath A, Jonsson B, Strandell T. Circulation in healthy old men, studied by right heart catheterization at rest and during exercise in supine and sitting position. *Acta Med Scand*. 1964;176:425–446.

31. Granath A, Strandell T. Relationships between cardiac output, stroke volume and intracardiac pressures at rest and during exercise in supine position and some anthropometric data in healthy old men. *Acta Med Scand*. 1964;176:447–466.

32. Bevegard S, Holmgren A, Jonsson B. The effect of body position on the circulation at rest and during exercise, with special reference to the influence on the stroke volume. *Acta Physiol Scand*. 1960;49:279–298.

33. Kovacs G, Olschewski A, Berghold A, Olschewski H. Pulmonary vascular resistances during exercise in normal subjects: A systematic review. *Eur Respir J.* 2012;39(2):319–328.

34. Linehan JH, Haworth ST, Nelin LD, Krenz GS, Dawson CA. A simple distensible vessel model for interpreting pulmonary vascular pressure-flow curves. *J Appl Physiol* (1985). 1992;73(3):987–994.

35. Morris AH, Chapman RH, Gardner RM. Frequency of technical problems encountered in the measurement of pulmonary artery wedge pressure. *Crit Care Med.* 1984;12(3):164–170.

36. Gnaegi A, Feihl F, Perret C. Intensive care physicians' insufficient knowledge of right-heart catheterization at the bedside: Time to act? *Crit Care Med.* 1997;25(2):213–220.

37. Jacka MJ, Cohen MM, To T, Devitt JH, Byrick R. Pulmonary artery occlusion pressure estimation: How confident are anesthesiologists? *Crit Care Med.* 2002;30(6):1197–1203.

38. LeVarge BL, Pomerantsev E, Channick RN. Reliance on end-expiratory wedge pressure leads to misclassification of pulmonary hypertension. *Eur Respir J.* 2014;44(2):425–434.

39. Ryan JJ, Rich JD, Thiruvoipati T, Swamy R, Kim GH, Rich S. Current practice for determining pulmonary capillary wedge pressure predisposes to serious errors in the classification of patients with pulmonary hypertension. *Am Heart J.* 2012;163(4):589–594.

40. Houston BA, Tedford RJ. What we talk about when we talk about the wedge pressure. *Circ Heart Fail.* 2017;10(9). https://doi.org/10.1161/CIRCHEARTFAILURE.117.004450

41. Dickinson MG, Lam CS, Rienstra M, Vonck TE, Hummel YM, Voors AA, et al. Atrial fibrillation modifies the association between pulmonary artery wedge pressure and left ventricular end-diastolic pressure. *Eur J Heart Fail.* 2017;19(11):1483–1490.

42. Halpern SD, Taichman DB. Misclassification of pulmonary hypertension due to reliance on pulmonary capillary wedge pressure rather than left ventricular end-diastolic pressure. *Chest.* 2009;136(1):37–43.

43. Wright SP, Moayedi Y, Foroutan F, Agarwal S, Paradero G, Alba AC, et al. Diastolic pressure difference to classify pulmonary hypertension in the assessment of heart transplant candidates. *Circ Heart Fail.* 2017;10(9):e004077.

44. Tedford R, Vachiery J, De Marco T, Chazova I, Coughlan J, Guazzi M, et al. Pulmonary hypertension due to left heart Diseases. *JACC.* 2018 (in press).

45. Caravita S, Faini A, Deboeck G, Bondue A, Naeije R, Parati G, et al. Pulmonary hypertension and ventilation during exercise: Role of the pre-capillary component. *J Heart Lung Transplant.* 2017;36(7):754–762.

46. Jacobs W, Konings TC, Heymans MW, Boonstra A, Bogaard HJ, van Rossum AC, et al. Noninvasive identification of left-sided heart failure in a population suspected of pulmonary arterial hypertension. *Eur Respir J.* 2015;46(2):422–430.

47. Opotowsky AR, Ojeda J, Rogers F, Prasanna V, Clair M, Moko L, et al. A simple echocardiographic prediction rule for hemodynamics in pulmonary hypertension. *Circ Cardiovasc Imaging.* 2012;5(6):765–775.

48. Berthelot E, Montani D, Algalarrondo V, Dreyfuss C, Rifai R, Benmalek A, et al. A clinical and echocardiographic score to identify pulmonary hypertension due to HFpEF. *J Card Fail.* 2017;23(1):29–235.

49. Hoeper MM, Lee SH, Voswinckel R, Palazzini M, Jais X, Marinelli A, et al. Complications of right heart catheterization procedures in patients with pulmonary hypertension in experienced centers. *J Am Coll Cardiol.* 2006;48(12):2546–2552.

50. Gupta D, Karrowni W, Chatterjee K. Swan-Ganz catheters. In: Chatterjee K, Anderson M, Heistad D, editors. *Cardiology: An Illustrated Textbook.* New Delhi, India: Jaypee Brothers Medical Publishers; 2012. p. 503–516.

51. Martin UJ, Krachman S. Hemodynamic monitoring. In: Criner GJ, D'Alonzo GE, editors. *Critical Care Study Guide: Text and Review.* Philadelphia, PA: Springer-Verlag; 2002. p. 44–69.

52. Kern MJ, Sorajja P, Lim M. *The Cardiac Catheterization Handbook*. 6th ed. Oxford, UK: Elsevier Health Sciences; 2015.

53. Rich S, D'Alonzo GE, Dantzker DR, Levy PS. Magnitude and implications of spontaneous hemodynamic variability in primary pulmonary hypertension. *Am J Cardiol*. 1985;55(1):159–163.

54. Farber HW, Karlinsky JB, Faling LJ. Fatal outcome following nifedipine for pulmonary hypertension. *Chest*. 1983;83(4):708–709.

55. Aromatorio GJ, Uretsky BF, Reddy PS. Hypotension and sinus arrest with nifedipine in pulmonary hypertension. *Chest*. 1985;87(2):265–267.

56. Partanen J, Nieminen MS, Luomanmaki K. Death in a patient with primary pulmonary hypertension after 20 mg of nifedipine. *N Engl J Med*. 1993;329(11):812.

57. Sitbon O, Humbert M, Jagot JL, Taravella O, Fartoukh M, Parent F, et al. Inhaled nitric oxide as a screening agent for safely identifying responders to oral calcium-channel blockers in primary pulmonary hypertension. *Eur Respir J*. 1998;12(2):265–270.

58. Sitbon O, Humbert M, Jais X, Ioos V, Hamid AM, Provencher S, et al. Long-term response to calcium channel blockers in idiopathic pulmonary arterial hypertension. *Circulation*. 2005;111(23):3105–3111.

59. Montani D, Savale L, Natali D, Jais X, Herve P, Garcia G, et al. Long-term response to calcium-channel blockers in non-idiopathic pulmonary arterial hypertension. *Eur Heart J*. 2010;31(15):1898–1907.

60. Mitchell JH, Blomqvist G. Maximal oxygen uptake. *N Engl J Med*. 1971;284(18):1018–1022.

61. Provencher S, Herve P, Sitbon O, Humbert M, Simonneau G, Chemla D. Changes in exercise haemodynamics during treatment in pulmonary arterial hypertension. *Eur Respir J*. 2008;32(2):393–398.

62. Provencher S, Chemla D, Herve P, Sitbon O, Humbert M, Simonneau G. Heart rate responses during the 6-minute walk test in pulmonary arterial hypertension. *Eur Respir J*. 2006;27(1):114–120.

63. Malhotra R, Dhakal BP, Eisman AS, Pappagianopoulos PP, Dress A, Weiner RB, et al. Pulmonary vascular distensibility predicts pulmonary hypertension severity, exercise capacity, and survival in heart failure. *Circ Heart Fail*. 2016;9(6):e003011.

64. Kafi SA, Melot C, Vachiery JL, Brimioulle S, Naeije R. Partitioning of pulmonary vascular resistance in primary pulmonary hypertension. *J Am Coll Cardiol*. 1998;31(6):1372–1376.

65. Langleben D, Orfanos SE. Pulmonary capillary recruitment in exercise and pulmonary hypertension. *Eur Respir J*. 2018;51(3):1702559.

66. D'Andrea A, Naeije R, D'Alto M, Argiento P, Golia E, Cocchia R, et al. Range in pulmonary artery systolic pressure among highly trained athletes. *Chest*. 2011;139(4):788–794.

67. Saggar R, Sitbon O. Hemodynamics in pulmonary arterial hypertension: Current and future perspectives. *Am J Cardiol*. 2012;110(6 Suppl):9S–15S.

68. Chaouat A, Sitbon O, Mercy M, Poncot-Mongars R, Provencher S, Guillaumot A, et al. Prognostic value of exercise pulmonary haemodynamics in pulmonary arterial hypertension. *Eur Respir J*. 2014;44(3):704–713.

69. Badesch DB, Abman SH, Ahearn GS, Barst RJ, McCrory DC, Simonneau G, et al. Medical therapy for pulmonary arterial hypertension: ACCP evidence-based clinical practice guidelines. *Chest*. 2004;126(1 Suppl):35S–62S.

70. Bossone E, Rubenfire M, Bach DS, Ricciardi M, Armstrong WF. Range of tricuspid regurgitation velocity at rest and during exercise in normal adult men: Implications for the diagnosis of pulmonary hypertension. *J Am Coll Cardiol*. 1999;33(6):1662–1666.

71. Galie N, Hoeper MM, Humbert M, Torbicki A, Vachiery JL, Barbera JA, et al. Guidelines for the diagnosis and treatment of pulmonary hypertension: The Task Force for the Diagnosis and Treatment of Pulmonary Hypertension of the European Society of Cardiology (ESC) and the European Respiratory Society (ERS), endorsed by the International Society of Heart and Lung Transplantation (ISHLT). *Eur Heart J*. 2009;30(20):2493–2537.

72. Kovacs G, Maier R, Aberer E, Brodmann M, Scheidl S, Troster N, et al. Borderline pulmonary arterial pressure is associated with decreased exercise capacity in scleroderma. *Am J Respir Crit Care Med.* 2009;180(9):881–886.

73. Condliffe R, Kiely DG, Peacock AJ, Corris PA, Gibbs JS, Vrapi F, et al. Connective tissue disease-associated pulmonary arterial hypertension in the modern treatment era. *Am J Respir Crit Care Med.* 2009;179(2):151–157.

74. Herve P, Lau EM, Sitbon O, Savale L, Montani D, Godinas L, et al. Criteria for diagnosis of exercise pulmonary hypertension. *Eur Respir J.* 2015;46(3):728–737.

75. Naeije R, Saggar R, Badesch D, Rajagopalan S, Gargani L, Rischard F, et al. Exercise-induced pulmonary hypertension: Translating pathophysiological concepts into clinical practice. *Chest.* 2018.

76. Mathier M. The nuts and bolts of interpreting hemodynamics in pulmonary hypertension associated with diastolic heart failure. *Adv Pulm Hypertens J.* 2011;10:33–40.

77. Robbins IM, Hemnes AR, Pugh ME, Brittain EL, Zhao DX, Piana RN, et al. High prevalence of occult pulmonary venous hypertension revealed by fluid challenge in pulmonary hypertension. *Circ Heart Fail.* 2014;7(1):116–122.

78. Fox BD, Shimony A, Langleben D, Hirsch A, Rudski L, Schlesinger R, et al. High prevalence of occult left heart disease in scleroderma-pulmonary hypertension. *Eur Respir J.* 2013;42(4):1083–1091.

79. Fujimoto N, Borlaug BA, Lewis GD, Hastings JL, Shafer KM, Bhella PS, et al. Hemodynamic responses to rapid saline loading: The impact of age, sex, and heart failure. *Circulation.* 2013;127(1):55–62.

80. Andersen MJ, Olson TP, Melenovsky V, Kane GC, Borlaug BA. Differential hemodynamic effects of exercise and volume expansion in people with and without heart failure. *Circ Heart Fail.* 2015;8(1):41–48.

81. Naeije R, Vachiery JL, Yerly P, Vanderpool R. The transpulmonary pressure gradient for the diagnosis of pulmonary vascular disease. *Eur Respir J.* 2013;41(1):217–223.

82. Gerges C, Gerges M, Lang MB, Zhang Y, Jakowitsch J, Probst P, et al. Diastolic pulmonary vascular pressure gradient: A predictor of prognosis in "out-of-proportion" pulmonary hypertension. *Chest.* 2013;143(3):758–766.

83. Tampakakis E, Leary PJ, Selby VN, De Marco T, Cappola TP, Felker GM, et al. The diastolic pulmonary gradient does not predict survival in patients with pulmonary hypertension due to left heart disease. *JACC Heart Fail.* 2015;3(1):9–16.

84. Tedford RJ, Beaty CA, Mathai SC, Kolb TM, Damico R, Hassoun PM, et al. Prognostic value of the pre-transplant diastolic pulmonary artery pressure-to-pulmonary capillary wedge pressure gradient in cardiac transplant recipients with pulmonary hypertension. *J Heart Lung Transplant.* 2014;33(3):289–297.

85. Tampakakis E, Tedford RJ. Balancing the positives and negatives of the diastolic pulmonary gradient. *Eur J Heart Fail.* 2017;19(1):98–100.

86. Vachiery JL, Adir Y, Barbera JA, Champion H, Coghlan JG, Cottin V, et al. Pulmonary hypertension due to left heart diseases. *J Am Coll Cardiol.* 2013;62(25 Suppl):D100–D108.

87. Miller WL, Grill DE, Borlaug BA. Clinical features, hemodynamics, and outcomes of pulmonary hypertension due to chronic heart failure with reduced ejection fraction: Pulmonary hypertension and heart failure. *JACC Heart Fail.* 2013;1(4):290–299.

88. Chatterjee NA, Lewis GD. Characterization of pulmonary hypertension in heart failure using the diastolic pressure gradient: Limitations of a solitary measurement. *JACC Heart Fail.* 2015;3(1):17–21.

29

Haemodynamic evaluation of the heart transplant patient

KAVITHA MUTHIAH, CHRISTOPHER S. HAYWARD, ANDREW JABBOUR
AND PETER MACDONALD

INTRODUCTION

Heart transplantation (HT) is a therapeutic option for patients with advanced heart failure refractory to medical therapy. It confers both survival benefit and improvement in quality of life in patients with advanced cardiac disease. Patient selection for transplant candidacy is paramount given the scarcity of donor organs.

In the current era of heart transplantation, one-third of patients on the waiting list are bridged with durable mechanical assist devices in the form of a left ventricular assist device (LVAD), biventricular assist device or total artificial heart. In addition to supporting the failing ventricle, this option may be considered in a subset of patients to lower the trans-pulmonary gradient and enable transplant eligibility.

Right heart catheterisation enables haemodynamic evaluation, both to assess suitability for heart transplantation and to enable haemodynamic optimisation of heart failure. In addition, it allows assessment of the need for right ventricular support following left ventricular assist device implantation. Following heart transplantation, endomyocardial biopsy and coronary angiography are pivotal in assessing the presence and severity of cardiac rejection and coronary artery vasculopathy, respectively.

RIGHT HEART CATHETERISATION

Technique

Right heart catheterisation is an important test for assessing and maintaining transplant eligibility. It may be performed via several venous approaches: Internal jugular, femoral or peripheral access via antecubital veins. The standard approach in many transplant centres is via the right internal jugular approach. The technique is described in Chapter 28.

Measurements

Routine haemodynamic measurements are obtained, including the following: Right atrial pressure, right ventricular end-diastolic pressure, pulmonary artery pressure (systole, diastole, mean), pulmonary wedge pressure. Table 29.1 provides a list of haemodynamic measurements with normal reference ranges, and Figure 29.1a illustrates the characteristic appearance of pressure waves recorded in each chamber. Derived indices include cardiac output (CO), thermodilution, estimated Fick, cardiac index (CI), pulmonary vascular resistance (PVR), systemic vascular resistance (SVR), right ventricular stroke work index (RVSWI), transpulmonary gradient (TPG) and diastolic pulmonary gradient (DPG). Table 29.2 provides derived haemodynamic variables and normal reference ranges.

Pulmonary hypertension due to left heart disease is haemodynamically defined as mean pulmonary artery pressure ≥ 25 mmHg and mean pulmonary artery wedge pressure ≥ 15 mmHg. It is further classified according to PVR and DPG as isolated post-capillary pulmonary hypertension (DPG <7 mmHg and/or PVR ≤ 3 Wood units) and combined post-capillary and pre-capillary pulmonary hypertension (DPG ≥ 7 mmHg and/or PVR >3 Wood units).[1]

Pulmonary hypertension and elevated PVR should be considered a relative contraindication to cardiac transplantation when the PVR is >5 Wood units or the PVR index is >6 Wood units/m^2 or the TPG exceeds 15 mmHg.[2] If the systolic pulmonary arterial pressure is greater than 60 mmHg in conjunction with any one of the preceding three variables, the risk of right heart failure and early death post-transplant is increased. Up to 20% of early deaths post-transplant are attributable to right heart failure.[3] If the PVR can be reduced to <2.5 Wood units with a vasodilator but systemic systolic blood pressure falls to <85 mmHg, the patient remains at high risk of right heart failure and mortality after cardiac transplantation.[4]

It is advocated that right heart catheterisation be performed periodically until transplantation once transplant candidacy is established. The frequency should be guided by initial haemodynamics. A vasodilator challenge should be administered when the pulmonary systolic pressure is ≥ 50 mmHg and either the TPG is ≥ 15 or the PVR is >3 Wood units while maintaining a systemic systolic arterial blood pressure of >85 mmHg.[2]

Table 29.1 Haemodynamic values and normal range

Variable	Normal range
Right atrial pressure (mmHg)	
Mean	1–7
Right ventricular pressure (mmHg)	
Systolic	15–28
Diastolic	0–8
Pulmonary artery (mmHg)	
Systolic	15–25
Diastolic	8–15
Mean	10–20
Pulmonary artery wedge (mmHg)	
Mean	6–12
Cardiac output (L/min)	4–8

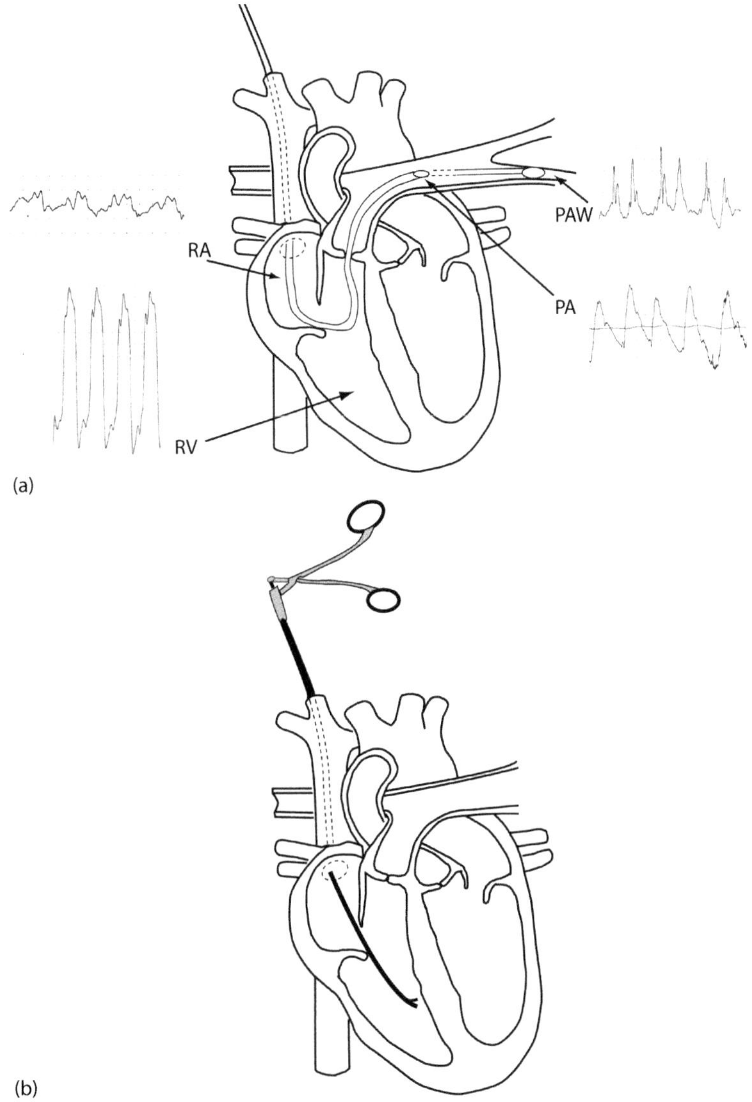

Figure 29.1 (a) Illustration of pressure tracings taken with a Swan-Ganz catheter and its anatomical placement in the pulmonary artery (*Abbreviations:* RA, right atrium; RV, right ventricle; PA, pulmonary artery; PAW, pulmonary artery wedge); (b) position and use of a bioptome. (Courtesy of R. Hawkins.)

VASODILATOR CHALLENGE

Vasodilators

GLYCERYL TRINITRATE

Glyceryl trinitrate (GTN) causes relaxation of vascular smooth muscle, which in turn leads to dilatation of both arterial and venous beds, although venous dilatation predominates over dilatation of the arterioles. Dilatation of the post-capillary vessels, including large veins, promotes peripheral pooling of blood and decreases venous return to the heart, reducing left ventricular end diastolic pressure and pulmonary artery wedge pressure (preload). This may in turn lead to a reduction in preload driven pulmonary hypertension. Arteriolar relaxation reduces systemic vascular resistance and arterial pressure (afterload).

A standard challenge protocol is as follows:

50 mg of GTN is added to 100 mL of 5% dextrose. The infusion is started at a rate of 10 mL/h

Table 29.2 Derived haemodynamic values and normal ranges

Variable	Formula	Normal range
Cardiac index	CO (L/min)/Body surface area (m^2)	2.8–4.2 L/min/m^2
Transpulmonary gradient	Mean PAP – Mean PAWP	<12 mmHg
Diastolic pulmonary gradient	DPAP – Mean PAWP	<7 mmHg
Pulmonary vascular resistance	(Mean PAP – Mean PAWP)/CO (L/min)	0.3–1.6 Wood Units
Systemic vascular resistance	(MAP – RAP)/CO (L/min)	9–20 Wood Units
Stroke volume index	(CI/HR) × 1000	33–47 mL/m^2/beat
Right ventricular stroke work index	SVI × (Mean PAP – RAP) × 0.0136	5–10 mmHg × mL/m^2

Abbreviations: CO, cardiac output; PAP, pulmonary artery pressure; PAWP, pulmonary artery wedge pressure; DPAP, diastolic pulmonary artery pressure; MAP, mean arterial pressure; RAP, right atrial pressure; CI, cardiac index; SVI, stroke volume index; HR, heart rate.

and increased at 5-minute intervals by 10 mL/h up to a rate of 50 mL/h. Blood pressure should be monitored every 2 minutes. If the TPG fails to fall below 12 mmHg, or the patient is already on oral nitrate therapy, challenging the patient with an alternative agent should be considered.

SODIUM NITROPRUSSIDE

Similar to glyceryl trinitrate, sodium nitroprusside causes relaxation of vascular smooth muscle and consequent dilatation of peripheral arteries and veins. Preferential veno-dilatation is less pronounced in comparison to GTN.

A standard challenge protocol is as follows:

50 mg of sodium nitroprusside is added to 100 mL of 5% dextrose. The infusion is started at a rate of 10 mL/h and increased at 5-minute intervals by 10 mL/h up to a rate of 40 mL/h. Blood pressure should be monitored every 2 minutes.

NITRIC OXIDE

Inhaled nitric oxide is a selective pulmonary vasodilator. It is delivered as a gas. It is rapidly inactivated when bound to haemoglobin and, as such, the effects remain local, thus minimising the risk of systemic hypotension. Its short half-life also permits rapid discontinuation, if necessary. It should be noted that selective pulmonary vasodilatation results in increased preload to the failing left ventricle. This is manifested as an elevation in pulmonary artery wedge pressure and may precipitate pulmonary oedema. As such, inhaled nitric oxide should be used with caution in the setting of left heart disease.

A standard challenge protocol is as follows:

Inhalation starting at 5–10 ppm increasing to 20 ppm. Timing of challenge is commenced when the level of 20 ppm is reached. Haemodynamic measurements are performed thereafter every 5 minutes for a duration of 10 minutes.

PROSTACYCLIN

Epoprostenol, also known as prostacyclin and PGI$_2$, causes direct vasodilatation of pulmonary and systemic arterial vascular beds, thus reducing both right and left ventricular afterload. Additionally, it is a potent endogenous inhibitor of platelet aggregation.

A standard challenge protocol is as follows:

500 µg epoprostenol is added to 100 mL buffer solution and injected into a 100 mL Baxter bag. The final solution will have a concentration of 5000 ng/mL. The infusion is started at 2 ng/kg/min and dose increased in increments of 2 ng/kg/min every 10–15 minutes. The dosing range during acute vasodilator testing is from 2 to 12 ng/kg/min.

NON-RESPONDERS TO ACUTE VASODILATOR

Patients who do not respond to an acute vasodilator challenge should be considered for admission for treatment with inotropes, diuretics and vasoactive agents such as inhaled nitric oxide alongside continuous haemodynamic monitoring.[1] Optimisation of volume status, in combination with inotropic support over 24–48 hours, may lead to an improvement in PVR.

LEFT VENTRICULAR ASSIST DEVICES

If pharmacological therapy fails to reverse pulmonary hypertension, mechanical circulatory support in the form of an LVAD to unload the ventricle should be considered. Several studies to date have shown this to be effective in normalising transpulmonary gradient and enabling transplant candidacy,[5-7] Improvement in haemodynamics is seen as early as 1 month post-LVAD implantation.[5]

Right heart catheterisation is important in risk stratification and in assessing the requirement for right ventricular support in patients undergoing LVAD implantation. Early post-LVAD mortality is due partly to development of right-sided heart failure.

Mechanisms of right ventricular failure post-LVAD

Following LVAD implantation, the interplay between ventricles changes. Decompression of the left ventricle with support causes a reduction in left ventricular end-diastolic pressure, which subsequently leads to a reduction in pulmonary pressure and improvement in right ventricular function. However, early post-LVAD implantation, the increased cardiac output from forward flow generated by the pump results in increased venous return, which may worsen pre-existing right ventricular failure. Additionally, excessive leftward shift of the interventricular septum from overaggressive decompression of the left ventricle decreases septal contribution to right ventricular contraction, potentially exacerbating right ventricular failure. Other causes of right ventricular failure post-LVAD implantation includes worsening of tricuspid regurgitation from increased venous return.

Risk prediction for right ventricular failure and requirement for right ventricular support

There are now several algorithms and risk prediction scores for the development of right ventricular failure post-LVAD support.[8-10] A combination of haemodynamic, echocardiographic and patient factors contribute to these risk prediction scores. These indices may be used to assess the need for permanent or temporary right ventricular support following LVAD. Scores are in part derived from haemodynamic measurements from right heart catheterisation (Table 29.3).[8, 11-13]

Table 29.3 Derived haemodynamic measurements from right heart catheterisation in predicting need for right ventricular support following left ventricular assist device therapy

Variable	Publication
Elevated RAP, >15 mmHg	Kormos et al.[11] Right ventricular failure in patients with the HeartMate II continuous-flow left ventricular assist device: incidence, risk factors, and effect on outcomes
RAP/mean PAWP >0.54	Soliman et al.[8] Derivation and validation of a novel right-sided heart failure model after implantation of continuous flow left ventricular assist devices
RAP/mean PAWP >0.63	Kormos et al.[11] Right ventricular failure in patients with the HeartMate II continuous-flow left ventricular assist device: incidence, risk factors, and effect on outcomes
RVSWI < 300 mmHg mL/m^2	Fukamachi et al.[12] Pre-operative risk factors for right ventricular failure after implantable left ventricular assist device insertion
PAPI < 1.85	Morine et al.[13] Pulmonary artery pulsatility index is associated with right ventricular failure after left ventricular assist device surgery

Abbreviations: RAP, right atrial pressure; PAWP, pulmonary artery wedge pressure; RVSWI, right ventricular stroke work index; PAPI, pulmonary artery pulsatility index, PAPI formula (systolic PAP – diastolic PAP)/RAP).

POST-TRANSPLANT SURVEILLANCE

Rejection of the transplanted heart in the form of cellular or antibody-mediated rejection and the development of cardiac allograft vasculopathy (CAV) contribute to morbidity and mortality post cardiac transplantation.

Endomyocardial biopsy

Endomyocardial biopsy is an established invasive clinical tool used for surveillance of cardiac allograft rejection. Performance of routine periodic right ventricular endomyocardial biopsy in the first post-transplant year is standard of care for rejection surveillance. An example of a surveillance regimen includes: Weekly biopsy in the first month; fortnightly in the subsequent two months; monthly until 6 months; 3 monthly thereafter up to a year. After the first year, there is more variability between institutions regarding the need for surveillance endomyocardial biopsy. While some institutions continue to perform surveillance endomyocardial biopsies at 6–12 monthly intervals, others only perform endomyocardial biopsy when there is clinical suspicion of rejection. Sustained ventricular tachycardia should be evaluated with both endomyocardial biopsy and coronary angiography.

Technique

The preferred access site for endomyocardial biopsy is the right internal jugular vein, since introduction of the flexible Stanford-Caves Schultz bioptome. Left internal jugular, femoral and subclavian access is also feasible. Biopsy specimens should be obtained from the interventricular septum. Sampling from the thin right ventricular free wall is high risk and should be avoided. Endomyocardial biopsy may be guided by fluoroscopy, echocardiography, or both, with continuous electrocardiographic monitoring. Biopsy performed for diagnosis of cardiomyopathy should be performed under both fluoroscopic and echocardiographic guidance, due to higher risk of myocardial perforation.

The procedure is generally performed without pre-medication. With the right internal jugular vein approach, venous puncture is performed under ultrasound guidance with infiltration of local anaesthesia. This is followed by the insertion of a 9 Fr sheath using the Seldinger technique. The bioptome

is advanced under fluoroscopic guidance into the right atrium. Using counterclockwise rotation, the bioptome is passed across the tricuspid valve towards the interventricular septum (Figure 29.1b). Contact of the bioptome with the myocardium generates ventricular ectopics. Resistance is felt when contact is made. The bioptome is then partially withdrawn, and with the jaws opened, readvanced to contact the myocardium. The jaws of the biopsy forceps are then closed and the bioptome withdrawn with the piece of myocardial tissue. The tissue is removed and placed in formalin for histopathological analysis. Five pieces of myocardium of 1–2 mm diameter are necessary for adequate sampling. Transplant recipients undergo endomyocardial biopsy numerous times, which leads to scarring of the interventricular septum with time. This increases the difficulty in obtaining adequate future tissue samples for histologic analysis.

Complications

In the contemporary era, serious complications associated with endomyocardial biopsy performed under imaging guidance are uncommon, under 1%.[14,15] These include perforation requiring pericardiocentesis or surgical patch, and damage to the tricuspid valve requiring surgical repair. Other complications related to the procedure include provocation of sustained atrial or ventricular arrhythmias, heart block requiring temporary pacing, tissue embolism and access-related complications such as pneumothorax or inadvertent arterial puncture. If atrial flutter is induced and sustained, a temporary pacing wire can be introduced to perform atrial overdrive pacing to restore sinus rhythm.

CORONARY ANGIOGRAPHY FOR CARDIAC ALLOGRAFT VASCULOPATHY

Cardiac allograft vasculopathy contributes to a significant proportion of deaths after cardiac transplantation, and its contribution to mortality increases with time from transplant. The prevalence is high – 20% at 3 years, 30% at 5 years and 45% at 8 years post-transplant.[16] Classical angina may be experienced in up to 50% of patients as the transplanted heart reinnervates. The characteristics that affect the risk of CAV development include: (i) donor characteristics:

higher age, male sex, higher body surface area, history of hypertension, history of infection, and (ii) recipient characteristics such as history of ischemic heart disease, LVAD implant before transplant, and history of infection. In addition, medication use such as azathioprine rather than mycophenolate mofetil, use of cyclosporine rather than tacrolimus, and use of OKT3 for induction therapy have been implicated as risk factors.[16]

Surveillance by coronary angiography or non-invasive techniques such as perfusion scanning with technetium-99 m sestamibi, stress echocardiography (usually with dobutamine) or computed tomographic coronary angiography is standard of care post-transplant. The last modality has been shown to be a reliable non-invasive imaging alternative to coronary angiography, with excellent sensitivity, specificity and negative predictive value for detection of CAV.[17]

There are important morphological differences between coronary artery disease in transplanted versus native hearts. The main differences are illustrated in Figure 29.2.[18] CAV has protean presentations.[2] The pathophysiology associated with early disease is thought to represent an inflammatory vasculitis, portending poorer outcomes. When CAV occurs beyond the second post-transplant year it is typically more indolent. Rapidly progressive or fulminant CAV, defined as a lesion greater than 70% within one year of a benign angiogram, has poor prognosis. As such, the speed of CAV development and the time after transplantation are the primary determinants of adverse outcomes.

Recommended nomenclature for CAV is listed in Table 29.4,[19] and considers both angiographic parameters and graft function.

Coronary angiography is relatively insensitive in detecting early disease and can be misleading when the disease is diffuse. Intravascular ultrasound (IVUS) has greater sensitivity in detecting early CAV. Numerous reports have shown that significant changes in intimal thickness, intimal area, intimal index and vessel area (all detectable by IVUS) can occur in the initial year after transplant. The present recommendation, however, does not advocate the routine use of IVUS for CAV surveillance, as

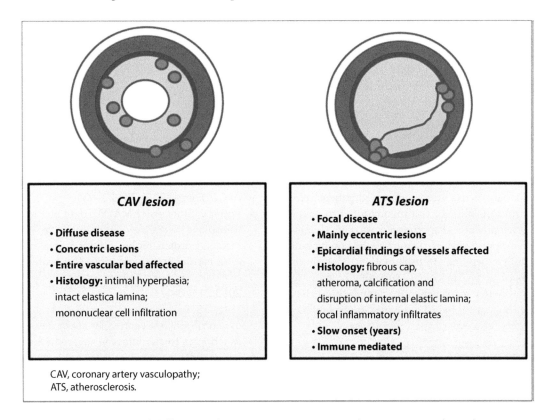

CAV lesion
- Diffuse disease
- Concentric lesions
- Entire vascular bed affected
- Histology: intimal hyperplasia; intact elastica lamina; mononuclear cell infiltration

ATS lesion
- Focal disease
- Mainly eccentric lesions
- Epicardial findings of vessels affected
- Histology: fibrous cap, atheroma, calcification and disruption of internal elastic lamina; focal inflammatory infiltrates
- Slow onset (years)
- Immune mediated

CAV, coronary artery vasculopathy;
ATS, atherosclerosis.

Figure 29.2 Morphological differences between coronary artery disease in transplanted versus native hearts. (Adapted from Angelini, A. et al., *Virchows Archiv.*, 464, 627, 2014.)

Table 29.4 Recommended nomenclature for cardiac allograft vasculopathy (CAV)

ISHLT CAV0 (Not significant)	No detectable angiographic lesion
ISHLT CAV1 (Mild)	Angiographic left main (LM) <50%, or primary vessel with maximum lesion of <70%, or any branch stenosis <70% (including diffuse narrowing) without allograft dysfunction
ISHLT CAV2 (Moderate)	Angiographic LM <50%; a single primary vessel ≥, or isolated branch stenosis ≥70% in branches of 2 systems, without allograft dysfunction
ISHLT CAV3 (Severe)	Angiographic LM ≥50%, or 2 or more primary vessels ≥70% stenosis, or isolated branch stenosis ≥70% in all 3 systems; or ISHLT CVA1 or CAV2 with allograft dysfunction (LVEF ≤ 45% in the presence of regional wall motion abnormalities or evidence of restrictive physiology)

Source: Mehra, M.R. et al., J. Heart Lung Transplant., 29, 717, 2010.

benefit of early detection is limited to prognostication rather than intervention. It may be used at any point in the transplant process for excluding significant disease when the angiogram appears ambiguous. However, it is unlikely that IVUS will define flow-limiting epicardial disease that is not demonstrated by a high-quality coronary angiogram.

Percutaneous coronary intervention with drug-eluting stents is recommended for CAV and offers short-term palliation for appropriate discrete lesions of significance. Surgical revascularisation is also an option in highly selected patients with lesions amenable to surgical revascularisation. A cohort of patients may be considered for retransplantation in the absence of contraindications.

SUMMARY

The future seems bright for the heart transplant patient. Intensive preliminary assessment with various modalities has greatly improved patient selection and suitability for transplantation. Progress in the development and appropriate use of mechanical cardiac support devices can improve haemodynamic instability pending transplantation. Continuing advances in pharmacology, surveillance monitoring and better management of complications have proven successful in reducing post-transplantation mortality rates over the past twenty years.

REFERENCES

1. Galie N, Humbert M, Vachiery JL, et al. 2015 ESC/ERS Guidelines for the diagnosis and treatment of pulmonary hypertension: The Joint Task Force for the Diagnosis and Treatment of Pulmonary Hypertension of the European Society of Cardiology (ESC) and the European Respiratory Society (ERS): Endorsed by: Association for European Paediatric and Congenital Cardiology (AEPC), International Society for Heart and Lung Transplantation (ISHLT). The European Respiratory Journal 2015;46:903–975.
2. Mehra MR, Canter CE, Hannan MM, et al. The 2016 International Society for Heart Lung Transplantation listing criteria for heart transplantation: A 10-year update. The Journal of Heart and Lung Transplantation: 2016;35:1–23.
3. Stobierska-Dzierzek B, Awad H, Michler RE. The evolving management of acute right-sided heart failure in cardiac transplant recipients. Journal of the American College of Cardiology 2001;38:923–931.
4. Butler J, Stankewicz MA, Wu J, et al. Pre-transplant reversible pulmonary hypertension predicts higher risk for mortality after cardiac transplantation. The Journal of Heart and Lung Transplantation: 2005;24:170–177.
5. Kutty RS, Parameshwar J, Lewis C, et al. Use of centrifugal left ventricular assist device as a bridge to candidacy in severe heart failure with secondary pulmonary hypertension. European Journal of Cardio-thoracic Surgery: Official Journal of the European Association for Cardio-thoracic Surgery 2013;43:1237–1242.

6. Mikus E, Stepanenko A, Krabatsch T, et al. Reversibility of fixed pulmonary hypertension in left ventricular assist device support recipients. *European Journal of Cardio-thoracic Surgery*: 2011;40:971–977.

7. Gupta S, Woldendorp K, Muthiah K, et al. Normalisation of haemodynamics in patients with end-stage heart failure with continuous-flow left ventricular assist device therapy. *Heart, Lung & Circulation* 2014;23:963–969.

8. Soliman OI, Akin S, Muslem R, et al. Derivation and validation of a novel right-sided heart failure model after implantation of continuous flow left ventricular assist devices: The EUROMACS (European Registry for Patients with Mechanical Circulatory Support) right-sided heart failure risk score. *Circulation* 2018;137:891–906.

9. Matthews JC, Koelling TM, Pagani FD, Aaronson KD. The right ventricular failure risk score a pre-operative tool for assessing the risk of right ventricular failure in left ventricular assist device candidates. *Journal of the American College of Cardiology* 2008;51:2163–2172.

10. Fitzpatrick JR, 3rd, Frederick JR, Hsu VM, et al. Risk score derived from pre-operative data analysis predicts the need for biventricular mechanical circulatory support. *The Journal of Heart and Lung Transplantation* 2008;27:1286–1292.

11. Kormos RL, Teuteberg JJ, Pagani FD, et al. Right ventricular failure in patients with the HeartMate II continuous-flow left ventricular assist device: Incidence, risk factors, and effect on outcomes. *The Journal of Thoracic and Cardiovascular Surgery* 2010;139:1316–1324.

12. Fukamachi K, McCarthy PM, Smedira NG, Vargo RL, Starling RC, Young JB. Preoperative risk factors for right ventricular failure after implantable left ventricular assist device insertion. *The Annals of Thoracic Surgery* 1999;68:2181–2184.

13. Morine KJ, Kiernan MS, Pham DT, Paruchuri V, Denofrio D, Kapur NK. Pulmonary artery pulsatility index is associated with right ventricular failure after left ventricular assist device surgery. *Journal of Cardiac Failure* 2016;22:110–116.

14. Isogai T, Yasunaga H, Matsui H, et al. Hospital volume and cardiac complications of endomyocardial biopsy: A retrospective cohort study of 9508 adult patients using a nationwide inpatient database in Japan. *Clinical Cardiology* 2015;38:164–170.

15. Saraiva F, Matos V, Goncalves L, Antunes M, Providencia LA. Complications of endomyocardial biopsy in heart transplant patients: A retrospective study of 2117 consecutive procedures. *Transplantation Proceedings* 2011;43:1908–1912.

16. Stehlik J, Edwards LB, Kucheryavaya AY, et al. The registry of the International Society for Heart and Lung Transplantation: Twenty-eighth adult heart transplant report–2011. *The Journal of Heart and Lung Transplantation*: 2011;30:1078–1094.

17. Wever-Pinzon O, Romero J, Kelesidis I, et al. Coronary computed tomography angiography for the detection of cardiac allograft vasculopathy: A meta-analysis of prospective trials. *Journal of the American College of Cardiology* 2014;63:1992–2004.

18. Angelini A, Castellani C, Fedrigo M, et al. Coronary cardiac allograft vasculopathy versus native atherosclerosis: Difficulties in classification. *Virchows Archiv* 2014;464:627–635.

19. Mehra MR, Crespo-Leiro MG, Dipchand A, et al. International Society for Heart and Lung Transplantation working formulation of a standardized nomenclature for cardiac allograft vasculopathy-2010. *The Journal of Heart and Lung Transplantation* 2010;29:717–727.

30

Trans-septal cardiac catheterisation

DAVID W. M. MULLER

INTRODUCTION

The recent proliferation of novel therapies for structural heart disease and treatment of complex cardiac arrhythmias has led to a resurgence in interest in safe techniques to access the left atrium. Techniques for directly measuring left atrial pressure by trans-septal puncture were described as early as 1959,[1] but became less necessary with the introduction of balloon-tipped catheters to measure the pulmonary arterial wedge pressure,[2] a reliable estimate of the left atrial pressure in most circumstances, and Doppler echocardiography, which obviated the need for direct pressure measurement to document valve stenosis severity. The first intervention performed using trans-septal catheterisation was balloon mitral valvuloplasty,[3] but it was not until ablation procedures for accessory pathways and atrial fibrillation became a dominant approach to arrhythmia management[4] that the technique began to grow exponentially. It has now become an essential component of treatment for multiple interventions including transcatheter mitral valve repair and replacement, left atrial appendage closure, closure of para-valvular mitral prosthetic leaks, and atrial septostomy.

ANATOMY OF THE ATRIAL SEPTUM

Embryologically, the atrial septum develops as a thin septum primum on the left atrial (LA) side, extending from the posterolateral aspect of the LA to the endocardial cushion. A thicker septum secundum subsequently forms superiorly on the right atrial (RA) side. The component of the septum not covered by the septum secundum forms the fossa ovalis. Resorption of the septum primum superiorly forms the ostium secundum. The septum secundum overlaps the ostium secundum, creating a channel (foramen ovale), which is held open by the higher right-sided cardiac pressures. This allows venous return of maternally-oxygenated blood from the abdomen and lower limbs to be shunted directly to the left side of the heart, limiting flow in the developing pulmonary circulation. At birth, the fall in intra-thoracic pressure results in a reduction in pulmonary vascular resistance and a reduction in RA pressure. Increasing pulmonary venous return to the left atrium increases the LA pressure. The foramen ovale closes and, in the majority of individuals, the two septa become fused. In approximately 25% of the population, the opening closes but does not fuse, resulting in a persistent channel (patent foramen ovale). Transient increases in right-sided pressure (as occurs with straining or coughing) result in a brief opening of the channel, and a very small right-to-left intra-cardiac shunt. This shunt is insufficient to affect cardiac function, but can allow passage of thrombus, air, or other foreign matter to the left atrium (LA), potentially resulting in cerebral or systemic artery occlusion (paradoxical embolism).

Other important structures related to the fossa ovalis include the aortic knuckle (torus aorticus), which lies antero-superiorly, and the coronary sinus, which lies antero-inferiorly (Figure 30.1a). The Eustachian valve, which lies on the anterior rim of the inferior vena cava (IVC), helps direct pre-natal blood flow from the IVC towards the foramen ovale and away from the right ventricle.

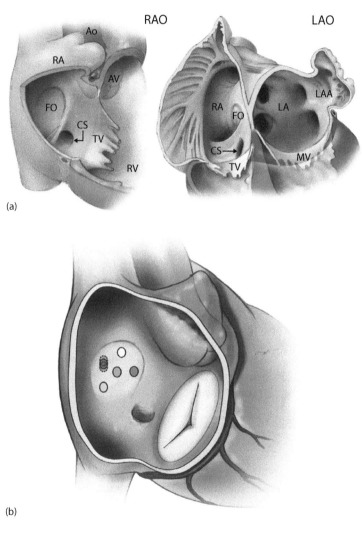

Figure 30.1 (a) Anatomy of the atrial septum. (*Abbreviations:* Ao, aorta; AR, aortic root; AV, aortic valve; CS, coronary sinus; FO, fossa ovalis; LA, left atrium; LAA, left atrial appendage; LAO, left anterior oblique; MV, mitral valve; PA, pulmonary artery; RA, right atrium; RAO, right anterior oblique; RV, right ventricle, TV, tricuspid valve.) (b) Optimal site of septal puncture according to specific trans-septal interventions. Red: MitraClip, paravalvular leak closure (a higher crossing site is recommended for medial leaks, and a lower crossing site is recommended for lateral leaks). Yellow: trans-septal patent foramen ovale closure; Blue: diagnostic studies, percutaneous left ventricular assist device placement, atrial septostomy. Green: left atrial appendage closure. Orange: pulmonary vein interventions. (Reproduced from Alkhouli, M., et al., *J. Am. Coll. Cardiol. Intv.*, 9, 2465, 2016. With permission.)

It may remain prominent into adult life. Its size and shape are variable, with some persisting as mobile structures that project into the RA.

TRANS-SEPTAL PUNCTURE TECHNIQUE

Prior to the procedure, any previous imaging of the septum and atria should be evaluated to identify anomalies such as a large PFO or septal aneurysm, a prominent Eustachian valve, septal thickening (e.g. lipomatous septal hypertrophy or previous atrial septal defect repair), or congenital abnormalities such as a left sided superior vena cava (SVC). The presence of thrombus in the left atrial appendage, or attached to the atrial walls should also be excluded. Bowing of the septum to the right or left should be noted. The procedure is best performed from the right femoral vein. Although technically more challenging, it can also be performed from the left femoral vein, internal jugular vein or hepatic vein.[5]

Trans-septal puncture has traditionally been performed using fluoroscopic guidance with a pigtail placed in the aortic root to minimise the risk of inadvertent aortic puncture. Access to transoesophageal and intra-cardiac echocardiography has now largely replaced fluoroscopic guidance because of the need to accurately determine the site of puncture for specific interventions. Ultrasound imaging also reduces the likelihood of atrial perforation and puncture of the aorta. An accurate puncture can greatly facilitate left atrial interventions. While a puncture in the centre of the fossa ovalis is acceptable for some interventions such as balloon mitral valvuloplasty and ideal for atrial septostomy, a puncture that is too anterior or too posterior will complicate other interventions. Likewise, access through a patent foramen ovale, though useful for diagnostic studies, is rarely appropriate for interventional procedures. The optimal site for septal puncture depends not only on the intervention, but also the pathology. Transcatheter mitral repair using MitraClip is best performed posteriorly 3.5–4.0 cm above the plane of the mitral annulus for secondary (functional) mitral regurgitation (MR), but higher (4.0–4.5 cm) for primary (degenerative) MR. A higher puncture is also required for medial jets than lateral jets. The same is true for closure of mitral prosthetic paravalvular leaks. Similarly, the orientation of the left atrial appendage can influence the optimal puncture site. The orifice of the appendage lies anteriorly, so an infero-posterior puncture is usually favoured. Conversely, ablation of the pulmonary veins, which lie posteriorly, can be facilitated by a more anterior septal puncture (Figure 30.1b).

TRANS-SEPTAL PUNCTURE EQUIPMENT

The Mullins technique for trans-septal puncture uses a sheath, dilator and a pre-shaped needle. The traditional fixed-curve Mullins sheath is available in a number of shapes and curvatures, primarily to facilitate LA ablation procedures. The standard sheath is 6–8 Fr and is 59 cm long with a 67 cm dilator. Additional flexibility and control of direction can be achieved by using a steerable sheath (Agilis, St Jude Medical, Saint Paul, MN, USA). Trans-septal needles (Brockenborough, Medtronic, Minneapolis, Minnesota or the BRK series of shaped needles from St Jude Medical, Saint Paul, MN, USA) are used to puncture the septum. The standard needle is 71 cm in length with a 21-gauge tip and a stylet to prevent perforation of the sheath during introduction of the needle. If a steerable sheath is used, a longer needle is required. The BRK series includes a number of shapes including the relatively shallow curve of the BRK needle and the greater curve of the BRK-1. The curvature of the needle can also be increased or decreased manually. The standard shape is appropriate when left atrial hypertension causes the septum to bulge into the RA, but greater curves are often required when the septum bulges to the left or is aneurysmal, or for interventions performed from the left femoral vein. The needles have a pointer at the hub indicating the direction of the curve.

When very accurate septal puncture is required, or is difficult to achieve with standard techniques, application of radiofrequency energy to the needle tip can facilitate septal puncture. This may be performed using a surgical diathermy unit applied to the proximal end of a standard needle, or a dedicated radiofrequency needle (Baylis Medical, Montreal, Canada). To minimise the risk of atrial perforation, a guidewire is sometimes used following introduction of the needle into the LA. The SafeSept wire (Pressure Products, San Pedro, California) is a 0.014 in nitinol wire with a J-tip that is advanced into the LA after needle puncture of the septum, providing a rail for safe passage of the needle. Alternatively, a 0.014 in angioplasty guidewire can be used.

TRANS-SEPTAL PROCEDURE

After femoral access is obtained, a 0.032 in J-tipped wire is advanced to the SVC. The Mullins sheath and introducer are advanced over the wire, the wire is removed and the sheath flushed. The needle and its stylet are then introduced. The needle is allowed to rotate during its passage to the SVC to minimise the risk of perforation of the sheath. The needle is advanced under fluoroscopy until it is 1–1.5 cm from the introducer tip. The stylet can be then removed, and the needle carefully flushed and attached to the pressure manifold. Vigorous aspiration of the needle can introduce air into the sheath. If this occurs, the needle must be removed and the sheath reflushed.

Once the needle is in the SVC, attention is turned to the echocardiographic images. Transoesophageal echocardiography allows simultaneous biplane imaging in the bicaval and short-axis views. The needle is rotated postero-medially (clockwise) towards 4–5 o'clock (12 o'clock being directly anterior and 6 o'clock being directly posterior) and the system is withdrawn into the RA. Once the echo images show tenting of the septum, appropriate measurements are made to confirm the correct site of puncture (Figure 30.2), and the needle is advanced into the LA. Puncture of the septum is confirmed by two-dimensional (2D) or 3D echo and by recognising a change in pressure waveform from a right atrial to a left atrial trace. If any doubt remains, dye can be injected through the needle to confirm that the tip is in the LA. Thereafter, the sheath assembly is advanced over the needle into the LA, and the needle is withdrawn. As soon as the sheath is securely positioned in the LA, anticoagulation should be given to maintain an activated clotting time (ACT) of 250–350 seconds depending on the complexity and likely duration of the planned intervention. If a larger delivery sheath is needed for the intervention, the trans-septal sheath can be exchanged over a wire placed in the left upper pulmonary vein. Occasionally, it is necessary to dilate the septum to allow passage of very large bore delivery sheaths.

POTENTIAL COMPLICATIONS

Although complications of trans-septal puncture are infrequent and mostly avoidable, they can be life-threatening. Embolisation of thrombus or air can occur if due attention is not paid to flushing the sheath and maintaining adequate

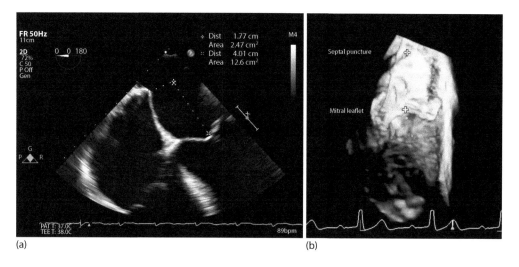

(a) (b)

Figure 30.2 **(a)** Transoesophageal image guidance for trans-septal puncture prior to MitraClip implantation. The atrial septum is tented towards the left atrium at a height of 4.01 cm above the coaptation zone of the mitral leaflets in a patient with severe mitral regurgitation secondary to leaflet tethering. **(b)** En face view of the atrial septum from the left atrial side. 3D echo measurement of septal puncture height above the mitral annulus.

anticoagulation. Stroke and transient cerebral ischaemic episodes occur in 0.5% of cases.[6] Embolisation of air into the right coronary artery can lead to transient inferior ST segment elevation but a similar syndrome can occur without apparent right coronary embolisation. This is thought to be a neurally mediated, Bezold-Jarisch-like event and usually responds to the administration of IV fluids and atropine.[7]

Cardiac perforation due to puncture of the right or left atrial free wall, or inadvertent injury to the left atrial appendage, can lead to cardiac tamponade.[8] An unusual cause of tamponade may occur with a low, posterior puncture in which the trans-septal needle exits the RA, traverses through peri-cardiac tissues in the extra-cardiac space, and enters the left atrium. In this situation, tamponade may not occur until the catheter is withdrawn at the completion of the procedure.

Following the use of large diameter trans-septal delivery sheaths, a defect may persist in the atrial septum, leading to an intra-cardiac shunt. The direction and extent of the shunt depends on the relative pressures in the left and right atria. The defect is rarely large enough to cause hypoxia due to a large right to left shunt, but a persistent communication between the atria may allow thromboembolic complications associated with systemic embolism. When very large defects remain after a trans-septal intervention, consideration should be given to closing the defect.[9]

CONCLUSIONS

Once the domain of a relatively small number of physicians interested in cardiovascular haemodynamics, trans-septal catheterisation is now a critically important skill and integral part of the electrophysiology and structural heart disease laboratories. Mitral valve and left atrial interventions depend on accurate site of septal puncture and are greatly facilitated by intra-procedural echocardiographic imaging. With due attention to technique, complications of septal puncture should be infrequent and rarely life-threatening.

REFERENCES

1. Ross J, Jr., Braunwald E, Morrow AG. Transseptal left atrial puncture; new technique for the measurement of left atrial pressure in man. *Am J Cardiol 1959*;3(5):653–655.
2. Swan HJ, Ganz W, Forrester J, Marcus H, Diamond G, Chonette D. Catheterization of the heart in man with use of a flow-directed balloon-tipped catheter. *N Engl J Med 1970*;283(9):447–451.
3. Lock JE, Khalilullah M, Shrivastava S, Bahl V, Keane JF. Percutaneous catheter commissurotomy in rheumatic mitral stenosis. *N Engl J Med 1985*;313(24):1515–1518.
4. Bonanno C, Paccanaro M, La Vecchia L, Ometto R, Fontanelli A. Efficacy and safety of catheter ablation versus antiarrhythmic drugs for atrial fibrillation: A meta-analysis of randomized trials. *J Cardiovasc Med (Hagerstown) 2010*;11(6):408–418.
5. Punamiya K, Beekman RH, Shim D, Muller DW. Percutaneous transhepatic mitral commissurotomy. *Cathet Cardiovasc Diagn 1996*;39(2):204–206.
6. Dagres N, Hindricks G, Kottkamp H, Sommer P, Gaspar T, Bode K, et al. Complications of atrial fibrillation ablation in a high-volume center in 1,000 procedures: Still cause for concern? *J Cardiovasc Electrophysiol 2009*;20(9):1014–1019.
7. Hildick-Smith DJ, Ludman PF, Shapiro LM. Inferior ST-segment elevation following transseptal puncture for balloon mitral valvuloplasty is atropine-responsive. *J Invasive Cardiol 2004*;16(1):1–2.
8. Holmes DR, Jr., Nishimura R, Fountain R, Turi ZG. Iatrogenic pericardial effusion and tamponade in the percutaneous intracardiac intervention era. *JACC Cardiovasc Interv 2009*;2(8):705–717.
9. Alkhouli M, Sarraf M, Holmes DR. Iatrogenic atrial septal defect. *Circ Cardiovasc Interv 2016*;9(4):e003545.

Percutaneous carotid interventions

31

Advances in stent technology

SMRITI SARAF AND PAUL BHAMRA-ARIZA

INTRODUCTION

First-generation drug-eluting stents (DES) were developed to combat high rates of in stent restenosis (ISR) (50%–60%) and target vessel revascularisation (TVR) (30%–50%) associated with bare metal stents (BMS).[1,2] The early DES was essentially a BMS platform with a drug carrier (polymer) responsible for storing a 'therapeutic agent' and enabling it to diffuse locally into the vascular tissue. The 'therapeutic agent' reduces neointimal hyperplasia induced by stent implantation. The stent platform was constructed from 316 L stainless steel with stent strut thickness ranging from 130 to 140 μm. Advantages of steel include its excellent mechanical properties, corrosion resistance and biocompatibility.[3] The first commercially available DES was the Cypher* stent (Cordis Corporation, Johnson & Johnson, USA) launched in 2003 (sirolimus-eluting), followed by the Taxus* stent (paclitaxel-eluting) in 2004 (Boston Scientific Corporation, USA). Although first-generation DES reduced restenosis across virtually all lesion and patient subsets, their safety has been limited by suboptimal polymer biocompatibility, local drug toxicity, and delayed stent endothelialisation leading to late and very late stent thrombosis[4] (ST). The permanent presence of polymers has been associated with local inflammation, impaired arterial healing and re-endothelialisation.[5] As a result, first generations DES are no longer used with any regularity.

Advances in stent platform construction and polymer biocompatibility have led to the emergence of second- and third-generation DES, which have in turn led to improved long-term clinical outcomes. In 2008, the zotarolimus-eluting stent (ZES) (Medtronic Vascular, USA) and the everolimus-eluting stent (EES) became commercially available, and are referred to as 'second-generation' DES. The second-generation DES has a stent platform composed of a cobalt-chromium (CoCr) alloy that gives rise to greater radial strength relative to thickness, thus allowing for thinner stent struts. Thinner struts and improved stent designs with fewer connectors improved stent flexibility and deliverability, and thinner struts led to a significant reduction in angiographic and clinical restenosis after coronary artery stenting.[6] When compared to first-generation DES, second-generation stents demonstrated superior re-endothelialisation performance and reduced ST rates.[7]

Third-generation DES are characterised by further refinements to the stent platform. The Resolute-ZES (strut thickness 91 μm), for example, consists of a single CoCr wire used to form a continuous sinusoidal shape that is then wrapped in a cylindrical form and laser-fused in specific locations to optimise deliverability and radial strength.[8] Platinum-chromium (PtCr) has also been used as an alloy to improve radial strength and to allow for a reduction in strut thickness.[9] The reduction in the number of connectors used in stents to improve deliverability and to a lesser extent, the reduction in stent strut thickness have led to a reduction in longitudinal axial strength. This in turn can increase the risk of longitudinal deformity resulting in longitudinal compression or shrinking and potential malapposition.[10] Benchmark testing has confirmed stents with two connectors have less longitudinal strength when exposed to compressing or elongating forces than those with more connectors.[11]

Despite advances in polymers, eluents and refinements in stent platforms, DES continue to have significant limitations. The persistent metal scaffold alters the vessel architecture and results in reduced compliance of the vessel. The residual foreign body disturbs normal vasomotion and promotes chronic inflammation, both of which contribute to late and very late ST. Most of these limitations can be overcome by use of bioresorbable stents. These stents are composed of a rigid scaffold that dissolves over time, leaving no metallic residue behind within the coronary artery. The bioresorbable vascular scaffold (BVS) is linked either by poly-lactide bridges or magnesium alloy and has a polymer coating that elutes the antiproliferative drug over 31 days.[11] The ABSORB BVS is linked by poly-lactide bridges and degrades by bulk erosion, and resorbs by a natural process. The water in surrounding vascular cells and blood penetrates the polymer matrix and the stent struts become more porous, resulting in replacement of the scaffold by proteoglycan. In the final step, lactic acid is converted to lactate and broken down to water and carbon dioxide via the Krebs cycle process. In the Absorb cohort A study,[12] complete dissolution of the everolimus coated scaffold struts was observed using optical coherence tomography over a 2-year period. The structure and functional integrity of the vessel was fully restored to a normal architecture with infiltration of smooth muscle cells. There was evidence of late luminal enlargement and late expansive remodelling resulting in less incidence of ST. Furthermore, due to bioresorption of the scaffold, permanent jailing of side branches and overhang at coronary ostia is prevented, making future revascularisation (percutaneous or surgical) easier at the site of previous stent implantation. As the stent scaffold disintegrates over time, imaging using multislice computed tomography or magnetic resonance imaging (MRI) is also more accurate due to lack of metal artefact.[13] Recent long-term data have highlighted an increased risk of late or very late scaffold thrombosis when compared to conventional DES.[12]

WHY WERE STENTS INVENTED?

Coronary angioplasty revolutionised the way coronary artery disease is managed. Although this proved to be a highly effective treatment, outcomes were compromised by the high rate of abrupt vessel closure resulting from acute arterial recoil and coronary artery dissection in the short term, and restenosis in the longer term. Coronary stents were therefore developed to overcome these problems, by acting as a scaffold within the artery to seal any potential dissection flap and prevent late recoil.

BASIC STRUCTURE OF THE CORONARY STENT

The conventional DES consist of three components: a metallic platform, polymer coating, and anti-proliferative drug. Stents were designed as a vascular scaffold to treat balloon angioplasty related dissections and acute vessel occlusion, and to reduce vascular recoil. Early BMS were made of 316 L stainless steel due to excellent mechanical properties and corrosion resistance, but other materials have later included CoCr alloy, or nickel-chromium alloy. Stainless steel has the disadvantage of being poorly visible on fluoroscopy and non-MRI compatible. Furthermore, there are concerns over the release of nickel, chromate and molybdenum ions, which may result in immune reactions and inflammatory responses and promote ISR.[13]

Newer alloys other than those containing stainless steel can allow for thinner struts while maintaining radial force. CoCr alloys have better radial strength and radio-opacity, and most stents are currently made from chromium with cobalt or platinum struts. PtCr alloys are twice as dense as CoCr alloys, and so have better radio-opacity under fluoroscopy. This in turn has allowed the development of stents with thinner stent struts and overall improved deliverability.

Coronary stents can be either balloon-expandable or self-expanding, although the latter is less commonly used in clinical practice. The balloon-expandable stent is crimped and pre-mounted on a balloon and expanded by inflation of the balloon, whose diameter determines the size of the expanded stent. The self-expanding stent is made of a coil or mesh configuration that is constrained within an outer sheath. When the sheath is withdrawn, the stent springs open to a predetermined size. Advantages include reduced stent strut malapposition with self-alignment of the stent struts to the vascular wall, thus facilitating strut healing and, in the case of DES, optimal drug delivery to the vessel wall. Disadvantages of self-expanding stents include reduced radial strength, which can be of some limitation, specifically in calcified lesions. Furthermore, in comparison to balloon-expandable stents they exhibit reduced trackability, which limits their use in tortuous and calcified vessels.

Different configurations were used to create different stent designs ranging from wire coils, slotted tubes, and a modular design. Wire coil stents consisted of a single coiled wire to form a sleeve around a balloon. This offered the advantage of great flexibility but poor radial strength. More recently, Medtronic has modified this such that the single wire is arranged in a sinusoidal pattern that winds in a helical fashion from one end of the stent to the other and is fused to adjacent loops at regular intervals. Slotted-tube stents were made from tubes of metal from which a stent design was laser-cut. The drawback of this design was poor flexibility due to the rigid structure, and consequently these are no longer routinely used in clinical practice. Modular stents have overcome the problems of inflexibility of slotted tube stents. The modular design consists of a series of rings with peaks or crowns fused with each other at various intervals. Stent design may be described as open cell or closed cell depending on the arrangement of connectors. An open cell design describes construction where some or all the internal inflection points of the rings are not fused or connected. This allows for better flexibility, conformability and consequent deliverability with side branch access. A closed cell design consists of sequential rings in which all internal inflection points are connected with regular peak-to-peak connections. This provides uniform cell expansion and uniformity in drug elution at the expense of increased rigidity and reduced deliverability in the presence of tortuous anatomy (Figure 31.1). Choice of metallic alloy,

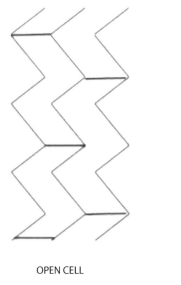

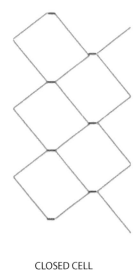

OPEN CELL   CLOSED CELL

Figure 31.1 Stent design showing open cell and closed cell patterns.

strut thickness, arrangement of connectors and consequent stent geometry therefore affect stent strength and deliverability. A reduction in the number of connectors leads to improved flexibility and conformability, but with a consequential reduction in longitudinal strength. Alternatively, increasing flexibility by reducing the number of connectors reduces the potential for strut fracture.

Another important component of the modern DES is the polymer. This is a drug carrier molecule that stores a therapeutic agent (drugs that essentially inhibit smooth muscle activation and replication, the main processes involved in ISR), as well as allowing the drug to diffuse into the vascular tissue in a controlled fashion. Polymers have been reported to result in an inflammatory effect leading to thrombosis.[14] To overcome this problem, newer stents have been designed to be polymer-free or to use bioresorbable polymers in the hope that as a polymer degrades, endothelial healing improves, and so polymer-free or bioresorbable stent designs may reduce the future risk of ISR or acute ST.

Important characteristics of the stent

1. Flexibility is defined as the amount of force required to bend an expanded stent to a given amount. Flexibility is related to trackability, which describes the ease with which an under-deployed stent is passed distally through a coronary artery to the target lesion.
2. Conformability is defined as the stent's ability to adapt to the natural curvature of the coronary artery.
3. Radial strength describes the ability of a stent to resist deformation and maintain the vessel lumen under a compressive load following stent deployment. Choice of metallic alloy, stent strut thickness and stent geometry influence radial strength. Radial strength is an important consideration when treating heavily calcified coronary lesions.
4. Longitudinal strength describes the resistance of the stent to compression or elongation along its long axis when exposed to pushing or pulling forces. Forward pressure on an angioplasty balloon or guide catheter, particularly when not coaxial with the stent, applies a force to a localised point on the proximal circumference of the stent, potentially resulting in forward compression of stent hoops and distortion

of the proximal end of the stent, with lumen compromise.
5. Radio-opacity describes the fluoroscopic visibility of the implanted stent, which is dependent on strut thickness and metallic alloy. Thinner struts are less visible than thicker struts. Visibility of 316 L stainless steel can be improved with radiopaque markings such as platinum and gold but this has been associated with intimal hyperplasia and local vessel wall inflammation, with high rates of restenosis. Newer stent materials such as CoCr or PtCr alloys have allowed development of thinner stent struts with a greater density but similar strength to stainless steel.

BARE METAL STENTS

As previously outlined, BMS can be considered as vascular scaffolds to treat balloon angioplasty-related dissections, acute vessel occlusions, and to reduce coronary artery recoil. The North American Stress Restenosis Study (STRESS) confirmed the advantage of BMS over balloon angioplasty—there was a lower angiographic restenosis rate (31.6% vs. 42.1%) and a lower target vessel revascularisation rate (TVR) (10.2% vs. 15.4%).[15] The Benestent Group compared implantation of the Palmaz-Shatz BMS to balloon angioplasty in patients with stable angina, and also confirmed the advantages of BMS over balloon angioplasty. There was a significant reduction in restenosis (22% vs. 32%) and TVR (13.1% vs. 22.9%).[16]

Despite the advantages of BMS over balloon angioplasty in preventing vessel recoil, the incidence of ISR was still a significant barrier to the long-term success of percutaneous coronary intervention (PCI).[17,18] The physical action of stretching and traumatising the endothelium after stent deployment results in an inflammatory process, which promotes platelet adhesion, mild luminal thrombus formation and fibrin deposition within the stent.[19] Following the development of thrombus, a focal inflammatory cellular infiltrate consisting of polymorphonuclear leukocytes and macrophages demarginates from the circulation and from the vasa vasorum, resulting in the stimulation of growth factors and cytokines, which activate smooth muscle cells in the media of the arterial wall, smooth muscle cell proliferation, and matrix formation (proteoglycans/collagen type III). Completion of vascular repair and re-endothelialisation normally occurs approximately 3–4 months after BMS implantation. In about 20%–40% of cases, smooth muscle cell activation leads to an untoward, excessive intimal hyperplasia, which can result in ISR and need for repeat revascularisation.[20–22]

FIRST-GENERATION DES

A restenosis rate of at least 20% with BMS prompted development of DES, where anti-proliferative agents delivered at the site of vessel injury could reduce ISR by inhibiting neointimal hyperplasia. Permanent polymer coatings are large molecules that are sub-classified into nonbiodegradable and biodegradable polymers. Their role is to act as a 'carrier' to control the release kinetics of the anti-proliferative drug that acts to minimise neointimal growth. The structure of the first generation DES was based on a stainless steel platform with strut thickness of 130–140 μm. Two widely-used DES were the Cypher (Cordis Corporation, Johnson & Johnson, USA) and Taxus (Boston Scientific Corporation, USA).

Sirolimus-eluting stent (SES)

Sirolimus has been shown to be a novel inhibitor of cellular proliferation, inhibiting cell proliferation in the G1 to S phase of the cell cycle.[23] The physical properties of sirolimus lend itself well to delivering local drug therapy: Sirolimus is very lipid-soluble and therefore almost no drug is released into the bloodstream during stent placement at the lesion site, and after stent implantation the diffusion gradient favours elution into tissue, again limiting the amounts of circulating free sirolimus.[24] Paclitaxel inhibits cell proliferation and migration by disturbing cellular microtubule organisation.[25] In contrast to sirolimus, which distributes equally within the vascular layers, paclitaxel accumulates in the adventitia,[26] which may limit its role in the prevention of ISR. In addition, the transmural diffusion coefficient of sirolimus is more than twice as high as the respective value of paclitaxel.[26] Penetration of paclitaxel into the vascular wall is also dependent on the presence of thrombotic material and its diffusion has been shown to be impaired in the presence of thrombus, with a direct dependency on its red blood cell count.[27] These drugs were

incorporated within a permanent polymer and coated onto the surface of the stainless steel platform; 80% of sirolimus is released within 30 days compared to 10% of paclitaxel being released over 2 weeks post-stent deployment, although 90% of it remains in the polymer forever.[28,29]

The first randomised trial comparing SES to BMS was the RAVEL study (Randomised study with the sirolimus-eluting Bx Velocity balloon-expandable stent trial),[28] which demonstrated 0% binary restenosis in the SES group in comparison to 26% in the BMS group at 6 months. There were also significant reductions in major adverse cardiac events (MACE)—5.8% MACE in the SES arm versus 27% in the BMS arm at 1 year ($p < 0.001$). The efficacy of SES was tested in more complex coronary disease with the SIRIUS trial (SIRolimUS-coated Bx Velocity balloon-expandable stent in the treatment of patients with de novo coronary artery lesions), which included diabetic patients.[30] Target lesion revascularisation (TLR) was reduced in diabetic patients from 22.3% in the BMS group to 6.9% in the SES group ($p < 0.01$) and in non-diabetic patients from 14.1% to 2.99% ($p < 0.001$). MACE in the diabetic group with BMS was 25% compared to 9.2% in the SES group, and 16.5% in the non-diabetic group with BMS compared to 6.5% in the SES group. The E-SIRUS trial compared BMS to SES in coronary artery diameters of 2.5–3.0 mm and lengths of 15–32 mm.[31] At 8 months follow up the minimum luminal diameter was significantly higher with SES than with BMS (2.22 mm vs. 1.33 mm $p < 0.001$) and the rate of restenosis was much higher with BMS vs. SES (42% vs. 5.9% $p < 0.0001$) confirming SES were better for longer and smaller diameter coronary vessels.

Paclitaxel-eluting stent (PES)

The main landmark PES trials were the TAXUS I-V trials. TAXUS I was the first randomised controlled trial (RCT) comparing TAXUS DES (using a slow release formulation) to an equivalent BMS.[32] At 12 months the MACE was not significantly different between the two groups, with significant improvements in minimal luminal diameter and diameter stenosis in the PES group. In addition, intravascular ultrasound measurements suggested significant improvements in normalised neointimal hyperplasia in the TAXUS group (14.8 vs. 21.6 mm³ in the control group). TAXUS II compared two different formulations of the PES/DES slow release (SR) formulation or moderate release (MR) formulation with BMS in patients undergoing PCI for non-complex coronary disease.[33] At 5 years the TLR rate was 10.3% for the SR group and 4.5% for the MR group, compared with 18.4% for the control groups ($p < 0.001$).[34] Five-year rates of MACE were 27.6%, 20.4% and 15.1% for the control, SR group and MR group. By the protocol definition, 8 cases of ST were reported in 7 patients during the 5-year follow up (2 in the control group, 3 in the SR group, 3 in the MR group).[34] Overall rates of definite or probable ST using Academic Research Consortium definitions were similar between the control (0.8%) and SR (2.3%; $P =$ NS) groups. One patient with a MR stent suffered from 2 STs at 317 days and 557 days after the index procedure. No ST occurred after 2 years with the PES stents, in contrast to 2 very late ST in the control group.[34] The MR formulation was as effective as or more effective than the SR formulation, with equivalent safety events, thereby establishing a clear safety margin. The TAXUS III trial compared the use of two SR PES for the treatment of BMS ISR.[35] As it was a small trial with limited relevance no further details are included. TAXUS IV confirmed the safety and effectiveness of SR PES for the treatment of de novo coronary artery disease compared to BMS.[36] The 5-year follow-up data[37] confirm lower rates of TVR in PES compared to BMS (16.9% vs. 27.4%, $p < 0.0001$) and less MACE (32.8% BMS vs. 24.0% PES, $p = 0.0001$ at 5 years). ST was comparable for PES and BMS (2.1% vs. 2.2%, $p = 0.87$). TAXUS V[38] studied patients undergoing revascularisation with SR PES with more complex coronary anatomy (78% of lesions were type B2/C) including longer lesions as well as a range of coronary artery stent sizes (2.25–4.0 mm DES) as in daily practice.[38] One-third of patients were type 2 diabetic. Compared with BMS, PES reduced the 9-month TLR from 15.7% to 8.6%; ($p < 0.001$). In the short term, there appeared to be no significant difference in MACE (5.5% vs. 5.7%) or ST at 9 months (0.7% in both groups).

Comparison of SES and PES (Table 31.1)

There is no doubt that development of DES was a milestone in stent technology. First-generation DES were reported to have better efficacy, with lower rates of ISR and target vessel revascularisation

than BMSs, with a reduction in the rate of TVR by 60%–70%.[39] Long-term data comparing the efficacy of SES and PES in patients with coronary disease showed no significant difference in rates of TLR and MACE. However, the overall rate of definite ST at 5 years was 4.6% for SES and 4.1% for PES ($p = 0.74$), and very late ST occurred at an annual rate of 0.65% per year with no significant difference between stent types.[40]

Studies in 2006 showed first-generation DES to be potentially associated with an increased risk of ST, although it is accepted some of these studies were methodologically flawed.[41,42] Neither was a true meta-analysis, since the data used were collated from papers and presentations rather than 'patient-level' information. The definitions of ST varied among the included studies to such an extent that a coherent a meta-analysis was invalid. However, autopsy studies following use of first-generation DES showed a heightened inflammatory response that is associated with a local hypersensitivity reaction and eosinophilic infiltration.[4] Despite delayed arterial healing and a similar incidence of late ST in first-generation coronary DES obtained at autopsy, the underlying composition of the neointima associated with SES and PES implants is different.[43] In patients with SES, greater inflammation involving eosinophils, lymphocytes, and giant cells (hypersensitivity reaction) results in positive re-modelling and malapposition. In contrast, excessive para-strut fibrin and malapposition was associated with PES implants. It is thought synthetic polymers are associated with inflammatory responses and local toxicity.[4,14] Coronary inflammation contributes to delayed re-endothelialisation of the stent and destruction of the medial vessel wall layers, promoting positive remodelling that contributes to delayed vascular healing.[4] Delayed endothelialisation of stent struts and the coronary artery wall promotes platelet adhesion and aggregation, which may eventually cause thrombus formation.[44]

Concerns over use of first-generation DES led to a reduction in DES usage in 2007, and the recommended use of dual anti-platelet therapy for 1 year or longer to avoid late ST. Following the controversy of first-generation DES and the perceived increased risk of ST, strict definitions of ST by the Academic Research Consortium were developed in December 2006. Later studies confirmed the incidence of ST did not differ significantly

Table 31.1 Trials comparing sirolimus versus paclitaxel drug eluting stents (for abbreviations see abbreviations list)

Trial	Design	Primary end point	Result
REALITY[48] (n = 1386)	Prospective multicentre trial Randomised trial comparing SES and PES in stable or unstable (recent MI within 72 hours contraindicated) patients	In-lesion Binary Stenosis using QCA at 8 months	No difference in restenosis in SES (9.6%) vs. PES (11.1%); (p = 0.31)
SIRTAX (n = 1012)	Randomised controlled single blinded trial comparing SES or PES in unstable or stable patients	Composite end point of MACE and TLR at 9 months	MACE was 6.2% in the SES group vs. 10.8% in the PES (p = 0.009), the difference was driven by lower rate of TLR in the SES group compared to the PES group (3.8% vs. 8.3%, p = 0.03)
SORTOUT II (n = 2098)	Randomised blinded trial in unselected patients	Composite end point of MACE, acute MI, TLR and TLV	No difference in MACE (9.3% SES vs. 11.2% PES), p = 0.16. No difference in stent thrombosis rates (2.5% SES vs. 2.9% PES)
TAXi (n = 202)	Prospective randomised trial comparing SES with PES	MACE & TLR	MACE at 7 months was 45 in PES vs. 6 5 SES (p = 0.8). TLR was 1% in PES vs. 3% in SES
ISAR-Diabetes (n = 250)	Prospective randomised study of PES or SES to prevent restenosis in diabetic patients	In segment late luminal loss on repeat angiography	PES was associated with higher rate of in segment late luminal loss (mean difference of 0.24 mm) as well as an increased risk of angiographic restenosis
ISAR-Smart 3 (n = 360)	Prospective randomised trial comparing SES with PES in patients undergoing PCI is small coronary vessels (<2.8 mm)	In stent late luminal loss on follow-up angiography	In-stent late luminal loss in PES was 0.32 mm (upper 95% boundary, 0.42 mm) which was greater than that in the SES group, failing to show non inferiority of the PES compared to the SES

between patients with DES and those with BMS in RCT.[45] Another meta-analysis of 9 randomised trials found that after one year, ST was more common with SES and PES when compared to BMS, although both DES were associated with a marked reduction TLR, and at 4 years there were no significant differences in the cumulative event rates of death or MI.[46] In a pooled analysis of 1748 patients consisting of 4 randomised trials comparing SES and BMS, no significant differences in MI, death or ST were found between the two groups.[47] Neither SES nor PES are any longer used in the US, Europe or Australia due to advances in stent technology, which has led to the development of second- and third-generation DES with new biocompatible polymer coatings, less toxic anti-proliferative drugs and state-of-the-art thin strut CoCr metal alloys. Further evolution of intracoronary stents includes the development of bioabsorbable stents and the concept of biodegradable polymers to minimise inflammation and local toxicity.

SECOND-GENERATION DES

Zotarolimus (formerly known as ABT-578) is a synthesised rapamycin analogue developed specifically for intravascular stents.[48] The first zotarolimus-eluting stent (E-ZES, Endeavor, Medtronic Inc., Santa Rosa, CA, USA) used a polymer consisting of a phospholipid portion, that mimics the outer membrane of red blood cells for biocompatibility, and a lauryl methacrylate (LMA monomer), that provides a hydrophobic region to confer stability and adhesion to the stent surface.[49] Due to concerns over higher rates of late lumen loss with E-ZES when compared to first-generation DES,[50,51] refinements to the E-ZES included a new biocompatible polymer called a BioLinx polymer. The Endeavor Resolute (R-ZES, Medtronic Inc., Santa Rosa, CA, USA) shares the same CoCr alloy platform as the E-ZES. However the newer polymer led to better drug-release kinetics; E-ZES elutes the zotarolimus in 1 week, whereas the R-ZES takes 60 days to elute 85% of the zotarolimus and 180 days to elute it completely.[52] E-ZES have been shown to be non-inferior to PES in the short term,[51] but in the long-term improved rates of cardiac death, MI and very late ST have been demonstrated in patients treated with E-ZES.[53] E-ZES and SES have been shown to have better long term safety over PES[54] and comparable rates of definite or probable ST at 3 years (Table 31.1).[55]

Everolimus is an analog of sirolimus used in both second- and third-generation DES. Different coronary stents have been developed using everolimus as an anti-proliferative agent. The Xience V (Abbott Vascular, Santa Clara, CA, USA) consists of a CoCr platform with thin stent struts (81 um). The polymer consists of two layers – a thin primer adhesion layer of poly (n-butyl methacrylate) and a drug reservoir of polymer (vinylidene fluoride-co-hexafluoropropylene). Approximately 80% of the drug is eluted in the first 30 days and 100% by four months.[56] The Promus Element plus and Promus-premier DES (Boston Scientific Corporation, USA) use the same drug and polymer as the Xience V but have a different stent platform. The PtCr platform is stronger than stainless steel and comparable to CoCr, enabling a reduction in strut thickness while maintaining radial strength and simultaneously improving radio-opacity. The Promus Element plus has been further modified to include additional connectors on the proximal two segments of the stent in an effort to address concerns of reduced axial strength and potential risk of longitudinal stent deformation.[10]

The early SPIRIT trials confirmed superiority of EES (Xience V) over PES with respect to target vessel failure and MACE due to fewer MI and ischemic TLR events but no significant difference in the cumulative rates of definite or probable ST.[57,58] Criticisms of SPIRIT II and III were that the trials were not powered to demonstrate superiority for clinical endpoints, and the protocol-mandated performance of routine follow-up angiography may have artificially raised rates of TLR; therefore SPIRIT IV randomised 3690 patients with coronary artery disease to receive EES or PES without routine follow-up angiography.[59] This demonstrated superiority of EES over PES with lower rates of target-lesion MI and ST. The SORTOUT IV trial enrolled 2774 patients to compare EES to SES.[60] The trial demonstrated EES to be non-inferior to SES with no significant differences in MACE at 3 years. However, there was a lower rate of late definite ST, which suggests the EES platform may be safer than the first generation SES.

THIRD-GENERATION DES (TABLE 31.2)

The clinical studies outlined above confirm an excellent safety and efficacy profile for the CoCr EES. The PtCr everolimus-eluting stent (PtCr-EES)

Table 31.2 Trials comparing third generation drug eluting stents (for abbreviations see abbreviations list)

Trial	Design	Primary end point	Result
Endeavour IV[53] (n = 1548)	RCT comparing E-ZES with PES	Composite of target vessel failure[a]	6.6% for E-ZES versus 7.2% for PES (p non inferiority <0.001) 5 year follow-up data confirmed lower incidence of MI/death in E-ZES and lower rates of very late ST, late MI
ZEST[61] (n = 2645)	RCT (single blind) comparing E-ZES with SES and PES	Composite of target vessel failure[a]	No difference in primary end point between E-ZES and SES. Less MACE when E-ZES compared to PES (10.2% vs. 14.1%, p for superiority 0.01). Incidence of ST lower in SES (E-ZES vs. SES vs. PES 0.7 vs. 0% vs. 0.8% respectively, p = 0.02)
PROTECT[55] (n = 8709)	RCT comparing E-ZES vs. SES	ST (definite, probable)	No difference at 3 years 4 year data: 1.6% in E-ZES vs. 2.6% in SES
SPIRIT III[57] (n = 1002)	Prospective, RCT EES vs. PES	Angiographic restenosis (In-segment LL at 8 months)	In-segment LL was lower in EES vs. PES (0.14 mm vs. 0.28 mm, P < 0.001 for non-inferiority and p = 0.004 for superiority)
SPIRIT IV[59] (n = 3690)	Prospective, RCT EES vs. PES	Composite of target vessel failure[a]	Target lesion failure was significantly lower in EES vs. PES (4.2% vs. 6.8%, HR 0.62, 95% CI 0.46-0.82, p = 0.001 for superiority) ST lower with EES vs. PES (0.29% vs. 1.06%, HR 0.27, 95% CI 0.11 to 0.67, P = 0.003)
SORTOUT IV[60] (n = 2774)	Randomised multicentre, single-blind, noninferiority trial comparing the EES with SES	Composite of target vessel failure[a] and ST	EES was found to be noninferior to the SES Primary end point occurred in 7.2% EES vs. 7.6% SES (hazard ratio, 0.94; 95% confidence interval, 0.71-1.23) Rate of definite ST was lower in EES group (0.2% vs. 1.4%; HR: 0.15, 95% CI 0.04 to 0.50)
HOST-ASSURE[64] (n = 3775)	Noninferiority trial, comparing (PtCr)-EES to 2nd generation CoCr-ZES in all-comers undergoing PCI	Composite of target vessel failure[a]	PtCr-EES was noninferior to CoCr-ZES (2.9% PtCr-EES vs. 2.9% CoCr-ZES (superiority p = 0.98, noninferiority p = 0.0247)
DUTCH PEERS[65] (n = 1788)	Randomised, single-blind, multicentre, non-inferiority trial comparing (PtCr)-EES to 3rd generation R-ZES	Target-vessel failure[a]	Absolute risk difference 0.88%, 95% CI −1.24% to 3.01%, upper limit of one-sided 95% CI 2.69%; non-inferiority p = 0.006 Definite ST occurred in 0.3% R-ZES vs. 0.7% (PtCr)-EES (p = 0.34)

a Target vessel failure – composite endpoint of cardiac death, myocardial infarction, and *ischemia driven* target vessel revascularisation.

uses the same anti-proliferative agent and polymer but with a novel PtCr scaffold. PLATINUM found no significant difference in clinical outcomes in patients undergoing PCI with a novel PtCr-EES compared with a CoCr everolimus-eluting stent (CoCr-EES).[62,63] PtCr-EES stents have been shown to be comparable in efficacy to the second generation R-RES in all comers undergoing PCI with no significant differences in TLF or ST (Table 31.2).[64] DUTCH PEERS further underlined the equivalence of the PtCr-EES and the third-generation R-ZES in an all-comers population.[65] Almost 60% of patients presented with ST-segment elevation MI or non-ST-segment elevation MI. No significant difference was seen between stent groups in the primary endpoint of target vessel failure or ST at 12 months. The Xience Sierra (Abbott Vascular, Santa Clara, CA, USA) is the newest iteration of an EES with an optimised multilink design (stent strut thickness measures 81 µm) that allows a smoother profile for crossing stenotic lesions. The stent strut thickness measures 81 µm and has the added advantage of greater flexibility and excellent stent expansion capability. For example, a 3.5 mm Sierra DES can be expanded to 5.5 mm without distorting strut architecture.

BIODEGRADABLE POLYMER-FREE STENTS (BP-DES) AND POLYMER-FREE DES

The theoretical advantage of biodegradable polymers (BP-DES) is that when the polymer disappears there no longer exists a potential chronic inflammatory stimulus, thereby potentially reducing the risk of late ST. The BioMatrix (Biosensors Inc, Newport Beach, CA) stent is a thin, stainless steel, laser-cut, tubular stent with 16.3%–18.4% metal surface area which has a bioresorbable polymer applied only to the abluminal (outer) surface. The anti-proliferative drug biolimus A9 (BA9) is highly lipophilic and transfers into the vessel wall over a period of 1 month. When compared to the durable polymer sirolimus stent, no significant difference in the composite endpoint of MI/death/TVR was noted.[66] Differences in favour of biolimus, including a lower rate of very late ST for as long as five years (0.7% vs. 2.5%, RR 0.26, 95% CI 0.10–0.68), may reflect a late safety advantage of a biodegradeable polymer.[66] The SYNERGY stent (Boston Scientific Corp., Natick, Massachusetts, USA) consists of a thin-strut PtCr stent platform that delivers

everolimus from an ultrathin bioabsorbable poly (DL-lactide-co-glycolide) (PLGA) polymer applied to the abluminal surface. Endothelialisation is complete within 28 days of implantation in a swine coronary artery model[67] and polymer reabsorption is complete within 4 months.[66] The EVOLVE trials confirmed the SYNERGY stent to be non-inferior to the durable polymer used in the PROMUS Element everolimus-eluting stent (EES) in terms of TLF and ST.[68,69] Other examples of DES with biodegradable polymers that have shown non-inferiority to conventional DES include the Orsiro stent (Biotronik AG, Bülach, Switzerland),[70] and the NOBORI Biolimus-Eluting Stent (Terumo Corporation, Tokyo, Japan).[71] The Orsiro stent is an ultrathin hybrid drug-eluting stent. It has a strut thickness of only 60 µm, with a double helix design that makes it highly flexible and deliverable. There is a passive coating of PROBIO, which seals the metal surface of the stent and prevents interaction with the surrounding structures, and the active coating of Biolute delivers the sirolimus drug, which gradually degrades over 2 years. The limus drug load is 1.4 µg/mm². The Bioflow V trial compared the Orsiro DES to the Xience stent, and demonstrated reduced TLF rates with Orsiro at 12 months (6.2% vs. 9.6% ($p = 9\ 0.04$), and reduced incidence of ST (0.5% vs. 0.7%).[72]

The Ultimaster Stent is a thin-strut, CoCr, biodegradable-polymer, sirolimus-eluting coronary stent. It has an open cell two-link design with a stent strut thickness of 80 micron resulting in greater flexibility without compromising radial force. The polymer DL-lactide-co-caprolactone degrades over a period of 3–4 months and the drug is coated on the abluminal side preventing delamination. In the Century II multicentre trial, Ultimaster was compared to the Xience stent in 194 patients and no significant difference was noted in clinical outcomes at 1 year between the two arms.[73]

Meta-analysis data suggests BP-DES are not superior to newer generation durable polymer DES for either efficacy or safety outcomes. When compared with CoCr everolimus eluting stents, BP-DES were associated with increase in myocardial infarction (MI) and death beyond the one year landmark point, which was attenuated in a sensitivity analysis restricted to trials at low risk of bias (rate ratio 1.48, 0.96–2.09).[74] Limitations of the study include no head-to-head comparison of any two BP-DES, so all estimates are based on indirect comparison only. A more recent meta-analysis demonstrated BP-DES significantly reduced late lumen loss and had lower rates of late ST when compared to conventional DES, with no clear benefit on mortality, MI, TLR and TVR rates.[75] Future randomised trials are required to evaluate whether any one BP-DES is superior to another.

Polymer-free DES should theoretically improve vessel healing and endothelialisation. This is achieved by incorporating drugs into a microporous or nanoporous surface of the metallic stent. The YUKON ChoiceDES (Translumina, Germany) has a modified stent surface containing micropores to enable the adsorption of different organic substances. The coating solution fills the pores completely and creates a uniform layer after evaporation of the solvent. After the drug is fully released, the microporous PEARL Surface favours the adhesion of endothelial cells. The stent platform allows for individualisation of the type and amount of anti-proliferative drug according to patient and lesion complexity. For example, the combination of rapamycin and probucol without use of a polymer (Dual-DES) has been compared to permanent polymer DES (SES, Cypher) and (ZES, Endeavor),[76] Probucol is a potent liposoluble antioxidant and has been shown to reduce neointimal hyperplasia, the dominant cause of ISR. Binary restenosis in the Dual-DES group was significantly lower than that in the ZES group but comparable with that in the SES group. Similarly, TLR with Dual-DES (6.8%) was significantly lower than ZES (13.6%; $p = 0.001$) but not different to that of SES (7.2%; $P = 0.83$). This trial was not powered to detect differences in rare clinical events, and follow up was only available for one year.[76]

The BioFreedom stent (Biosensors Inc., Newport Beach, CA, USA) uses a stainless steel BioFlex II stent platform with a textured abluminal surface onto which BA9 in solvent is applied. The antiproliferative agent is directly released from a mechanically modified textured surface without a polymer, thereby preventing polymer-associated tissue responses. Recently, the Bio Freedom stent has been compared to an uncoated BMS (Gazelle™) in patients with a bleeding risk using a 1-month period of dual anti-platelet therapy. Patients receiving the Bio Freedom stent experienced a 50% reduction in the need for repeat revascularisation and 29% reduction in risk of cardiac death, MI or ST,[77] thus highlighting the potential application of reduced period of double antiplatelet therapy in this high-risk population subset with the benefits of drug elution but without the drawbacks of a polymer.

BIOABSORBABLE STENTS

Until recently, bioabsorbable (BVS) scaffolds were considered to have revolutionised the treatment of coronary artery disease. Conventional DES had already been shown to provide a rigid scaffold preventing vessel recoil and negative remodelling alongside local drug delivery to inhibit neointimal growth. However, the additional properties of disappearing stent scaffold theoretically offered a number of advantages over conventional stents, including improved long-term vessel healing and remodelling, restoration of vasomotor function of the treated segment, and the hope this would translate into a reduced risk of late and very late ST. Other advantages include avoidance of permanent 'jailing' of side branches and stent strut protrusion where ostial coronary disease has been targeted, and improved assessment with cardiac imaging (lack of artefact from stent struts), and the ability to undergo future coronary bypass grafting.

The first BVS was the Igaki-Tamai stent (Kyoto Medical Planning Co., Ltd. Kyoto, Japan). This was a self-expanding stent but despite promising results was discontinued as it required an 8Fr-guiding catheter for implantation and heated contrast dye at 80° for expansion. The most widely used BVS are the Absorb (Abbott Vascular, Santa Clara, CA, USA) and the DESolve scaffold (Elixir Medical Corporation, Sunnyvale, California, USA). Other BVS include the REVA stent (REVA Medical, San Diego, CA, USA), Ideal BVS (Xenogenics Corporation, MA, USA) and the Dreams scaffold (*Biotronik* AG, Bülach, Switzerland).

The Absorb stent consists of a balloon-expandable poly-L-lactide (PLLA) scaffold coated with a thin bioabsorbable poly-D, L-lactide, and is coated with Everolimus. Platinum radio-opaque markers at each end of the radiolucent scaffold allow visualisation of the stent during angiography. The scaffold has a strut thickness of 150 μm and has undergone a number of iterations to address concerns regarding mechanical integrity.[78] Initial studies with Absorb confirmed full resorption of the polymeric struts, with return of vasomotion in the scaffolded area and comparable levels of MACE when compared to an Everolimus-Eluting metallic Stent.[79] In addition, intracoronary imaging demonstrated late luminal enlargement (late gain). The luminal area enlargement between 6 months and 2 years was due to a decrease in plaque size without change in vessel size.[79] Initial short-term data based on four randomised trials comparing the Absorb BVS versus an Everolimus-Eluting Metallic Stent in patients with coronary artery disease demonstrated comparable efficacy when a patient-oriented composite endpoint (all-cause mortality, all MI, or all revascularisation) and a device-oriented composite endpoint of TLF (cardiac mortality, target vessel-related MI (TV-MI), or ischaemia-driven TLR) were used.[80] However, a larger meta-analysis using six trials found that patients treated with a BVS had a higher risk of definite or probable ST than those treated with a metallic stent (OR 1.99 [95% CI 1.00–3.98]; $p = 0.05$), with the highest risk between 1 and 30 days after implantation (3.11 [1.24–7.82]; $p = 0.02$).[12] The GHOST-EU (Gauging coronary Healing with biOesorbable Scaffolding platforms in EUrope) registry was a retrospective, multicentre, randomised registry conducted at 10 European centres in which 'real-world' patients undergoing PCI with BVS were studied.[81] Approximately one-third of patients had suffered a MI, 25% of patients were diabetic, 50% of patients had 'complex disease,' and multi-vessel disease was present in 34.8% of patients. At 6 months, the incidence of cardiac death was 1%, target vessel MI 2%, TLR 2.5%, TVR 4% and cumulative incidence of TLF at 6 months was 4.4%, and diabetes was noted to be the only independent predictor of TLF (HR: 2.4, 95% CI: 1.28–4.53, $p = 0.006$). Overall, the authors concluded Absorb BVS was associated with acceptable rates of TLF at 30 days and 6 months, considering the complexity of the patients and lesions treated. However, again signals of scaffold thrombosis were higher than expected (1.5% of patients at 30 days and 2.1% at six months).[81]

Long-term follow up data from ABSORB III[82] confirmed TV-MI is increased with BVS compared with EES (8.6% vs. 5.9%; HR: 1.47; 95% CI: 1.02 to 2.11; $p = 0.03$), due to an increase in MI related to device thrombosis (1.9% vs. 0.6% EES; HR: 3.26; 95% CI: 1.13 to 9.35; $p = 0.02$). Device thrombosis (including those cases not resulting in TV-MI) was also found to be higher with BVS compared with EES between 1 and 3 years, and cumulative through 3 years. In comparison, no patient developed very late ST after EES. Before 1 year, scaffold thrombosis

events clustered in very small vessels (those with reference diameter <2.25 mm), whereas between 1 and 3 years scaffold thrombosis events clustered in vessels more appropriately sized for the device (reference diameter ≥2.25 mm). Alarmingly, patients with scaffold thrombosis in both periods were on double antiplatelet therapy at the time of the event. Similarly, the AIDA trial[83] has highlighted similar concerns with respect to scaffold thrombosis. The AIDA trial was a single blind, multicentre, investigator-initiated, non-inferiority, randomised clinical trial that included 1845 unselected CAD patients with 2446 lesions assigned to either BVS or EES therapy. Exclusion criteria included lesions more than 70 mm in length, a reference vessel diameter of less than 2.5 mm or more than 4.0 mm (estimated visually), bifurcation lesions for which use of two stents or scaffolds was planned, and ISR. The primary endpoint was target vessel failure the composite of cardiac death, TV-MI or TVR at 2 years. Device thrombosis at 2 years was a main secondary endpoint. Patients were reasonably complex in the sense that 50% had complex coronary anatomy and 54% presented with an acute coronary syndrome at admission (including one-fourth of participants with ST-segment elevation MI). The 2-year data was released early owing to safety concerns. The main findings were at 2-year follow-up, and BVS were associated with a risk of target vessel failure comparable to that of EES but had an approximately 3.5 times higher risk of thrombosis and a higher risk of TV-MI as compared to EES. Furthermore, almost one-third of BVS thromboses occurred in the period beyond 1 year after implantation. There was no interaction between device thrombosis and vessel size, as suggested by ABSORB III, and stent post-dilation was not seen to be associated with scaffold thrombosis. These findings have also been confirmed by a large meta-analysis (5583 patients). Compared with metallic EES, the risk of target lesion failure was higher with Absorb BVS (9.6 vs. 7.2%; absolute risk difference +2.4%; risk ratio 1.32, 95% CI: 1.10–1.59) and the risk of ST was higher with Absorb BVS (2.4 vs. 0.7%; absolute risk difference +1.7%; risk ratio 3.15; 95% CI: 1.87–5.30).

Multiple factors are hypothesised to be involved in late/very late scaffold thrombosis. The natural breakdown of the scaffold structure by bulk erosion during the first 6 months is essential to restoration of normal vasomotion with BVS. However, optical coherence tomography has demonstrated that late scaffold discontinuities are common, but rarely associated with clinical adverse events.[84] Such natural discontinuities, when filled with neointimal tissue, do not protrude into the lumen and are of no clinical consequence.[85] However, suboptimal implantation techniques and limitations of the BVS (post-dilatation beyond the recommended value) can result in excessive polymer stretching, or elongation can prevent the scaffold from breaking down normally, leaving macroscopic space-occupying structures protruding into the lumen, either at the time of implantation, or at any time due to excessive biomechanical cyclic stress.[85] Malapposition, acute disruption, under-deployment, device-vessel mismatch, incomplete coverage of lesion (geographical miss) or overlap can lead to alterations in laminar flow.[86] Low endothelial shear stress reduces the endothelial expression of nitric oxide, prostacyclin I2 and tissue plasminogen activator, promoting a prothrombotic state.[86] Low endothelial shear stress may increase the risk of scaffold thrombosis by inhibiting endothelial cell proliferation and slowing re-endothelialisation of the scaffold.[86] Endothelial shear stress peaks over the strut surface edges and promotes platelet activation and release thromboxane A2 and adenosine diphosphate, and subsequent activation of the coagulation cascade. Polymer resorption may not be complete in humans as late as 4 years after device implantation, as evidenced by Fourier transformation and spectroscopic thrombus aspirate analysis,[87] and thrombogenicity of the breakdown products and/or the extracellular matrix replacing the strut void may also increase the risk of scaffold thrombosis. Because of the increased risk of late scaffold thrombosis, Abbott has discontinued the normal commercial sale of BVS in Europe and restricted its usage to centres only participating in ongoing registry studies.

The Magmaris stent (Biotronik AG, Bülach, Switzerland) is the first resorbable magnesium scaffold that has shown promising data. The Biosolve II study was a prospective, multicentre first-in-man trial evaluating the efficacy and safety of this resorbable stent in 123 patients with two de novo lesions in two separate coronary arteries.[88] The primary endpoint of the study was in-segment late lumen loss at 6 months, and the secondary endpoint was a composite of target lesion failure, TLR, MI or ST at 2 years. Ninety-five percent of the magnesium is resorbed at 12 months, and results have demonstrated 0% incidence of ST at 2 years follow up.

CONCLUSION

The trials described above confirm the superior efficacy and safety of second-generation DES over first-generation DES. Further refinements in stent platforms, delivery systems and polymer-free stents have led to the development of third-generation DES that offer improved radial strength as well as efficacy and safety through reduced late loss and low rates of ST. However, DES continue to have certain limitations, with risks of late and very late ST, potential stent fracture, incomplete endothelialisation, and abnormal vasomotion secondary to the residual metal scaffold that result in rigidity of the vessel. BVS have been developed to overcome some of these limitations. It was thought BVS were completely resorbed over a 2–3 year period and would hence reduce the risk of late or very late ST. Initial studies suggested vasomotion of the vessel improves, with evidence of late luminal enlargement and late expansive remodelling resulting in restoration of normal architecture of the vessel. Long-term data have now given a signal of late scaffold thrombosis. Further data from large studies are awaited to determine the safety and efficacy of these novel stents to justify their use in clinical practice.

ABBREVIATIONS

BMS	bare metal stents
BP-DES	biodegradable polymers drug eluting stents
BVS	biovascular scaffold
CoCr	cobalt-chromium
DES	drug eluting stent
EES	everolimus-eluting stent
ISR	instent restenosis
LST	late stent thrombosis
MACE	major adverse cardiac event
MI	myocardial infarction
MR	moderate release
PCI	percutaneous coronary intervention
QCA	quality control analysis
RCT	randomised clinical trial
SES	sirolimus-eluting stent
SR	slow release
ST	stent thrombosis

TLF	target lesion failure
TLR	target lesion revascularisation
TVR	target vessel revascularisation
TV-MI	recurrent target vessel myocardial infarction
PES	paclitaxel-eluting stent
PCI	percutaneous coronary intervention
PtCr	platinum chromium
ZES	zotarolimus-eluting stent

REFERENCES

1. Cassese S, Byrne RA, Tada T, Pinieck S, Joner M, Ibrahim T, et al. Incidence and predictors of restenosis after coronary stenting in 10,004 patients with surveillance angiography. *Heart*. 2014;100(2):153–159.

2. Kirtane AJ, Gupta A, Iyengar S, Moses JW, Leon MB, Applegate R, et al. Safety and efficacy of drug-eluting and bare metal stents: Comprehensive meta-analysis of randomized trials and observational studies. *Circulation*. 2009;119(25):3198–3206.

3. AL-Mangour B, Mongrain R, Yue S. Coronary stents fracture: An engineering approach (review). *Mater Sci Appl*. 2013; 4(10):16.

4. Virmani R, Guagliumi G, Farb A, Musumeci G, Grieco N, Motta T, et al. Localized hypersensitivity and late coronary thrombosis secondary to a sirolimus-eluting stent: Should we be cautious? *Circulation*. 2004;109(6):701–705.

5. Lüscher TF, Steffel J, Eberli FR, Joner M, Nakazawa G, Tanner FC, et al. Drug-eluting stent and coronary thrombosis: Biological mechanisms and clinical implications. *Circulation*. 2007;115(8):1051–1058.

6. Kastrati A, Mehilli J, Dirschinger J, Dotzer F, Schühlen H, Neumann F-J, et al. Intracoronary stenting and angiographic results: Strut thickness effect on restenosis outcome (ISAR-STEREO) trial. *Circulation*. 2001;103(23):2816–2821.

7. Huang KN, Grandi SM, Filion KB, Eisenberg MJ. Late and very late stent thrombosis in patients with second-generation drug-eluting stents. *Can J Cardiol*. 2013;29(11):1488–1494.

8. Lee SWL, Chan MPH, Chan KKW. Acute and 16-month outcomes of a new stent: The first-in-man evaluation of the Medtronic S9 (Integrity) stent. *Catheter Cardiovasc Interv*. 2011;78(6):898–908.

9. Menown IA, Noad R, Garcia E, Meredith I. The platinum chromium element stent platform: From alloy, to design, to clinical practice. *Adv Therapy*. 2010;27(3):129–141.

10. Hanratty C, Walsh S. Longitudinal compression: A "new" complication with modern coronary stent platforms – time to think beyond deliverability? *EuroIntervention*. 2011;7(7):872–877.

11. Ormiston JA, Webber B, Webster MWI. Stent longitudinal integrity: Bench insights into a clinical problem. *JACC Cardiovasc Interv*. 2011;4(12):1310–1317.

12. Cassese S, Byrne RA, Ndrepepa G, Kufner S, Wiebe J, Repp J, et al. Everolimus-eluting bioresorbable vascular scaffolds versus everolimus-eluting metallic stents: A meta-analysis of randomised controlled trials. *Lancet*. 2016;387(10018):537–544.

13. Koster R, Vieluf D, Kiehn M, Sommerauer M, Kahler J, Baldus S, et al. Nickel and molybdenum contact allergies in patients with coronary in-stent restenosis. *Lancet*. 2000;356(9245):1895–1897.

14. van der Giessen WJ, Lincoff AM, Schwartz RS, van Beusekom HM, Serruys PW, Holmes DR, Jr., et al. Marked inflammatory sequelae to implantation of biodegradable and nonbiodegradable polymers in porcine coronary arteries. *Circulation*. 1996;94(7):1690–1697.

15. Fischman DL, Leon MB, Baim DS, Schatz RA, Savage MP, Penn I, et al. A randomized comparison of coronary-stent placement and balloon angioplasty in the treatment of coronary artery disease. Stent Restenosis Study Investigators. *N Engl J Med*. 1994;331(8):496–501.

16. Serruys PW, de Jaegere P, Kiemeneij F, Macaya C, Rutsch W, Heyndrickx G, et al. A comparison of balloon-expandable-stent implantation with balloon angioplasty in patients with coronary artery disease. Benestent Study Group. *N Engl J Med*. 1994;331(8):489–495.

17. Chen MS, John JM, Chew DP, Lee DS, Ellis SG, Bhatt DL. Bare metal stent restenosis is not a benign clinical entity. *Am Heart J.* 2006;151(6):1260–1264.

18. Hsieh IC, Hsieh MJ, Chang SH, Wang CY, Lee CH, Lin FC, et al. Clinical and angiographic outcomes after intracoronary bare-metal stenting. *PLOS ONE.* 2014;9(4):e94319.

19. Virmani R, Farb A. Pathology of in-stent restenosis. *Curr Opin Lipidol.* 1999;10(6):499–506.

20. Bonaa KH, Mannsverk J, Wiseth R, Aaberge L, Myreng Y, Nygard O, et al. Drug-eluting or bare-metal stents for coronary artery disease. *N Engl J Med.* 2016;375(13):1242–1252.

21. Akiyama T, Moussa I, Reimers B, Ferraro M, Kobayashi Y, Blengino S, et al. Angiographic and clinical outcome following coronary stenting of small vessels: A comparison with coronary stenting of large vessels. *J Am Coll Cardiol.* 1998;32(6):1610–1618.

22. Elezi S, Kastrati A, Neumann FJ, Hadamitzky M, Dirschinger J, Schomig A. Vessel size and long-term outcome after coronary stent placement. *Circulation.* 1998;98(18):1875–1880.

23. Javier AF, Bata-Csorgo Z, Ellis CN, Kang S, Voorhees JJ, Cooper KD. Rapamycin (sirolimus) inhibits proliferating cell nuclear antigen expression and blocks cell cycle in the G1 phase in human keratinocyte stem cells. *J Clin Invest.* 1997;99(9):2094–2099.

24. Abizaid A. Sirolimus-eluting coronary stents: A review. *Vasc Health Risk Manag.* 2007;3(2):191–201.

25. Rowinsky EK, Donehower RC. Paclitaxel (taxol). *N Engl J Med.* 1995;332(15):1004–1014.

26. Levin AD, Vukmirovic N, Hwang CW, Edelman ER. Specific binding to intracellular proteins determines arterial transport properties for rapamycin and paclitaxel. *Proc Natl Acad Sci U S A.* 2004;101(25):9463–9467.

27. Hwang CW, Levin AD, Jonas M, Li PH, Edelman ER. Thrombosis modulates arterial drug distribution for drug-eluting stents. *Circulation.* 2005;111(13):1619–1626.

28. Morice MC, Serruys PW, Sousa JE, Fajadet J, Ban Hayashi E, Perin M, et al. A randomized comparison of a sirolimus-eluting stent with a standard stent for coronary revascularization. *N Engl J Med.* 2002;346(23):1773–1780.

29. Serruys PW, Kutryk MJ, Ong AT. Coronary-artery stents. *N Engl J Med.* 2006;354(5):483–495.

30. Moses JW, Leon MB, Popma JJ, Fitzgerald PJ, Holmes DR, O'Shaughnessy C, et al. Sirolimus-eluting stents versus standard stents in patients with stenosis in a native coronary artery. *N Engl J Med.* 2003;349(14):1315–1323.

31. Schofer J, Schluter M, Gershlick AH, Wijns W, Garcia E, Schampaert E, et al. Sirolimus-eluting stents for treatment of patients with long atherosclerotic lesions in small coronary arteries: Double-blind, randomised controlled trial (E-SIRIUS). *Lancet.* 2003;362(9390):1093–1099.

32. Grube E, Silber S, Hauptmann KE, Mueller R, Buellesfeld L, Gerckens U, et al. TAXUS I: Six- and twelve-month results from a randomized, double-blind trial on a slow-release paclitaxel-eluting stent for de novo coronary lesions. *Circulation.* 2003;107(1):38–42.

33. Colombo A, Drzewiecki J, Banning A, Grube E, Hauptmann K, Silber S, et al. Randomized study to assess the effectiveness of slow- and moderate-release polymer-based paclitaxel-eluting stents for coronary artery lesions. *Circulation.* 2003;108(7):788–794.

34. Silber S, Colombo A, Banning AP, Hauptmann K, Drzewiecki J, Grube E, et al. Final 5-year results of the TAXUS II trial: A randomized study to assess the effectiveness of slow- and moderate-release polymer-based paclitaxel-eluting stents for de novo coronary artery lesions. *Circulation.* 2009;120(15):1498–1504.

35. Tanabe K, Serruys PW, Grube E, Smits PC, Selbach G, van der Giessen WJ, et al. TAXUS III Trial: In-stent restenosis treated with stent-based delivery of paclitaxel incorporated in a slow-release polymer formulation. *Circulation.* 2003;107(4):559–564.

36. Stone GW, Ellis SG, Cox DA, Hermiller J, O'Shaughnessy C, Mann JT, et al. One-year clinical results with the slow-release, polymer-based, paclitaxel-eluting TAXUS stent: The TAXUS-IV trial. *Circulation*. 2004;109(16):1942–1947.

37. Ellis SG, Stone GW, Cox DA, Hermiller J, O'Shaughnessy C, Mann T, et al. Long-term safety and efficacy with paclitaxel-eluting stents: 5-year final results of the TAXUS IV clinical trial (TAXUS IV-SR: Treatment of De Novo Coronary Disease Using a Single Paclitaxel-Eluting Stent). *JACC Cardiovasc Interv*. 2009;2(12):1248–1259.

38. Stone GW, Ellis SG, Cannon L, Mann JT, Greenberg JD, Spriggs D, et al. Comparison of a polymer-based paclitaxel-eluting stent with a bare metal stent in patients with complex coronary artery disease: A randomized controlled trial. *JAMA*. 2005;294(10):1215–1223.

39. Stettler C, Wandel S, Allemann S, Kastrati A, Morice MC, Schomig A, et al. Outcomes associated with drug-eluting and bare-metal stents: A collaborative network meta-analysis. *Lancet*. 2007;370(9591):937–948.

40. Raber L, Wohlwend L, Wigger M, Togni M, Wandel S, Wenaweser P, et al. Five-year clinical and angiographic outcomes of a randomized comparison of sirolimus-eluting and paclitaxel-eluting stents: Results of the Sirolimus-Eluting Versus Paclitaxel-Eluting Stents for Coronary Revascularization LATE trial. *Circulation*. 2011;123(24):2819–2828, 6 p following 28.

41. Nordmann AJ, Briel M, Bucher HC. Mortality in randomized controlled trials comparing drug-eluting vs. bare metal stents in coronary artery disease: A meta-analysis. *Eur Heart J*. 2006;27(23):2784–2814.

42. Camenzind E SP, Wijns W, editors. Safety of drug-eluting stents: A metaanalysis of 1st generation DES programs. *World Congress of Cardiology*. 2006; Barcelona.

43. Nakazawa G, Finn AV, Vorpahl M, Ladich ER, Kolodgie FD, Virmani R. Coronary responses and differential mechanisms of late stent thrombosis attributed to first-generation sirolimus- and paclitaxel-eluting stents. *J Am Coll Cardiol*. 2011;57(4):390–398.

44. Joner M, Finn AV, Farb A, Mont EK, Kolodgie FD, Ladich E, et al. Pathology of drug-eluting stents in humans: Delayed healing and late thrombotic risk. *J Am Coll Cardiol*. 2006;48(1):193–202.

45. Mauri L, Hsieh WH, Massaro JM, Ho KK, D'Agostino R, Cutlip DE. Stent thrombosis in randomized clinical trials of drug-eluting stents. *N Engl J Med*. 2007;356(10):1020–1029.

46. Stone GW, Moses JW, Ellis SG, Schofer J, Dawkins KD, Morice MC, et al. Safety and efficacy of sirolimus- and paclitaxel-eluting coronary stents. *N Engl J Med*. 2007;356(10):998–1008.

47. Spaulding C, Daemen J, Boersma E, Cutlip DE, Serruys PW. A pooled analysis of data comparing sirolimus-eluting stents with bare-metal stents. *N Engl J Med*. 2007;356(10):989–997.

48. Garcia-Touchard A, Burke SE, Toner JL, Cromack K, Schwartz RS. Zotarolimus-eluting stents reduce experimental coronary artery neointimal hyperplasia after 4 weeks. *Eur Heart J*. 2006;27(8):988–993.

49. Buellesfeld L, Grube E. ABT-578-eluting stents. *Herz*. 2004;29(2):167–170.

50. Kandzari DE, Leon MB, Popma JJ, Fitzgerald PJ, O'Shaughnessy C, Ball MW, et al. Comparison of zotarolimus-eluting and sirolimus-eluting stents in patients with native coronary artery disease: A randomized controlled trial. *J Am Coll Cardiol*. 2006;48(12):2440–2447.

51. Leon MB, Mauri L, Popma JJ, Cutlip DE, Nikolsky E, O'Shaughnessy C, et al. A randomized comparison of the Endeavor zotarolimus-eluting stent versus the TAXUS paclitaxel-eluting stent in de novo native coronary lesions: 12-month outcomes from the ENDEAVOR IV trial. *J Am Coll Cardiol*. 2010;55(6):543–554.

52. Waseda K, Ako J, Yamasaki M, Koizumi T, Sakurai R, Hongo Y, et al. Impact of polymer formulations on neointimal proliferation after zotarolimus-eluting stent

with different polymers: insights from the RESOLUTE trial. *Circ Cardiovasc Interv.* 2011;4(3):248–255.

53. Kirtane AJ, Leon MB, Ball MW, Bajwa HS, Sketch Jr MH, Coleman PS, et al. The "final" 5-year follow-up from the ENDEAVOR IV trial comparing a zotarolimus-eluting stent with a paclitaxel-eluting stent. *JACC Cardiovasc Interv.* 2013;6(4):325–333.

54. Leon MB, Nikolsky E, Cutlip DE, Mauri L, Liberman H, Wilson H, et al. Improved late clinical safety with zotarolimus-eluting stents compared with paclitaxel-eluting stents in patients with de novo coronary lesions: 3-year follow-up from the ENDEAVOR IV (Randomized Comparison of Zotarolimus- and Paclitaxel-Eluting Stents in Patients With Coronary Artery Disease) trial. *JACC Cardiovasc Interv.* 2010;3(10):1043–1050.

55. Camenzind E, Wijns W, Mauri L, Kurowski V, Parikh K, Gao R, et al. Stent thrombosis and major clinical events at 3 years after zotarolimus-eluting or sirolimus-eluting coronary stent implantation: A randomised, multicentre, open-label, controlled trial. *The Lancet.* 2012;380(9851):1396–1405.

56. Windecker S, Jüni P. The drug-eluting stent saga. *Circulation.* 2009;119(5):653–656.

57. Stone GW, Midei M, Newman W, Sanz M, Hermiller JB, Williams J, et al. Comparison of an everolimus-eluting stent and a paclitaxel-eluting stent in patients with coronary artery disease: A randomized trial. *JAMA.* 2008;299(16):1903–1913.

58. Caixeta A, Lansky AJ, Serruys PW, Hermiller JB, Ruygrok P, Onuma Y, et al. Clinical follow-up 3 years after everolimus- and paclitaxel-eluting stents: A pooled analysis from the SPIRIT II (A Clinical Evaluation of the XIENCE V Everolimus Eluting Coronary Stent System in the Treatment of Patients With De Novo Native Coronary Artery Lesions) and SPIRIT III (A Clinical Evaluation of the Investigational Device XIENCE V Everolimus Eluting Coronary Stent System [EECSS] in the Treatment of Subjects With De Novo Native Coronary Artery Lesions) randomized trials. *JACC Cardiovasc Interv.* 2010;3(12):1220–1228.

59. Stone GW, Rizvi A, Newman W, Mastali K, Wang JC, Caputo R, et al. Everolimus-eluting versus paclitaxel-eluting stents in coronary artery disease. *N Engl J Med.* 2010;362(18):1663–1674.

60. Okkels Jensen L, Thayssen P, Hansen HS, Christiansen EH, Tilsted HH, Krusell LR, et al. Randomized comparison of everolimus-eluting and sirolimus-eluting stents in patients treated with percutaneous coronary intervention: The Scandinavian Organization for Randomized Trials With Clinical Outcome IV (SORT OUT IV). *Circulation.* 2012;125(10):1246–1255.

61. Park D-W, Kim Y-H, Yun S-C, Kang S-J, Lee S-W, Lee C-W, et al. Comparison of zotarolimus-eluting stents with sirolimus- and paclitaxel-eluting stents for coronary revascularization: The ZEST (comparison of the efficacy and safety of zotarolimus-eluting stent with sirolimus-eluting and paclitaxel-eluting stent for coronary lesions) randomized trial. *J Am Coll Cardiol.* 2010;56(15):1187–1195.

62. Stone GW, Teirstein PS, Meredith IT, Farah B, Dubois CL, Feldman RL, et al. A prospective, randomized evaluation of a novel everolimus-eluting coronary stent: The PLATINUM (a Prospective, Randomized, Multicenter Trial to Assess an Everolimus-Eluting Coronary Stent System [PROMUS Element] for the Treatment of Up to Two de Novo Coronary Artery Lesions) trial. *J Am Coll Cardiol.* 2011;57(16):1700–1708.

63. Meredith IT, Teirstein PS, Bouchard A, Carrié D, Möllmann H, Oldroyd KG, et al. Three-year results comparing platinum-chromium PROMUS element and cobalt-chromium XIENCE V everolimus-eluting stents in de novo coronary artery narrowing (from PLATINUM Trial). *Am J Cardiol.* 2014;113(7):1117–1123.

64. Park KW, Kang S-H, Kang H-J, Koo B-K, Park B-E, Cha KS, et al. A randomized comparison of platinum chromium-based everolimus-eluting stents versus cobalt chromium-based Zotarolimus-Eluting stents in all-comers receiving percutaneous coronary intervention: HOST–ASSURE (harmonizing optimal strategy for treatment of coronary artery

stenosis–safety & effectiveness of drug-eluting stents & anti-platelet regimen), a randomized, controlled, noninferiority trial. *J Am Coll Cardiol.* 2014;63(25, Part A):2805–2816.

65. von Birgelen C, Sen H, Lam MK, Danse PW, Jessurun GAJ, Hautvast RWM, et al. Third-generation zotarolimus-eluting and everolimus-eluting stents in all-comer patients requiring a percutaneous coronary intervention (DUTCH PEERS): A randomised, single-blind, multicentre, non-inferiority trial. *The Lancet.* 2014;383(9915):413–423.

66. Serruys PW, Farooq V, Kalesan B, de Vries T, Buszman P, Linke A, et al. Improved safety and reduction in stent thrombosis associated with biodegradable polymer-based biolimus-eluting stents versus durable polymer-based sirolimus-eluting stents in patients with coronary artery disease: Final 5-year report of the LEADERS (Limus Eluted From A Durable Versus ERodable Stent Coating) randomized, noninferiority trial. *JACC Cardiovasc Interv.* 2013;6(8):777–789.

67. Foss A, Chen YL, Marks A, Lange J, Lind D, Knapp D, Allocco DJ, Dawkins KD. Characterisation of in vivo poly(DL-lactic-co-glycolic acid) degradation from a drug coated stent. *EuroIntervention.* 2012;8 Supplement N.

68. Meredith IT, Verheye S, Dubois CL, Dens J, Fajadet J, Carrie D, et al. Primary endpoint results of the EVOLVE trial: A randomized evaluation of a novel bioabsorbable polymer-coated, everolimus-eluting coronary stent. *J Am Coll Cardiol.* 2012;59(15):1362–1370.

69. Kereiakes DJ, Meredith IT, Windecker S, Lee Jobe R, Mehta SR, Sarembock IJ, et al. Efficacy and safety of a novel bioabsorbable polymer-coated, everolimus-eluting coronary stent: The EVOLVE II Randomized Trial. *Circ Cardiovasc Interv.* 2015;8(4).

70. Windecker S, Haude M, Neumann FJ, Stangl K, Witzenbichler B, Slagboom T, et al. Comparison of a novel biodegradable polymer sirolimus-eluting stent with a durable polymer everolimus-eluting stent: Results of the randomized BIOFLOW-II trial. *Circ Cardiovasc Interv.* 2015;8(2):e001441.

71. Natsuaki M, Kozuma K, Morimoto T, Kadota K, Muramatsu T, Nakagawa Y, et al. Final 3-year outcome of a randomized trial comparing second-generation drug-eluting stents using either biodegradable polymer or durable polymer: NOBORI biolimus-eluting versus XIENCE/PROMUS everolimus-eluting stent trial. *Circ Cardiovasc Interv.* 2015;8(10).

72. Kandzari DE, Mauri L, Koolen JJ, Massaro JM, Doros G, Garcia-Garcia HM, et al. Ultrathin, bioresorbable polymer sirolimus-eluting stents versus thin, durable polymer everolimus-eluting stents in patients undergoing coronary revascularisation (BIOFLOW V): A randomised trial. *Lancet.* 2017;390(10105):1843–1852.

73. Orvin K, Carrie D, Richardt G, Desmet W, Assali A, Werner G, et al. Comparison of sirolimus eluting stent with bioresorbable polymer to everolimus eluting stent with permanent polymer in bifurcation lesions: Results from CENTURY II trial. *Catheter Cardiovasc Interv.* 2016;87(6):1092–1100.

74. Bangalore S, Toklu B, Amoroso N, Fusaro M, Kumar S, Hannan EL, et al. Bare metal stents, durable polymer drug eluting stents, and biodegradable polymer drug eluting stents for coronary artery disease: Mixed treatment comparison meta-analysis. *BMJ.* 2013;347:f6625.

75. Lupi A, Gabrio Secco G, Rognoni A, Lazzero M, Fattori R, Sheiban I, et al. Meta-analysis of bioabsorbable versus durable polymer drug-eluting stents in 20,005 patients with coronary artery disease: An update. *Catheter Cardiovasc Interv.* 2014;83(6):E193–206.

76. Byrne RA, Mehilli J, Iijima R, Schulz S, Pache J, Seyfarth M, et al. A polymer-free dual drug-eluting stent in patients with coronary artery disease: A randomized trial vs. polymer-based drug-eluting stents. *Eur heart J.* 2009;30(8):923–931.

77. Urban P, Meredith IT, Abizaid A, Pocock SJ, Carrie D, Naber C, et al. Polymer-free drug-coated coronary stents in patients at high bleeding risk. *N Engl J Med.* 2015;373(21):2038–2047.

78. Onuma Y, Serruys PW, Gomez J, de Bruyne B, Dudek D, Thuesen L, et al. Comparison of in vivo acute stent recoil between the bioresorbable everolimus-eluting coronary scaffolds (revision 1.0 and 1.1) and the metallic everolimus-eluting stent. *Catheter Cardiovasc Interv.* 2011;78(1):3–12.

79. Serruys PW, Ormiston JA, Onuma Y, Regar E, Gonzalo N, Garcia-Garcia HM, et al. A bioabsorbable everolimus-eluting coronary stent system (ABSORB): 2-year outcomes and results from multiple imaging methods. *Lancet*. 2009;373(9667):897–910.

80. Stone GW, Gao R, Kimura T, Kereiakes DJ, Ellis SG, Onuma Y, et al. 1-year outcomes with the Absorb bioresorbable scaffold in patients with coronary artery disease: A patient-level, pooled meta-analysis. *Lancet*. 2016;387(10025):1277–1289.

81. Capodanno D, Gori T, Nef H, Latib A, Mehilli J, Lesiak M, et al. Percutaneous coronary intervention with everolimus-eluting bioresorbable vascular scaffolds in routine clinical practice: Early and midterm outcomes from the European multicentre GHOST-EU registry. *EuroIntervention*. 2015;10(10):1144–1153.

82. Kereiakes DJ, Ellis SG, Metzger C, Caputo RP, Rizik DG, Teirstein PS, et al. 3-year clinical outcomes with everolimus-eluting bioresorbable coronary scaffolds: The ABSORB III trial. *J Am Coll Cardiol*. 2017;70(23):2852–2862.

83. Wykrzykowska JJ, Kraak RP, Hofma SH, van der Schaaf RJ, Arkenbout EK, AJ IJ, et al. Bioresorbable scaffolds versus metallic stents in routine PCI. *N Engl J Med*. 2017;376(24):2319–2328.

84. Onuma Y, Serruys PW, Muramatsu T, Nakatani S, van Geuns RJ, de Bruyne B, et al. Incidence and imaging outcomes of acute scaffold disruption and late structural discontinuity after implantation of the absorb Everolimus-Eluting fully bioresorbable vascular scaffold: Optical coherence tomography assessment in the ABSORB cohort B Trial (A Clinical Evaluation of the Bioabsorbable Everolimus Eluting Coronary Stent System in the Treatment of Patients With De Novo Native Coronary Artery Lesions). *JACC Cardiovasc Interv*. 2014;7(12):1400–1411.

85. Stone GW, Granada JF. Very late thrombosis after bioresorbable scaffolds: Cause for concern? *J Am Coll Cardiol*. 2015;66(17):1915–1917.

86. Sotomi Y, Suwannasom P, Serruys PW, Onuma Y. Possible mechanical causes of scaffold thrombosis: Insights from case reports with intracoronary imaging. *EuroIntervention*. 2017;12(14):1747–1756.

87. Raber L, Brugaletta S, Yamaji K, O'Sullivan CJ, Otsuki S, Koppara T, et al. Very late scaffold thrombosis: Intracoronary imaging and histopathological and spectroscopic findings. *J Am Coll Cardiol*. 2015;66(17):1901–1914.

88. Haude M, Ince H, Abizaid A, Toelg R, Lemos PA, von Birgelen C, et al. Sustained safety and performance of the second-generation drug-eluting absorbable metal scaffold in patients with de novo coronary lesions: 12-month clinical results and angiographic findings of the BIOSOLVE-II first-in-man trial. *Eur Heart J*. 2016;37(35):2701–2719.

Facilitated coronary interventions: Adjuncts to balloon dilatation

DAVID W. M. MULLER

INTRODUCTION

By far the greatest contribution to the welfare of patients undergoing percutaneous vascular interventional procedures in the recent past has been the development of the endoluminal stent. Improvements in stent profile, tracking and deliverability, and drug-elution characteristics are such that stents can be placed in almost any sized epicardial coronary artery with the prospect of an excellent initial clinical outcome and reduced need for repeat intervention. However, there remain subsets of patients with complex coronary or peripheral disease for whom conventional approaches remain challenging. This chapter deals with devices that have a role in selected patients when used alone or prior to coronary stenting.

DIRECTIONAL ATHERECTOMY

The directional atherectomy catheter was developed as a means of removing atheromatous tissue from the coronary artery wall. It was expected that this would optimise the initial improvement in luminal dimensions, reduce the potential for coronary dissection and abrupt closure, and

improve long-term clinical outcome by reducing the incidence of restenosis. The catheter is an over-the-wire system that consists of a metal housing assembly that is open on one side, with an inflatable balloon attached to the external surface of the contralateral side (Figure 32.1). Within the housing is a cup-shaped cutting tool that is attached to a rotating shaft. When activated by a hand-held motor drive unit, the cutting blade rotates at 2000 rpm. Tissue is resected by advancing the cutting blade forwards while the housing is held in place against the vessel wall by inflation of the balloon to 10–15 psi (0.5–1 atm). Atheromatous tissue is pushed forwards into a cone-shaped collecting chamber in front of the metal housing. After each passage of the cutting blade, the balloon is deflated, the device is rotated through 90°, the balloon is reinflated, and the blade is withdrawn to its starting position. This sequence is repeated 6–8 times before the entire device is removed and the nose cone is cleared of the retrieved tissue. During a typical passage of the device, 8–10 mg of atheroma may be retrieved from the collecting chamber. If residual disease is apparent by repeat angiography or intravascular imaging, further resection can be

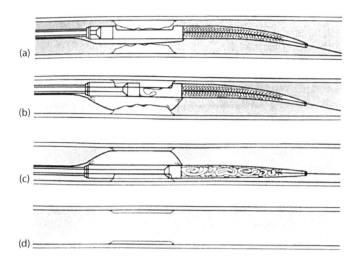

Figure 32.1 The directional atherectomy catheter. After inflation of the balloon (a), the rotating blade is advanced forwards (b), excising tissue and pushing it forwards into the collecting chamber at the distal end of the device. The balloon is then deflated, the device is rotated (c) and the process repeated until sufficient atheroma has been removed (d).

performed to remove as much tissue as possible. Low-pressure balloon inflation with a slightly oversized angioplasty balloon is usually required to optimise the angiographic result.

The major advantage of directional coronary atherectomy (DCA) over conventional balloon angioplasty was that a larger initial lumen could be achieved.[1,2] Tissue resection might also be particularly useful in avoiding side branch closure in bifurcation lesions by minimising plaque redistribution across the origin of the side branch ('snow-plough effect'); it was also an effective treatment for ostial lesions in large arteries. The extent of lumen enlargement was comparable to that achieved by coronary stenting[3,4] and one study suggested that aggressive debulking might achieve long-term results that are equal to, or better than, those of coronary stenting.[4] However, use of the device was limited by the fact that it is bulky, relatively inflexible and required the use of 9.5–10 Fr guiding catheters. Randomised trials of directional atherectomy and balloon angioplasty also failed to show a reduction in restenosis rates and the need for target lesion revascularisation, or improvement, in event-free survival, even when atherectomy was performed aggressively to optimise the initial angiographic result.[1] Indeed, in one study,[5] the 1-year mortality and myocardial infarction rates were higher in patients treated by DCA than in those treated by conventional balloon angioplasty.

Debulking prior to coronary stenting was also evaluated as a means of reducing the incidence of restenosis, but also showed no consistent benefit.[6-8] As a consequence, DCA has largely been replaced as a tool for optimising coronary interventions.

Directional atherectomy does, however, have a role in peripheral artery disease. The Silverhawk directional atherectomy system (Fox Hollow Technologies, Redwood City, CA) is Food and Drug Administration-approved. Several large registries[9,10] have reported favourable outcomes and suggest this might be a useful intervention, particularly where stenting is inadvisable, such as in the common femoral, distal superficial femoral and popliteal arteries. One multicentre registry enrolled 1,258 patients with symptomatic lower limb atherosclerosis. A procedural success rate of 98% was achieved with a 6-month target lesion revascularisation (TLR) rate of 90%, and 12-month TLR rate of 80%.[10] A second multicentre registry showed a 12-month primary patency rate of 78% in a population of 800 patients.[9] However, a recent randomised comparison showed that treatment of superficial femoral artery stenoses by paclitaxel eluting balloon and stenting was superior to stenting alone and to directional atherectomy with bailout stenting, with a lower 6-month diameter stenosis, and a lower binary restenosis rate (23% vs. 52% vs. 54%, respectively, $p < 0.017$).[11]

ROTATIONAL ATHERECTOMY

Debulking and plaque modification can also be achieved by percutaneous rotational atherectomy (PTRA). The original rota-system (Boston Scientific, Natick, MA) introduced in 1988, achieves this by the action of a diamond-encrusted, olive-shaped burr that rotates at speeds up to 200,000 rpm (Figure 32.2). Rotation of the burr is driven by an air-nitrogen gas turbine. As the burr is advanced over a specialised wire into contact with the lesion, the plaque surface is ablated by abrasion, forming micro-particulate debris (<5 μm diameter) that passes through the myocardial capillaries into the general circulation. The burrs are available in 0.25 mm increments, from 1.25 to 2.5 mm for use in the coronary arteries. Larger sizes are available for use in peripheral arteries. The very high rotation speed (140,000–180,000 rpm) almost eliminates friction between the device and the 0.09 in guidewire, which allows it to be passed readily through tortuous, calcified coronary segments. The heat generated by the high rotation speed is limited by infusion of a saline solution through the catheter sheath. The coronary system is compatible with a 6 Fr guiding catheter.

Although the PTRA catheter was designed to remove tissue as a means of improving the initial and late outcomes of balloon angioplasty, its greatest value is in the treatment of heavily calcified lesions. Severe coronary calcification remains one of the most common indications for referral for coronary bypass surgery and occurs in 5%–10% of patients undergoing percutaneous coronary intervention (PCI). Inadequate lesion preparation in calcified lesions can result in coronary dissection, failure to cross with a stent, and incomplete stent expansion. Abrasion and tissue ablation occur maximally where the atheromatous tissue is densely fibrotic and calcified. The burr has relatively little effect on adjacent normal elastic tissue or soft plaque. The mechanism of action of the device almost certainly includes not only tissue ablation, but also release of fibrotic contractures and disruption of calcified plaque by the formation of microfissures, thereby allowing subsequent balloon dilatation of the lesion. Indeed, some lesions cannot be dilated or stented without initial treatment by rotational atherectomy.

A major limitation of PTRA is the formation of sufficient microparticulate matter to cause sludging of flow in the myocardial microcirculation. 'Slow' or 'no-flow' occurs in up to 10% of patients treated with rotational atherectomy and may cause non-Q wave or Q-wave myocardial infarction. It occurs most commonly after treatment of long, heavily calcified lesions in large coronary arteries. In addition to capillary plugging by microemboli, coronary epicardial or microcirculatory spasm may also play a role. The frequency of this complication can be reduced by meticulous attention to technique. First, the initial burr size should be small, particularly in diffusely diseased or heavily calcified arteries. The burr should be engaged with the lesion for relatively short periods (~30 seconds) before retraction to allow flushing and distal passage of any particulate debris. The burr should be advanced very slowly with a constant rotation speed. A fall in rotation speed of more than 5000 rpm is associated with an increased risk of vessel wall injury (dissection and heat injury), and the formation of larger particles and poor distal flow. Various medical cocktails have been used to minimise the risk of poor distal flow. These include nitroglycerine (4 mg/L), verapamil (10 mg/L) and heparin (5000 IU/L) in the infusion solution. If

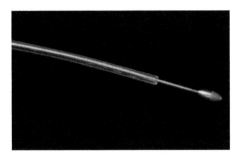

Figure 32.2 The rotational atherectomy catheter. The diamond-tipped burr rotates at up to 200,000 rpm and abrades fibrocalcific plaques forming a fine slurry of microparticulates.

no-reflow does occur, it can usually be treated by a combination of intracoronary verapamil (100–1000 µg in increments of 100–300 µg) and nitroglycerine (in incremental doses of 150–300 µg). Manual perfusion by vigorously flushing saline or autologous blood into the coronary artery also seems to improve flow. More refractory cases may require use of adenosine, a glycoprotein IIb/IIIa antagonist, or an intra-aortic balloon pump to improve distal perfusion.

Other important complications of PTRA include extensive coronary dissection, perforation, and transient heart block. Great care needs to be taken in treating highly angulated lesions to minimise this risk. The system has changed little since its introduction. The 0.09-in guidewire remains difficult to use in tortuous calcified vessels with poor torqueing and tracking capabilities. It is often necessary to cross complex lesions with a conventional angioplasty wire, and exchange this for the rota-wire using a micro-catheter. Efforts are currently underway to improve the performance of the wire, and ease of use of the rota-system.

PTRA has become a niche device indicated for non-dilatable coronary stenoses. Randomised comparisons of rotational atherectomy with balloon angioplasty showed little benefit of debulking over conventional angioplasty, with disappointingly high restenosis rates.[12,13] Rotational atherectomy has also been proposed as a means of treating in-stent restenosis, but data supporting this approach are not strong.[14] Nonetheless, PTRA prior to stenting plays a very valuable role in the management of densely fibrotic or calcified lesions. Whether debulking prior to stenting reduces the incidence of restenosis remains to be determined. In one study,[13] use of aggressive PTRA prior to bare-metal stenting (burr:artery ratio >0.80) resulted in a lower restenosis rate than stenting after less aggressive debulking (30.9% vs. 50.0%, $p < 0.05$), but this strategy was associated with a higher incidence of procedural complications. More recent data have confirmed the role of PTRA as a means of preparing heavily calcified lesions for subsequent stenting, rather than as a means of reducing restenosis.[15,16] This is also reflected in the latest European guidelines for PCI, which give PTRA for preparation of heavily calcified lesions a Class IIa (level of evidence C) recommendation.[17]

An alternative to the Boston Scientific PTRA system is the Diamondback 360 Orbital Atherectomy system (Cardiovascular System, Inc, St Paul, MN), which has a unique, eccentrically mounted design that increases the ablation diameter with increasing rotational speed. It has a single-sized, diamond-tipped burr (1.25 mm), with an electrically-driven rotation speed of 80,000–120,000 rpm. The eccentricity of the burr allows treatment of larger diameter arteries than would otherwise be possible. The system is Food and Drug Administration approved and commercially available in the USA and in Japan. Coronary orbital atherectomy has been evaluated in the ORBIT I and II trials[18,19] with relatively low complication and TLR rates. Orbital atherectomy has also been used peripherally.[20] The Orbital Atherectomy System for Treating Peripheral vascular Stenosis (OASIS), reported a low incidence of complications including dissection (2%), perforation (2%) and distal embolism (2%).[20]

CUTTING BALLOON ANGIOPLASTY

Given that much of the benefit of rotational atherectomy involves plaque modification rather than debulking, attention has again turned to modifying fibro-calcific lesions to facilitate stent placement by cutting balloon angioplasty. The Flextome™ Cutting Balloon™ device (Boston Scientific, Marlborough, MA, USA) was introduced in 1991 and consists of a non-compliant balloon with 3 or 4 micro-blades placed longitudinally on the outer surface of the balloon. Expansion of the balloon incises the lesion, allowing subsequent balloon expansion at lower dilatation pressures than would otherwise be necessary.[21] The device has been used both in calcified coronary lesions,[21] in aorto-ostial stenosis,[22] and in in-stent stenoses to prevent balloon slippage.[23] The largest trial of the Cutting Balloon™,[24] showed no difference in restenosis rate when compared with balloon angioplasty. The major limitation of the device is its relative rigidity, making it unsuitable for very tortuous arteries or angulated lesions.

Other devices developed for lesion preparation include the AngioSculpt scoring balloon (Spectranetics, Colorado Springs, CO, USA).[25,26] This has three nitinol wires that spiral around the external balloon surface, providing greater flexibility than the Cutting Balloon™. Several registries have shown better acute results following use of the scoring balloon prior to stent implantation than PTCA before stent implantation.[25,26] However, this has not translated into better long-term arterial patency.[26] The recently introduced OPN balloon (Swiss Interventional Systems, Frauenfeld, Switzerland) has a twin-layered construction that provides a rated burst pressure of 35 atm to pre-dilate calcified lesions or optimise stent expansion. The Chocolate balloon (QT Vascular Ltd, Singapore) has a 'pillows and channeling grooves' design achieved using a nitinol constraining wire structure on a semi-compliant balloon. It is said to provide uniform balloon expansion, reducing the potential for dissection at high pressures. To date, neither the OPN balloon, nor the Chocolate balloon, has been evaluated in a prospective study.

ULTRASONIC ABLATION DEVICES

Therapeutic ultrasound is based on delivery of high-energy, low-frequency ultrasound from an external piezo-electric crystal to the tip of a relatively inflexible catheter. Rapid oscillation of the ultrasound emitters generates sound waves that cause cyclic cavitation (bubble formation) and implosion in adjacent fluids and tissues. Cavity implosion generates local pressures equivalent to those used in balloon angioplasty. This is believed to be the primary mechanism of action of the device; other mechanisms include a mechanical effect of the device itself and heat generation. In vitro studies suggest that ultrasound energy may be used to ablate atheromatous plaque including fibro-calcific disease. However, clinical studies suggest that the greatest value of the device is in creating micro-fractures in calcific plaque. Ultrasound energy has also been used to dissolve fresh thrombus. Following ultrasound ablation, the vast majority of the remaining particulate debris is <10 μ in diameter and passes readily through the coronary microcirculation.[27] An additional potential benefit seen in some studies[28] is vasodilatation, and an increase in epicardial coronary flow and myocardial perfusion.

The Coronary Lithoplasty System (Shockwave Medical, Fremont, CA, USA) received CE Mark approval in 2017. It consists of a semi-compliant balloon supporting a series of unfocused emitters of ultrasound energy.[29] After low-pressure balloon inflation, multiple pulses are delivered, followed by further balloon dilatation to the nominal balloon pressure. A multicentre registry (DISRUPT CAD) showed fractures of calcified coronary lesions by optical coherence tomography (OCT), with the greatest frequency of fractures in the most heavily calcified lesions.[29] There were no apparent adverse consequences of lithoplasty. One of the limitations of the system is its relative inflexibility. Comparisons of lithoplasty with rotational atherectomy and cutting balloons have not yet been performed. It is likely to prove valuable in large arteries (which cannot be adequately treated by PTRA) or in smaller vessels that remain resistant to balloon dilatation after PTRA with a 1.5 mm burr.

TRANSLUMINAL EXTRACTION ATHERECTOMY

Several devices developed for atheroma removal were shown to be most effective in removing thrombotic material and the loose gruel of degenerated saphenous vein grafts.[30] They have been less effective in removing the fibro-calcific disease of native coronary artery disease. The transluminal extraction catheter (TEC) (Interventional Technologies Inc., San Diego, USA) was one such device. It consisted of a cone-shaped head with two cutting blades and a central hollow aspiration channel through which excised debris is removed. The cutting head was driven by a battery-operated hand-held motor drive unit and rotated at 750 rpm. Excised tissue was collected in a vacuum bottle connected to the aspiration channel. The devices were available in 0.5 Fr increments from 5.5 to 7.5 Fr and were used over a specialised 0.014 in wire that had a 0.021 in ball at its tip to limit the extent of travel of the device. Like directional atherectomy catheters, the TEC catheter required a 10 Fr guiding catheter to provide adequate support during passage of the device and to allow adequate contrast opacification of the segment being treated. The procedure was limited by the maximum size of the device (7.5 Fr), with the majority of lesions having a significant residual narrowing that required adjunctive balloon dilatation and stent implantation. Widespread use of the device was limited by the fact that distal embolisation and no-reflow occurred with a similar frequency to that of balloon dilatation and stenting alone, and that in treated saphenous vein grafts, restenosis and late total occlusion occurred disappointingly frequently.[31] The company was acquired by Boston Scientific in 2001 and its development was ultimately discontinued.

Other mechanical thrombectomy devices include the Angiojet Rheolytic Thrombectomy system (Medrad Interventional/Possis Medical, Inc. Minneapolis, MN),[32] which aspirates thrombus and loose plaque material by directing a high velocity jet of saline from the catheter tip, backwards to the aspiration port of the catheter. This creates a very high negative pressure zone (−600 mmHg) and powerful suction at the catheter tip. The device has been used predominantly as an adjunct to stenting in acute myocardial infarction. In one study of 501 patients, use of the device prior to stenting was associated with more frequent ST-segment resolution and a reduction in the 6-month major adverse cardiovascular event rate compared to infarct artery stenting alone.[32]

LASER FACILITATED ANGIOPLASTY

Devices designed to deliver laser energy to a catheter tip are largely of historical interest. The systems were expensive, cumbersome and of doubtful efficacy. Laser energy is typically generated by stimulation of a liquid, solid or gaseous medium. This results in excitation of atoms and subsequent release of photons with specific wavelengths ranging from approximately 300 nm to >10,000 nm. The characteristics of the electromagnetic energy generated by these devices depend on its wavelength, pulse repetition rate, and duration of the pulse (pulse width). Excimer lasers produce energy from a gaseous medium (xenon-chlorine) with a wavelength of 308 nm, have a relatively small penetration depth (30–50 μm), and produce little thermal injury. The dominant mechanism of action is via the formation of a vapour bubble that implodes, generating a photoacoustic effect on surrounding tissues. Solid-state lasers in the mid-infrared range, such as the holmium:YAG laser, have a higher ablation threshold and penetration depth than excimer lasers.

Although the initial enthusiasm for laser-facilitated angioplasty was dampened by disappointing results from randomised clinical trials,[33,34] improvements in device technology led to a resurgence in interest in laser energy and its application to several specific patient subgroups. In particular, the development of a laser guidewire has been of value in the treatment of chronic total occlusions (CTOs). The Spectranetics excimer laser wire is a steerable 0.018 in wire that consists of 12 optical fibres with a shapeable tip. In one series, 56% of chronic total occlusions were crossed with this wire after failure of a conventional guidewire.[35] It should be noted, however, that the results of 'conventional' angioplasty for chronic total occlusions have improved considerably since the introduction of wires and catheters specifically designed for CTOs. Use of these latter wires may provide greater success rates to those achieved with laser wires, at a considerably lower cost. Another recent application of laser angioplasty has been as a means of facilitating stent expansion in heavily calcified stenoses. In one study,[36] contrast injection during laser angioplasty resulted in greater plaque fracture and a larger final stent diameter than laser angioplasty alone.

There are two additional non-coronary interventional procedures for which laser energy has a potential role. Extraction of permanent pacemaker leads appears to be greatly facilitated by the use of a purpose-designed laser sheath. This can be passed distally over the pacemaker lead to ablate fibrotic adhesions between the lead and the underlying myocardium, thereby allowing safe removal of the leads, and in many instances, obviating the need for surgical extraction. Transmyocardial laser revascularisation (TMR) and percutaneous endomyocardial revascularisation (PMR) have also been advocated as treatments for refractory angina in patients with severe, non-operable coronary artery disease. Initially, CO_2 or holmium:YAG lasers were used to create channels from the epicardial surface, through the ischaemic myocardium to the left ventricular cavity as a means of providing an alternative vascular conduit.[37] More recently, catheters have been designed and tested clinically as a means of applying the same concept percutaneously from the endocardial surface.[38] Several series have reported substantial symptomatic improvements in patients treated in this manner, although few have consistently demonstrated objective evidence of resolution of the underlying ischaemia. Histological studies have shown that the new channels invariably thrombose rapidly but that this is associated with a local inflammatory response and neovascularisation with the formation of small capillary channels.[39] A recent meta-analysis of trans-myocardial laser suggested that the risks associated with the intervention outweigh any potential benefit.[40]

INTRACORONARY RADIATION

For almost two decades, recurrent narrowing or restenosis was a major limitation of coronary angioplasty and related interventions. Multiple trials of drug therapies failed to show any reduction in the incidence of restenosis after balloon angioplasty of uncomplicated lesions.[41] Coronary stenting improved the long-term clinical outcome in these patients but, as the boundaries of eligibility for stenting were stretched to include long lesions in diffusely diseased arteries, lesions in small calibre arteries, and chronic total occlusions, restenosis re-emerged as an ongoing limitation of percutaneous coronary interventions. Brachytherapy, or endoluminal radiation therapy, appeared initially to have a significant impact on the extent of post-angioplasty and in-stent restenosis.

Two primary types of ionising radiation were used in clinical and experimental trials. Beta sources, such as ^{32}P, ^{90}Sr, ^{90}Y, and ^{188}Re, emit electrons with a broad distribution of energies, typically in the 0.2–2.5 MeV range. Gamma sources, including ^{192}Ir and ^{125}I, produce high-energy photons that have a much greater tissue penetration than the electrons released from beta sources. Both beta and gamma radiation occur naturally and are emitted during the transition of unstable radioisotopes to more stable, lower energy states. Beta sources have the advantage that the electrons emitted interact strongly with adjacent tissues and therefore act locally with little penetration to other tissues. Shielding requirements are limited and, since high activity sources can be used, the time required to deliver the calculated radiation dose to the treated site (dwell time) is short. In contrast, gamma sources deliver photons that interact weakly with tissues, penetrate deeply beyond the treated tissues, and require far more shielding than is provided in conventional catheterisation laboratories to protect staff and other hospital personnel. The lower activity of the gamma emitters used clinically also necessitated long dwell times during which all personnel needed to leave the catheterisation laboratory.

Although clearly more user-friendly, beta radiation had limitations. The lower depth of penetration of beta radiation resulted in the potential for variable circumferential dosing for eccentric lesions or non-centred catheter sources. Beta sources were not suitable for very large non-coronary arteries or saphenous vein grafts, and, since beta radiation is efficiently blocked by metal, did not provide optimal inhibition of neointimal hyperplasia after stent implantation. Some of these limitations were overcome by selecting delivery modalities other than a central catheter or ribbon. Radioisotope-filled balloons are not limited by centering or distance issues and the use of stents coated with a radiation source appeared to avert the shielding effects of the stent metal. However, unlike other delivery systems, use of isotope-filled balloons exposed the patient and operator to the risk of leakage or radioisotope spill in the event of balloon rupture or during preparation of the balloon. Similarly, as discussed below, data from clinical trials showed that radioisotope-coated stents had their own unique limitations.

Endovascular radiation was first shown to inhibit neointimal hyperplasia many years ago.[42] Several models of restenosis were used to examine the efficacy of both beta and gamma radiation. Although there was some variability in the results of the published trials, the majority showed a significant degree of inhibition of intimal hyperplasia at doses of 15–20 Gray (Gy). Some studies showed that high-dose radiation also caused inhibition of endothelial cell proliferation and an absence of endothelial covering at the treated sites,[43] increasing the potential for late thrombotic occlusion at the site of angioplasty or stent implantation because of failure of the injured site to heal.

Much of the initial clinical evaluation of endovascular radiation was performed with ^{192}Ir (gamma) radiation sources. The first randomised clinical trial of intracoronary gamma radiation enrolled 55 patients with post-angioplasty or in-stent restenosis.[44] Actively treated patients received between 8 and 30 Gy of gamma radiation delivered from a catheter-based array of radioactive seeds. At follow-up, the angiographic restenosis rate was reduced from 54% in the control group to 17%. One-year event-free survival was 85% in the treated group compared with 52% in the untreated group.[44] Similar magnitudes of benefit were observed in another randomised gamma study, the GAMMA-1[45] trial.

Data from several non-randomised trials suggested that catheter-based beta radiation was as effective as gamma radiation for the prevention of restenosis.[46,47] However, the results from observational studies of radioisotope-impregnated stents were disappointing.[48,49] Stents covered with beta-emitters such as ^{32}P had several obvious advantages including low toxicity to the operator, a short treatment period, and uniform circumferential delivery without attenuation of the dose by the stent metal. However, very low-dose radiation seemed to promote intimal hyperplasia after arterial injury, resulting in relatively little intimal hyperplasia within the stented segment, but with stenoses proximal or distal to the treated segment giving the artery an appearance referred to as the 'candy-wrapper' effect.[48]

As clinical experience with these devices increased, the reported incidence of complications also rose. Thrombotic occlusion occurred late after stent implantation, presumably because of incomplete stent endothelialisation. Failure of wound healing also lead to aneurysm formation. As a consequence, intracoronary radiation was very quickly replaced by the use of drug-eluting stents once these became available.

DISTAL PROTECTION DEVICES

Although sound in principle, debulking of atheromatous lesions with any of the above devices does have risks. Embolisation of atheromatous debris may occur during any of these procedures,[50] and probably also occurs frequently during apparently uncomplicated balloon dilatation and stent procedures.[51] Distal embolisation is particularly likely to occur during percutaneous interventions in degenerated vein grafts in which it commonly causes poor flow, myocardial infarction and profound haemodynamic compromise. During carotid or vertebral interventions, even minor episodes of distal embolisation may cause profound neurological complications, and following renal artery interventions, atheroembolism may result in deterioration of already compromised renal function.

Recognition of the clinical importance of distal atheroembolism after vascular interventions has led to the design and development of a number of distal protection devices.[52] Broadly speaking, these devices may be classified as passive filters or systems designed to capture material by arterial occlusion and to retrieve it by active aspiration. The PercuSurge Guardwire Distal Protection Device (Medtronic, Minneapolis, MN) (Figure 32.3) consists of a 0.014 or 0.018-in steerable wire on a nitinol hypotube.[53,54] Arterial occlusion is achieved by inflation of a low-pressure elastomeric balloon. Prior to deflation and removal, a catheter (Export, Medtronic, Minneapolis, MN) with a 1 mm aspiration port is advanced to a point immediately proximal to the balloon and 50–60 mL of blood, containing the captured debris, is aspirated. Several small series have been reported[53,54] and suggest that particulate matter typically falls in the 50–200 μ range, although particles in excess of 3 mm in diameter have been retrieved. The device was evaluated in 801 patients in the SVG Angioplasty Free of Emboli Randomized (SAFER) trial.[55] The 30-day major adverse cardiac event (MACE) rate was lower in the protected group (9.6% vs. 16.5%, $p = 0.001$) driven mostly by a reduction in rates of myocardial infarction and no-reflow.[55] The system was also evaluated in the context of acute ST-elevation myocardial infarction. The Enhanced Myocardial Efficacy and Recovery by Aspiration of Liberalized Debris (EMERALD) trial randomly assigned 501 patients to intervention with or without distal protection and aspiration.[56] The study showed no improvement in success of reperfusion, infarct size or event-free survival in spite of successful retrieval of debris in the majority of patients treated.[56] The devices have several potential limitations. These include the potential for the occlusion balloon to cause arterial injury or distal embolism, the

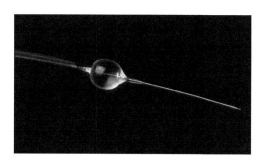

Figure 32.3 The PercuSurge distal protection device. Particulate matter, which is captured by a low inflation pressure balloon, can be retrieved by aspiration through a large lumen monorail catheter. Particles up to several millimetres in diameter can be retrieved in this manner.

risks of end-organ ischaemia during the period of balloon occlusion, and a reduction in precision of stent deployment because contrast angiography cannot be performed with the balloon inflated.

Several passive filters have been designed as alternatives to the balloon occlusion systems.[57–59] They have the apparent advantages of allowing perfusion during distal protection, and perhaps, of limiting arterial trauma during the time the device is in position. Each system consists of a retractable membrane that has a series of 50, 100, or 200 µm diameter holes. Atheromatous debris has been retrieved from coronary, renal and carotid arteries and from saphenous vein grafts during a variety of interventions. It has become clear that even routine, apparently uncomplicated coronary balloon angioplasty procedures can lead to embolisation of atheromatous debris. Whether this results in myocardial injury and an adverse long-term outcome remains controversial.[52] Although current guidelines give a class 1 recommendation (level of evidence B) to the use of embolic protection devices in saphenous vein graft interventions, recent data have been somewhat conflicting with some studies suggesting a benefit to distal protection,[60] and others suggesting no benefit.[61,62] A recent meta-analysis of distal protection in the setting of acute myocardial infarction also showed that although TIMI 3 flow and myocardial blush scores were better in the distal protection group, no significant difference was apparent in major adverse events.[63]

CONCLUSIONS

Multiple adjuncts to balloon angioplasty have been evaluated over the recent past. With few exceptions, most of the interventions have been disappointing, or superseded by current generation drug-eluting stents. There remains a need for technologies to facilitate treatment of heavily calcified lesions. While these are reliably treated by rotational atherectomy in most instances, difficulties are still encountered in crossing severe stenoses with the rota-wire, and in treating bulky calcific lesions in large arteries. Future technologies may address these limitations.

REFERENCES

1. Baim DS, Cutlip DE, Sharma SK, Ho KK, Fortuna R, Schreiber TL, et al. Final results of the balloon vs optimal atherectomy trial (BOAT). *Circulation*. 1998;97(4):322–331.

2. Topol EJ, Leya F, Pinkerton CA, Whitlow PL, Hofling B, Simonton CA, et al. A comparison of directional atherectomy with coronary angioplasty in patients with coronary artery disease. The CAVEAT study group. *N Engl J Med*. 1993;329(4):221–227.

3. Adelman AG, Cohen EA, Kimball BP, Bonan R, Ricci DR, Webb JG, et al. A comparison of directional atherectomy with balloon angioplasty for lesions of the left anterior descending coronary artery. *N Engl J Med*. 1993;329(4):228–233.

4. Tsuchikane E, Sumitsuji S, Awata N, Nakamura T, Kobayashi T, Izumi M, et al. Final results of the stent versus directional coronary atherectomy randomized trial (START). *J Am Coll Cardiol*. 1999;34(4):1050–1057.

5. Elliott JM, Berdan LG, Holmes DR, Isner JM, King SB, Keeler GP, et al. One-year follow-up in the coronary angioplasty versus excisional atherectomy trial (CAVEAT I). *Circulation*. 1995;91(8):2158–2166.

6. Bramucci E, Angoli L, Merlini PA, Barberis P, Laudisa ML, Colombi E, et al. Adjunctive stent implantation following directional coronary atherectomy in patients with coronary artery disease. *J Am Coll Cardiol*. 1998;32(7):1855–1860.

7. Gruberg L, Mehran R, Dangas G, Hong MK, Mintz GS, Kornowski R, et al. Effect of plaque debulking and stenting on short- and long-term outcomes after revascularization of chronic total occlusions. *J Am Coll Cardiol*. 2000;35(1):151–156.

8. Stankovic G, Colombo A, Bersin R, Popma J, Sharma S, Cannon LA, et al. Comparison of directional coronary atherectomy and stenting versus stenting alone for the treatment of de novo and restenotic coronary artery narrowing. *Am J Cardiol*. 2004;93(8):953–958.

9. McKinsey JF, Zeller T, Rocha-Singh KJ, Jaff MR, Garcia LA. Lower extremity revascularization using directional atherectomy: 12-month prospective results of the definitive le study. *JACC Cardiovasc Interv*. 2014;7(8):923–933.

10. Ramaiah V, Gammon R, Kiesz S, Cardenas J, Runyon JP, Fail P, et al. Midterm outcomes from the TALON registry: Treating peripherals with Silverhawk: Outcomes collection. *J Endovasc Ther*. 2006;13(5):592–602.

11. Ott I, Cassese S, Groha P, Steppich B, Hadamitzky M, Ibrahim T, et al. Randomized comparison of paclitaxel-eluting balloon and stenting versus plain balloon plus stenting versus directional atherectomy for femoral artery disease (ISAR-STATH). *Circulation.* 2017;135(23):2218–2226.

12. Safian RD, Feldman T, Muller DW, Mason D, Schreiber T, Haik B, et al. Coronary angioplasty and rotablator atherectomy trial (CARAT): Immediate and late results of a prospective multicenter randomized trial. *Catheter Cardiovasc Interv.* 2001;53(2):213–220.

13. Whitlow PL, Bass TA, Kipperman RM, Sharaf BL, Ho KK, Cutlip DE, et al. Results of the study to determine rotablator and transluminal angioplasty strategy (STRATAS). *Am J Cardiol.* 2001;87(6):699–705.

14. vom Dahl J, Dietz U, Haager PK, Silber S, Niccoli L, Buettner HJ, et al. Rotational atherectomy does not reduce recurrent in-stent restenosis: Results of the angioplasty versus rotational atherectomy for treatment of diffuse in-stent restenosis trial (ARTIST). *Circulation.* 2002;105(5):583–588.

15. Abdel-Wahab M, Richardt G, Joachim Buttner H, Toelg R, Geist V, Meinertz T, et al. High-speed rotational atherectomy before paclitaxel-eluting stent implantation in complex calcified coronary lesions: The randomized ROTAXUS (rotational atherectomy prior to taxus stent treatment for complex native coronary artery disease) trial. *JACC Cardiovasc Interv.* 2013;6(1):10–19.

16. Barbato E, Carrie D, Dardas P, Fajadet J, Gaul G, Haude M, et al. European expert consensus on rotational atherectomy. *Euro Interv.* 2015;11(1):30–36.

17. Windecker S, Kolh P, Alfonso F, Collet JP, Cremer J, Falk V, et al. ESC/EACTS guidelines on myocardial revascularization: The task force on myocardial revascularization of the European Society of Cardiology (ESC) and the European Association for Cardio-Thoracic Surgery (EACTS) developed with the special contribution of the European Association of Percutaneous Cardiovascular Interventions (EAPCI). *Eur Heart J.* 2014;35(37):2541–2619.

18. Bhatt P, Parikh P, Patel A, Chag M, Chandarana A, Parikh R, et al. Long-term safety and performance of the orbital atherectomy system for treating calcified coronary artery lesions: 5-year follow-up in the ORBIT I trial. *Cardiovasc Revasc Med.* 2015;16(4):213–216.

19. Genereux P, Bettinger N, Redfors B, Lee AC, Kim CY, Lee MS, et al. Two-year outcomes after treatment of severely calcified coronary lesions with the orbital atherectomy system and the impact of stent types: Insight from the ORBIT II trial. *Catheter Cardiovasc Interv.* 2016;88(3):369–377.

20. Safian RD, Niazi K, Runyon JP, Dulas D, Weinstock B, Ramaiah V, et al. Orbital atherectomy for infrapopliteal disease: Device concept and outcome data for the OASIS trial. *Catheter Cardiovasc Interv.* 2009;73(3):406–412.

21. Barath P, Fishbein MC, Vari S, Forrester JS. Cutting balloon: A novel approach to percutaneous angioplasty. *Am J Cardiol.* 1991;68(11):1249–1252.

22. Kurbaan AS, Kelly PA, Sigwart U. Cutting balloon angioplasty and stenting for aorto-ostial lesions. *Heart.* 1997;77(4):350–352.

23. Kurbaan AS, Foale RA, Sigwart U. Cutting balloon angioplasty for in-stent restenosis. *Catheter Cardiovasc Interv.* 2000;50(4):480–483.

24. Mauri L, Bonan R, Weiner BH, Legrand V, Bassand JP, Popma JJ, et al. Cutting balloon angioplasty for the prevention of restenosis: Results of the Cutting Balloon Global Randomized Trial. *Am J Cardiol.* 2002;90(10):1079–1083.

25. de Ribamar Costa J, Jr., Mintz GS, Carlier SG, Mehran R, Teirstein P, Sano K, et al. Nonrandomized comparison of coronary stenting under intravascular ultrasound guidance of direct stenting without predilation versus conventional predilation with a semi-compliant balloon versus predilation with a new scoring balloon. *Am J Cardiol.* 2007;100(5):812–817.

26. Miyazaki T, Latib A, Ruparelia N, Kawamoto H, Sato K, Figini F, et al. The use of a scoring balloon for optimal lesion preparation prior to bioresorbable scaffold implantation: A comparison with conventional balloon predilatation. *EuroIntervention.* 2016;11(14):e1580–e1588.

27. Rosenschein U, Bernstein JJ, DiSegni E, Kaplinsky E, Bernheim J, Rozenzsajn LA. Experimental ultrasonic angioplasty: Disruption of atherosclerotic plaques and

thrombi in vitro and arterial recanalization in vivo. *J Am Coll Cardiol.* 1990;15(3):711–717.

28. Fischell TA, Abbas MA, Grant GW, Siegel RJ. Ultrasonic energy. Effects on vascular function and integrity. *Circulation.* 1991;84(4):1783–1795.

29. Ali ZA, Brinton TJ, Hill JM, Maehara A, Matsumura M, Karimi Galougahi K, et al. Optical coherence tomography characterization of coronary lithoplasty for treatment of calcified lesions: First description. *JACC Cardiovasc Imaging.* 2017;10(8):897–906.

30. Braden GA, Xenopoulos NP, Young T, Utley L, Kutcher MA, Applegate RJ. Transluminal extraction catheter atherectomy followed by immediate stenting in treatment of saphenous vein grafts. *J Am Coll Cardiol.* 1997;30(3):657–663.

31. Safian RD, Grines CL, May MA, Lichtenberg A, Juran N, Schreiber TL, et al. Clinical and angiographic results of transluminal extraction coronary atherectomy in saphenous vein bypass grafts. *Circulation.* 1994;89(1):302–312.

32. Migliorini A, Stabile A, Rodriguez AE, Gandolfo C, Rodriguez Granillo AM, Valenti R, et al. Comparison of angiojet rheolytic thrombectomy before direct infarct artery stenting with direct stenting alone in patients with acute myocardial infarction. The JETSTENT trial. *J Am Coll Cardiol.* 2010;56(16):1298–1306.

33. Appelman YE, Piek JJ, Strikwerda S, Tijssen JG, de Feyter PJ, David GK, et al. Randomised trial of excimer laser angioplasty versus balloon angioplasty for treatment of obstructive coronary artery disease. *Lancet.* 1996;347(8994):79–84.

34. Reifart N, Vandormael M, Krajcar M, Gohring S, Preusler W, Schwarz F, et al. Randomized comparison of angioplasty of complex coronary lesions at a single center. Excimer laser, rotational atherectomy, and balloon angioplasty comparison (ERBAC) study. *Circulation.* 1997;96(1):91–98.

35. Hamburger JN, Gijsbers GH, Ozaki Y, Ruygrok PN, de Feyter PJ, Serruys PW. Recanalization of chronic total coronary occlusions using a laser guide wire: A pilot study. *J Am Coll Cardiol.* 1997;30(3):649–656.

36. Lee T, Shlofmitz RA, Song L, Tsiamtsiouris T, Pappas T, Madrid A, et al. The effectiveness of excimer laser angioplasty to treat coronary in-stent restenosis with peri-stent calcium as assessed by optical coherence tomography. *EuroIntervention.* 2018. doi:10.4244/EIJ-D-18-00139.

37. Allen KB, Dowling RD, Fudge TL, Schoettle GP, Selinger SL, Gangahar DM, et al. Comparison of transmyocardial revascularization with medical therapy in patients with refractory angina. *N Engl J Med.* 1999;341(14):1029–1036.

38. Lauer B, Junghans U, Stahl F, Kluge R, Oesterle SN, Schuler G. Catheter-based percutaneous myocardial laser revascularization in patients with end-stage coronary artery disease. *J Am Coll Cardiol.* 1999;34(6):1663–1670.

39. Gassler N, Wintzer HO, Stubbe HM, Wullbrand A, Helmchen U. Transmyocardial laser revascularization. Histological features in human nonresponder myocardium. *Circulation.* 1997;95(2):371–375.

40. Briones E, Lacalle JR, Marin-Leon I, Rueda JR. Transmyocardial laser revascularization versus medical therapy for refractory angina. *Cochrane Database Syst Rev.* 2015(2):CD003712

41. Popma JJ, Califf RM, Topol EJ. Clinical trials of restenosis after coronary angioplasty. *Circulation.* 1991;84(3):1426–1436.

42. Friedman M, Felton L, Byers S. The antiatherogenic effect of iridium-192 upon the cholesterol-fed rabbit. *J Clin Invest.* 1964;43:185–192.

43. Carter AJ, Laird JR, Bailey LR, Hoopes TG, Farb A, Fischell DR, et al. Effects of endovascular radiation from a beta-particle-emitting stent in a porcine coronary restenosis model. A dose-response study. *Circulation.* 1996;94(10):2364–238.

44. Teirstein PS, Massullo V, Jani S, Popma JJ, Mintz GS, Russo RJ, et al. Catheter-based radiotherapy to inhibit restenosis after coronary stenting. *N Engl J Med.* 1997;336(24):1697–1703.

45. Leon MB, Teirstein PS, Moses JW, Tripuraneni P, Lansky AJ, Jani S, et al. Localized intracoronary gamma-radiation therapy to inhibit the recurrence of restenosis after stenting. *N Engl J Med.* 2001;344(4):250–256.

46. Waksman R, Bhargava B, White L, Chan RC, Mehran R, Lansky AJ, et al. Intracoronary beta-radiation therapy

inhibits recurrence of in-stent restenosis. *Circulation*. 2000;101(16):1895–1898.

47. King SB, 3rd, Williams DO, Chougule P, Klein JL, Waksman R, Hilstead R, et al. Endovascular beta-radiation to reduce restenosis after coronary balloon angioplasty: Results of the beta energy restenosis trial (BERT). *Circulation*. 1998;97(20):2025–2030.

48. Albiero R, Adamian M, Kobayashi N, Amato A, Vaghetti M, Di Mario C, et al. Short- and intermediate-term results of ³²P radioactive beta-emitting stent implantation in patients with coronary artery disease: The Milan dose-response study. *Circulation*. 2000;101(1):18–26.

49. Wardeh AJ, Kay IP, Sabate M, Coen VL, Gijzel AL, Ligthart JM, et al. Beta-particle-emitting radioactive stent implantation. A safety and feasibility study. *Circulation*. 1999;100(16):1684–1689.

50. Abbo KM, Dooris M, Glazier S, O'Neill WW, Byrd D, Grines CL, et al. Features and outcome of no-reflow after percutaneous coronary intervention. *Am J Cardiol*. 1995;75(12):778–782.

51. Tardiff BE, Califf RM, Tcheng JE, Lincoff AM, Sigmon KN, Harrington RA, et al. Clinical outcomes after detection of elevated cardiac enzymes in patients undergoing percutaneous intervention. IMPACT II investigators. Integrilin (eptifibatide) to Minimize Platelet Aggregation and Coronary Thrombosis-II. *J Am Coll Cardiol*. 1999;33(1):88–96.

52. Topol EJ, Yadav JS. Recognition of the importance of embolization in atherosclerotic vascular disease. *Circulation*. 2000;101(5):570–580.

53. Carlino M, De Gregorio J, Di Mario C, Anzuini A, Airoldi F, Albiero R, et al. Prevention of distal embolization during saphenous vein graft lesion angioplasty. Experience with a new temporary occlusion and aspiration system. *Circulation*. 1999;99(25):3221–3223.

54. Webb JG, Carere RG, Virmani R, Baim D, Teirstein PS, Whitlow P, et al. Retrieval and analysis of particulate debris after saphenous vein graft intervention. *J Am Coll Cardiol*. 1999;34(2):468–475.

55. Baim DS, Wahr D, George B, Leon MB, Greenberg J, Cutlip DE, et al. Randomized trial of a distal embolic protection device during percutaneous intervention of saphenous vein aorto-coronary bypass grafts. *Circulation*. 2002;105(11):1285–1290.

56. Stone GW, Webb J, Cox DA, Brodie BR, Qureshi M, Kalynych A, et al. Distal microcirculatory protection during percutaneous coronary intervention in acute ST-segment elevation myocardial infarction: A randomized controlled trial. *JAMA*. 2005;293(9):1063–1072.

57. Cura FA, Escudero AG, Berrocal D, Mendiz O, Trivi MS, Fernandez J, et al. Protection of distal embolization in high-risk patients with acute ST-segment elevation myocardial infarction (PREMIAR). *Am J Cardiol*. 2007;99(3):357–363.

58. Guetta V, Mosseri M, Shechter M, Matetzky S, Assali A, Almagor Y, et al. Safety and efficacy of the filter wire EZ in acute ST-segment elevation myocardial infarction. *Am J Cardiol*. 2007;99(7):911–915.

59. Teramoto R, Sakata K, Miwa K, Matsubara T, Yasuda T, Inoue M, et al. Impact of distal protection with filter-type device on long-term outcome after percutaneous coronary intervention for acute myocardial infarction: Clinical results with Filtrap. *J Atheroscler Thromb*. 2016;23(12):1313–1323.

60. Iqbal MB, Nadra IJ, Ding L, Fung A, Aymong E, Chan AW, et al. Embolic protection device use and its association with procedural safety and long-term outcomes following saphenous vein graft intervention: An analysis from the British Columbia Cardiac Registry. *Catheter Cardiovasc Interv*. 2016;88(1):73–83.

61. Brennan JM, Al-Hejily W, Dai D, Shaw RE, Trilesskaya M, Rao SV, et al. Three-year outcomes associated with embolic protection in saphenous vein graft intervention: Results in 49 325 senior patients in the Medicare-linked National Cardiovascular Data Registry CATHPCI Registry. *Circ Cardiovasc Interv*. 2015;8(3):e001403.

62. Paul TK, Bhatheja S, Panchal HB, Zheng S, Banerjee S, Rao SV, et al. Outcomes of saphenous vein graft intervention with and without embolic protection device: A comprehensive review and meta-analysis. *Circ Cardiovasc Interv*. 2017;10(12):e005538.

63. Jin B, Dong XH, Zhang C, Li Y, Shi HM. Distal protection devices in primary percutaneous coronary intervention of native coronary artery lesions: A meta-analysis of randomized controlled trials. *Curr Med Res Opin*. 2012;28(6):871–876.

33

Catheter-based reperfusion in acute myocardial infarction

MING-YU (ANTHONY) CHUANG, RICHARD BROGAN AND DEREK P. CHEW

INTRODUCTION

Significant advances in catheter-based technology and techniques have been made in the last two decades. Within current practice, primary percutaneous coronary intervention (PCI) is now the reperfusion strategy of choice in most patients presenting with acute coronary syndrome (ACS) with high-risk features. Furthermore, next-generation pharmaco-therapeutic agents and novel strategies have provided new ways to address the pathophysiology underlying acute coronary culprit lesions. This chapter provides an overview of the current status of primary PCI with emphasis on important practical and technical issues for health professionals treating patients with ACS.

MODE OF ARTERIAL ACCESS

There is now robust evidence in favour of the radial approach as the default access in patients with ACS undergoing primary PCI. The MATRIX trial, the largest randomised trial to compare radial and femoral access, randomised 8404 patients (48% ST-elevation myocardial infarction [STEMI], 52% non-STEMI) to either trans-radial or trans-femoral access and showed that radial access was associated with lower risk of major bleeding and access-related complications. Subsequent meta-analyses also confirmed these findings.[1-4] Contrary to earlier belief, radial access in the hands of experienced operators was also found not to be associated with increased radiation exposure.[5] Based on these data, radial access is now the recommended access of choice unless there are compelling reasons for femoral access, such as primary PCI in the context of cardiogenic shock (CS) or during the resuscitation of cardiac arrest where the potential need for higher calibre mechanical support devices such as intra-aortic balloon pump (IABP) use is high.[6,7]

CHOICE OF STENT

Coronary stenting is the technique of choice during primary PCI, and second-generation drug-eluting stents (DES) now represent the standard-of-care in contemporary clinical practice.[6,7] Compared with balloon angioplasty, PCI using bare-metal stent (BMS) is associated with lower risk of recurrent myocardial infarction (MI) and target vessel revascularisation (TVR),[8,9] but continues to be associated with a significant risk of in-stent stenosis.[10] In a meta-analysis of 6,298 patients (11 trials) comparing first-generation DES (paclitaxel, sirolimus) and BMS, DES was associated with a significantly lower rate of target vessel restenosis (hazard ratio [HR] = 0.57, 95% confidence interval [95%CI] = 0.50–0.66, $p < 0.001$), but at a cost of increased risk of stent thrombosis (SR); (HR = 2.81, 1.28–6.19, $p = 0.04$).[11] These findings led to the development of second-generation DES with newer anti-proliferative drugs (zotarolimus, everolimus), and improved stent design including thinner struts and biocompatible polymers.[12] Second-generation DES now have robust evidence demonstrating superior safety and efficacy compared with BMS and first-generation DES, with three recent trials in particular (EXAMINATION, COMFORTABLE AMI, NORSTENT) highlighting the lower risks of ST and recurrent MI.[13–17]

The EXAMINATION trial is a single-blinded, multi-centre, randomised trial that compared second-generation everolimus-eluting stent (EES; Xience) with BMS in patients presenting with STEMI. Compared with BMS, EES was associated with significantly lower rates of ST (0.5 vs. 2.5%, $p = 0.019$) with no difference in recurrent MI and bleeding.[16] At 5-year follow-up, EES continues to be associated with a significant lower rate of TVR, as well as a lower rate of all-cause mortality.[17] The COMFORTABLE AMI trial was a single-blinded, multi-centre, randomised trial that compared biolimus-eluting stent (BES) with BMS, and also demonstrated lower rates of TVR (HR = 0.28; 95%CI = 0.13–0.59; $p < 0.001$),

TVR re-infarction (HR = 0.20, 95%CI = 0.06–0.69, $p = 0.01$) with a trend towards lower risk of ST (0.9% vs. 2.1%; HR = 0.42, 95%CI = 0.15–1.19, $p = 0.10$).[14,15] Similarly, the NORSTENT trial randomly assigned 9013 patients with stable and unstable coronary artery disease (~31% ACS undergoing PCI) to either second-generation DES (everolimus, zotarolimus) or BMS. At 6 years, DES was associated with significantly lower rates of repeat revascularisation (HR = 0.76, 95%CI = 0.69–0.85, $p < 0.001$) and definite ST (0.8 vs. 1.2%, $p = 0.0498$), with no difference in recurrent MI, all-cause mortality and major bleeding.[13]

Based on these data, the European Society of Cardiology (ESC) has updated its 2017 guideline recommending second-generation DES in primary PCI over BMS (Class I, Level A).[6] Current evidence suggests there is no significant difference in outcomes between the second-generation stents.[18]

Lastly, in patients at high bleeding risk, a polymer-free and carrier-free drug-coated stent (BioFreedom; biolimus-A9 drug-coated stent) has recently been shown to have superior safety and efficacy compared to BMS when used with only 1 month of dual antiplatelet therapy in the LEADERS-FREE trial.[19] However, only ~10% of patients included in this trial had ACS as the indication for PCI; therefore, the applicability of these data to primary PCI may be limited. Trials are currently underway comparing second-generation DES with BioFreedom stents in patients who cannot tolerate more than 1 month of dual antiplatelet therapy (Resolute Onyx – ClinicalTrials.gov Identifier: NCT03344653; Synergy – ClinicalTrials.gov Identifier: NCT02605447).

PHARMACOTHERAPY IN PRIMARY PCI

Patients undergoing primary PCI should receive a combination of aspirin, a P2Y12 inhibitor and a parenteral anticoagulant. Choosing the optimal combination of platelet inhibitors and anticoagulant to balance the risks of ischemia and bleeding is essential to improve patient outcomes in primary PCI. In this section, we summarise the current evidence of pharmacotherapy in primary PCI. The recommended dosages of antiplatelet and anticoagulation therapies are presented in Table 33.1.

Table 33.1 Recommended dosages of antiplatelet and anticoagulation therapies in primary percutaneous coronary intervention

	Standard dose	Stage 4 CKD[a]	Stage 5 CKD[b]
Antiplatelet therapies			
Aspirin	Loading dose of 150–300 mg orally followed by a maintenance dose of 75–100 mg/day	No adjustment required	No adjustment required
Ticagrelor	Loading dose of 180 mg orally, followed by a maintenance dose of 90 mg twice per day	No adjustment required	Not recommended
Prasugrel	Loading dose of 60 mg orally, followed by a maintenance dose of 10 mg/day. If body weight <60 kg, reduce maintenance dose to 5 mg/day. Contraindicated if previous stroke/transient ischemic attack	No adjustment required	Not recommended
Clopidogrel	Loading dose of 300–600 mg orally followed by a maintenance dose of 75 mg/day	No adjustment required	No information available
Abciximab	Bolus of 0.25 mg/kg intravenously and 0.125 µg/kg/min infusion for 12 h	Caution; consider bleeding risk	Caution; consider bleeding risk
Eptiibatide	Double follow of 18 µg/kg intravenously (10 minutes interval) followed by an infusion of 2 µg/kg/min for up to 18 h	Reduce infusion dose to 1 µg/kg/min	Not recommended
Tirofiban	25 µg/kg over 3 min intravenously followed by a maintenance infusion of 0.15 µg/kg/min for up to 18 h	Reduce infusion rate to 50%	Not recommended
Anticoagulant therapies			
Unfractionated heparin	70–100 IU/kg intravenous bolus with no glycoprotein IIb/IIIa inhibitors. 50–70 IU/kg intravenous bolus with glycoprotein IIb/IIIa inhibitors	No adjustment required	No adjustment required
Enoxaparin	1 mg/kg subcutaneously or 0.5 mg/kg intravenously followed by 1 mg/kg twice a day	1 mg/kg per day	Not recommended
Bivalirudin	0.75 mg/kg intravenous bolus with 1.75 mg/kg/h infusion for up to 4 h after procedure	Reduce infusion rate to 1 mg/kg/h	Reduce infusion rate to 0.25 mg/kg/h

Source: Ibanez, B. et al., *Rev. Esp. Cardiol. (Engl. Ed.)*, 70, 1082, 2017; Chew, D.P. et al., *Heart Lung Circ.*, 25, 895–951, 2016.
[a] Estimated glomerular filtration rate 15–30 mL/min/1.73 m^2.
[b] Estimated glomerular filtration rate 15 mL/min/1.73 m^2.

Platelet inhibition

Aspirin has a robust evidence base in primary PCI and an oral dose of 150–300 mg of aspirin should be given as soon as possible following ACS diagnosis.[20] However, while the peri-procedural aspirin use is unlikely to be challenged, the incremental benefit of longer-term aspirin among patients treated with potent P2Y12 inhibition is currently under investigation (GLOBAL LEADERS trial, ClinicalTrials.gov Identifier: NCT01813435).

For P2Y12 inhibition in primary PCI, the preferred agents are prasugrel and ticagrelor (over clopidogrel).[6,7] These agents have more a rapid onset of action, greater potency and have superior outcomes compared to clopidogrel.[6,21,22] In the TRITON-TIMI 38 study, prasugrel was more effective than clopidogrel when added to aspirin for reducing the rate of ischaemic events (current MI, stroke and death) but was associated with an increased risk of major bleeding and no difference in overall mortality.[21] Prasugrel, however, is contraindicated in patients with previous stroke/transient ischemic attack (TIA) and is generally not recommended in patients aged ≥ 75 years or low body weight (≤ 60 kg), as it is associated with more harm than benefit due to an increased risk of bleeding. The efficacy of ticagrelor in the context of primary PCI was demonstrated in the PLATO study, which randomised 18,624 patients with an ACS to either ticagrelor or clopidogrel with ~60% of patients undergoing PCI.[22] Compared to clopidogrel, ticagrelor was associated with significantly lower rates of death from any cause, death from a vascular cause, MI, and ST but a higher rate of non-coronary artery bypass graft (CABG) related major bleed. Of note, this benefit over clopidogrel did not emerge until after 30 days. Clopidogrel has not been directly evaluated in any large outcome studies in the setting of primary PCI, therefore it should only be used if neither of the two agents is available,[6,7] though its incremental benefit over aspirin in the context of fibrinolysis was examined in CLARITY TIMI 25. Subsequent secondary meta-analyses of patients undergoing PCI from an early study have confirmed the benefit of clopidogrel. Cangrelor is a potent, intravenous, reversible P2Y12 inhibitor with a rapid onset and offset of action (duration of action = 1–2 hours). It has been assessed in three randomised, controlled trials (RCTs) against clopidogrel loading or placebo.[23–25] A meta-analysis of these three trials showed a modest relative reduction in peri-procedural ischemic events

(death, recurrent MI, urgent revascularisation and ST at 48 hours) (odds ratio [OR] = 0.87, 95%CI = 0.78–0.99, $p = 0.0007$), with a relative increase in the rate of major bleeding (OR = 1.38, 95%CI = 1.03–1.85, $p = 0.029$).[26] The fact that cangrelor has not been compared against the more potent P2Y12 inhibitors (prasugrel or ticagrelor) limits the applicability of these results to current practice. However, cangrelor may still have a role as a peri-procedural antiplatelet agent in patients not adequately loaded with oral P2Y12 inhibition. Currently, cangrelor is not approved for clinical use in Australia.

There is little evidence to guide when the P2Y12 inhibitor should be initiated in patients with ACS undergoing primary PCI. The ATLANTIC trial randomised 1,862 patients with STEMI to receive ticagrelor either 'pre-hospital' or 'immediately before angiography'.[27] It observed no differences in terms of primary outcome (primary outcome defined as a >70% resolution of ST-segment elevation before PCI or TIMI 3 flow before intervention), as well as rates of major adverse cardiovascular events and major bleeding. Reinforcing these observations in patients with non-ST elevation ACS, the ACCOAST trial studied, earlier 'pre-treatment' with prasugrel 30 mg at the time of diagnosis (before angiography) compared to 60 mg at the time of PCI following angiography did not reduce ischaemic events, but did increase bleeding events, especially in those requiring CABG.[28] In interpreting these results, the higher rate of CABG and medical management in this population should be considered. These results argue against 'field-initiation' of P2Y12 inhibition. In summary, a P2Y12 inhibitor should be initiated soon after ACS diagnosis, but consideration should be given to other factors such as 'ischaemic versus bleeding risk', the likelihood of needing CABG (e.g. patients with diabetes or extensive electrocardiogram (ECG) changes) and time to angiography.[6,7]

The three glycoprotein IIb/IIIa (GP IIb/IIIa) inhibitors approved for clinical use in ACS are abciximab (a recombinant monoclonal antibody fragment), tirofiban (a peptidomimetic molecule) and eptifibatide (a cyclic peptide). A 2013 Cochrane Review found that when administered during primary PCI, GP IIb/IIIa inhibition is associated with a relative reduction in 30-day death and MI (OR = 0.66, 95%CI = 0.60–0.72), but with an increased risk of severe bleeding (OR = 1.39, 95%CI = 1.21–1.61).[29] However, no trials have been conducted assessing the efficacy of GP IIb/IIIa when added to more potent P2Y12 inhibitors (ticagrelor, prasugrel). Therefore, routine use of GP IIb/IIIa inhibitors is not recommended and its use should be reserved for selected patients with high ischemic risk or with thrombotic complications during PCI (e.g. no reflow).[6,7]

Anticoagulation

Anticoagulation options for primary PCI include unfractionated heparin (UFH), enoxaparin, and bivalirudin.

Heparin is an indirect thrombin inhibitor. Although there has been no placebo-controlled trial evaluating UFH in the context of primary PCI, its use is still recommended as there is a large body of experience with UFH. Enoxaparin is a low molecular weight heparin that principally inhibits factor Xa. The ATOLL trial randomised 910 patients presenting with STEMI to receive either enoxaparin or UFH before primary PCI, and showed that enoxaparin was not associated with a reduction in death or MI and bleeding.[30] A later meta-analysis of 23 PCI trials (including both randomised and observation studies, including 30,966 patient, of which 33% underwent primary PCI) reported a relative risk reduction (RR) in mortality associated with enoxaparin (RR = 0.66, 95%CI = 0.57–0.76, $p < 0.001$) with lower rates of major bleeding (RR = 0.80, 95%CI = 0.68–0.95, $p = 0.009$).[31] Based on these data, both enoxaparin and UFH are recommended in patients with ACS undergoing primary PCI.[6,7]

Bivalirudin is a direct thrombin inhibitor that antagonises the actions of thrombin independently of antithrombin. In the context of primary PCI in ACS, bivalirudin has been compared to UHF in seven RCTs totalling ~20,000 patients (with and without GP IIb/IIIa inhibitor use).[32–38] A meta-analysis of six of these trials showed that bivalirudin was associated with a modest reduction in all-cause mortality, cardiac mortality and major bleeding, but higher rates of ST.[33] The benefit of reduction in major bleeding, however, appears to be modulated by the: (1) type of vascular access (less benefit if radial access), (2) type of P2Y12 inhibitor used (less benefit if ticagrelor or prasugrel used) and (3) concurrent GP IIb/IIIa use (less benefit if GP IIb/IIIa used as bailout-therapy only). To better reflect contemporary practice, the 2017 VALIDATE-SWEDEHEART trial randomised 6,006 patients presenting with STEMI or non-STEMI to receive either bivalirudin or heparin (all undergoing PCI, receiving a potent P2Y12 inhibitor [ticagrelor, prasugrel or cangrelor], without the planned use of glycoprotein IIb/IIIa inhibitor, and with predominantly radial-artery access).[32] In this study, no differences were observed between the treatment arms in terms of all-cause death, MI, major bleed and definite ST. Based on these data, bivalirudin may be considered in patients with ACS undergoing primary PCI, especially in patients at high bleeding risk or who have a contraindication to heparin (e.g. those with heparin-induced thrombocytopenia).[6,7]

Fondaparinux was associated with potential harm in the setting of primary PCI in the OASIS-6 trial and is not recommended.[39] With increasing use of oral anticoagulation within the community, evidence informing the use of combination anticoagulation and antiplatelet therapy is evolving. In the acute setting, in general, anticoagulation should be suspended immediately after primary PCI and consideration for the intermediate and longer-term use of triple therapy (aspirin, P2Y12 inhibition and oral anticoagulant) or dual therapy (a combination these) should be based on judicious consideration of the coronary risks, the separate indication for anticoagulation, e.g. mechanical valves[6,7] and the patient's bleeding risk.

THROMBUS ASPIRATION IN PRIMARY PCI

Percutaneous coronary intervention has been shown to significantly increase vessel patency rate compared to thrombolysis.[40,41] However, even following the restoration of infarct-related vessel patency, incomplete myocardial reperfusion can still be detected in a significant proportion of patients.[42] It is hypothesized that this phenomenon can be attributed to distal embolisation of atherothrombotic material with subsequent microvascular obstruction.[43] Given that incomplete reperfusion has been strongly linked to larger infarct size, worse left ventricular (LV) systolic function and subsequent inferior clinical outcome, substantial efforts have been made to improve myocardial reperfusion after primary PCI. This led to the development of thrombus aspiration (TA) devices that may limit distal embolisation and microvascular obstruction, reduce rates of ST,[44,45] and allow for better visualisation of plaque and facilitation of direct stenting.[46]

Devices and technique

While many different commercially available manual TA devices are available (Table 33.2), they generally operate on similar mechanisms, and comparative studies do not demonstrate differences between the devices.[47,48] Most of the manual TA devices are 6-Fr compatible and contain two lumina: a smaller lumen for the guide wire and a large lumen for aspiration. The larger aspiration lumen is connected proximally to a syringe, which enables the operator to aspirate athero-thrombotic material manually while manoeuvring the distal catheter through the coronary lesion. The distal end of the device consists of an atraumatic tip with a radiopaque marker. When performing TA, pre-aspiration coronary injections should be minimised to reduce the chance of distal embolisation. The aspiration catheter is manoeuvred back and forth through the culprit lesion while negative pressure is maintained in the proximal syringe. When retracting the device, the guide catheter should be fully engaged with the coronary ostium and the syringe, pressure must be kept negative to avoid systemic embolisation of thrombus.[49]

The only mechanical TA device available on the market is the AngioJet® (Boston Scientific, USA). The AngioJet® operates by using a backward-travelling saline jet at the catheter tip to fragment and aspirate thrombus though catheter holes. Of note, because of its size, the AngioJet® can only be used in large coronary arteries with a diameter greater than 2 mm.

Trial evidence

In total, 24 trials involving 22,096 patients have been conducted comparing routine TA versus conventional PCI in ACS.[49] While initial small-scale randomised and observational studies suggested benefit,[50-52] three large-scale, investigator-initiated, open-label, randomised controlled trials involving 18,306 patients have failed to demonstrate a consistent benefit (TAPAS, TASTE and TOTAL trials).[49,53-56] The important study characteristics of these trials are summarised in Table 33.3. A meta-analysis of individual patient data from these three trials was published in 2017 by the Thrombectomy Trialists Collaboration.[57] It revealed that routine TA during STEMI did not reduce the incidence of 30-day all-cause death (HR = 0.85, 95%CI = 0.71–1.01, $p = 0.06$), cardiovascular death (HR = 0.84, 95%CI = 0.70–1.01, $p = 0.06$), and new congestive heart failure (HR = 1.10, 95%CI = 0.87–1.40, $p = 0.44$). There was also no significant difference in recurrent MI, ST, heart failure or TVR at 1-year. From the safety standpoint, there was a non-significant increase in the risk of 30-day stroke and TIA (HR = 1.43, 95%CI = 0.98–2.1, $p = 0.06$). In the subgroup analysis, patients with high thrombus burden (defined by TIMI thrombus ≥ 3) appeared to derive a greater cardiovascular benefit (fewer cardiovascular deaths) but at a cost of greater risk of stroke/TIA. Similarly, a meta-analysis of seven trials comparing mechanical TA with routine primary PCI concluded that mechanical TA did not reduce adverse cardiac events and was associated with a trend toward increased risk of stroke (1.3% vs. 0.4%, $p = 0.07$).[58] Based on these findings, major clinical guidelines have recommended against routine used of TA[6,7,59] (Table 33.4 and Figure 33.1).

Selective thrombus aspiration

It is important to note that the majority of the trials assessing TA in primary PCI used a strategy of

Table 33.2 Commercially available thrombus aspiration devices

Manual thrombus aspiration devices	Mechanical thrombus aspiration devices
Eliminate™ (Terumo, Japan)	AngioJet® (Boston Scientific, USA)
Export® (Medtronic, USA)	
QuickCat™ (Spectranetics, USA)	

Table 33.3 Important characteristics and findings of the TAPAS, TASTE and TOTAL trials

	TAPAS (2008)[53]	TASTE (2013)[54,55]	TOTAL (2015)[56]
Trial design	Single-centre RCT	Multi-centre registry-based RCT	Multi-centre RCT
Number screened	1.161	12.005	N/A
Number randomised	1,071	7,244	10,732
Patient population	STEMI	STEMI	STEMI
Intervention	Export®	Eliminate™ and Export®	Export®
Primary outcome	Myocardial blush grade	30-day all-cause mortality	Composite outcome (cardiovascular death, recurrent MI, cardiogenic shock, HF with NYHA class IV)
Time of randomisation	Before angiogram	After angiogram	Before angiogram
Predilatation in TA group	Precluded	Allowed	6%
Direct stenting facilitated by TA (%)	62	15	17
Drug eluting stent use (%)	0	49	45
Effective thrombus retrieval (%)	73	NA	70
Outcome			
30-day stroke	NA	=	↑
30-day mortality	=	=	=
1-year mortality	↓	=	=
1-year recurrent myocardial infarction	=	=	=
1-year target-vessel revascularisation	=	=	=
Limitations	• Small sample size • No data on stroke • No data on new-onset heart failure	• Not powered to detect survival difference <25%	

Source: Mahmoud, K.D. and Zijlstra, F., Nat. Rev. Cardiol., 13, 418–428, 2016.
Abbreviations: N/A, not available; RCT, randomised controlled trial; STEMI, St-elevation myocardial infarction; MI, myocardial infarction; HF, heart failure; NYHA, New York Heart Association class; TA, thrombus aspiration.

Table 33.4 Guideline recommendations for thrombus aspiration in acute coronary syndrome

Guideline	Recommendations	Grade and level of recommendation
2017 European Society of Cardiology[6]	Routine use of thrombus aspiration is not recommended	III, B
2016 Cardiac Society of Australia and New Zealand[7]	Thrombus aspiration can be considered when large thrombus burden impairs achievement of a satisfactory PCI result	N/A
2015 American College of Cardiology/American Heart Association[59]	Routine aspiration thrombectomy before primary percutaneous coronary intervention is not useful	III, A

Abbreviations: N/A, not available; PCI, percutaneous coronary intervention.

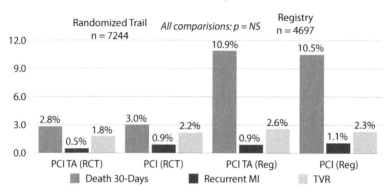

Figure 33.1 Randomised and registry data from the Primary outcomes of the Thrombus Aspiration during ST-Segment Elevation Myocardial Infarction (TASTE) trial comparing routine thrombus aspiration versus conventional primary percutaneous intervention (30-day mortality, recurrent myocardial infarction and target vessel revascularisation). No significant differences in outcomes were observed in all outcomes between routine thrombus aspiration versus conventional primary percutaneous intervention.

'routine TA' rather than 'selective TA'. Intuitively, more benefit is to be expected of TA in patients with a high thrombus burden and easily accessible lesion over a severely calcified tortuous vessel or distal lesion. While there is a lack of evidence, a carefully performed TA may still be a valuable technique in selected patients and provide the interventionalist with technical advantage in lesion visualisation and intra-procedural decision-making.

CULPRIT VERSUS COMPLETE REVASCULARISATION

ACS and multivessel disease frequently co-exist, with approximately 40%–65% of patients presenting with ST-elevation myocardial infarction (STEMI) having significant stenosis in one or more non-infarct related arteries (IRAs).[60–62] Revascularisation of the IRA in STEMI restores blood supply to a previously ischaemic region, reducing cell death and preserving viable myocardium, and improves outcome.[63] In the setting of co-existing multivessel disease, revascularisation of a stenotic non-IRA may theoretically: (1) improve blood supply to the remaining myocardium, (2) prevent subsequent ACS events by treating atherosclerotic plaque(s) that may be rendered unstable by the pro-inflammatory insult associated with index ACS, and (3) reduce the risk of future symptomatic ischaemia.[49,64,65] Complete revascularisation involves revascularisation of all non-IRA that contains a clinically significant stenosis either at the index procedure (single-stage) or in a second intervention (multistage). However, intervention on a non-IRA is associated with an increased risk of procedural-related complications, including peri-procedural MI, contrast-induced nephropathy, stent-related complications (ST, stent re-stenosis) and additional bleeding risk when performed as a staged procedure. Previous international guidelines have recommended intervention on only the 'IRA' vessel (i.e. culprit).[66,67] However, more recent data suggest that simultaneous intervention on both IRA and non-IRA (i.e. non-culprit) can be performed safely and may improve outcome.

Trial evidence

Seven trials were published between 2004 and 2014 comparing complete versus culprit-only revascularisation.[68–75] Key trial characteristics are summarised in Table 33.5. All of the trials are limited by a relatively small number of participants, with the largest trials being CvLPRIT ($n = 296$),[68] DANAMI-3PRIMULTI ($n = 627$),[70] and PRAMI ($n = 461$).[73] Of the three

Table 33.5 Important trial characteristics evaluating culprit versus complete revascularisation in acute coronary syndrome

Trial	Trial design	Sample size	Definition of significant stenosis	Timing of complete revascularisation
CvLPRIT 2015[68]	Multi-centre RCT	150/146	>70% diameter stenosis in 1 plane or >50% in 2 planes	At index procedure, unless operator decided for clinical reasons that the procedure needed to be staged. In the cases of staged intervention, it was mandated that the non-culprit lesions be treated during the index admission
DANAMI-3-PRIMULTI 2015[70]	Multi-centre RCT	314/313	>50% stenosis visually in arteries >2 mm diameter and FFR ≤0.8 or >90% stenosis visually regardless FFR measurement	Staged intervention 48 hours after index procedure but deform discharge
PRAGUE-13 2015	Multi-centre RCT	106/108	>70% stenosis	Staged intervention for the non-culprit artery(ies) between days 3 and 40 after the index procedure
Zhang 2015[74]	Not defined	215/213	Between 75% and 90% stenosis	Staged intervention for the non-culprit lesions between days 7 and 10 after the index procedure
PRAMI 2013[73]	Multi-centre RCT	234/231	Stenosis ≥50%	At index procedure
Dambrink and Ghani 2010[69]	Single-centre RCT	80/41	50%–90% diameter stenosis in 1 view + FFR <0.75 or >90% stenosis regardless of FFR	'Early' staged intervention (median 7.5 days)
HELP AMI 2004[71]	Multi-centre RCT	53/17	Not defined	At index procedure

Abbreviations: RCT, randomised controlled trial; FFR, fractional flow reserve.

trials, DANAMI-3-PRIMULTI was the only one that used fractional-flow-reserved (FFR) to assess the haemodynamic significance of stenosis in non-IRAs; and CvLPRIT and PRAMI required complete revascularisation at the time of index procedure.

A 2017 Cochrane Review of these trials reported that complete and culprit-only revascularisation strategies did not differ significantly in short-term all-cause mortality, cardiovascular mortality, non-fatal MI, repeat revascularisation, or long-term all-cause mortality.[75] There were, however, lower rates of long-term cardiovascular mortality, non-fatal MI and unplanned repeat revascularisation although these positive findings should be interpreted with caution due to limited sample size. A subgroup analysis of the timing of revascularisation (single-staged vs. multi-staged) showed that complete revascularisation performed during the index procedure was associated with significantly lower rates of late unplanned repeat revascularisation and non-fatal MI, while no difference was observed if performed in a multi-staged fashion. Pooled effect estimates are summarised in Table 33.6. A similar result was also found in another meta-analysis.[76] For safety outcomes, there were no significant differences in the risk of acute kidney injury,

stroke or bleeding between the two strategies. It is important to note, however, that the recent CULPRIT-SHOCK study reported increased in adverse events and mortality for patients undergoing multi-vessel PCI with CS. These data imply the need to consider the patients' haemodynamic stability when deciding on a strategy of complete revascularisation by percutaneous means.

Summary and ongoing trials

Overall, current evidence suggests that multivessel revascularisation can be performed safely and may reduce the risk of recurrent ischaemia. However, the quality of the evidence is low. Large, high-quality RCTs are required to draw firm conclusions regarding long-term cardiovascular benefit. The optimal timing for revascularisation and the utility of FFR also remains to be fully elucidated. Based on current data, major guidelines recommend that complete revascularisation should be considered in patients presenting with ACS with multivessel disease during index admission (see Table 33.7).

There are six ongoing trials as of December 2017: COCUA (ClinicalTrials.gov Identifier: NCT01180218), COMPARE ACUTE (ClinicalTrials

Table 33.6 Effect estimates extracted from 2017 Cochrane review of trials comparing culprit versus complete revascularisation in acute coronary syndrome

Outcome	Relative effect/hazard ratio (95% confidence interval)	Number of participants
Short-term all-cause mortality (<30 days after index intervention)	0.65 (0.18–2.37)	696
Short-term cardiovascular mortality (<30 days after index intervention)	0.33 (0.03–3.18)	627
Short-term myocardial infarction (≥1 year after the intervention)	1.74 (0.52–5.9)	627
Short-term revascularisation (<30 days after index intervention)	0.53 (0.2–1.45)	696
Long-term all-cause mortality (≥1 year after the intervention)	0.80 (0.58–1.11)	2417
Long-term cardiovascular mortality (≥1 year after the intervention)	0.50 (0.32–0.79)	2229
Long-term myocardial infarction (≥1 year after the intervention)	0.62 (0.44–0.89)	2099
Long-term revascularisation (≥1 year after the intervention)	0.47 (0.39–0.57)	2616

Source: Ong, P. et al., *Int. J. Cardiol.*, 250, 16–20, 2018.

Table 33.7 Major guideline recommendations for complete versus culprit revascularisation in non-shocked patient with ST-elevation myocardial infarction and non-ST elevation myocardial infarction

Guideline	Recommendations	Grade and level of recommendation
2017 European Society of Cardiology[6]	Routine revascularisation of non-infarct related artery lesions should be considered in STEMI patients with multi-vessel disease before hospital discharge	IIa, A
2016 Cardiac Society of Australia and New Zealand[7]	Stenosed coronary arteries in patients with multi-vessel disease at the time of primary PCI, rather than infarct-related artery stenosis alone, may lessen onset of recurrent ischaemia, although the number of objective late cardiovascular events in these trials was small	Nil
2015 American College of Cardiology/ American Heart Association (ACC/ AHA)[78]	PCI of a non-infarct artery may be considered in selected patients with STEMI and multivessel disease and who are haemodynamically stable, either at the time of primary PCI or as a planned, staged procedure	IIb, B

Abbreviations: PCI, Percutaneous coronary intervention; STEMI, ST elevation myocardial infarction.

gov Identifier: NCT01399736), COMPLETE (ClinicalTrials.gov Identifier: NCT01740479), ASSIST-CMR (ClinicalTrials.gov Identifier: NCT01818960), CROSS-AMI (ClinicalTrials.gov Identifier: NCT01179126), and FIT (ClinicalTrials.gov identifier: NCT01160900).

SPECIFIC PATIENT GROUPS

Cardiogenic shock

CS complicating MI occurs in approximately 5%–10% of patients[79] and continues to be associated with very high early mortality.[80,81] In addition to standard medical therapy including invasive blood pressure monitoring and inotropic/vasopressor therapy, the 1999 SHOCK trial established the basis for emergency invasive management in CS.[63] Since then, a number of strategies and devices have been developed in an attempt to further improve outcomes in these patients, including intraortic balloon pump (IABP) counterpulsation (see Chapter 35), the Impella® device and upfront complete revascularisation.[82–85] Left ventricular assist device (LVAD) and extracorporeal membrane oxygenation (ECMO) are discussed here.

Introduced nearly five decades ago, IABP is now routinely used in clinical practice as an adjunct treatment for MI complicated by CS on the basis that it is associated with enhanced coronary blood flow, increased organ perfusion and decreased systemic inflammation.[86] However, the 2012 IABP-SHOCK II trial (Intraaortic balloon pump in CS II) cast doubt on the established practice and showed that IABP counterpulsation does not improve outcome nor does it limit infarct size.[87] A later 2015 Cochrane Review also reported similar results.[88] Consequently, the latest guidelines recommend against 'routine' use of IABP in CS.[6,7,89] However, IABP may still be considered for haemodynamic support in selected patients, e.g. severe mitral insufficiency or ventricular septal defect.[6]

As a consequence of the negative findings of IABP, other mechanical circulatory support (MCS) devices have gathered increasing interest.[85] One of the devices that has been trialled in a sizable randomised trial is the Impella® device. The Impella® device is inserted via a standard 9 Fr femoral sheath, and consists of an axial pump on a pigtail catheter that crosses the aortic valve, with the intention to unload the left ventricle (LV) by continuously drawing blood from the LV and delivering it into the ascending aorta (non-pulsatile) with flow rates up to 4.0 L/minute.[82,90] While the device theoretically provides superior haemodynamic support compared to IABP, it has failed, so far, to demonstrate superior short-term survival compared to IABP in the 'IMPRESS in Severe Shock trial'.[90] At present, no MCS devices have been shown to improve survival in CS (including LVAD and ECMO).[82,83]

The finding of the potential benefit of complete revascularisation in STEMI complicated by CS was further investigated in the CULPRIT-SHOCK trial.[84] The CULPRIT-SHOCK trial is a multicentre, open-label, randomised, controlled trial that randomised 685 patients with CS in a 1:1 fashion to either: (1) complete revascularisation with immediate PCI to all lesions including chronic total occlusions, or (2) culprit-only revascularisation with the option of staged non-IRA revascularisation. At 30-days, culprit-only revascularisation was associated with significantly lower risk of death (HR = 0.83, 95%CI = 0.72–0.98, p = 0.03) and a trend towards less severe renal failure requiring renal replacement therapy (HR = 0.71, 95%CI = 0.49–1.03, p = 0.07), with no significant difference in recurrent MI, heart failure admission, stroke or bleeding.

Elderly/multiple competing non-cardiac risks

Chronological age in isolation should not determine suitability for routine invasive strategy; rather, other factors should also be taken into consideration such as estimated life expectancy, co-morbidity burden, quality of life (QoL), and patient value and preferences.[91] With lower rates of intracranial bleeding but the potential for access complications, primary PCI rather than fibrinolysis is the preferred strategy when reperfusion is being considered for STEMI in the elderly. Further research is necessary to develop a robust method to objectively quantify non-cardiac co-morbidities to inform decision-making regarding selecting patients with numerous co-morbidities for reperfusion.

Saphenous vein grafts, previous bypass grafts

Several large studies suggest that patients with previous bypass surgery presenting with MI have more advanced coronary disease and increased morbidity and mortality[92,93] but few have focused on primary PCI. In the GUSTO trial, 35% of patients with previous CABG had saphenous vein culprit lesions. Patients with saphenous graft occlusions responded poorly to thrombolytic therapy.[94] However, PCI to saphenous grafts is associated with a risk of plaque embolisation and no-reflow phenomenon, with worse clinical outcome compared with native artery PCI.[93,95–98] A number of embolic protection devices have demonstrated ischemic benefit in randomised trials and the 2011 ACCF/AHA guidelines recommend use of embolic protection devices during saphenous vein graft intervention whenever feasible (*Medtronic*: PercuSurge GuardWire, TriActiv system, Spider FXTM, Interceptor PLUS; *Boston Scientific*: FilterWire EX; *MedNova*: CardioShield).[78] Covered stent[99–101] and adjunctive glycoprotein IIb/IIIa antagonist[102–104] do not provide benefit, and their use is not recommended.[78]

SYSTEMS CONSIDERATION

Primary PCI is the preferred reperfusion strategy of choice in patients with STEMI within 12 hours of symptom onset and the absence of absolute contraindication.[6,7] However, choice of reperfusion strategy (i.e. considering initial fibrinolysis and transfer) requires consideration of expected delays in providing primary PCI, time from symptom onset to first medical contact (FMC), extent of ischaemic myocardium, presence of haemodynamic compromise, and bleeding risk from fibrinolytic therapy. It is well established that if the time to treatment is similar, primary PCI is superior to fibrinolysis in reducing mortality, recurrent MI or stroke.[105–108] However, if primary PCI cannot be performed in a timely fashion, the extent to which the PCI-related time delay diminishes the advantages of PCI over fibrinolysis is not well established. Earlier studies have calculated time delays that may mitigate the benefit of PCI over fibrinolysis as 60 minutes,[109] 110 minutes[110] and 120 minutes.[111] However, these studies predated routine coronary artery stenting and routine early angiography and stenting for patients who have undergone fibrinolysis. This was addressed in the 2013 STREAM trial, where STEMI patients without the possibility of immediate primary PCI (within 1 hour) were randomised to either 'immediately fibrinolysis followed by routine early angiography' or 'transfer to primary PCI (median delay to primary PCI = 78 minutes)'.[112] This study showed no differences in clinical outcomes between the two treatment strategies. Based on these data, current guidelines generally recommend primary PCI over fibrinolysis if it can be performed within 90–120 minutes of FMC; and for patients who have undergone fibrinolysis, early routine coronary angiography is indicated (with immediate transfer to a PCI-capable hospital).[6,7]

Strategies to reduce time to reperfusion and pre-hospital logistics of care

An effective reperfusion strategy requires extensive health service provision extending to all aspects of STEMI care, from FMC through to effective PCI operator proficiency. Coordinated protocol with planned decision-making that incorporates ambulance services, first responder physicians, emergency and cardiology departments are critical to achieving acceptable targets. It should be emphasised that the ambulance service has a critical role in the early diagnosis, triage and treatment of these patients.[113,114] Strategies that can effectively shorten time to reperfusion include:

1. *Early and pre-hospital ECG*: All patients presenting with suspected ACS should receive a 12-lead ECG and have it interpreted within 10 minutes of FMC.[6,7] Pre-hospital ECG is recommended as it reduces door-to-balloon time.[115]
2. *Pre-hospital activation of catheterisation laboratory*: When a STEMI diagnosis is made in the pre-hospital setting, the catheterisation laboratory should be activated immediately, as it reduces door-to-balloon time.[116–118]
3. *Bypassing emergency department (ED) on arrival in a PCI centre*: For patients triaged to a primary PCI strategy, direct admission to the catheterisation lab reduces FMC-to-wire crossing by up to 20 minutes.[119]
4. *Pre-hospital fibrinolysis*: For patients triaged for a fibrinolytic strategy, a maximal delay time from STEMI diagnosis to fibrinolytic bolus administration should be ≤10 minutes.[6]

Risk estimation during acute coronary syndrome

Accurate estimation of bleeding and ischemic risks in patients presenting with ACS is essential to help guide decision-making regarding: (1) choice of anti-thrombotic therapies, and (2) timing and appropriateness of invasive management. Several studies of ACS care have demonstrated a mismatch between physician assessments of ischaemic and bleeding risks and those derived from validated risk models.[120–122] This mismatch may contribute to the misapplication of evidence-based guideline recommendations that are not optimal for individual patient needs.[123,124] While there are currently no data to suggest that routine use of validated risk-stratification tools improve patient outcomes, major clinical guidelines universally recommend early assessment of ischaemic and bleeding risk using these tools.[6,7] For ischemic risk, the Global Registry of Acute Cardiac Events (GRACE) is recommended over the Thrombolysis In Myocardial Infarction (TIMI) score as it has superior discriminatory power.[6,7,120,125,126] For bleeding risk, the ACUITY and CRUSADE scores may be used, with the latter being the most discriminatory.[127,128]

Performance measures

There remains discordance between guideline recommendations and actual clinical care around the world.[7,58,129] To reduce this variation in practice and to improve quality of care, it is recommended that health systems should establish measurable quality indicators, as well as systems to measure and audit these indicators. Integrating continuous audit/feedback systems within work routines and patient flows are strongly recommended. This serves as a foundation for quality assurance initiatives and provides continuous data for new innovations to improve patient care. Suggested quality and outcome indicators can be found in recently published guidelines.[6,7]

AREAS FOR FUTURE RESEARCH AND CONCLUSION

Primary PCI is the reperfusion modality of choice and is the accepted standard of care in STEMI and non-STEMI. However, important areas of uncertainty persist and require further exploration. Specific areas of future research include: (1) strategies to reduce ischaemic-reperfusion injury, (2) refinement of acute and long-term anti-thrombotic and anticoagulation regimens, and (3) strategies and devices for management of patients in CS.

ACKNOWLEDGEMENT

We acknowledge Dr M Szpytma for assistance in drafting of the manuscript.

REFERENCES

1. Karrowni W, Vyas A, Giacomino B, Schweizer M, Blevins A, Girotra S, et al. Radial versus femoral access for primary percutaneous interventions in ST-segment elevation myocardial infarction patients: A meta-analysis of randomized controlled trials. *JACC Cardiovasc Interv.* 2013;6(8):814–823.
2. Ferrante G, Rao SV, Juni P, Da Costa BR, Reimers B, Condorelli G, et al. Radial versus femoral access for coronary interventions across the entire spectrum of patients with coronary artery disease: A meta-analysis of randomized trials. *JACC Cardiovasc Interv.* 2016;9(14):1419–1434.
3. Ando G, Capodanno D. Radial access reduces mortality in patients with acute coronary syndromes: Results from an updated trial sequential analysis of randomized trials. *JACC Cardiovasc Interv.* 2016;9(7):660–670.
4. Bavishi C, Panwar SR, Dangas GD, Barman N, Hasan CM, Baber U, et al. Meta-analysis of radial versus femoral access for percutaneous coronary interventions in non-ST-segment elevation acute coronary syndrome. *Am J Cardiol.* 2016;117(2):172–178.
5. Rigattieri S, Sciahbasi A, Drefahl S, Mussino E, Cera M, Di Russo C, et al. Transradial access and radiation exposure in diagnostic and interventional coronary procedures. *J Invasive Cardiol.* 2014;26(9):469–474.
6. Ibanez B, James S, Agewall S, Antunes MJ, Bucciarelli-Ducci C, Bueno H, et al. ESC guidelines for the management of acute myocardial infarction in patients presenting with ST-segment elevation. *Rev Esp Cardiol (Engl Ed).* 2017;70(12):1082.
7. Chew DP, Scott IA, Cullen L, French JK, Briffa TG, Tideman PA, et al. National Heart Foundation of Australia & Cardiac Society of Australia and New Zealand: Australian Clinical Guidelines for the Management of Acute Coronary Syndromes 2016. *Heart Lung Circ.* 2016;25(9):895–951.
8. Nordmann AJ, Hengstler P, Harr T, Young J, Bucher HC. Clinical outcomes of primary stenting versus balloon angioplasty in patients with myocardial infarction: A meta-analysis of randomized controlled trials. *Am J Med.* 2004;116(4):253–262.
9. Stone GW, Grines CL, Cox DA, Garcia E, Tcheng JE, Griffin JJ, et al. Comparison of angioplasty with stenting, with or without abciximab, in acute myocardial infarction. *N Engl J Med.* 2002;346(13):957–966.
10. Bates ER. Balancing the evidence base on coronary stents. *N Engl J Med.* 2016;375(13):1286–1288.
11. De Luca G, Dirksen MT, Spaulding C, Kelbaek H, Schalij M, Thuesen L, et al. Drug-eluting vs bare-metal stents in primary angioplasty: A pooled patient-level meta-analysis of randomized trials. *Arch Intern Med.* 2012;172(8): 611–621; discussion 21–22.
12. Iqbal J, Gunn J, Serruys PW. Coronary stents: Historical development, current status and future directions. *Br Med Bull.* 2013;106:193–211.
13. Bonaa KH, Mannsverk J, Wiseth R, Aaberge L, Myreng Y, Nygard O, et al. Drug-eluting or bare-metal stents for coronary artery disease. *N Engl J Med.* 2016;375(13):1242–1252.
14. Raber L, Kelbaek H, Ostojic M, Baumbach A, Heg D, Tuller D, et al. Effect of biolimus-eluting stents with biodegradable polymer vs bare-metal stents on cardiovascular events among patients with acute myocardial infarction: The COMFORTABLE AMI randomized trial. *JAMA.* 2012;308(8):777–787.
15. Raber L, Kelbaek H, Taniwaki M, Ostojic M, Heg D, Baumbach A, et al. Biolimus-eluting stents with biodegradable polymer versus bare-metal stents in acute myocardial infarction: Two-year clinical results of the COMFORTABLE AMI trial. *Circ Cardiovasc Interv.* 2014;7(3):355–364.

16. Sabate M, Cequier A, Iniguez A, Serra A, Hernandez-Antolin R, Mainar V, et al. Everolimus-eluting stent versus bare-metal stent in ST-segment elevation myocardial infarction (EXAMINATION): 1 year results of a randomised controlled trial. *Lancet.* 2012;380(9852):1482–1490.

17. Sabate M, Brugaletta S, Cequier A, Iniguez A, Serra A, Jimenez-Quevedo P, et al. Clinical outcomes in patients with ST-segment elevation myocardial infarction treated with everolimus-eluting stents versus bare-metal stents (EXAMINATION): 5-year results of a randomised trial. *Lancet.* 2016;387(10016):357–366.

18. Piccolo R, Stefanini GG, Franzone A, Spitzer E, Blochlinger S, Heg D, et al. Safety and efficacy of resolute zotarolimus-eluting stents compared with everolimus-eluting stents: A meta-analysis. *Circ Cardiovasc Interv.* 2015;8(4).

19. Urban P, Meredith IT, Abizaid A, Pocock SJ, Carrie D, Naber C, et al. Polymer-free drug-coated coronary stents in patients at high bleeding risk. *N Engl J Med.* 2015;373(21):2038–2047.

20. Antithrombotic Trialists C. Collaborative meta-analysis of randomised trials of antiplatelet therapy for prevention of death, myocardial infarction, and stroke in high risk patients. *BMJ.* 2002;324(7329):71–86.

21. Wiviott SD, Braunwald E, McCabe CH, Montalescot G, Ruzyllo W, Gottlieb S, et al. Prasugrel versus clopidogrel in patients with acute coronary syndromes. *N Engl J Med.* 2007;357(20):2001–2015.

22. Wallentin L, Becker RC, Budaj A, Cannon CP, Emanuelsson H, Held C, et al. Ticagrelor versus clopidogrel in patients with acute coronary syndromes. *N Engl J Med.* 2009;361(11):1045–1057.

23. Bhatt DL, Lincoff AM, Gibson CM, Stone GW, McNulty S, Montalescot G, et al. Intravenous platelet blockade with cangrelor during PCI. *N Engl J Med.* 2009;361(24):2330–2341.

24. Harrington RA, Stone GW, McNulty S, White HD, Lincoff AM, Gibson CM, et al. Platelet inhibition with cangrelor in patients undergoing PCI. *N Engl J Med.* 2009;361(24):2318–2329.

25. Bhatt DL, Stone GW, Mahaffey KW, Gibson CM, Steg PG, Hamm CW, et al. Effect of platelet inhibition with cangrelor during PCI on ischemic events. *N Engl J Med.* 2013;368(14):1303–1313.

26. Steg PG, Bhatt DL, Hamm CW, Stone GW, Gibson CM, Mahaffey KW, et al. Effect of cangrelor on periprocedural outcomes in percutaneous coronary interventions: A pooled analysis of patient-level data. *Lancet.* 2013;382(9909):1981–1992.

27. Montalescot G, van't Hof AW, Lapostolle F, Silvain J, Lassen JF, Bolognese L, et al. Prehospital ticagrelor in ST-segment elevation myocardial infarction. *N Engl J Med.* 2014;371(11):1016–1027.

28. Montalescot G, Bolognese L, Dudek D, Goldstein P, Hamm C, Tanguay JF, et al. Pretreatment with prasugrel in non-ST-segment elevation acute coronary syndromes. *N Engl J Med.* 2013;369(11):999–1010.

29. Bosch X, Marrugat J, Sanchis J. Platelet glycoprotein IIb/IIIa blockers during percutaneous coronary intervention and as the initial medical treatment of non-ST segment elevation acute coronary syndromes. *Cochrane Database Syst Rev.* 2013(11):CD002130.

30. Montalescot G, Zeymer U, Silvain J, Boulanger B, Cohen M, Goldstein P, et al. Intravenous enoxaparin or unfractionated heparin in primary percutaneous coronary intervention for ST-elevation myocardial infarction: The international randomised open-label ATOLL trial. *Lancet.* 2011;378(9792):693–703.

31. Silvain J, Beygui F, Barthelemy O, Pollack C, Jr., Cohen M, Zeymer U, et al. Efficacy and safety of enoxaparin versus unfractionated heparin during percutaneous coronary intervention: Systematic review and meta-analysis. *BMJ.* 2012;344:e553.

32. Erlinge D, Omerovic E, Frobert O, Linder R, Danielewicz M, Hamid M, et al. Bivalirudin versus heparin monotherapy in myocardial infarction. *N Engl J Med.* 2017;377(12):1132–1142.

33. Shah R, Rogers KC, Matin K, Askari R, Rao SV. An updated comprehensive meta-analysis of bivalirudin vs heparin use in primary percutaneous coronary intervention. *Am Heart J.* 2016;171(1):14–24.

34. Han Y, Guo J, Zheng Y, Zang H, Su X, Wang Y, et al. Bivalirudin vs heparin with or without tirofiban during primary percutaneous coronary intervention in acute myocardial infarction: The Bright randomized clinical trial. *JAMA.* 2015;313(13):1336–1346.

35. Stone GW, Witzenbichler B, Guagliumi G, Peruga JZ, Brodie BR, Dudek D, et al. Bivalirudin during primary PCI in acute myocardial infarction. *N Engl J Med.* 2008;358(21):2218–2230.

36. Steg PG, van't Hof A, Hamm CW, Clemmensen P, Lapostolle F, Coste P, et al. Bivalirudin started during emergency transport for primary PCI. *N Engl J Med.* 2013;369(23):2207–2217.

37. Shahzad A, Kemp I, Mars C, Wilson K, Roome C, Cooper R, et al. Unfractionated heparin versus bivalirudin in primary percutaneous coronary intervention (heat-PPCI): An open-label, single centre, randomised controlled trial. *Lancet.* 2014;384(9957):1849–1858.

38. Valgimigli M, Frigoli E, Leonardi S, Rothenbuhler M, Gagnor A, Calabro P, et al. Bivalirudin or unfractionated heparin in acute coronary syndromes. *N Engl J Med.* 2015;373(11):997–1009.

39. Yusuf S, Mehta SR, Chrolavicius S, Afzal R, Pogue J, Granger CB, et al. Effects of fondaparinux on mortality and reinfarction in patients with acute ST-segment elevation myocardial infarction: The OASIS-6 randomized trial. *JAMA.* 2006;295(13):1519–1530.

40. Lincoff AM, Topol EJ. Illusion of reperfusion. Does anyone achieve optimal reperfusion during acute myocardial infarction? *Circulation.* 1993;88(3):1361–1374.

41. Kampinga MA, Nijsten MW, Gu YL, Dijk WA, de Smet BJ, van den Heuvel AF, et al. Is the myocardial blush grade scored by the operator during primary percutaneous coronary intervention of prognostic value in patients with ST-elevation myocardial infarction in routine clinical practice? *Circ Cardiovasc Interv.* 2010;3(3):216–223.

42. Stone GW, Peterson MA, Lansky AJ, Dangas G, Mehran R, Leon MB. Impact of normalized myocardial perfusion after successful angioplasty in acute myocardial infarction. *J Am Coll Cardiol.* 2002;39(4):591–597.

43. Crea F, Camici PG, Bairey Merz CN. Coronary microvascular dysfunction: An update. *Eur Heart J.* 2014;35(17):1101–1111.

44. Sianos G, Papafaklis MI, Daemen J, Vaina S, van Mieghem CA, van Domburg RT, et al. Angiographic stent thrombosis after routine use of drug-eluting stents in ST-segment elevation myocardial infarction: The importance of thrombus burden. *J Am Coll Cardiol.* 2007;50(7):573–583.

45. Napodano M, Dariol G, Al Mamary AH, Marra MP, Tarantini G, D'Amico G, et al. Thrombus burden and myocardial damage during primary percutaneous coronary intervention. *Am J Cardiol.* 2014;113(9):1449–1456.

46. Alak A, Lugomirski P, Aleksova N, Jolly SS. A meta-analysis of randomized controlled trials of conventional stenting versus direct stenting in patients with acute myocardial infarction. *J Invasive Cardiol.* 2015;27(9):405–409.

47. Vlaar PJ, Svilaas T, Vogelzang M, Diercks GF, de Smet BJ, van den Heuvel AF, et al. A comparison of 2 thrombus aspiration devices with histopathological analysis of retrieved material in patients presenting with ST-segment elevation myocardial infarction. *JACC Cardiovasc Interv.* 2008;1(3):258–264.

48. Frobert O, Calais F, James SK, Lagerqvist B. ST-elevation myocardial infarction, thrombus aspiration, and different invasive strategies. A taste trial substudy. *J Am Heart Assoc.* 2015;4(6):e001755.

49. Mahmoud KD, Zijlstra F. Thrombus aspiration in acute myocardial infarction. *Nat Rev Cardiol.* 2016;13(7):418–428.

50. Burzotta F, Trani C, Romagnoli E, Mazzari MA, Rebuzzi AG, De Vita M, et al. Manual thrombus-aspiration improves myocardial reperfusion: The randomized evaluation of the effect of mechanical reduction of distal embolization by thrombus-aspiration in primary and rescue angioplasty (Remedia) trial. *J Am Coll Cardiol.* 2005;46(2):371–376.

51. Mangiacapra F, Wijns W, De Luca G, Muller O, Trana C, Ntalianis A, et al. Thrombus aspiration in primary percutaneous coronary intervention in high-risk patients with ST-elevation myocardial infarction: A real-world registry. *Catheter Cardiovasc Interv.* 2010;76(1):70–76.

52. Sardella G, Mancone M, Canali E, Di Roma A, Benedetti G, Stio R, et al. Impact of thrombectomy with EXPort catheter in infarct-related artery during primary percutaneous coronary intervention (Expira Trial) on cardiac death. *Am J Cardiol.* 2010;106(5):624–629.

53. Svilaas T, Vlaar PJ, van der Horst IC, Diercks GF, de Smet BJ, van den Heuvel AF, et al. Thrombus aspiration during primary percutaneous coronary intervention. *N Engl J Med.* 2008;358(6):557–567.

54. Frobert O, Lagerqvist B, Olivecrona GK, Omerovic E, Gudnason T, Maeng M, et al. Thrombus aspiration during ST-segment elevation myocardial infarction. *N Engl J Med.* 2013;369(17):1587–1597.

55. Jolly SS, Cairns JA, Yusuf S, Rokoss MJ, Gao P, Meeks B, et al. Outcomes after thrombus aspiration for ST elevation myocardial infarction: 1-year follow-up of the prospective randomised total trial. *Lancet.* 2016;387(10014):127–135.

56. Jolly SS, Cairns JA, Yusuf S, Meeks B, Pogue J, Rokoss MJ, et al. Randomized trial of primary PCI with or without routine manual thrombectomy. *N Engl J Med.* 2015;372(15):1389–1398.

57. Jolly SS, James S, Dzavik V, Cairns JA, Mahmoud KD, Zijlstra F, et al. Thrombus aspiration in ST-segment-elevation myocardial infarction: An individual patient meta-analysis: Thrombectomy trialists collaboration. *Circulation.* 2017;135(2):143–152.

58. Kumbhani DJ, Bavry AA, Desai MY, Bangalore S, Bhatt DL. Role of aspiration and mechanical thrombectomy in patients with acute myocardial infarction undergoing primary angioplasty: An updated meta-analysis of randomized trials. *J Am Coll Cardiol.* 2013;62(16):1409–1418.

59. Writing Committee M, Drozda JP, Jr., Ferguson TB, Jr., Jneid H, Krumholz HM, Nallamothu BK, et al. 2015 ACC/AHA focused update of secondary prevention lipid performance measures: A report of the American college of cardiology/American Heart Association task force on performance measures. *Circ Cardiovasc Qual Outcomes.* 2016;9(1):68–95.

60. Dziewierz A, Siudak Z, Rakowski T, Zasada W, Dubiel JS, Dudek D. Impact of multivessel coronary artery disease and noninfarct-related artery revascularization on outcome of patients with ST-elevation myocardial infarction transferred for primary percutaneous coronary intervention (from the Eurotransfer Registry). *Am J Cardiol.* 2010;106(3):342–347.

61. Jo HS, Park JS, Sohn JW, Yoon JC, Sohn CW, Lee SH, et al. Culprit-lesion-only versus multivessel revascularization using drug-eluting stents in patients with ST-segment elevation myocardial infarction: A Korean acute myocardial infarction registry-based analysis. *Korean Circ J.* 2011;41(12):718–725.

62. Sorajja P, Gersh BJ, Cox DA, McLaughlin MG, Zimetbaum P, Costantini C, et al. Impact of multivessel disease on reperfusion success and clinical outcomes in patients undergoing primary percutaneous coronary intervention for acute myocardial infarction. *Eur Heart J.* 2007;28(14):1709–1716.

63. Hochman JS, Sleeper LA, Webb JG, Sanborn TA, White HD, Talley JD, et al. Early revascularization in acute myocardial infarction complicated by cardiogenic shock. Shock investigators. Should we emergently revascularize occluded coronaries for cardiogenic Shock. *N Engl J Med.* 1999;341(9):625–634.

64. Avanzas P, Arroyo-Espliguero R, Cosin-Sales J, Aldama G, Pizzi C, Quiles J, et al. Markers of inflammation and multiple complex stenoses (pancoronary plaque vulnerability) in patients with non-ST segment elevation acute coronary syndromes. *Heart.* 2004;90(8):847–852.

65. Kubo T, Imanishi T, Kashiwagi M, Ikejima H, Tsujioka H, Kuroi A, et al. Multiple coronary lesion instability in patients with acute myocardial infarction as determined by optical coherence tomography. *Am J Cardiol.* 2010;105(3):318–322.

66. O'Gara PT, Kushner FG, Ascheim DD, Casey DE, Jr., Chung MK, de Lemos JA, et al. 2013 ACCF/AHA guideline for the management of ST-elevation myocardial infarction: a report of the American

College of Cardiology Foundation/ American Heart Association Task Force on Practice Guidelines. Circulation. 2013;127(4):e362-425.

67. Task Force on the management of STEMI, Steg PG, James SK, Atar D, Badano LP, Blomstrom-Lundqvist C, et al. ESC guidelines for the management of acute myocardial infarction in patients presenting with ST-segment elevation. *Eur Heart J.* 2012;33(20):2569–2619.

68. Gershlick AH, Khan JN, Kelly DJ, Greenwood JP, Sasikaran T, Curzen N, et al. Randomized trial of complete versus lesion-only revascularization in patients undergoing primary percutaneous coronary intervention for STEMI and multivessel disease: The CvLPRIT trial. *J Am Coll Cardiol.* 2015;65(10):963–972.

69. Ghani A, Dambrink JH, van't Hof AW, Ottervanger JP, Gosselink AT, Hoorntje JC. Treatment of non-culprit lesions detected during primary PCI: Long-term follow-up of a randomised clinical trial. *Neth Heart J.* 2012;20(9):347–353.

70. Engstrom T, Kelbaek H, Helqvist S, Hofsten DE, Klovgaard L, Holmvang L, et al. Complete revascularisation versus treatment of the culprit lesion only in patients with ST-segment elevation myocardial infarction and multivessel disease (Danami-3-Primulti): An open-label, randomised controlled trial. *Lancet.* 2015;386(9994):665–671.

71. Di Mario C, Mara S, Flavio A, Imad S, Antonio M, Anna P, et al. Single vs multivessel treatment during primary angioplasty: Results of the multicentre randomised HEpacoat for cuLPrit or multivessel stenting for Acute Myocardial Infarction (HELP AMI) Study. *Int J Cardiovasc Intervent.* 2004;6(3–4):128–133.

72. Politi L, Sgura F, Rossi R, Monopoli D, Guerri E, Leuzzi C, et al. A randomised trial of target-vessel versus multi-vessel revascularisation in ST-elevation myocardial infarction: Major adverse cardiac events during long-term follow-up. *Heart.* 2010;96(9):662–667.

73. Wald DS, Morris JK, Wald NJ, Chase AJ, Edwards RJ, Hughes LO, et al. Randomized trial of preventive angioplasty in myocardial infarction. *N Engl J Med.* 2013;369(12):1115–1123.

74. Zhang J, Wang Q, Yang H, Ma L, Fu X, Hou W, et al. [Evaluation of different revascularization strategies for patients with acute myocardial infarction with lesions of multiple coronary arteries after primary percutaneous coronary intervention and its economic evaluation]. *Zhonghua Wei Zhong Bing Ji Jiu Yi Xue.* 2015;27(3):169–174.

75. Bravo CA, Hirji SA, Bhatt DL, Kataria R, Faxon DP, Ohman EM, et al. Complete versus culprit-only revascularisation in ST elevation myocardial infarction with multivessel disease. *Cochrane Database Syst Rev.* 2017;5:CD011986.

76. Gaffar R, Habib B, Filion KB, Reynier P, Eisenberg MJ. Optimal Timing of complete revascularization in acute coronary syndrome: A systematic review and meta-analysis. *J Am Heart Assoc.* 2017;6(4). doi:10.1161/JAHA.116.005381.

77. Ong P, Camici PG, Beltrame JF, Crea F, Shimokawa H, Sechtem U, et al. International standardization of diagnostic criteria for microvascular angina. *Int J Cardiol.* 2018;250:16–20.

78. Levine GN, Bates ER, Blankenship JC, Bailey SR, Bittl JA, Cercek B, et al. 2015 ACC/AHA/SCAI Focused Update on Primary Percutaneous Coronary Intervention for Patients With ST-Elevation Myocardial Infarction: An Update of the 2011 ACCF/AHA/SCAI Guideline for Percutaneous Coronary Intervention and the 2013 ACCF/AHA Guideline for the Management of ST-Elevation Myocardial Infarction. *J Am Coll Cardiol.* 2016;67(10):1235–1250.

79. Goldberg RJ, Spencer FA, Gore JM, Lessard D, Yarzebski J. Thirty-year trends (1975 to 2005) in the magnitude of, management of, and hospital death rates associated with cardiogenic shock in patients with acute myocardial infarction: A population-based perspective. *Circulation.* 2009;119(9):1211–1219.

80. Reyentovich A, Barghash MH, Hochman JS. Management of refractory cardiogenic shock. *Nat Rev Cardiol.* 2016;13(8):481–492.

81. Brogan RA, Alabas O, Almudarra S, Hall M, Dondo TB, Mamas MA, et al. Relative survival and excess mortality following primary percutaneous coronary intervention for ST-elevation myocardial infarction. *Eur Heart J Acute Cardiovasc Care.* 2017:2048872617710790.

82. Werdan K, Gielen S, Ebelt H, Hochman JS. Mechanical circulatory support in cardiogenic shock. *Eur Heart J.* 2014;35(3):156–167.

83. Gilani FS, Farooqui S, Doddamani R, Gruberg L. Percutaneous Mechanical support in cardiogenic shock: A review. *Clin Med Insights Cardiol.* 2015;9(Suppl 2):23–28.

84. Thiele H, Akin I, Sandri M, Fuernau G, de Waha S, Meyer-Saraei R, et al. PCI strategies in patients with acute myocardial infarction and cardiogenic shock. *N Engl J Med.* 2017;377(25):2419-32.

85. Sandhu A, McCoy LA, Negi SI, Hameed I, Atri P, Al'Aref SJ, et al. Use of mechanical circulatory support in patients undergoing percutaneous coronary intervention: Insights from the National Cardiovascular Data Registry. *Circulation.* 2015;132(13):1243–1251.

86. Thiele H, Allam B, Chatellier G, Schuler G, Lafont A. Shock in acute myocardial infarction: The cape horn for trials? *Eur Heart J.* 2010;31(15):1828–1835.

87. Patel MR, Smalling RW, Thiele H, Barnhart HX, Zhou Y, Chandra P, et al. Intra-aortic balloon counterpulsation and infarct size in patients with acute anterior myocardial infarction without shock: The Crisp AMI randomized trial. *JAMA.* 2011;306(12):1329–1337.

88. Unverzagt S, Buerke M, de Waha A, Haerting J, Pietzner D, Seyfarth M, et al. Intra-aortic balloon pump counterpulsation (IABP) for myocardial infarction complicated by cardiogenic shock. *Cochrane Database Syst Rev.* 2015(3):CD007398.

89. Chew DP, Scott IA, Cullen L, French JK, Briffa TG, Tideman PA, et al. Corrigendum to 'National Heart Foundation of Australia & Cardiac Society of Australia and New Zealand: Australian Clinical Guidelines for the Management of Acute Coronary Syndromes 2016'. *Heart Lung Circ.* 2016;25: 898–952. *Heart Lung Circ.* 2017;26(10):1117.

90. Ouweneel DM, Eriksen E, Sjauw KD, van Dongen IM, Hirsch A, Packer EJ, et al. Percutaneous mechanical circulatory support versus intra-aortic balloon pump in cardiogenic shock after acute myocardial infarction. *J Am Coll Cardiol.* 2017;69(3):278–287.

91. Saunderson CE, Brogan RA, Simms AD, Sutton G, Batin PD, Gale CP. Acute coronary syndrome management in older adults: Guidelines, temporal changes and challenges. *Age Ageing.* 2014;43(4):450–455.

92. Davis KB, Alderman EL, Kosinski AS, Passamani E, Kennedy JW. Early mortality of acute myocardial infarction in patients with and without prior coronary revascularization surgery: A coronary artery surgery study registry study. *Circulation.* 1992;85(6):2100–2109.

93. Blachutzik F, Achenbach S, Troebs M, Roether J, Nef H, Hamm C, et al. Angiographic findings and revascularization success in patients with acute myocardial infarction and previous coronary bypass grafting. *Am J Cardiol.* 2016;118(4):473–476.

94. White HD, Van de Werf FJ. Thrombolysis for acute myocardial infarction. *Circulation.* 1998;97(16):1632–1646.

95. Bundhoo SS, Kalla M, Anantharaman R, Morris K, Chase A, Smith D, et al. Outcomes following PCI in patients with previous CABG: A multi centre experience. *Catheter Cardiovasc Interv.* 2011;78(2):169–176.

96. Hindnavis V, Cho SH, Goldberg S. Saphenous vein graft intervention: A review. *J Invasive Cardiol.* 2012;24(2):64–71.

97. Garg P, Kamaruddin H, Iqbal J, Wheeldon N. Outcomes of primary percutaneous coronary intervention for patients with

previous coronary artery bypass grafting presenting with STsegment elevation myocardial infarction. *Open Cardiovasc Med J.* 2015;9:99–104.

98. Brilakis ES, Rao SV, Banerjee S, Goldman S, Shunk KA, Holmes DR, Jr., et al. Percutaneous coronary intervention in native arteries versus bypass grafts in prior coronary artery bypass grafting patients: A report from the National Cardiovascular Data Registry. *JACC Cardiovasc Interv.* 2011;4(8):844–850.

99. Stone GW, Goldberg S, O'Shaughnessy C, Midei M, Siegel RM, Cristea E, et al. 5-year follow-up of polytetrafluoroethylene-covered stents compared with bare-metal stents in aortocoronary saphenous vein grafts the randomized BARRICADE (Barrier Approach to Restenosis: Restrict Intima to Curtail Adverse Events) trial. *JACC Cardiovasc Interv.* 2011;4(3):300–309.

100. Turco MA, Buchbinder M, Popma JJ, Weissman NJ, Mann T, Doucet S, et al. Pivotal, randomized U.S. study of the Symbiottrade mark covered stent system in patients with saphenous vein graft disease: Eight-month angiographic and clinical results from the Symbiot III trial. *Catheter Cardiovasc Interv.* 2006;68(3):379–388.

101. Stankovic G, Colombo A, Presbitero P, van den Branden F, Inglese L, Cernigliaro C, et al. Randomized evaluation of polytetra-fluoroethylene-covered stent in saphenous vein grafts: The Randomized Evaluation of polytetrafluoroethylene COVERed stent in Saphenous vein grafts (RECOVERS) Trial. *Circulation.* 2003;108(1):37–42.

102. Mak KH, Challapalli R, Eisenberg MJ, Anderson KM, Califf RM, Topol EJ. Effect of platelet glycoprotein IIb/IIIa receptor inhibition on distal embolization during percutaneous revascularization of aortocoronary saphenous vein grafts. EPIC Investigators. Evaluation of IIb/IIIa platelet receptor antagonist 7E3 in Preventing Ischemic Complications. *Am J Cardiol.* 1997;80(8):985–988.

103. Roffi M, Mukherjee D, Chew DP, Bhatt DL, Cho L, Robbins MA, et al. Lack of benefit from intravenous platelet glycoprotein IIb/IIIa receptor inhibition as adjunctive treatment for percutaneous interventions of aortocoronary bypass grafts: A pooled analysis of five randomized clinical trials. *Circulation.* 2002;106(24):3063–3067.

104. Ellis SG, Lincoff AM, Miller D, Tcheng JE, Kleiman NS, Kereiakes D, et al. Reduction in complications of angioplasty with abciximab occurs largely independently of baseline lesion morphology. EPIC and EPILOG Investigators. Evaluation of 7E3 for the Prevention of Ischemic Complications. Evaluation of PTCA To Improve Long-term Outcome with abciximab GPIIb/IIIa Receptor Blockade. *J Am Coll Cardiol.* 1998;32(6):1619–1623.

105. Zijlstra F, Hoorntje JC, de Boer MJ, Reiffers S, Miedema K, Ottervanger JP, et al. Long-term benefit of primary angioplasty as compared with thrombolytic therapy for acute myocardial infarction. *N Engl J Med.* 1999;341(19):1413–1419.

106. Keeley EC, Boura JA, Grines CL. Primary angioplasty versus intravenous thrombolytic therapy for acute myocardial infarction: A quantitative review of 23 randomised trials. *Lancet.* 2003;361(9351):13–20.

107. Widimsky P, Budesinsky T, Vorac D, Groch L, Zelizko M, Aschermann M, et al. Long distance transport for primary angioplasty vs immediate thrombolysis in acute myocardial infarction. Final results of the randomized national multicentre trial--PRAGUE-2. *Eur Heart J.* 2003;24(1):94–104.

108. Andersen HR, Nielsen TT, Rasmussen K, Thuesen L, Kelbaek H, Thayssen P, et al. A comparison of coronary angioplasty with fibrinolytic therapy in acute myocardial infarction. *N Engl J Med.* 2003;349(8):733–742.

109. Nallamothu BK, Bates ER. Percutaneous coronary intervention versus fibrinolytic therapy in acute myocardial infarction: Is timing (almost) everything? *Am J Cardiol.* 2003;92(7):824–826.

110. Betriu A, Masotti M. Comparison of mortality rates in acute myocardial infarction treated by percutaneous coronary intervention versus fibrinolysis. *Am J Cardiol.* 2005;95(1):100–101.

111. Boersma E, Primary Coronary Angioplasty vs. Thrombolysis G. Does time matter? A pooled analysis of randomized clinical trials comparing primary percutaneous coronary intervention and in-hospital fibrinolysis in acute myocardial infarction patients. *Eur Heart J.* 2006;27(7):779–788.

112. Armstrong PW, Gershlick AH, Goldstein P, Wilcox R, Danays T, Lambert Y, et al. Fibrinolysis or primary PCI in ST-segment elevation myocardial infarction. *N Engl J Med.* 2013;368(15):1379–1387.

113. Terkelsen CJ, Sorensen JT, Maeng M, Jensen LO, Tilsted HH, Trautner S, et al. System delay and mortality among patients with STEMI treated with primary percutaneous coronary intervention. *JAMA.* 2010;304(7):763–771.

114. Huber K, De Caterina R, Kristensen SD, Verheugt FW, Montalescot G, Maestro LB, et al. Pre-hospital reperfusion therapy: A strategy to improve therapeutic outcome in patients with ST-elevation myocardial infarction. *Eur Heart J.* 2005;26(19):2063–2074.

115. Hutchison AW, Malaiapan Y, Cameron JD, Meredith IT. Pre-hospital 12 lead ECG to triage ST elevation myocardial infarction and long term improvements in door to balloon times: The first 1000 patients from the MonAMI project. *Heart Lung Circ.* 2013;22(11):910–916.

116. Savage ML, Poon KK, Johnston EM, Raffel OC, Incani A, Bryant J, et al. Pre-hospital ambulance notification and initiation of treatment of ST elevation myocardial infarction is associated with significant reduction in door-to-balloon time for primary PCI. *Heart Lung Circ.* 2014;23(5):435–443.

117. Fordyce CB, Al-Khalidi HR, Jollis JG, Roettig ML, Gu J, Bagai A, et al. Association of rapid care process implementation on reperfusion times across multiple st-segment-elevation myocardial infarction networks. *Circ Cardiovasc Interv.* 2017;10(1). doi:10.1161/CIRCINTERVENTIONS.116.004061.

118. Stowens JC, Sonnad SS, Rosenbaum RA. Using EMS dispatch to trigger STEMI alerts decreases door-to-balloon times. *West J Emerg Med.* 2015;16(3):472–480.

119. Bagai A, Jollis JG, Dauerman HL, Peng SA, Rokos IC, Bates ER, et al. Emergency department bypass for ST-Segment-elevation myocardial infarction patients identified with a prehospital electrocardiogram: A report from the American Heart Association Mission: Lifeline program. *Circulation.* 2013;128(4):352–359.

120. Chew DP, Junbo G, Parsonage W, Kerkar P, Sulimov VA, Horsfall M, et al. Perceived risk of ischemic and bleeding events in acute coronary syndromes. *Circ Cardiovasc Qual Outcomes.* 2013;6(3):299–308.

121. Yan AT, Yan RT, Tan M, Fung A, Cohen EA, Fitchett DH, et al. Management patterns in relation to risk stratification among patients with non-ST elevation acute coronary syndromes. *Arch Intern Med.* 2007;167(10):1009–1016.

122. Scott IA, Derhy PH, O'Kane D, Lindsay KA, Atherton JJ, Jones MA, et al. Discordance between level of risk and intensity of evidence-based treatment in patients with acute coronary syndromes. *Med J Aust.* 2007;187(3):153–159.

123. Yan RT, Yan AT, Tan M, McGuire DK, Leiter L, Fitchett DH, et al. Underuse of evidence-based treatment partly explains the worse clinical outcome in diabetic patients with acute coronary syndromes. *Am Heart J.* 2006;152(4):676–683.

124. Chew DP, Juergens C, French J, Parsonage W, Horsfall M, Brieger D, et al. An EXAMINATION of clinical intuition in risk assessment among acute coronary syndromes patients: Observations from a prospective multi-center international observational registry. *Int J Cardiol.* 2014;171(2):209–216.

125. Fox KA, Dabbous OH, Goldberg RJ, Pieper KS, Eagle KA, Van de Werf F, et al. Prediction of risk of death and myocardial infarction in the six months after presentation with acute coronary syndrome: Prospective multinational observational study (GRACE). *BMJ.* 2006;333(7578):1091.

126. Fox KA, Fitzgerald G, Puymirat E, Huang W, Carruthers K, Simon T, et al. Should patients with acute coronary disease be stratified for management according to their risk? Derivation, external validation and outcomes using the updated GRACE risk score. *BMJ Open.* 2014;4(2):e004425.

127. Mehran R, Pocock SJ, Nikolsky E, Clayton T, Dangas GD, Kirtane AJ, et al. A risk score to predict bleeding in patients with acute coronary syndromes. *J Am Coll Cardiol.* 2010;55(23):2556–2566.

128. Subherwal S, Bach RG, Chen AY, Gage BF, Rao SV, Newby LK, et al. Baseline risk of major bleeding in non-ST-segment-elevation myocardial infarction: The CRUSADE (Can Rapid risk stratification of Unstable angina patients Suppress ADverse outcomes with Early implementation of the ACC/AHA Guidelines) Bleeding Score. *Circulation.* 2009;119(14):1873–1882.

129. Fox KA, Goodman SG, Klein W, Brieger D, Steg PG, Dabbous O, et al. Management of acute coronary syndromes. Variations in practice and outcome; findings from the Global Registry of Acute Coronary Events (GRACE). *Eur Heart J.* 2002;23(15):1177–1189.

34

Percutaneous carotid interventions

TARANEH AMIR-NEZAMI AND ANTHONY GRABS

INTRODUCTION

The aging population of vasculopath patients in the past decades is the main drive for increasing burden of both coronary and non coronary atherosclerotic disease which share the same traditional risk factors for development and progression.

As a result of advanced age, medical comorbidities and their impact on patient fitness for open surgical procedures, most clinicians focus has been diverted on to the less invasive percutaneous therapeutic interventions that are safer alternative to open surgery.

Continuing advances in endovascular techniques and technology have allowed the application of endovascular interventions in different vascular beds (cervical carotid, renal, visceral, aortic and Iliofemoral arteries), to the extent that the endovascular approach is now considered first management for both coronary and non-coronary atherosclerotic disease, as it carries less cardiovascular morbidity and mortality in high-risk surgical patients. Many patients with coronary artery disease, however, have concomitant atherosclerotic disease in other arterial beds that may preclude diagnostic or therapeutic endovascular procedures, and some asymptomatic patients with cerebrovascular, aortic or iliofemoral atherosclerotic or non-atherosclerotic disease will be first identified during a cardiac catheter planning

or in peri-procedure time. As a result, a multidisciplinary team approach involving the cardiologist, the vascular surgeon and the interventional radiologist is now the mainstay of medical management for this group of patients.

Occasionally, iliac or femoral stenotic disease may need to be addressed in order to gain safe access for those cardiac interventions requiring larger size femoral access, such as transfemoral aortic valve replacement (TAVI), or in patients in whom transradial access is prohibited. This may entail endovascular reconstruction (angioplasty with or without stenting) or a hybrid procedure with femoral cut-down for endartrectomy and patch angioplasty.

The focus of this chapter is on the available evidence, indications and technical aspects of the carotid artery stenting, an intervention that is commonly performed by both vascular surgeons and interventional cardiologists.

CAROTID ANGIOPLASTY AND STENTING: AN EVOLVING INTERVENTION

Atherosclerotic carotid artery disease involving the origin of the internal carotid artery and the distal common carotid artery is a frequent clinical problem associated with a significant risk of debilitating stroke. Multiple major randomised controlled trials and registries have compared different management modalities such as best medical therapy (BMT) and carotid endarterectomy (CEA). These trials include symptomatic patients (ECST, NASCET trials[1,2]) and asymptomatic patients (ACAS, ACST trials[3,4]) with extracranial carotid artery disease. On the basis of published evidence, there is no question that CEA in the hands of experienced operators remains the best option for treating carotid artery disease under most circumstances.[5]

The concept of treating carotid bifurcation disease using endovascular means is not new. However, due to fear of cerebral embolisation there was substantial initial reluctance to accept and adopt these evolving techniques with an uncertain outcome, explaining the slow transition to modern carotid artery stenting (CAS).[6,7] Unpredictable outcomes with CAS in studies performed during the early CAS era (before 2000) were caused by poor patient selection and limited technology and operator skills, and the results of studies undertaken during this period were unreliable.[8-12]

Innovations such as routine use of stent and embolic protection devices (EPDs), the introduction of dedicated endovascular products for carotid intervention (different shape and length of introducers and guiding catheters, low-profile guide wires and balloons with monorail technology), and implementation of new antiplatelet drugs have contributed significantly to the improvement of CAS techniques and its outcome over time.[7] Thus, in today's modern practice, an improved understanding of patient selection in line with technical and technological advances has made carotid intervention safer and more controlled.[6]

Endovascular treatment of carotid disease has been compared with open carotid surgery or endarterectomy in a number of randomised controlled trials (RCT) and in worldwide series.

EVA-3S, SPACE, ICSS and CREST are the most influential of the contemporary RCTs to influence practice in average-risk patients.[13-19] Many interpretations have been made of these RCTs data by different clinicians, and include the following important observations (Table 34.1).

- CAS was associated with nearly a twofold higher risk of procedural death/stroke in symptomatic patients.

- The 30-day death/stroke/myocardial infarction rates (MI) were similar between CEA/CAS (using CREST definition of MI) for symptomatic and asymptomatic patients.
- The 30-day death/stroke rate was higher after CAS in patients older than 70, but the death/stroke rate in patients who had CAS and were <70 years of age was similar to the CEA group.[19,20,21]
- Successful CAS was durable, as the long-term stroke risks were similar to CEA.
- Recurrent stenosis was higher following CAS, but this was not associated with increased ipsilateral stroke risk.[22]

There is no doubt that CAS in its current form has an acceptable safety profile in some clinical situations, and that many patients have and will benefit from it. The question is, when can CAS be used instead of CEA?[5]

Based on these data, it would be acceptable to offer CAS to symptomatic patients who pose a prohibitive surgical risk, or to patients with major anatomic risk for CEA. The latter group includes patients with surgically inaccessible high lesions, patients with hostile neck from radiation therapy, complex previous neck surgery, or cervical stomas, and patients with contralateral recurrent laryngeal nerve palsy, or those with recurrent stenosis following previous endarterectomy.[23]

Medically high-risk patients also refers to patients with severe cardiopulmonary disorders precluding general anaesthesia or a prolonged supine surgical procedure.

The European Society of Vascular Surgery (ESVS) has recently published updated guidelines for management of atherosclerotic carotid and vertebral artery disease, which provides a comprehensive evidence-based document to guide clinical practice in the management of cerebrovascular disease. Figure 34.1 represents the algorithm detailing management of symptomatic and asymptomatic carotid disease.[24]

The 2017 ESVS guidelines recommend carotid endarterectomy in patients reporting carotid territory symptoms within the preceding 6 months and who have a 70%–99% carotid stenosis, provided the documented procedural death/stroke rate is <6%. CEA should also be considered in symptomatic patients with 50%–69% carotid stenosis.[24]

Table 34.1 Thirty-day risks following carotid artery endarterectomy (CEA) and carotid artery stenting (CAS) in trials that randomised >500 recently symptomatic patients into EVA-3S, SPACE, ICSS, and CREST

30 day risk	EVA-3S [13]		SPACE[17]		ICSS[18]		CREST[14]	
	CEA	CAS	CEA	CAS	CEA	CAS	CEA	CAS
	n = 262	n = 261	n = 589	n = 607	n = 857	n = 853	n = 653	n = 668
Death	1.2%	0.8%	0.9%	1.0%	0.8%	2.3%		
Any stroke	3.5%	9.2%	6.2%	7.2%	4.1%	7.7%	3.2%	5.5%
Ipsilateral stroke			5.1%	6.4%	3.5%	6.8%		
Disabling stroke	0.4%	2.7%	2.9%	4.1%	2.3%	2.0%	0.9%	1.2%
Death/any stroke	3.9%	9.6%	6.5%	7.4%	4.7%	8.5%	3.2%	6.0%
Disabling stroke/death	1.5%	3.4%	3.8%	5.1%	3.2%	4.0%		
Clinical MI	0.8%	0.4%			0.5%	0.4%		
Death/stroke/MI					5.2%	8.5%	5.4%	6.7%
Cranial nerve injury	7.7%	1.1%			5.3%	0.1%	5.1%	0.5%

Source: Reprinted with permission from Elsevier, *Eur. J. Vasc. Endovasc. Surg.*, 55, Naylor, AR. et al., Editor's choice–management of atherosclerotic carotid and vertebral artery disease: 2017 Clinical Practice Guidelines of the European Society for Vascular Surgery (ESVS), 3–81.

Abbreviation: MI, myocardial infarction.

When revascularisation is indicated in patients with carotid territory symptoms within the preceding 6 months and who are high risk for surgery and are aged <70 years, CAS may be considered as an alternative to endarterectomy, provided the documented procedural death/stroke rate is <6%.[24]

Recommendations derived from multiple professional organisations, including the American Heart Association, have repeatedly advised that only 'highly selected' asymptomatic patients should undergo CEA, but they never defined what 'highly selected' means.[25,26]

The 2017 ESVS guidelines define 'highly selected' asymptomatic patients as those with 'higher risk for stroke' on BMT. CAS may be considered in selected asymptomatic patients who have been deemed by the multidisciplinary team to be 'high-risk for surgery' and who have an asymptomatic 60%–99% stenosis in the presence of one or more imaging characteristics that may be associated with an increased risk of late ipsilateral stroke, provided documented procedural risks are <3% and the patient's life expectancy exceeds 5 years.[24]

Patients with the following clinical and imaging features are considered 'higher-risk for stroke' on BMT and will benefit from revascularisation:

- Silent infarction on CT/MRI
- Stenosis progression
- Plaque characteristics: Large plaque area, large juxta-luminal black area on computerised plaque analysis, plaque echolucency, intraplaque haemorrhage on MRI
- Impaired cerebral vascular reserve
- Spontaneous embolisation on transcranial doppler (TCD) monitoring[24]

In summary, with the current modern endovascular technology and careful patient selection in the hands of an experienced operator, CAS may be considered an alternative to carotid endaterectomy only in a certain subgroup of patients.[7]

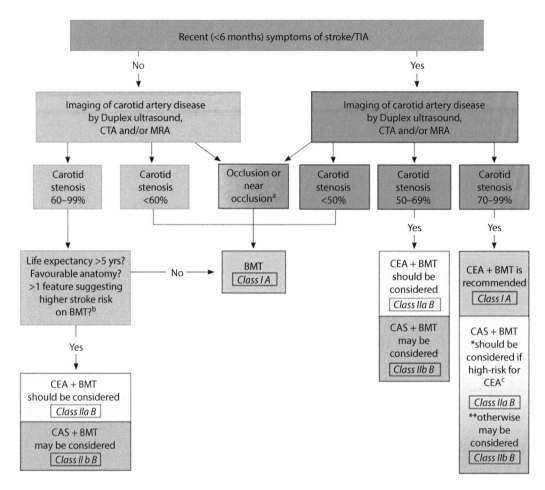

Figure 34.1 Algorithm detailing management strategies in patients with symptomatic and asymptomatic atherosclerotic extracranial carotid artery stenoses. Green boxes denote Level I recommendations, yellow boxes denote level IIa and IIb recommendations. (*Abbreviations:* BMT, best medical therapy; CAS, carotid artery stenting; CEA, carotid endarterectomy; CTA, computed tomography angiography; MRA, magnetic resonance angiography; TIA, transient ischaemic attack.) (a) Post-stenotic internal carotid artery narrowed to the point of near occlusion. (b) Clinical/imaging features that might be associated with an increased risk of late stroke on BMT in asymptomatic patients. (c) Clinical/imaging features that might make a patient 'high risk for CEA'. * denotes recommendation for CAS in symptomatic patients with 70%–99% stenoses deemed 'high-risk for CEA'. ** denotes recommendation for CAS in symptomatic patients with 70%–99% stenoses deemed 'average risk for CEA'. Reprinted with permission from Elsevier Ltd, Management of atherosclerotic carotid and vertebral disease. (From Naylor, AR. et al., *Eur. J. Vasc. Endovasc. Surg.*, 55, 3–81, 2018.)

PRE-PROCEDURE CHECKLIST FOR CAROTID ARTERY STENTING

A pre-procedural overview of the respective anatomical imaging is mandatory for safe planning and delivery of the CAS procedure. The most recent pre-operative vascular imaging (CTA or MRA) is used for this purpose. Essential imaging information required for CAS includes: Anatomical evaluation of the carotid index lesion and vessels proximal and distal to it, assessment of any aortic, arch and supra-aortic trunks, existing disease or tortuosity in access vessels (iliofemoral disease), identification of any important anatomical variation of the arch and its major vessels (e.g. bovine arch, type III arch), estimation of the internal carotid artery (ICA) and common carotid artery (CCA) diameters, and lesion length.

Certain anatomical features such as shaggy aorta, severe arch atherosclerotic disease or tortuosity, diffuse common carotid artery disease or tortuosity, severe angulation of the carotid bifurcation or distal ICA, significant iliofemoral stenotic disease precluding access, mobile thrombus, and vulnerable carotid plaque are considered unsuitable anatomy and relative contraindications for carotid endovascular interventions.

Absolute contraindications for carotid stenting are: significant contraindication to angiography, angiographically visible intraluminal thrombus and carotid artery occlusion.[27]

Patient's medical management should be optimised by the clinician prior to the procedure to ensure that patient is on dual antiplatelet therapy (aspirin 100 mg and clopidogrel 75 mg daily) at least 5 days prior to the planned CAS. It is recommended that antihypertensive medication be withheld on the day of the procedure.[23]

Another critical pre-procedural requirement is to ensure that the patient understands the nature of the procedure and is able to maintain supine position during the procedure and to follow instructions for neurocognitive assessment. Major disabling ipsilateral stroke and dementia are contraindication for carotid stenting.

CHOICE OF EMBOLIC PROTECTION DEVICES AND CAROTID STENT

Several embolic protection devices (EPDs) including the distal filter, distal occlusion balloon, and proximal protection devices with flow stasis or reversal are available. Selection of the appropriate type of EPD depends on lesion characteristics and anatomic considerations.[7]

Different outcomes have been reported for use of EPDs during CAS, explaining the ongoing debate concerning the routine use of EPDs for CAS.[7]

According to the ICSS sub-study that analysed data from centres using filter-type EPDs in most patients, filter-protected CAS was associated with increased new MRI ischaemic lesions, but this observation did not seem to translate to worse cognitive function.[28] Proximal protection devices appear to have a lower microembolic burden.[29]

There are no RCTs to determine whether protection devices reduce the risk of post-CAS stroke, but a systematic review concluded that embolic protection was associated with significantly fewer procedural strokes than unprotected CAS.[30,19]

Given the perceived benefits of stenting (better primary lumen result, less embolisation, fewer problems with dissection and restenosis) and the technical limitations of percutaneous transluminal angioplasty, the primary intention in most endovascular carotid treatments is to place a dedicated carotid stent.[6]

In general, self-expanding stents should be chosen over balloon-expandable stents because of the potential for crush injury of the latter. A variety of self-expanding, tapered or straight stents mostly constructed of Nitinol are available for use with the respective embolic protection devices (Acculink, Xact, Wallstent, Precise, Protégé, and others).[23] A new generation of carotid stents with braided Nitinol design and internal dual layer micromesh technology (Casper stent, MicroVention Inc., a subsidiary of Terumo), which provides sustained embolic protection and prevents plaque prolapse, is now available.

Flexibility and scaffolding are the two main characteristics that drive stent choice. Closed-cell stents with smaller free cell area and greater percentage of wall coverage offer better scaffolding and reduce embolisation risk.[7] In today's practice, self-expanding, closed-cell, tapered carotid stents are frequently used. Tapered configuration of the stent permits coverage of the carotid lesion from the distal CCA into the ICA.[6]

A systematic review by Schnaudigel et al. demonstrated that use of embolic protection devices and closed-cell designed stents have significantly reduced the incidence of new ipsilateral diffusion-weighted imaging lesions,[31] supporting the recommendation for routine use of closed-cell stents and EPD in CAS.

TECHNICAL ASPECTS OF CAROTID ARTERY STENTING

Extracranial angiography and carotid cannulation can, in general, be performed using conventional coronary angioplasty equipment; however, dedicated carotid stents and EPDs are needed for CAS. The procedure is performed in the supine position, with the patient awake for ongoing neurocognitive assessment using a squeezable squeaky toy in the patient's contralateral hand.

Continuous haemodynamic and cardiac monitoring are essential during the procedure.

The femoral artery is the most common access site for performing CAS; however, brachial, radial and direct carotid approaches are alternatives in cases with certain anatomical features.[19]

After femoral arterial access is obtained, the patient is fully anticoagulated using intravenous unfractionated heparin. The activated clotting time (ACT) is monitored regularly thereafter to ensure the ACT remains at 250 seconds or longer during the procedure. Arch aortography with attention to its major vessels is performed using a dedicated catheter (e.g. pigtail). Extreme care to prevent embolisation of air or thrombus must be taken at all times using a power injector.

A long diagnostic catheter (e.g. a simple-curve catheter like the vertebral, or a reversed-angle catheter such as Vitek, or a Simmons catheter) is then used to cannulate the common carotid artery and perform a selective baseline carotid and vertebral angiography. The number of angiograms should be kept to a minimum but should include projections (e.g. left anterior oblique) that display the carotid bifurcation, and others that show the distribution of the intracranial vessels.

Different techniques (exchange, coaxial or probing) are described for carotid lesion access. Lesion anatomy, operator experience and choice of EPD are the main factors influencing choice of carotid access technique.[19]

An exchange technique, by which the ipsilateral external carotid artery (ECA) is cannulated under roadmap guidance with a selective guiding catheter over a 0.035" hydrophilic guide wire, is frequently used. This wire is subsequently exchanged for a stiff and high-torque exchange wire like the Supra Core with its distal floppy tip parked in the distal branch of the ECA. A long (90 cm) guiding sheath (Destination or Shuttle) of appropriate size (6 Fr or 7 Fr depending on the desired stent profile) is then gently advanced over the stiff wire to within 2–3 cm of the carotid bifurcation.

A pre-intervention selective angiogram is obtained next, with the carotid bifurcation at the centre of the field of view. With use of quantitative vevessel analysis and computerised calibration, measurements such as ICA and CCA diameter, along with lesion length, are obtained from this angiogram. This information will assist selection of the appropriate-size EPD (to fit the ICA) and would be essential in choosing a suitably sized, tapered carotid stent.

After completion of the angiographic evaluation, decision must be made about the use of EPD.

The internal carotid artery lesion is then crossed using a 0.014" guidewire that is a fixed or mobile component of the distal embolic protection device (most commonly used), usually with road-mapping guidance.[7]

The EPD is placed into a straight and non-diseased segment of the distal extracranial ICA (before its petrous segment). Position of the distal filter device should be monitored throughout the entire procedure.

Once EPD placement is completed, angiography is repeated in a new position that includes the tip of the carotid sheath in the inferior part and the EPD in the superior aspect of the field of view.[6]

Occasionally, predilatation of the lesion is needed prior to stent placement in order to avoid snow-ploughing and to permit safe passage of the stent delivery system (most carotid stents have 6 Fr or 7 Fr compatible delivery systems). This might be achieved by using a 3–4 mm diameter coronary balloon of 0.014" profile.[6,19]

The carotid stent of choice is delivered and advanced over the existing 0.014" wire using road-mapping guidance. The stent is deployed across the lesion in the internal carotid artery, commonly extending back into the common carotid artery across the bifurcation. Most operators prefer to deploy the carotid stent without use of road map and instead use the bony landmarks of the reference image. Figure 34.2 shows pre- and post-carotid stent angiography using a Wallstent.

Following stent placement and prior to retrieval of the EPD, a completion angiogram is acquired in multiple planes to evaluate the result. The carotid stent may need post-dilatation to optimise its expansion and achieve adequate wall apposition; however, aggressive ballooning should be avoided as it carries high risk of embolisation. Most clinicians are happy to accept some degree of stenosis (less than 30%), as most Nitinol stents continue to expand after deployment.[19]

If a decision is made to post-dilate the stent, this is done with a rapid exchange, short balloon of appropriate size based on the ICA diameter (usually 5 × 20 mm), maintaining the balloon within the stent to avoid potential risk of dissection.

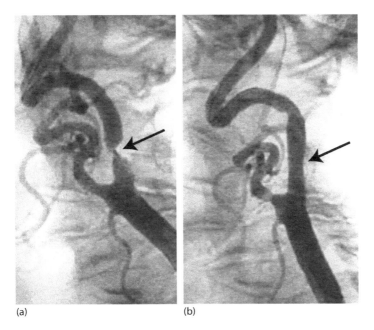

(a)   (b)

Figure 34.2 Carotid angiography pre (a) and post-stenting after deployment (b) of a 10 × 30 mm Wallstent across the origin of the external carotid artery.

Distention of the carotid sinus after ballooning and stenting is often associated with vagal responses, resulting in a reflex bradycardia and hypotension. This can be managed using intravenous atropine or glycopyrrolate and, if necessary, by infusion of inotropic agents. It may take 24–48 hours before the carotid sinus adapts to the radial force of the stent, hence post-CAS haemodynamic monitoring is essential.[23]

ICA vasospasm occasionally occurs due to wire and filter manipulation, and is managed by careful repositioning or removal of the wire and filter, completion of the procedure in a timely manner and intra-arterial administration of a small dose of nitroglycerin via the long sheath.[7] Luminal plaque protrusion (through the stent interstices) or flow-limiting ICA dissection should be managed with gentle repeat angioplasty and further stent placement for double scaffolding.[19]

Incidence of distal cerebral embolisation varies and may be affected by operator experience and patient selection. Advanced patient age and unfavourable or difficult arch anatomy are some of the known predictors for embolic stroke. Options available for treatment of an embolic event include catheter-directed thrombolysis (using urokinase or tissue plasminogen activator), thrombus maceration,

aspiration thrombectomy, snare removal, and administration of glycoprotein IIb/IIIa receptor inhibitor (e.g. Abciximb), all with variable results. Presently, prevention remains the best option for avoiding the disastrous consequences of distal cerebral embolisation.[32–34]

After retrieval of the EPD, a final angiogram is performed, with attention to both extra- and intracranial carotid circulation, looking for any complications (e.g. kink, distal embolisation).

Femoral access site haemostasis is usually achieved using a closure device; however, in those patients with a diseased femoral artery it is best to exchange the long sheath for a short sheath of the same size and apply manual compression once the ACT is less than 180 seconds.[23]

Post-procedure care and follow-up

Following carotid artery stenting, patients should be transferred to the neurovascular ward or high-dependency unit for close monitoring of any neurologic or haemodynamic complications. This is generally continued for 24–48 hours, and in the absence of complications or haemodynamic compromise, patients may be discharged in 48 hours.

Patients are advised to continue dual antiplatelet therapy for at least 4 weeks, which is the presumed timeframe for stent endothelialisation. After this, lifelong single antiplatelet therapy with a daily dose of aspirin is necessary.

Blood pressure should be monitored after discharge and patients are directed to return to the emergency department should they develop severe headache or any neurologic symptoms.[19]

Patient follow-up is scheduled at 1 month, 6 months and annually thereafter for clinical and imaging assessment with a carotid duplex ultrasound.[22]

REFERENCES

1. Group ECSTC. Randomised trial of endarterectomy for recently symptomatic carotid stenosis: Final results of the MRC European Carotid Surgery Trial (ECST). *Lancet.* 1998;351(9113):1379–1387.
2. Ferguson G, Eliasziw M, Barr H, Clagett G, Barnes R, Wallace M et al. The North American symptomatic carotid endarterectomy trial: Surgical results in 1415 patients. *Stroke.* 1999;30(9):1751–1758.
3. Benavente O, Moher D, Pham B. Executive Committee for the Asymptomatic Carotid Atherosclerosis Study. Endarterectomy for asymptomatic carotid artery stenosis. *JAMA.* 1995;273(18):1421–1428.
4. Halliday A, Harrison M, Hayter E, Kong X, Mansfield A, Marro J et al. 10-year stroke prevention after successful carotid endarterectomy for asymptomatic stenosis (ACST-1): A multicentre randomised trial. *Lancet.* 2010;376(9746):1074–1084.
5. Leal I, Orgaz A, Doblas M, Criado E. Selection of patients for carotid endarterectomy versus carotid artery stenting. In: Stanley J, Veith F, Wakefield T, editors. *Current Therapy in Vascular and Endovascular Surgery.* 5th ed. Philadelphia, PA: Elsevier Saunders; 2014: 40–42.
6. Cleveland TJ. Techniques of carotid percutaneous transluminal angioplasty and stenting. In: Thompson M, Morgan R, editors. *Endovascular Intervention for Vascular Disease: Principle and Practice.* New York: Informa Healthcare; 2008: 173–183.
7. Cao P, De Rango P. Carotid artery stenting. In: Cronenwett J, Johnston K, Rutherford R, editors. *Rutherford's Vascular Surgery.* 8th ed. Philadelphia, PA: Elsevier Health Sciences; 2014: 1544–1566.
8. Naylor AR, Bolia A, Abbott RJ, Pye IF, Smith J, Lennard N et al. Randomized study of carotid angioplasty and stenting versus carotid endarterectomy: A stopped trial. *J Vasc Surg.* 1998;28(2):326–334.
9. Alberts M. Results of a multicenter prospective randomized trial of carotid artery stenting vs. carotid endarterectomy. *Stroke.* 2001;32:325.
10. CAVATAS Investigators. Endovascular versus surgical treatment in patients with carotid stenosis in the Carotid and Vertebral Artery Transluminal Angioplasty Study (CAVATAS): A randomised trial. *Lancet.* 2001;357(9270):1729–1737.
11. Brooks W, McClure R, Jones M, Coleman T, Breathitt L. Carotid angioplasty and stenting versus carotid endarterectomy: Randomized trial in a community hospital. *J Am Coll Cardiol.* 2001;38(6):1589–1595.
12. Brooks W, McClure R, Jones M, Coleman T, Breathitt L. Carotid angioplasty and stenting versus carotid endarterectomy for treatment of asymptomatic carotid stenosis: A randomized trial in a community hospital. *Neurosurgery.* 2004;54(2):318–325.
13. Mas J, Trinquart L, Leys D, Albucher J, Rousseau H, Viguier A et al. Endarterectomy versus angioplasty in patients with symptomatic severe carotid stenosis (EVA-3S) trial: Results up to 4 years from a randomised, multicentre trial. *Lancet Neurol.* 2008;7(10):885–892.
14. Silver F, Mackey A, Clark W, Brooks W, Timaran C, Chiu D et al. Safety of stenting and endarterectomy by symptomatic status in the carotid revascularization endarterectomy versus stenting trial (CREST). *Stroke.* 2011;42(3):675–680.
15. Moore W, Kempczinski R, Nelson J, Toole J. Recurrent carotid stenosis: Results of the asymptomatic carotid atherosclerosis study. *Stroke.* 1998;29(10):2018–2025.
16. Mas J, Chatellier G. Endarterectomy versus stenting in patients with severe symptomatic stenosis. *N Engl J Med.* 2006;355:1660–1671.

17. SPACE Collaborators. 30 day results from the SPACE trial of stent-protected angioplasty versus carotid endarterectomy in symptomatic patients: A randomised non-inferiority trial. *Lancet.* 2006;368(9543):1239–1247.

18. ICSS Investigators. Carotid artery stenting compared with endarterectomy in patients with symptomatic carotid stenosis (International Carotid Stenting Study): An interim analysis of a randomised controlled trial. *Lancet.* 2010;375(9719):985–997.

19. Naylor AR, Macdonald S. Extracranial cerebrovascular disease. In: Beard J, Gains P, editors. *Vascular and Endovascular Surgery; Companion to Specialist Surgical Practice,* 5th ed. London, UK: Saunders Elsevier; 2014:160–186.

20. Brott T, Hobson R, Howard G, Roubin G et al. Stenting versus endarterectomy for treatment of carotid-artery stenosis. *N Engl J Med.* 2010;363(1):11–23.

21. Carotid Stenting Trialists' Collaboration (CSTC). Short-term outcome after stenting versus endarterectomy for symptomatic carotid stenosis: A preplanned meta-analysis of individual patient data. *Lancet.* 2010;376(9746):1062–1073.

22. Economopoulos K, Sergentanis T, Tsivgoulis G, Mariolis A et al. Carotid artery stenting versus carotid endarterectomy: A comprehensive meta-analysis of short-term and long-term outcomes. *Stroke.* 2011;42(3):687–692.

23. Chaer R, Schneider P. Technical aspect of percutaneous carotid angioplaty and stenting for arteriosclerotic disease. In: Stanley J, Veith F, Wakefield T editors. *Current Therapy in Vascular and Endovaccular Surgery,* 5th ed. Philadelphia, PA: Elsevier Saunders; 2014: 43–46.

24. Naylor AR, Ricco J-B, De Borst G, Debus S, de Haro J, Halliday A et al. Editor's choice–management of atherosclerotic carotid and vertebral artery disease: 2017 clinical practice guidelines of the European Society for Vascular Surgery (ESVS). *Eur J Vasc Endovasc Surg.* 2018;55(1):3–81.

25. Meschia J, Bushnell C, Boden-Albala B, Braun L, Bravata D, Chaturvedi S et al. Guidelines for the primary prevention of stroke. *Stroke.* 2014;45(12):3754–3832.

26. Goldstein L, Bushnell C, Adams R, Appel L et al. Guidelines for the primary prevention of stroke: A guideline for healthcare professionals from the American Heart Association/American Stroke Association. *Stroke.* 2011;42:517–584.

27. Bladin C and The carotid stenting guidelines committee. Guidelines for patient selection and performance of carotid artery stenting. *Intern Med J.* 2011;41(4): 344–347.

28. Bonati L, Jongen L, Haller S, Zwenneke Flach H et al. New ischaemic brain lesions on MRI after stenting or endarterectomy for symptomatic carotid stenosis: Substudy of the ICSS. *Lancet Neuro.* 2010;9:353–362.

29. Schmidt A, Diederich KW, Scheinert S, Bräunlich S et al. Effect of two different neuroprotection systems on microembolization during carotid artery stenting. *J Am Coll Cardiol.* 2004; 44:1966–1969.

30. Garg N, Karagiorgos N, Pisimisis GT, Sohal DP, Longo GM, Johanning JM et al. Cerebral protection devices reduce periprocedural strokes during carotid angioplasty and stenting: A systematic review of the current literature. *J Endovasc Ther.* 2009;16(4):412–427.

31. Schnaudigel S, Gröschel K, Pilgram SM, Kastrup A et al. New brain lesions after carotid stenting versus carotid endarterectomy, a systematic review of the literature. *Stroke.* 2008; 39: 1911–1919.

32. Cremonesi A, Setacci C, Bignamini A, Bolognese L et al. Carotid artery stenting: First consensus document of the ICCS-SPREAD Joint Committee. *Stroke.* 2006; 37: 2400–2409.

33. Schneider PA. Management of the complications of carotid interventions. In: Schneider PA, Bohannon T, Silva M, editors. *Carotid Interventions:* CRC Press; 2004: 275–283.

34. Schillinger M, Gschwendtner M, Reimers B, Trenkler J et al. Does carotid stent cell design matter? *Stroke.* 2008;39: 905–909.

35

The intra-aortic balloon pump: Principles and use

ANTHONY NICHOLSON

INTRODUCTION

The intra-aortic balloon pump (IABP) is a device used to provide temporary circulatory support during times of actual or potential cardiac dysfunction and is the most frequently used circulatory-assist device for critically ill cardiac patients available today.[1-5] A catheter with an elongated balloon is inserted into the femoral artery and the catheter tip is positioned in the descending thoracic aorta. Circulatory support is provided by counterpulsation, whereby the intra-aortic balloon (IAB) is inflated in early diastole and deflated in early systole, resulting in an increase in coronary artery blood flow and cardiac output, and a reduction in cardiac afterload, cardiac workload and left ventricular myocardial oxygen demand.[6-10]

HISTORY

In 1968, Kantrowitz described the first clinically successful use of an IABP.[11] Since then, many developments have occurred. Newer models are smaller, lighter and able to support patients during transport. Improvements in electronics have resulted in ease of use, increased automation and more sophisticated alarm systems. Improvements have also been made in balloon design, particularly in regard to insertion and removal, which can both be performed without surgical assistance. This has resulted in increased use, portability and availability, as surgical expertise and the operating theatre environment are no longer necessary.[2,4,5,12]

To date, however, and despite documented improvements in myocardial energetics and confirmed benefits following use of IABP after acute myocardial infarction with cardiogenic shock, IABP counterpulsation has not resulted in improved survival outcomes for some groups of patients.[1,13–18] Yet, and despite the introduction of other mechanical circulatory support devices, the IABP remains the device of choice in the setting of high-risk percutaneous coronary intervention (PCI) patients presenting with myocardial infarction and cardiogenic shock, and for those likely to require coronary artery bypass surgery.[2,12,19,20]

INDICATIONS

The use of an IABP is aimed at:

1. Improving coronary artery blood flow
2. Increasing myocardial oxygen delivery as a result of increased aortic root and coronary perfusion pressures
3. Decreasing myocardial oxygen consumption by reduction of left ventricular (LV) afterload

Other effects of IAB pumping include a decrease in LV systolic wall tension, decreased LV end-systolic and end-diastolic volumes, reduced preload, and increased cardiac output.[3,8,9,10]

The IABP is used to rest the myocardium in patients with potentially reversible severe heart failure,[5] and in other patients whose myocardium may benefit from rest, improved oxygen delivery and decreased myocardial oxygen demand, or in patients with compromised left ventricular function subjected to a temporary insult from cardiac surgery or PCI.[7,21–24]

There is increased prophylactic use of the IABP prior to cardiac surgery, especially in patients with severely compromised ventricular function (i.e. those in whom left ventricular ejection fraction [LVEF] <30%) who are considered high risk.[25] Associated with this is a trend towards presurgical insertion of an IAB in patients where perioperative use is indicated; published studies have not demonstrated any significant improvement in outcomes in these patients.[1,20,22,26] Results from the Benchmark Survey suggest that the most frequent indications for use of the IABP, in increasing order, are: in association with cardiac catheterisation, cardiogenic shock, weaning from cardiopulmonary bypass, perioperative use in high-risk patients and for refractory unstable angina. These account for approximately 80% of all IABP insertions.[27]

Specific indications for use of IABP:

1. Left ventricular failure or cardiogenic shock
2. Myocardial infarction
3. Refractory unstable angina
4. Failure to wean from heart-lung machine
5. Post cardiac transplant
6. As a bridge to cardiac transplantation
7. High risk patients undergoing PCI
8. Those in whom PCI has failed and are subsequently unstable
9. High risk patients undergoing non-cardiac surgery requiring general anaesthesia
10. Papillary muscle rupture

CONTRAINDICATIONS

Contraindications to IABP use can be either absolute or relative, which in part depend on patient circumstances/status and clinical judgement.[3,6,9]

Absolute contraindications include:

1. Irreversible brain damage
2. End-stage heart disease, unless as support until transplantation
3. Dissecting aortic or thoracic aneurysms, as there is risk of further dissection

Relative contraindications include:

1. Aortic incompetence, as counterpulsation may worsen the patient's condition by increasing myocardial workload
2. Severe peripheral vascular disease, which may hinder balloon insertion

CARDIOVASCULAR PHYSIOLOGY

Aspects of cardiovascular physiology relevant to IABP therapy are presented in the following.

Cardiac cycle

The cardiac cycle (see Chapter 14) begins electrical activity initiated from the sino-atrial node in the right atrium. In response to this electrical activity, the myocardium of the ventricles contracts. The first phase is the period of **isovolumetric contraction**.[28,29]

At the beginning of isovolumetric contraction, the mitral valve closes, the left ventricle is full of blood, and the left ventricular pressure increases without a change in left ventricular volume because the aortic valve is closed. When left ventricular pressure exceeds that within the aortic root, the aortic valve opens. This marks the end of isovolumetric contraction, at which point the phase of **rapid ejection** begins, and blood rushes out of the left ventricle into the aorta. As the left ventricle continues to contract, the ventricular and aortic pressures attain their maximum values, the peak systolic pressures. The period of **reduced ejection** follows on immediately from the rapid ejection period, and the left ventricular volume continues to fall. Ventricular pressure also falls during this period, until ventricular pressure falls below that of the aorta, causing the aortic valve to close. This marks the end of **ventricular systole**.[28,29]

Ventricular diastole commences with closure of the aortic valve and a low left ventricular blood volume, followed by a period of **isovolumetric relaxation,** when left ventricular pressure falls with no change in left ventricular volume because the mitral valve is closed. When pressure in the left ventricle falls below left atrial pressure, the mitral valve opens and the phase of **rapid filling** begins, when blood rapidly enters the left ventricle from the left atrium. This is followed by a period of **reduced ventricular filling** that continues until atrial systole, at which time the atrial muscle contracts and completes left ventricular filling. Atrial contraction contributes 25%–30% of ventricular filling volume in the normal heart.[28–30] The temporal relationships between the electrocardiogram (ECG) and the pressure changes in the left ventricle and aorta are shown in Figure 35.1.

Haemodynamics and contractility

The efficiency with which the heart pumps blood is dependent on many factors, some of which can be influenced by the IABP. Clinically the effectiveness of the heart, as a pump, is assessed by measuring the **cardiac output** (CO).[28–30] The CO is dependent on heart rate (HR) and stroke volume (SV), as represented by the formula:

$$CO = HR \times SV \qquad (35.1)$$

Stroke volume is the volume of blood ejected by the heart during each systole and is influenced by preload, afterload and myocardial contractility. It can be calculated from the difference between left ventricular end-diastolic volume (LVEDV) and left ventricular end-systolic volume (LVESV):

$$SV = LVEDV - LVESV \qquad (35.2)$$

Preload refers to the degree of stretch of the myocardium at the point of ventricular contraction and is best represented by the LVEDV, which depends on the amount of blood returning to the heart. Clinically, the left ventricular preload is assessed by measurement of the **left ventricular end-diastolic pressure** (LVEDP), the filling pressure of the left side of the heart. LVEDP can be estimated by measurement of **pulmonary artery wedge pressure** (PAWP).[28,29]

Afterload is the wall stress of the myocardium during left ventricular ejection and is generally referred to as the load against which the myocardium exerts its contractile force, i.e. the impedance to left ventricular ejection. It is a major determinant of myocardial oxygen consumption.[28,29] An approximation of afterload, useful for clinical assessment, is made by measuring **mean arterial pressure** (MAP), or preferably, if CO is measured, by calculation of the **systemic vascular resistance** (SVR), where:

$$SVR = (MAP - CVP)/CO \qquad (35.3)$$

and CVP is the **central venous pressure**—a measure of the filling pressure of the right side of the heart (vascular resistance is expressed either in Wood units or as dynes-sec-cm^{-5}).

The other contributor to SV, and hence CO, is **contractility**, an intrinsic property of myocardium, which reflects the mechanical work performed by the heart. Contractility is dependent on many factors, including preload, afterload, heart rate, sympathetic and parasympathetic stimulation, and clinically, administration of drugs that can directly alter myocardial contractility. Clinically, the most frequently used indicator of myocardial contractility is the **ejection fraction** (EF). This can be estimated either by echocardiography or ventriculography. The ejection fraction is normally about 65%–75% of left ventricular blood volume.[28,29]

Coronary blood supply

During the normal cardiac cycle, oxygenated blood is delivered to the myocardium and peripheral tissues.

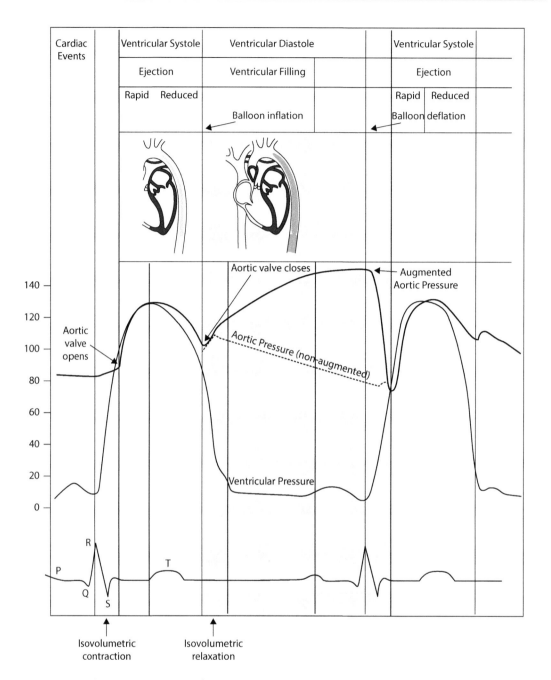

Figure 35.1 Graphic representation of temporal changes in left ventricular and aortic pressures during two cardiac cycles and the associated electrocardiographic signals. Also displayed are the periods of IAB inflation and deflation relative to intrinsic pressure changes. Similar haemodynamic changes occur in the right heart.

In contrast to other organs, the majority of myocardial blood supply is delivered during diastole, when the muscular tissue is relaxed. Coronary blood flow is dependent on the pressure difference in diastole between the aortic root and the LV.

Due to the high metabolic demands placed upon it, the heart normally extracts 65%–70% of delivered oxygen.[28,29] The balance between oxygen delivered to the heart and oxygen utilisation needs to be closely regulated and is referred to as oxygen supply and demand. Any decrease in supply or increase in demand without compensatory mechanisms being invoked can be detrimental to the myocardium.

Oxygen demand will increase with increases in HR, preload, afterload, and contractility; oxygen supply can decrease due to decreases in coronary blood flow arising from tachycardia, diastolic hypotension, increased preload, hypocapnia or coronary spasm. Decreased oxygen delivery may also occur due to anaemia or decreased 2,3 DPG.[28,29]

THE INTRA-AORTIC BALLOON PUMP

The IABP is a ventricular assist device used when the myocardium is unable to provide sufficient cardiac output to maintain oxygen delivery adequate for basal metabolic demands. The pump provides augmentation to the body's intrinsic cardiac output, so by definition can only work properly if some effective myocardial activity is present.

The IABP consists of three parts: An elongated balloon mounted on a catheter, a gas delivery module and a control console. The catheter has two lumina and is usually inserted via the femoral artery. The central lumen, which runs the full length of the catheter, is attached to a standard pressure transducer mounted on or near the pump console. This permits measurement of aortic blood pressure. The second larger lumen carries the driving gas for the balloon, which is usually helium. This lumen ends distally by emptying into an elongated balloon that surrounds the catheter; it is this that inflates to assist the left ventricle. The balloon is made of either polyurethane or Cardiothane-51, which have low thrombogenic surface properties and reliable durability.

Originally, carbon dioxide was used as the shuttle gas but now helium is used exclusively. Helium has a lower molecular weight and density, which together with a much higher viscosity to density ratio result in faster balloon inflation and deflation.[7,9] The significantly lower density of helium contributes greatly to its ability to maintain a laminar flow at higher flow rates than carbon dioxide, which more readily becomes turbulent. Helium, however, has a very low solubility in blood, which creates greater problems when balloons rupture as it tends to form large bubbles that are poorly absorbed and act as large emboli. Any bubbles that do form tend to remain stable and cause prolonged vessel obstruction.[32] The low molecular weight of helium also results in diffusion of very small amounts of gas through the balloon membrane. This slow gas leakage is not of clinical significance but means that the balloon needs to be refilled; most balloon pumps automatically refill the balloon to compensate for this, in some cases as frequently as every 2 hours. Just as helium leaks out of the balloon, water vapour tends to leak into the balloon and accumulate in the delivery tubing. Significant accumulation of condensate can impair gas shuttling, and for this reason most pumps have a collection and purging system to deal with this problem.[11,31]

MECHANISM OF AUGMENTATION

When implementing IAB pumping there are two major considerations to achieve maximum benefit:

Timing: The points in the cardiac cycle when the balloon is inflated and deflated, and
Triggering: The signal used to trigger balloon inflation and deflation

Ventricular assistance using the IABP is often referred to as **counterpulsation** because, with proper timing, the balloon is deflated while the ventricle is contracting and inflated while the ventricle is in diastole, i.e. it cycles counter to the cardiac cycle. Counterpulsation relies on phasic displacement of blood, equal in volume to that of the inflated balloon, within a fixed intravascular space.[1,5] Hence, balloon inflation improves myocardial oxygen delivery by an increase in coronary artery blood flow through augmentation of diastolic blood pressure, which increases **coronary perfusion pressure**. Balloon deflation decreases myocardial oxygen demand by lowering the aortic end-diastolic pressure (AEDP). This decreases afterload, which enables the left ventricle to deliver blood into the aorta at a lower pressure so that less work is performed to achieve ejection, as well as allowing an increase in SV.[3,6,9,10,18]

The mechanism for balloon assistance is related to the timing of balloon inflation and deflation and associated changes in aortic volume and pressure. An understanding of balloon events and effects is made easier by starting with the beginning of diastole. Appearance of the dicrotic notch (DN) on the arterial waveform at the end of the T-wave on the ECG (Figure 35.1) indicates the beginning of diastole. Ideally, balloon inflation occurs at the DN, which represents the closure of the aortic valve. Balloon inflation increases the total volume contained within the aorta. As a result of this sudden increase in aortic volume and the relative rigidity of the aorta, there is a sudden increase in aortic pressure. As a result, blood already contained within the aorta is displaced superiorly and inferiorly and there is an increase in both coronary perfusion pressure and systemic perfusion pressure. With proper balloon timing, this augmented diastolic arterial pressure is higher than the patient's native systolic arterial pressure (which is overridden), hence the term **augmentation**.[3,6,9,10,18]

The balloon remains inflated until the beginning of the next systole. At this point, the balloon is rapidly deflated to create a relative negative pressure. With correct timing this causes a fall in aortic pressure just as the left ventricle is generating sufficient pressure to open the aortic valve and begin ventricular ejection. This means that the required ventricular-generated pressure is reduced, which subsequently reduces oxygen demand. The reduction in afterload allows the ventricle to empty more effectively, which increases SV, and which in turn may lead to a decrease in preload. These effects combine to improve CO.[3,6,9,10,18]

In summary, the major benefits of IAB counterpulsation are:

1. Increased myocardial oxygen delivery
2. Decreased myocardial oxygen demand
3. Decreased afterload
4. Decreased preload
5. Increased cardiac output

CHANGES TO THE ARTERIAL WAVEFORM

Figure 35.2a shows the pressure waveform recorded from the proximal descending aorta via an IAB and from a peripheral artery. Despite clear features common to both traces, there are several notable differences between the two waveforms. The systolic peak of the radial trace is greater and narrower than that from the aorta, and the diastolic hump following the DN is generally more marked in the radial trace.

Figure 35.2b shows the radial artery waveform during IABP augmentation, at an augmentation ratio of 1:2, where the balloon inflates at every second cardiac cycle, i.e. 2:1 counterpulsation. This ratio is chosen initially to assist with selection of the most effective timing of inflation and deflation. Features of this trace include the marked and sudden increase in diastolic pressure at the expected point of the DN; this is the **peak diastolic pressure** (PDP). Also highlighted are the **assisted peak systolic pressure** (APSP), the **balloon aortic end diastolic pressure** (BAEDP), and the **patient aortic end diastolic pressure** (PAEDP).

PDP is the increase in diastolic pressure due to balloon inflation (augmentation), which should be greater than the native PSP. APSP is the systolic pressure generated by the myocardium immediately following balloon deflation. With correct timing this pressure should be less than PSP, as there is a reduction in afterload associated with balloon deflation.

BAEDP is the lowest pressure in the cardiac cycle that results from balloon deflation, while the PAEDP is the lowest pressure in the cardiac cycle due to intrinsic myocardial activity. Correct timing will cause the BAEDP to be lower than the PAEDP by 10–15 mmHg.[9,10]

As shown in Figure 35.2b, the three main goals to aim for with IAB pumping that indicate good

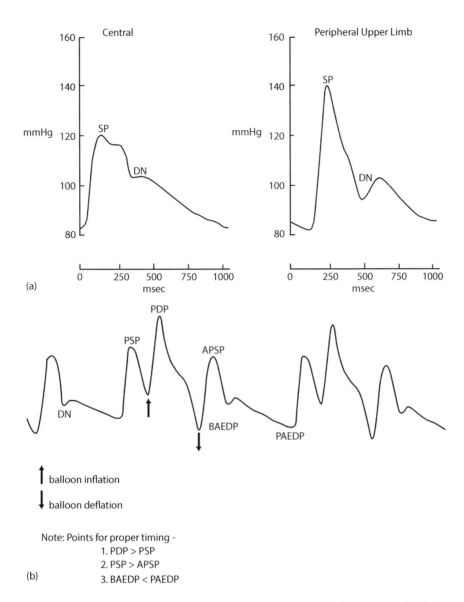

Figure 35.2 **(a)** Diagram showing shape characteristics of pressure waveforms recorded from a central artery (e.g. proximal descending thoracic aorta) at left, and from a peripheral artery (e.g. radial artery) at right. Note the increase in systolic peak (SP) and the more pronounced dicrotic notch (DN) in the peripheral trace. **(b)** Example of radial artery pressure trace during IAB augmentation at an assist ratio of 1:2. Features to note include: peak systolic pressure (PSP), which should be greater than the assisted peak systolic pressure (APSP); the peak diastolic pressure (PDP); the balloon aortic end diastolic pressure (BAEDP), which should be less than the patient aortic end diastolic pressure (PAEDP); and the dicrotic notch (DN).

timing of inflation and deflation are: 1. PDP > PSP; 2. PSP > APSP, and 3. BAEDP < PAEDP.

TIMING

Optimal timing is determined by assessment of the haemodynamic response to counterpulsation.[10] Where possible, it is better to use the IAB central lumen aortic pressure trace to fine-tune the timing, rather than the radial artery trace. There is less distortion of the aortic trace, which makes timing more accurate and there is less delay in the pressure signal. Quaal stated that the time delay to the dicrotic notch due to differences in pulse

wave velocity and blood flow velocity is the same, 40–50 msec, for the IAB central lumen, the subclavian and radial arteries.[32] Despite this, the aortic trace is preferred for adjusting the timing of the IABP, as it is a more accurate reflection of cardiac and pressure events. The differences can be observed when both a radial arterial trace and the balloon aortic trace are available.

Timing errors

EARLY INFLATION

With early inflation, the balloon is inflated well before the DN (Figure 35.3a). This results in premature

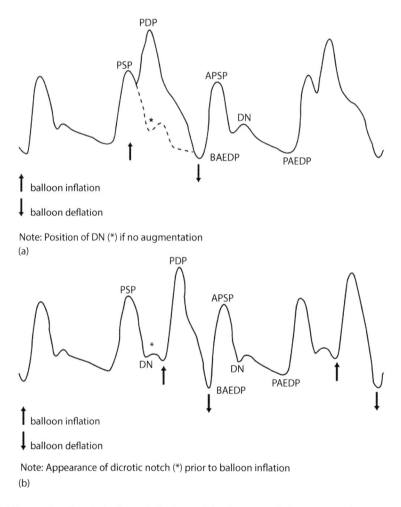

balloon inflation
balloon deflation
Note: Position of DN (*) if no augmentation
(a)

balloon inflation
balloon deflation
Note: Appearance of dicrotic notch (*) prior to balloon inflation
(b)

Figure 35.3 (a) Example of early balloon inflation, with absence of dicrotic notch (DN). Representative traces of timing errors are all displayed at a ratio of 1:2. (*Abbreviations:* PSP, peak systolic pressure; PDP, peak diastolic pressure; BAEDP, balloon-assisted end-diastolic pressure; APSP, assisted peak systolic pressure; PAEDP, patient aortic end diastolic pressure.) (b) With late inflation, the balloon is inflated well after the dicrotic notch (DN), which is clearly visible between the PSP and the PDP (peak diastolic pressure).

closure of the aortic valve, which reduces SV and CO, with an increase in LVEDV. If this situation persists, myocardial work and oxygen consumption will increase, which is likely to worsen the patient's condition.

LATE INFLATION

In this situation, the balloon is inflated well after the DN, which is clearly visible between PSP and the augmented PDP (Figure 35.3b). In this instance the balloon inflates after the aorta is maximally filled with blood, so that the increase in volume and subsequent pressure is less than it could be, which results in a diminution in augmented coronary and peripheral perfusion.

EARLY DEFLATION

Early deflation will result in the BAEDP reaching its nadir well before the beginning of the next systole. This will let the pressure within the aorta rise again as the left ventricle is about to begin emptying (Figure 35.4a). The APSP will rise due to an

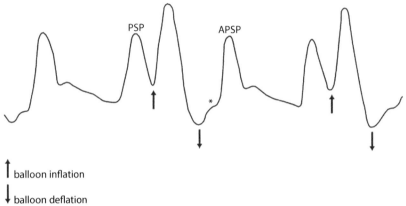

↑ balloon inflation

↓ balloon deflation

Note: Increase in end diastolic pressure before (*) next systole. May get APSP ≥ PSP (unassisted operation APSP < PSP)

(a)

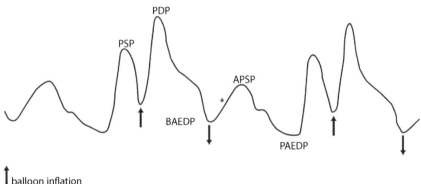

↑ balloon inflation

↓ balloon deflation

Note: Rate of rise of assisted peak systolic pressure (*) may be prolonged, and BAEDP ≥ PAEDP (unassisted operation BAEDP < PAEDP)

(b)

Figure 35.4 **(a)** If the IAB is deflated too early, prior to the next systolic ejection, there is often an increase in the end-diastolic pressure (*) with an associated increase in the assisted peak systolic pressure (APSP). (PSP, peak systolic pressure.) **(b)** With late deflation of the balloon, the left ventricle has to open the aortic valve at a higher pressure, which may result in an increase in the balloon-assisted end-diastolic pressure (BAEDP) and a decrease in the slope of the following systole (*). (*Abbreviations:* PDP, peak diastolic pressure; PAEDP, patient aortic end diastolic pressure.)

increase in afterload because of retrograde flow of blood, which fills the 'space' left by the deflated balloon.

LATE DEFLATION

With late deflation of the balloon, the LV has to open the aortic valve at a higher pressure, resulting in increased left ventricular work (Figure 35.4b). As the left ventricular work increases so does oxygen consumption, increasing the delivery demand. This is compounded by an associated decrease in CO due to increased afterload.

TRIGGERING MODES

ECG triggering

There are two patient-derived physiological signals used for balloon triggering, and one console-generated signal. Most commonly, pumping will be triggered using the patient's ECG, which is the default trigger mode on most IABPs. This signal may be established with direct skin leads from the patient to the console, or via a slave cable from the anaesthetic or other monitor to the appropriate input jack on the console. Choice between these two triggers is often dependent on circumstances at the time of balloon insertion.

The ability to apply IABP-specific patient ECG electrodes during surgery is limited, so that a slave signal is most commonly used. In most situations, this signal is adequate for reliable pumping, but the signal may be degraded at times requiring an alternative trigger. This is particularly the case with an intrinsically reduced signal strength from the patient. Apart from this situation, there is little difference with regard to triggering and pumping reliability between these two ECG sources.

When the heart is paced, either temporarily following surgery or with a permanent pacemaker, the appropriate trigger mode will need to be selected on the console. The exact type will depend on the individual IABP being used. All consoles have at least one pacing mode, designed to ignore/reject the pacing spike(s), and trigger from the ECG (T and R waves). Some consoles distinguish between atrial, ventricular or A-V sequential pacing. When slaving from another monitor while the heart is being paced, it is important to determine whether the pacing spike is suppressed or transmitted from the monitor to the IABP console. If the pacing spike is suppressed and the trigger mode is ECG with pacing, then the console will be aiming to detect a pacing spike. In this situation the pump may trigger irregularly and erratically due to inappropriate trigger selection. With a regular rhythm newer balloon pumps are capable of reliable triggering at heart rates up to 180 bpm.[3,10] It has been recommended that during periods of tachycardia (HR > 110–120 bpm) the IABP be set to inflate on every second beat; this allows for complete balloon filling on alternate beats rather than only partial filling for every beat.

Pressure triggering

Pressure triggering is most frequently achieved from the aortic pressure signal obtained via the IAB catheter. In this instance, the pressure transducer is connected directly to the balloon console. Alternatively, the pressure signal may be slaved from the anaesthetic monitor, which most often is derived from the radial artery. In either case, the size of the pulse pressure must be above a certain threshold to enable reliable triggering. In many newer machines, the pressure trigger mode detects both magnitude of the pressure increase with systole and the rate of rise, which helps to eliminate artefactual interference. The sensitivity with respect to pulse pressure size can generally be adjusted for very low output states. This triggering mode is less reliable than ECG triggering when the heart rate is very high, i.e. >150, or when the rhythm is irregular.[10]

Internal triggering

The internal asynchronous triggering mode is only used when there is no intrinsic myocardial activity, which means this mode is generally reserved for intraoperative use during cardiopulmonary bypass (CPB). The standard default rate for this mode is 80 inflations per minute but this is variable from as low as 10 per minute to as high as 120 per minute, depending on the particular model. It must be remembered that when using this mode there is **no** synchronisation between the balloon inflation/deflation cycle and activity of the heart. Consequently, internal triggering may worsen ventricular failure if used inappropriately.

Internal triggering is used during CPB to avoid thrombus formation on the balloon. This precaution is taken even though the patient is fully heparinised for bypass. Although the default internal trigger rate is 80 per minute, this is generally reduced to the minimum possible during bypass to minimally interfere with the surgery. The lowest rate available varies with the make of pump, from a low of 10 per minute up to about 32. If this frequency still results in surgical interference, then the balloon inflation volume may also be reduced.

BALLOON PRESSURE WAVEFORM

All IABP models currently available enable display of the waveform, which represents pressure changes within the balloon associated with inflation and deflation; this is referred to as the **balloon pressure waveform**.

This pressure trace has characteristic features, deviations from which can be used for trouble-shooting. A normal balloon pressure waveform is presented in Figure 35.5, features of which include: balloon pressure **baseline**; **rapid balloon inflation**; **peak inflation artefact** (pressure artefact); balloon pressure **plateau**; **rapid balloon deflation**; **deflation undershoot** (vacuum artefact); and the **console zero baseline**.[33]

The width of the balloon pressure waveform represents duration of balloon inflation and consequently will change with changes in heart rate.

The level of the balloon pressure plateau reflects the pressure within the aorta during balloon inflation. The balloon wall material is highly compliant so there is rapid pressure equalisation across the wall. This means that the plateau pressure should be within 10–15 mmHg of the PDP on the arterial

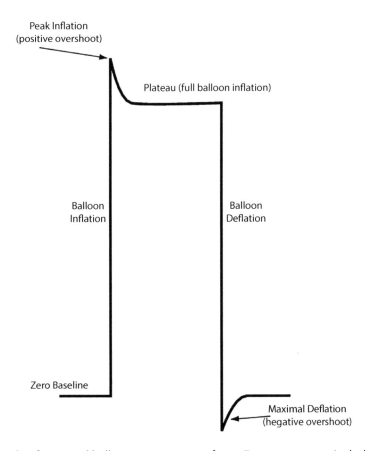

Figure 35.5 Example of a normal balloon pressure waveform. Features to note include balloon pressure baseline; rapid balloon inflation; peak inflation artefact (pressure artefact); balloon pressure plateau; rapid balloon deflation; deflation undershoot (vacuum artefact); and the console zero baseline.

trace. The level of the plateau pressure will change in response to changes in aortic pressure. During periods of relative hypertension, the plateau level will rise, reflecting the higher pressure needed to achieve full balloon inflation. Similarly, during periods of decreased aortic pressure the plateau level will fall.

Low balloon pressure baseline: Normally the baseline pressure is 5–10 mmHg, i.e. above zero. If the baseline value falls below this, likely causes include insufficient filling initially or loss of helium either through a leak in the circuit or normal diffusion of helium through the balloon wall.

High balloon pressure baseline: The baseline may rise in response to over-pressurisation of the gas system due to a kink in the tubing or the balloon. Otherwise, a baseline increase signifies overfilling, implying an internal fault.

High plateau pressure: With an increase in the plateau pressure there is also generally a change in shape of the BPW, where the plateau rises and becomes rounded. Causes for this include: a kink in the catheter; balloon occlusion; balloon not fully unwrapped or unsheathed if percutaneously inserted; balloon too large for the aorta; or the patient may be hypertensive.

BALLOON INSERTION

The preferred method of insertion is percutaneously into the femoral artery using the Seldinger technique. If difficulty is encountered in locating the artery, a surgical cutdown may be required. In either case, once localised, a sheath is inserted into the artery through which the fully deflated balloon is passed. To ensure complete deflation prior to insertion, the balloon should be fully evacuated using a 50 cc syringe and the one-way valve supplied with the balloon. It is crucial that the balloon not be inflated or unfurled prior to insertion, as this will make insertion impossible. Advancement of the balloon is over a guidewire, until the balloon catheter tip is just distal to (below) the origin of the subclavian artery. When in this position, the distal end of the balloon should be situated

close to, but above, the renal arteries.[34] It has been recommended that, where possible, the balloon be restricted to the descending thoracic aorta, as this usually has less atheromatous plaque than the abdominal aorta.[35] Complications associated with percutaneous insertion are most commonly related to puncture of an inappropriate site, or use of excessive force to advance the guidewire or balloon catheter.[36]

A recent development in balloon insertion and design is the sheathless balloon. This is also inserted percutaneously, but no guiding sheath is placed into the femoral artery. This results in less obstruction to blood flow in the affected femoral artery and a 30% reduction in cross-sectional area of the artery punctured. Reports to date are equivocal about the advantages of sheathless balloon catheters.[9,18,36,37]

Less frequently, IABs are inserted surgically. This technique involves suturing a Dacron graft side-arm onto the vessel wall, through which the balloon is passed. Most commonly, the femoral artery is used, although there are reports of antegrade insertion into the thoracic aorta at the time of cardiac surgery.[27,36]

BALLOON SIZES

The most commonly inserted balloon has a volume of 40 cc. This size is suitable for most adults, while a 30 or 34 cc balloon can be used in smaller patients. Paediatric balloons with volumes as low as 2.5 cc are also available. Rarely, very large patients require a 50 cc balloon. It is recommended that when inflated the balloon occupy between 75% and 95% of the aortic lumen.[9,18,37] This reduces the amount of direct contact between the balloon and the intimal surface of the aorta and results in less damage to both surfaces and to red blood cells. Two general principles regarding balloon size are: first, that the balloon lie between the subclavian artery and the renal arteries, and second, that the diameter be such that there is maximal volume displacement of blood on inflation without distension of the aorta. Studies have demonstrated that 90% of patients have aortic diameters in excess of 19 mm, and subsequently most balloon catheters have diameters between 14 and 16.5 mm when inflated.[18,37,38]

WEANING

Weaning is considered likely to be successful if the patient can maintain a cardiac index greater than 2 L/min/m², PAWP < 18 mmHg, and left ventricular stroke work index (LVSWI) > 20 g/m/m².[3,6,39] Pharmacological support is reduced prior to weaning, so that it may then be increased if necessary during the weaning process. The weaning process itself involves a reduction in the frequency of augmentation, by changing the pumping ratio from 1:1 to 1:2 in the first instance, and if this is well tolerated then reducing the ratio further. The degree to which the ratio may be reduced varies with different models, but in some instances it may not be sufficiently low to enable gradual weaning from counterpulsation. In these situations the volume to which the balloon is inflated may also be reduced gradually. The time frame for this will depend on how well the patient copes with each change in pump settings. Several hours should be allocated for each change.

COMPLICATIONS

The use of the IABP is fraught with a degree of morbidity and mortality. Death resulting directly as a consequence of balloon insertion and counterpulsation is reported to be less than 1%. Reported rates for complications vary from 5% to 35%, with significant complication rates reported to be between 10% and 20%, and permanent morbidity less than 5%.[14,27,35,40,41]

Mortality in patients who receive IABP support is in the range of 26%–50%, largely because of the nature of their cardiac problems that necessitated IABP use. Risk factors for mortality in patients receiving counterpulsation include advanced age, female gender, high New York Heart Association (NYHA) classification, preoperative glycerol trinitrate (GTN), operative or post-operative balloon insertion, and transthoracic insertion.[14,19,27,41–43] Despite the high mortality and the well-recognised risk factors, the IAB is inserted for compelling indications, so that identification of risk factors does not influence patient management, except to encourage removal of the device as soon as the cardiac status of the patient permits.

Several categories of complication associated with IABP therapy have been identified.[14,27,35,36,40,41] These include:

1. Trauma to the arterial wall during insertion
2. Limb ischaemia
3. Dislodged thrombus
4. Haematologic (thrombocytopaenia, haemolysis, haemorrhage)
5. Balloon leak or rupture
6. Infection

Limb ischaemia is the most common complication, occurring in 9%–25% of patients.[41,43,44] In the great majority of cases ischaemia resolves with balloon removal; however, in 1%–2% of cases ischaemia may persist and result in some degree of lower limb amputation.[41] Risk factors associated with limb ischaemia include severity of peripheral vascular disease, extent of myocardial failure, presence of significant longstanding hypertension, diabetes mellitus, female gender, smoking and duration of therapy.[27,35]

Infection associated with presence of the balloon catheter is the second most common complication (3%–4% incidence). Balloon rupture occurs in 1%–4% of cases, although a study cited by Baldyga[44] reported a mean incidence for 2 years of 9% and 10.1% with a range up to 17%. Balloon rupture and leakage is assumed to occur due to plaque abrasion. It is more likely to occur in patients with a history of hypertension, those who display a marked diastolic augmentation from the IABP, and in women.[41] Consequences of IAB rupture are gas embolism and vascular entrapment of the balloon. Gas embolism resulting in neurological sequelae is a very rare occurrence, even following balloon rupture.[41] Balloon entrapment may occur following slow leakage as well as sudden rupture. Rupture and leakage are often first detected by presence of blood in the shuttle gas tubing, although the gas leak alarm may sound, or an increased frequency in balloon refilling may be noted.[41]

SET-UP

The procedures involved in setting up for IAB pumping are similar for all models of IABP currently available. There will be slight differences depending on which particular unit is in use, but the following guidelines apply to all:

1. Open the helium cylinder and ensure the helium pressure is satisfactory.
2. Where possible, connect the IABP to mains power. Turn on power switch on the console.
3. After the catheter has been inserted into the patient and the one-way valve removed, connect the helium delivery hose to the console.
4. Establish an ECG signal from the patient to the console by connecting the ECG cable directly to the console, or indirectly by connecting the ECG cable to the anaesthetic monitor and then running a slave cable from the anaesthetic monitor to the console.
5. Connect the aortic pressure monitoring line to the nearby pressure transducer. This may be mounted onto the console, but for safety reasons is not recommended. Ensure that the pressure transducer has been zeroed to the patient's approximate mid-chest height. Use of a pressurised continuous flush device is recommended to avoid blood clotting within the central lumen and to ensure a good, reliable aortic pressure trace. Heparin, at a concentration of 4 IU/mL may also be added to the bag of flush. It is extremely important that the flush device be carefully set up to avoid air bubbles, which will dampen the trace and potentially form emboli within the patient.
6. Establish a reliable triggering mode. The ECG signal is the preferred triggering mode, but the arterial pressure may be used if there is a poor ECG signal or there is electrical interference from the electrocautery device during surgery.
7. Confirm console settings for initiation of pumping. These are:
   a. Inflation and deflation timing set to middle of their respective ranges
   b. Augmentation ratio 1:2, which allows for comparison between augmented and non-augmented beats
   c. Ensure there is a triggering signal (usually a flashing display) for each cardiac cycle of the selected triggering mode
   d. Where appropriate, ensure balloon inflation volume is zero
8. Fill the balloon; most consoles have an automated filling function.
9. Start pumping; in certain models it is necessary to increase the volume of helium delivered to the balloon until it is maximal, or until maximal augmentation is achieved.
10. Establish maximal augmentation by adjustment of both the time of inflation and time of deflation.
11. Increase augmentation ratio to 1:1 when satisfied with timing.

REFERENCES

1. Hou D, Yang F, Perfusion XH, Clinical application of intra-aortic balloon counterpulsation in high-risk patients undergoing cardiac surgery. *Perfusion.* 2018; 27;33(3):178–184.
2. Khera R, Cram P, Vaughan-Sarrazin M, Horwitz PA, Girotra S. Use of mechanical circulatory support in percutaneous coronary intervention in the United States. *Am J Cardiol.* 2016;117(1):10–16.
3. Krishna M, Zacharowski K. Principles of intra-aortic balloon pump counterpulsation. *Continu Educat Anaesthesia Critical Care Pain.* 2009;9(1):24–28.
4. Stretch R, Sauer CM, Yuh DD, Bonde P. National trends in the utilization of short-term mechanical circulatory support: Incidence, outcomes, and cost analysis. *J Am Coll Cardiol.* 2014;64(14):1407–1415.
5. Patel NJ, Patel N, Bhardwaj B, Golwala H, Kumar V, Atti V, et al. Trends in utilization of mechanical circulatory support in patients hospitalized after out-of-hospital cardiac arrest. *Resuscitation.* 2018;127:105–113.
6. Santa-Cruz RA, Cohen MG, Ohman EM. Aortic counterpulsation: A review of the hemodynamic effects and indications for use. *Cathet Cardiovasc Interv.* 2006;67(1):68–77.
7. Parissis H, Graham V, Lampridis S, Lau M, Hooks G, Mhandu PC. IABP: History-evolution-pathophysiology-indications: What we need to know. *J Cardiothorac Surg.* 2016; 11:122–134.
8. Annamalai SK, Buiten L, Esposito ML, Paruchuri V, Mullin A, Breton C, et al. Acute hemodynamic effects of intra-aortic balloon counterpulsation pumps in advanced heart failure. *J Card Fail.* 2017;23(8):606–614.
9. Turi ZG. Intra-aortic balloon counterpulsation. In *Critical Care Medicine: Principles of Diagnosis and Management in the Adult,*

Parrillo JE, Dellinger PR, editors, 3rd ed. Philadelphia, PA, Mosby Elsevier; 2008, 93–115.

10. Hanlon-Pena PM, Quaal SJ. Intra-aortic balloon pump timing: Review of evidence supporting current practice. *Am J Crit Care.* 2011;20(4):323–334.

11. Kantrowitz A. Origins of intraaortic balloon pumping. *Ann of Thorac Surg.* 1990;50(4):672–674.

12. Khera R, Cram P, Lu X, Vyas A, Gerke A, Rosenthal GE, et al. Trends in the use of percutaneous ventricular assist devices: Analysis of national inpatient sample data, 2007 through 2012. *JAMA.* 2015;175(6):941–950.

13. Craner RC, Carvajal T, Villablanca PA, Jahanyar J, Yang EH, Ramakrishna H. The increasing importance of percutaneous mechanical circulatory support in high-risk transcatheter coronary interventions: An evidence-based analysis. *J Cardiothorac Vasc Anesth.* 2018;32(3):1507–1524.

14. Pappalardo F, Ajello S, Thoracic MGJO, 2018. Contemporary applications of intra-aortic balloon counterpulsation for cardiogenic shock: A "real world" experience. *J Thorac Dis.* 2018;10(4):2125–2134.

15. Dahlslett T, Karlsen S, Grenne B, Cardiovascular BSJ, 2017. Intra-aortic balloon pump optimizes myocardial function during cardiogenic shock. *JACC Cardiovasc Imag.* 2018;11(3):512–514.

16. Rathod KS, Koganti S, Iqbal MB, Jain AK, Kalra SS, Astroulakis Z, et al. Contemporary trends in cardiogenic shock: Incidence, intra-aortic balloon pump utilisation and outcomes from the London Heart Attack Group. *Eur Heart J Acute Cardiovasc Care.* 2017;7(1):16–27.

17. Patterson T, Perera D, Redwood SR. Intra-aortic balloon pump for high-risk percutaneous coronary intervention. *Circulation Cardiovasc Interv.* 2014;7(5):712–720.

18. Trost JC, Hillis LD. Intra-aortic balloon counterpulsation. *Am J Cardiol.* 2006;97(9):1391–1398.

19. Kolte D, Khera S, Aronow WS, Mujib M, Palaniswamy C, Sule S, et al. Trends in incidence, management, and outcomes of cardiogenic shock complicating ST-elevation myocardial infarction in the United States. *J Am Heart Assoc.* 2014;3:e000590.

20. Böning A, Buschbeck S, Roth P, Scheibelhut C, Bödeker RH, Brück M, et al. IABP before cardiac surgery: Clinical benefit compared to intraoperative implantation. *Perfusion.* 2013;28(2):103–108.

21. Burgio G, Martucci G, Panarello G, Scarlata M, Pastore F, Pilato M, et al. Intra-aortic balloon counterpulsation in high-risk cardiac patients undergoing noncardiac surgery: A case series. *J Cardiothorac and Vasc Anesth.* 2016;30(2):428–431.

22. MacKay EJ, Patel PA, Gutsche JT, Weiss SJ, Augoustides JG. Contemporary clinical niche for intra-aortic balloon counterpulsation in perioperative cardiovascular practice: An evidence-based review for the cardiovascular anesthesiologist. *J Cardiothorac and Vasc Anesth.* 2017;31(1):309–320.

23. White JM, Ruygrok PN. Intra-aortic balloon counterpulsation in contemporary practice – where are we? *Heart Lung Circ.* 2015;24(4):335–341.

24. Lewis PA, Ward DA, Courtney MD. The intra-aortic balloon pump in heart failure management: Implications for nursing practice. *Aust Crit Care.* 2009;22(3):125–131.

25. Dietl CA, Berkheimer MD, Woods EL, Gilbert CL, Pharr WF, Benoit CH. Efficacy and cost-effectiveness of preoperative IABP in patients with ejection fraction of 0.25 or less. *Ann Thorac Surg.* 1996;62(2):401–409.

26. Poirier Y, Voisine P, Plourde G, Rimac G, Barria Perez A, Costerousse O, et al. Efficacy and safety of preoperative intra-aortic balloon pump use in patients undergoing cardiac surgery: A systematic review and meta-analysis. *Int J Cardiol.* 2016;207:67–79.

27. Ferguson JJ, Cohen M, Freedman RJ, Stone GW, Miller MF, Joseph DL, et al. The current practice of intra-aortic balloon counterpulsation: Results from the Benchmark Registry. *J Am Coll Cardiol.* 2001;38(5):1456–1462.

28. Crystal GJ, Heerdt PM. Cardiovascular physiology: Integrative function. In *Pharmacology and Physiology for Anesthesia: Foundations and Clinical Application,* Egan TA, Hemmings HC Jr, editors. Philadelphia, PA, Elsevier-Saunders; 2014, 366–389.

29. Katz, Arnold M. Physiology of the Heart, Wolters Kluwer Health, 2010. ProQuest Ebook Central, https://ebookcentral. proquest.com/lib/adelaide/detail. action?docID=2031935. 592 p.

30. Macciò S, Marino P. Role of the left atrium. In: Smiseth OA, Tendera M, editors. *Diastolic Heart Failure*. London, UK, Springer-Verlag; 2008, 53–70.

31. Shedlick RR, Maccioli GA. Physical and medical aspects of inflation gases: Helium vs carbon dioxide. In: Maccioli GA, editor. *Intra-aortic Balloon Pump Therapy*. Baltimore, MD, Williams & Wilkins 1997, 43–50.

32. Quaal SJ. Conventional timing using the arterial pressure waveform. In: Quaal SJ, editor. *Comprehensive Intraaortic Balloon Counterpulsation*, 2nd ed. St Louis, MO, 1993, 246–59.

33. Kalina J. Use of the balloon pressure waveform in conjunction with the augmented arterial pressure waveform. In: Quaal SJ, editor. *Comprehensive Intraaortic Balloon Counterpulsation*, 2nd ed. St Louis, MO, 1993, 295–308.

34. Sodhi N, Lasala JM. Mechanical circulatory support in acute decompensated heart failure and shock. *Interv Cardiol Clinics*. 2017;6(3):387–405.

35. Evaluation: Intra-aortic balloon pumps. *Health Dev*. 1997;26(5):184–216.

36. Parissis H, Soo A, Al-Alao B. Intra aortic balloon pump: Literature review of risk factors related to complications of the intraaortic balloon pump. *J Cardiothorac Surg*. 2011;6(1):147.

37. Tate DA. Physical and clinical aspects of intra-aortic balloon pump catheters. In: Maccioli GA editor. *Intra-Aortic Balloon Pump Therapy*. Baltimore, MD, Willams & Wilkins; 1997, 51–56.

38. de Waha S, Desch S, Eitel I, et al. Intra-aortic balloon counterpulsation: Basic principles and clinical evidence. *Vasc Pharmacol*. 2014;60(2):52–56.

39. Bueti G, Watson K. The Intra-aortic balloon pump. In: Taylor DA, Sherry SP, Sing RF, editors. *Interventional Critical Care: A Manual for Advanced Care Practitioners*, Cham, Switzerland, Springer; 2016, 147–159.

40. Lange SS. Complications associated with IABC. In: Quaal SJ, editor *Comprehensive Intraaortic Balloon Counterpulsation*, 2nd ed. St Louis, MO; 1993, 146–164.

41. Christenson JT, Cohen M, Ferguson JJ, et al. Trends in intraaortic balloon counterpulsation complications and outcomes in cardiac surgery. *Ann Thorac Surg*. 2002;74(4):1086–1090; discussion 1090–1091.

42. Bojar RM. *Manual of Perioperative Care in Adult Cardiac Surgery*, John Wiley & Sons, 2010. ProQuest Ebook Central. https:// ebookcentral.proquest.com/lib/adelaide/ detail.action?docID=624739. 834 p.

43. Burkhoff D. Intra-aortic balloon counterpulsation and other circulatory assist devices. In: Baim DS, editor. *Grossman's Cardiac Catheterization, Angiography, and Intervention*, Philadelphia, PA, Wolters Kluwer; 2005, 412–429.

44. Baldyga AP. Complications of intra-aortic balloon pump therapy. In: Maccioli GA, editor. *Intra-Aortic Balloon Pump Therapy*, Baltimore, MD, Williams & Wilkins; 1997, 127–161.

PART 6

Interventions for structural heart disease

36

Interventional transoesophageal echocardiography

MAYOORAN NAMASIVAYAM AND MARTIN SHAW

INTRODUCTION

The scope of interventional cardiology has evolved rapidly over the past few decades. Procedures once only feasible with open cardiac surgery, such as valve replacement or repair of inter-atrial septal defects, are now mainstream transcatheter procedures performed daily in interventional cardiology laboratories worldwide. This advancement has progressed concurrrently with the development of skills and technology to facilitate better visualisation of intracardiac structures during such procedures. In addition to fluoroscopy, the mainstay of this imaging work is done by echocardiography, which is easy to use, portable, widely available, radiation-free and relatively safe. While transthoracic echocardiography (TTE) and intracardiac echocardiography (ICE) are used to some extent within interventional cardiology, transoesophageal echocardiography (TEE) forms the basis from which most interventionalists visualise their instruments and targets during procedures.

As such, this chapter aims to provide an overview of the use of transoesophageal echocardiography during key cardiovascular interventions. More detailed review can be found in dedicated texts on interventional echocardiography.[1] All staff involved in cardiac interventions, from interventionalists and anaesthesiologists to nursing staff, radiographers and technicians should find this chapter adds to their understanding of transoesophageal echocardiography and its role in cardiovascular interventions.

PRINCIPLES OF TRANSOESOPHAGEAL ECHOCARDIOGRAPHY

TEE is a procedure whereby a flexible probe containing an ultrasound transducer is introduced into the patient's oesophagus to visualise the heart from behind. Its key advantages over TTE are the fact that it does not require ultrasound waves to pass through the chest wall or lung, thus improving imaging quality, particularly for posterior cardiac structures such as the left atrium and the mitral valve. TEE can be performed with light sedation, no sedation or under general anaesthesia. The latter is often the case in long procedures, but there is an increasing trend to use light sedation, hence operators should become familiar with the use of TEE under these conditions. Often TEE is performed by an imaging cardiologist, but in many centres, anaesthesiologists, intensivists and interventional cardiologists may also be the TEE operators during cardiac interventions.

Before performing TEE, previous echocardiographic or other cardiac imaging should be reviewed to plan the imaging sequence. Operators must also be aware that previous imaging may have missed particular diagnoses, thus TEE should also serve to confirm or question previous findings and add to the existing baseline knowledge of the case by expecting to find the unexpected. TEE is a relatively safe procedure, but staff should be aware of potential risks. There is an approximate risk of 1:1000 for oesophageal perforation, which is possibly the most serious risk, but other risks include trauma to the pharynx, aspiration pneumonia, tooth dislodgement or damage, and bleeding. Simple steps can be taken to minimise these risks, and when patients are consented for cardiac interventions requiring TEE, the risks of TEE should be explained to the patient. Patients who are scheduled for cardiac interventions requiring TEE should be screened for a history of any symptoms of dysphagia or, specifically, experiencing difficulty with food bolus passage through the oesophagus. A history of hematemesis, odynophagia or severe gastro-oesophageal reflux symptoms may also suggest problems within the oesophagus. If there is any concern for oesophageal or gastric stricture, malignancy, bleeding or ulceration, then further evaluation of the oesophagus and stomach with upper gastrointestinal video-endoscopy +/− barium swallow (for stricture) is recommended prior to intubation with a TEE probe to minimise the risk of trauma, bleeding and perforation.

If patients are awake or lightly sedated for the procedure, intubation is made easier with a spray of local anaesthetic to the posterior pharynx. The probe head is lubricated in gel and the probe is gently introduced over the tongue and then flexed into the posterior pharynx. Slight retroflexion once the probe is over the tongue helps the probe stay posterior and thus enter the oesophagus rather than the trachea. Any signs of tracheal intubation with the TEE probe (e.g. probe not showing any clear cardiac images and patient coughing excessively or experiencing respiratory distress) should lead to probe withdrawal. Once the probe is confirmed to be in the oesophagus, then image acquisition can commence.

Imaging in TEE is mainly done in the mid-oesophageal position but transgastric views taken from the stomach may be particularly helpful in certain circumstances.[2] The various structures of the heart are visualised by moving the probe to different levels within the oesophagus and changing the acquisition of viewing angle, which changes the ultrasound crystal array angle. Viewing can occur from 0° to 180°. At any position, the TEE probe can be flexed, retroflexed and moved laterally leftward or rightward to enhance imaging quality. Manipulations in oesophageal/gastric level are made by withdrawing or advancing the probe, while flexion, lateral position and viewing angle are controlled using a series of wheels and buttons on the probe. The presence of excessive air within the oesophagus or stomach will create a probe/air/tissue interface that reduces imaging quality. Particularly during long procedures, or when a large amount of high energy output mode imaging is performed, probe temperature will increase. Probe temperature should be monitored to avoid overheating the oesophagus, which increases risk of trauma and perforation.

IMAGING MODES IN ECHOCARDIOGRAPHY

Echocardiography uses high frequency sound wave transmission and reflection to identify various structures within the heart. Its common format is 2D imaging, which most operators would be familiar with. Doppler imaging, which allows for colour assessment to assess flow direction and velocity, can be employed to understand valve function and dysfunction, and to quantify gradients across valves using spectral Doppler. Increasingly, 3D imaging has been employed in interventional imaging due to its ability to spatially represent cardiac structures in a way that is analogous to direct visualisation (i.e. as though looking with one's own eyes directly into the heart). The use of a 3D probe also facilitates simultaneous multiplanar imaging in 2D, allowing the same structure to be viewed from two viewing angles simultaneously—another very useful technique during intervention.

SPECIFIC CASES (TEE)

Before review of specific cases, it is prudent to mention the brief overview that should occur before any procedure. All chambers and valves should be briefly assessed, and the patient should be assessed for pericardial effusion prior to commencement of the intervention. Post-procedure, this general sweep should also occur to ensure no post procedure effusion (that might suggest cardiac perforation) nor any damage to valves, and no change in ventricular function.

TRANS-SEPTAL PUNCTURE

Trans-septal puncture is a key step in any procedure requiring access to the left heart from a venous access approach. It is therefore used widely in left atrial appendage closure, atrial fibrillation ablation, left sided atrial flutter ablation, left sided accessory pathway ablation and mitral valve procedures, among other case types. The role of the imaging team is to facilitate a safe trans-septal approach that minimises risk of tamponade. The

recommended view for trans-septal puncture is the mid-oesophageal short axis view at 30°–60° and the bicaval view at 90°–110°.[3,4] We find using multi-planar imaging to show these two views of the inter-atrial septum simultaneously (using a 3D probe) is very helpful. Essentially, the puncture should be guided such that it crosses in the thinnest membranous part of the septum with avoidance of the aorta and avoidance of an excessively posterior approach that might lead to perforation. The interventionalist should be asked to 'tent' the inter-atrial septum prior to actually puncturing, in order for the imaging team to confirm whether this location will facilitate a safe approach and trajectory. Imaging during trans-septal puncture can also be used to direct access to the left atrium posteriorly, inferiorly or superiorly according to the needs of the intervention. Following trans-septal puncture, a quick sweep to check for pericardial effusion should occur. Figure 36.1 shows successful entry into the left atrium via trans-septal puncture, as confirmed by bubbles appearing in the left atrium upon injection by the interventionalist.

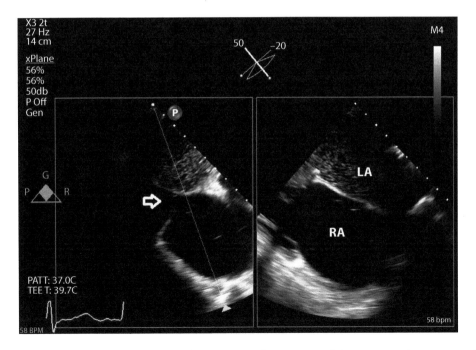

Figure 36.1 Multiplanar transoesophageal imaging confirms successful trans-septal puncture, with bubbles present on left side of septum upon injection. Arrow shows catheter (*Abbreviations:* LA, Left atrium; RA, Right atrium).

TRANSCATHETER MITRAL VALVE REPAIR AND REPLACEMENT

Various approaches to mitral valve repair using a percutaneous approach are available, including direct repair of leaflets, annuloplasty, annuloplasty-coronary sinus procedures and ventricular remodelling approaches. Mitral valve repair using the MitraClip device is an increasingly common procedure (see Chapter 30). This procedure, derived from the Alfieri method of surgically joining the anterior and posterior leaflet, requires careful visualisation of valve leaflets, and documentation of coaptation defects in the three anatomical planes.

TEE is crucial to identifying the mechanism of mitral regurgitation (MR), which alters slightly the approach to intervention. A higher trans-septal puncture (4–5 cm above the mitral valve annular plane) is recommended for degenerative MR, while a puncture 3.5–4 cm above the annular plane is recommended for functional MR.[4] Following trans-septal puncture, the use of the long axis 3 chamber view at 120° can be quite useful, in addition to the bicommissural view at 60°. 3D and multiplanar imaging should be employed where possible to guide clip positioning and orientation. 3D en-face imaging from a left atrial view shows clip orientation well in order to grasp the leaflets perpendicular to the line of coaptation (Figure 36.2a).

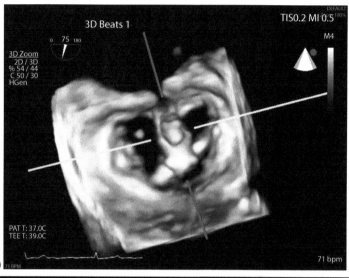

(a)

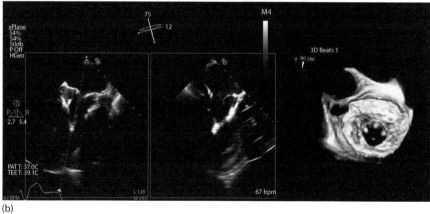

(b)

Figure 36.2 **(a)** Three-dimensional en-face view of MitraClip rotational orientation (tilted vertical line) appropriately perpendicular to line of coaptation (tilted horizontal line). **(b)** Multiplanar view of transcatheter mitral valve replacement in situ, with three-dimensional en-face view (from left atrium) on far right panel.

2D multiplanar imaging of the mitral valve is then used for the actual 'grasp'. Whenever the delivery system is advanced, the 3D en-face view should be reassessed to ensure optimal rotational alignment of the clip. Following placement of the clip, the degree of residual MR should be quantified as should be the degree of mitral stenosis. Evidence of leaflet tear or perforation should also be sought.

TEE can also be used to assist with transcatheter occlusion of periprosthetic mitral valve leak in surgical valves with periprosthetic regurgitation.[3,4] In addition to percutaneous repair techniques, transcatheter mitral valve replacement is also emerging as a means of effectively treating MR in non-surgical patients.[5] The Tendyne transcatheter mitral valve replacement[6] is one such device, and relies on good 3D transoesophageal imaging for deployment (Figure 36.2b).

PERCUTANEOUS MITRAL VALVE BALLOON VALVULOPLASTY

Percutaneous balloon mitral valvuloplasty is a useful therapy for rheumatic mitral valve stenosis (see Chapter 38). Prior to the procedure, the suitability of the mitral valve for ballooning using standard scoring systems, such as the Wilkins score,[7] should be assessed. The optimal view for suitability scoring, if available, is often the short axis view of the mitral valve in the parasternal window on TTE, rather than TEE. Intra-procedurally, prior to proceeding, the left atrial appendage should be checked for thrombus, which represents a contraindication to balloon valvuloplasty. The initial approach to balloon valvuloplasty is similar to the MitraClip procedure with a trans-septal puncture. Following this, TEE should guide optimal positioning of the balloon and should document the degree of stenosis and/or the creation of any significant regurgitation following ballooning. Short axis imaging from a transgastric approach can be useful.

TRANSCATHETER AORTIC VALVE IMPLANT/REPLACEMENT (TAVI/TAVR)

TAVI can be performed without TEE; however, TEE plays an important role in aiding deployment and assessing valve positioning and function, so many operators employ TEE during TAVI. The role of TEE is to coordinate with fluoroscopic imaging in order to provide the interventionalist with a more complete information set to plan and execute device deployment and confirm device function. The long axis view of the aortic valve in 120° allows good visualisation of the aortic and mitral valve, the left ventricular outflow tract and the proximal aorta. The short axis aortic valve view at 30° is useful in identifying locations of paravalvular leak. A mild degree of paravalvular leak can be expected on TEE following a successful TAVI; however, moderate or severe AR suggests a suboptimal result. The other key role of TEE is to help avoid injury to the mitral valve during instrumentation and deployment of the TAVI device. Visualisation of the aortic root for dissection or haematoma is also a valuable function of TEE. 3D imaging may also be used to assist with device sizing, using multiplanar annular and coronary height measurement.

ATRIAL SEPTAL DEFECT AND PATENT FORAMEN OVALE

TEE plays a vital role in atrial septal defect and patent foramen ovale closure. While some operators can close a patent foramen ovale without TEE, atrial septal defect closure requires echocardiographic imaging by TEE or ICE routinely. Echocardiography facilitates appropriate device sizing, deployment, and checking for apposition of both sides of the closure device. The TEE working views are as described for trans-septal puncture, and once again multiplanar and 3D imaging can prove useful. The primary focus during deployment is to ensure that there is a lip of the occlusion device on each side of the inter-atrial septum, in order to prevent device prolapse through the septal defect. A small amount of hub flow seen mid device is normal post deployment but flow around the device across the inter-atrial septum should raise concern for a suboptimal deployment. 3D imaging can be quite useful when multiple atrial septal defects are closed during a single procedure, in order to plan for potential device overlap when sizing (Figure 36.3).[8] Three-dimensional en-face and cross-sectional imaging can also confirm correct position of the occlusion device before its release.

LEFT ATRIAL APPENDAGE OCCLUSION DEVICE

TEE is central to successful percutaneous closure of the left atrial appendage using a closure device. Pre-operative TEE should be done to confirm the absence of thrombus and plan for device sizing and technical approach. Following trans-septal puncture

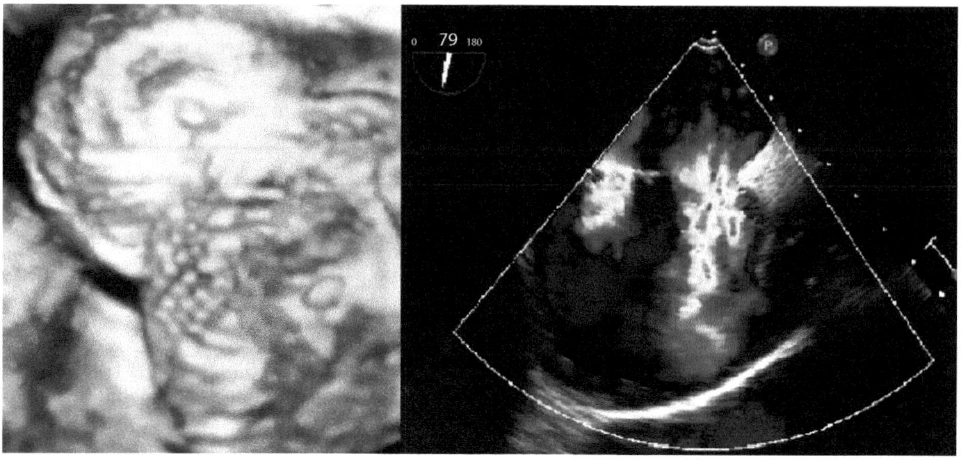

Figure 36.3 Three-dimensional view of double atrial septal defect occlusion device deployment showing overlap (left) that allowed successful simultaneous closure of two large atrial septal defects, as shown by Doppler imaging (right).

guidance, measurements of left atrial appendage depth and orifice diameter should occur at 4 standard views (0°, 45°, 90° and 135°) to confirm device sizing. It should be noted that as patients are fasted, their volume status may lead to underestimation of appendage size and, as such, fluid loading should be done prior to device implant sizing in order to reflect true baseline non-fasted state. This is when comparison to pre-operative imaging is valuable. Intra-procedurally, thrombus should be excluded again before instrumentation of the left atrium. Following deployment, TEE should confirm adequate device compression into the appendage and check for flow around the device into the appendage. The goal is for haemodynamic isolation of the left atrial appendage with no residual communication with the left atrium. A 6 week post-procedure TEE can be done to evaluate for residual flow around the device (of which flow less than 5 mm in maximal diameter is considered an acceptable result)

TRICUSPID VALVE REPAIR

Percutaneous tricuspid valve repair is an emerging technique using, at this early point in its development, either pledgetted sutures to convert the tricuspid valve into a bicuspid valve (Mitralign) or to employ the MitraClip in the tricuspid position. Dedicated tricuspid devices are also being evaluated. Optimal imaging is difficult, particularly the en-face view, but a combination of imaging at 0°, 30° and 160° in addition to rotation of 3D imagery to facilitate live 3D en-face views can combine to facilitate the procedure.

OTHER PROCEDURES

TEE can be valuable in confirming cannula positioning in extra-corporeal membrane oxygenation initiation, during electrophysiology ablation procedures for trans-septal puncture, alcohol septal ablation and to guide coronary sinus instrumentation. An important note is that during atrial fibrillation ablation, some operators prefer withdrawal of the TEE probe following confirmation of safe trans-septal puncture and lack of atrial appendage thrombus, in order to minimise the risk of oesophageal perforation during actual ablation.

OTHER ECHOCARDIOGRAPHIC MODALITIES

Pericardiocentesis is best guided by transthoracic imaging from the subcostal or apical approach depending on the largest window of fluid and operator preference. Similarly, endomyocardial biopsy can be guided by TTE when the samples are being taken in non-transplanted hearts for diagnostic purposes (we prefer using fluoroscopy alone in the post-transplant surveillance population). The bioptome tip should be seen to cross the tricuspid valve and target the mid interventricular septum.

Caution should be taken to ensure jaws are visible before the 'bite' and the interventionalist should also monitor fluoroscopy position to ensure the bioptome does not inadvertently prolapse into the right ventricular outflow tract. Post-procedure effusion should be excluded following biopsy. ICE can be used for a variety of procedures where TEE is helpful to facilitate echocardiographic views from within the heart itself. ICE can be beneficial in providing near-field imaging and avoiding the need for oesophageal intubation—particularly for procedures where sedation is minimal and procedure time is long.[9] It is less widely available and more expensive than TEE, provides less comprehensive imaging, and is less well developed but is nonetheless an important tool that can be used to good effect in certain situations.

CONCLUSIONS

TEE is a widely available and relatively safe, portable imaging modality with excellent temporal resolution, making it ideal to guide intracardiac interventions. Its development has progressed in parallel with advances in interventional cardiology, and the symbiosis of interventional cardiology and cardiac imaging will no doubt continue to flourish in the years to come. The future of interventional TEE is exciting. TEE can now be integrated with fluoroscopic imaging to provide hybrid imaging that can be of great use to the interventionalist.[10] As 3D imaging technology increases, we suspect the ability to guide and navigate the heart using real-time 3D imaging will become considerably easier and more accessible, facilitating wider interventional capability. Investigators are also working on merging echocardiographic and magnetic resonance imaging during intervention to facilitate even better imaging guidance, combining the strengths of both modalities.[11,12] Awareness of the key principles of TEE use can help those involved in cardiovascular interventions obtain the most from this powerful tool.

REFERENCES

1. Picard MH, Passeri JJ, Dal-Bianco JP. *Intraprocedural Imaging of Cardiovascular Interventions.* Cham, Switzerland: Springer; 2016.

2. Reeves ST, Finley AC, Skubas NJ, Swaminathan M, Whitley WS, Glas KE, et al. Basic perioperative transesophageal echocardiography examination: A consensus statement of the American Society of Echocardiography and the Society of Cardiovascular Anesthesiologists. *J Am Soc Echocardiogr.* 2013;26(5):443–456.

3. Pislaru SV, Michelena HI, Mankad SV. Interventional echocardiography. *Prog Cardiovasc Dis.* 2014;57(1):32–46.

4. Patrianakos A, Zacharaki A, Skalidis E, Hamilos M, Parthenakis F, Vardas P. The growing role of echocardiography in interventional cardiology: The present and the future. *Hellenic J Cardiol.* 2017;58(1):17–31.

5. Regueiro A, Granada JF, Dagenais F, Rodes-Cabau J. Transcatheter mitral valve replacement: Insights from early clinical experience and future challenges. *J Am Coll Cardiol.* 2017;69:2175–92.

6. Muller DW, Farivar RS, Jansz P, Bae R, Walters D, Clarke A, et al., Transcatheter mitral valve replacement for patients with symptomatic mitral regurgitation: A global feasibility trial. *J Am Coll Cardiol.* 2017;69:381–391.

7. Wilkins G, Weyman AE, Abascal V, Block P, Palacios I. Percutaneous balloon dilatation of the mitral valve: An analysis of echocardiographic variables related to outcome and the mechanism of dilatation. *Heart.* 1988;60(4):299–308.

8. Namasivayam M, Baron DW, Feneley MP. Transcatheter deployment of two atrial septal defect closure devices using 3-dimensional transoesophageal echocardiography guidance. *Intl J Cardiol.* 2016;207:231–232.

9. Hijazi ZM, Shivkumar K, Sahn DJ. Intracardiac echocardiography during interventional and electrophysiological cardiac catheterization. *Circulation.* 2009;119(4):587–596.

10. Faletra FF, Pedrazzini G, Pasotti E, Murzilli R, Leo LA, Moccetti T. Echocardiography-X-ray image fusion. *JACC Cardiovasc Imag.* 2016;9(9):1114–1117.

11. Sherwood V, Civale J, Rivens I, Collins DJ, Leach MO, ter Haar GR. Development of a hybrid magnetic resonance and ultrasound imaging system. *Biomed Res Intl.* 2014;2014, Article ID 914347, 16 pages.

12. Preiswerk F, Toews M, Cheng CC, Chiou Jr YG, Mei CS, Schaefer LF, et al. Hybrid MRI-ultrasound acquisitions, and scannerless real-time imaging. *Magn Reson Med.* 2017;78(3):897–908.

37

Interventions for congenital heart disease

DAVID W. M. MULLER

INTRODUCTION

The remarkable progress made recently in the design and development of devices for percutaneous coronary interventions has been paralleled by bioengineering triumphs that allow the treatment of a range of structural heart diseases, including congenital heart disorders. These procedures include closure of atrial and ventricular septal defects, patent ductus arteriosus and foramen ovale defects, and aorto-coronary fistulae. Balloon dilatation of valvular stenoses, closure of septal defects, and stenting of aortic coarctation are now routinely performed. This chapter deals with some of the interventions for congenital heart disease that are performed in adult cardiac catheterisation laboratories.

CLOSURE OF SEPTAL DEFECTS

Percutaneous management of congenital atrial and ventricular septal defects has been feasible for several decades. Some of the early prototypes were difficult to position and deploy, could not be retrieved once deployed, and had design defects that, in several instances, led to their recall. Of the devices currently available, the Amplatzer septal occlusion device (St. Jude Medical, Saint Paul, MN, USA) and the Occlutech device (Occlutech GmbH, Jena, Germany) appear to be the most robust, and most readily placed and retrieved.

Atrial septal defect (ASD)

Atrial septal defects may occur in the region of the foramen ovale (ostium secundum defects), at the junction of the superior vena cava and right atrium (sinus venosus defects), or as part of an endocardial cushion defect (ostium primum defect). The ostium secundum atrial septal defect (ASD) is the most common congenital defect encountered in adults. It accounts for approximately 7% of all congenital heart disease and for 30%–40% of all patients presenting with a congenital defect in adult life. ASDs occur more frequently in women than in men, with a female to male ratio of 1.5–2.0:1.[1] They can be multiple and can be associated with excessive mobility of the surrounding septum. Sinus venosus defects are commonly associated with anomalous drainage of the right upper and lower pulmonary veins into the right atrium. Ostium primum defects are usually associated with other developmental defects of the endocardial cushion (the fibrous structure that forms the tricuspid and mitral valve annuli), such as a cleft mitral valve and a membranous ventricular septal defect. Ostium primum and sinus venosus defects are not suitable for percutaneous closure since the accompanying abnormalities usually require surgical correction.

Isolated ASDs are commonly asymptomatic during the first three decades of life. Most often, they are diagnosed following a routine physical examination, a routine chest X-ray, or an echocardiogram performed for atypical symptoms. Approximately 70% of patients with an ASD are symptomatic by the 5th decade, but the morbidity and mortality of the condition rise quickly during the 6th decade. Almost 50% have at least mild pulmonary hypertension by the age of 40 years. Those few patients who develop severe pulmonary hypertension, with or without shunt reversal (Eisenmenger's syndrome), usually do so within several years of birth. When symptoms do occur, they usually consist of exertional fatigue, breathlessness, and palpitations. Ultimately, long-standing right ventricular volume overload and pulmonary hypertension may result in right heart failure, atrial arrhythmias, and stroke due to atrial thrombus formation or paradoxical embolism.

The functional significance of an ASD is determined in the cardiac catheterisation laboratory by oximetry studies (see Chapter 16) and calculation of the pulmonary to systemic flow ratio (Qp/Qs). The conventional criterion for closure of an ASD is a Qp/Qs ratio ≥1.5:1. However, closure is now typically recommended if there is echocardiographic evidence of right ventricular volume overload, regardless of the calculated shunt ratio. Surgical closure requires cardiopulmonary bypass, a right atriotomy, and primary closure or closure using a pericardial or synthetic patch. Although the mortality risk for otherwise healthy young patients is very low, the risk is higher in older patients with co-morbidities. The morbidity, cost, and inconvenience are also considerable for patients of any age.

Several devices have been designed for percutaneous treatment of septal defects.[2-7] The Amplatzer septal occlusion device (St. Jude Medical, Saint Paul, MN, USA) is a self-expanding, self-centering double disc made from 0.004 to 0.005 in nitinol (Figure 37.1).[5,6] The left atrial disc is 7 mm larger in diameter than the waist diameter, and the right atrial disc is 5 mm larger than the waist. Each disc

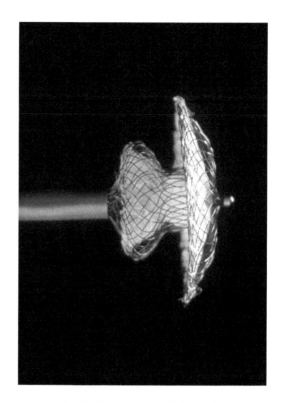

Figure 37.1 The Amplatzer atrial septal occlusion device shown with delivery sheath immediately prior to deployment.

has a central, thin polyester membrane that contributes to early closure of the defect and promotes endothelialisation. Devices are available in 1 mm increments with central waist sizes ranging from 4 to 38 mm. The device size is selected according to the size of the defect, with a central waist diameter 1–2 mm larger than the balloon-stretched diameter of the defect. Devices up to 20 mm can be deployed through an 8 Fr sheath; those between 20 and 26 mm require a 9 Fr sheath; those between 26 and 30 mm can be deployed through a 10 Fr sheath; and larger sizes require a 12 Fr delivery sheath.

Placement of atrial septal occlusion devices is most reliably performed using transoesophageal echocardiographic guidance but can also be performed using intra-cardiac echocardiography (ICE). Direct measurement of the defect by echocardiography underestimates the true size, but more accurate estimates can be made using a customised sizing balloon. A thorough initial assessment of the septum should be performed to ensure there are no associated congenital anomalies (such as anomalous pulmonary venous drainage) and

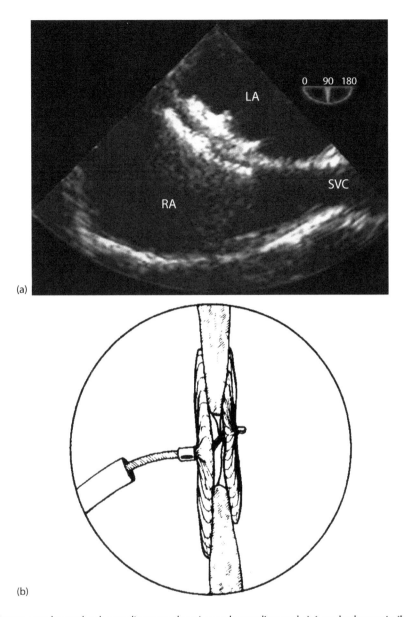

(a)

(b)

Figure 37.2 Transoesophageal echocardiogram showing echocardiograph **(a)** and schematic **(b)** of the Amplatzer septal occlusion device in situ. (Courtesy of AGA Medical Corporation, St. Jude Medical/Abbott.)

that there is only a single defect. Once the device has been deployed, correct positioning is confirmed by fluoroscopy and echocardiographic criteria before the delivery cable is unscrewed, leaving the device in situ (Figure 37.2). In the case of multiple defects, it may be necessary to place a second device. Post-operative care is as for coronary stenting and most patients can be discharged from hospital on the first post-operative day. Animal studies have shown that endothelialisation of the metal struts is usually complete within 3–4 months.[5] Daily antiplatelet therapy, and antibiotic prophylaxis for dental procedures, should be given for 6 months to minimise the risks of thrombus formation or infective endocarditis.

Worldwide experience with the Amplatzer device is extensive. Other devices used for ASD closure include the Occlutech device (Occlutech GmbH, Jena, Germany), the Gore Helex or GSO device (WL Gore & Associates, Newark, DE, USA) and the biodegradable Biostar device (BIO-STAR, NMT Medical, Boston, MA, USA). Complications following use of these devices have been infrequent but can include stroke, infective endocarditis, cardiac perforation, aortic erosion, and cardiac arrhythmias.[8] Atrial fibrillation (AF) occurs infrequently in the early post-operative period but, to date, has not been a significant long-term issue. However, late AF or flutter has been reported in as many as 50%–60% of patients after surgical ASD closure,[9] raising the possibility that very late atrial arrhythmias could still occur after percutaneous ASD closure.

Patent foramen ovale (PFO)

Similar devices are also available for closure of a PFO in patients with a history of paradoxical thrombo-embolism. After birth, the left-sided septum primum and the right-sided septum secundum, which overlap to form the atrial septum, typically fuse and prevent flow between the left and right atria. However, in 20% or more of the adult population, the foramen remains patent.[10,11] In some, this can be associated with excessive mobility of the septum. Excursion of the septum by more than 10 mm from the midline is denoted by the term septal aneurysm, an entity associated with an increased risk of recurrent cryptogenic stroke. Occasionally, septal aneurysms can be multiply-perforated (fenestrated). Neither the PFO nor the unfenestrated septal aneurysm is of any haemodynamic consequence. However, under certain circumstances, right-to-left shunting can occur. During the inspiration that follows straining or the Valsalva manoeuvre, a fall in intrathoracic pressure causes a rapid increase in venous blood return, a rise in right atrial pressure, and right atrial distention. If transient right-to-left shunting occurs, small thrombi or other material (air, fat, surgical glue) can cross from the venous to the arterial circulation, causing transient cerebral ischaemia or cerebral infarction, or infarction of other organ systems.

Paradoxical embolism through a PFO is almost always a diagnosis of exclusion. It is unusual to be able to make a definitive diagnosis, although thrombi straddling the atrial septum have occasionally been seen during transoesophageal echocardiography and post mortem studies.[12,13] Approximately 40% of strokes in the adult population are cryptogenic (i.e. no intracranial), carotid or cardiovascular cause can be found. In this group of patients, the incidence of PFO is considerably higher (>50%) than in the general population, particularly in patients younger than 40 years.[14] Most of these individuals do not have a history of deep venous thrombosis or pulmonary embolism, and few have a history or laboratory evidence of an underlying thrombotic disorder. Recurrent stroke may occur in spite of anticoagulation therapy, particularly if the PFO is associated with an atrial septal aneurysm.[15] Because of this risk of recurrence, and the risks associated with lifelong anticoagulant therapy, percutaneous PFO closure is now an accepted option in patients who have had an unequivocal neurological event and in whom no other cardiac or vascular cause can be found.[7,16]

Until recently, the evidence supporting PFO closure after cryptogenic stroke or systemic embolism was not strong. However, a series of three studies published in 2017 showed a consistent benefit of closure in reducing recurrent stroke.[17-19] The CLOSE trial[17] enrolled 663 patients with a PFO and atrial septal aneurysm or large inter-atrial shunt. The patients were randomised in a 1:1:1 ratio to closure using any of 11 devices approved in Europe, antiplatelet therapy or oral anticoagulation, and were followed for 5.3 ± 2.0 years. There were no recurrent strokes in the closure group, compared with an incidence of 6.0% in the antiplatelet group (hazard ratio 0.03, $p < 0.001$). New AF occurred in 4.6% of the closure group compared with 0.9% of the antiplatelet therapy group ($p = 0.02$), but atrial arrhythmias occurred infrequently after the first 4 post-operative weeks.[17] Adverse outcomes were numerically lower in the anticoagulation group compared with the antiplatelet group, but these differences were not statistically significant. Similarly, the REDUCE trial[19] showed a recurrent stroke rate of 5.4% in the medically-treated group compared with 1.4% in the group treated with the Gore HELEX device (HR 0.23, $p = 0.002$), and the 980 patient RESPECT trial[18] showed a hazard ratio of 0.55 ($p = 0.046$) in patients treated with the Amplatzer PFO septal occluder.

The Amplatzer PFO device is similar in design to the Amplatzer ASD occlusion device, with several modifications.[7,16] The PFO device has a larger right atrial disc (26 mm) than left atrial disc (18 mm) and has a narrow waist. A smaller device with equally sized discs (18 mm), and a larger device (35 mm diameter) are also available. The larger size is recommended for patients with a very redundant (aneurysmal) atrial septum. It is important in using any of the PFO devices that the catheter used to cross the septum (typically a Multipurpose diagnostic coronary catheter) passes through the foramen rather than through the membrane adjacent to the foramen. In the latter case, the device may fail to close the defect. Once the septum has been crossed appropriately, deployment of the device is straightforward, with sequential release of the left and right atrial discs on either side of the atrial septum. As for ASD closures, transoesophageal echocardiography (or ICE) is valuable for ensuring correct positioning of the device and complete closure of the foramen. However, it is not mandatory, as the PFO can almost always be crossed under fluoroscopic guidance using a 0.035 in guidewire, with deployment also guided by fluoroscopic landmarks.

Ventricular septal defect (VSD)

Defects of the ventricular septum are among the most common congenital cardiac anomalies seen clinically. Sub-pulmonary or 'supracristal' defects lie above a muscular ridge in the right ventricular outflow tract called the crista supraventricularis. Defects below the crista may be in the region of the membranous septum ('membranous' VSDs) or in the muscular portion of the septum ('muscular' VSDs). Membranous VSDs are the most common form; muscular VSDs are commonly multiple. Like atrial septal defects, VSDs are generally well tolerated, although severe pulmonary hypertension and shunt reversal (Eisenmenger's syndrome) may occur. Many children with congenital VSDs do not require treatment, since spontaneous closure often occurs during the first decade of life. However, defects that are still present at 8–10 years of age are unlikely to close spontaneously and should be closed if a functionally significant left-to-right shunt is detected. Surgical closure is generally well tolerated, but is associated with significant morbidity and mortality, especially if multiple muscular defects are present.[20]

The Amplatzer ventricular septal closure device is similar in concept to the ASD device but has a thicker waist and symmetrical right and left ventricular discs. Balloon sizing is usually not required, as sizing by transoesophageal echocardiography is more reliable than for sizing ASDs. Muscular defects can be closed using either a venous or an arterial approach. They are most readily crossed from the left ventricular side. In children, in whom use of large calibre sheaths in the femoral artery might lead to significant vascular injury, it is safest to pass a wire from the arterial side and to retrieve it through the femoral or internal jugular vein using a snare. The device can then be deployed from the right ventricular side without risk of arterial injury.[21] In adults, delivery from the arterial (left ventricular) side can be performed. This may also be necessary in children if the delivery sheath kinks when used from the right ventricular side. Closure of VSDs is technically more challenging than closure of atrial defects, having longer fluoroscopy and procedure times. However, the results are favourable with a low incidence of complications and a high closure rate.[21] Like many complex procedures, results are likely to be best in experienced hands.

PATENT DUCTUS ARTERIOSUS (PDA)

The same technology that has been used for atrial and ventricular septal defects has been used for closure of PDA defects. The ductus arteriosus connects the pulmonary artery to the descending aorta at the level of the origin of the subclavian artery. During fetal life, venous blood is shunted from the pulmonary artery through the ductus to the arterial circulation, bypassing the developing pulmonary circulation. After birth, the ductus usually closes to form the ligamentum arteriosum. In children in whom the ductus remains patent, a left-to-right shunt develops after birth, with oxygenated blood passing from the aorta to the pulmonary artery. Severe pulmonary hypertension may occur and cause shunt reversal and Eisenmenger's syndrome.

Closure of the ductus can be accomplished surgically or by transcatheter means, even in very small and pre-term infants.[22] A specifically designed Amplatzer device (Amplatzer Duct Occluder II) can be used for large defects (Figure 37.3).[23] The champagne cork-shaped device is deployed from the pulmonary arterial side. In adults, it is technically easier to cross the defect with an exchange wire from the aortic side and to then snare it from the pulmonary artery or internal jugular

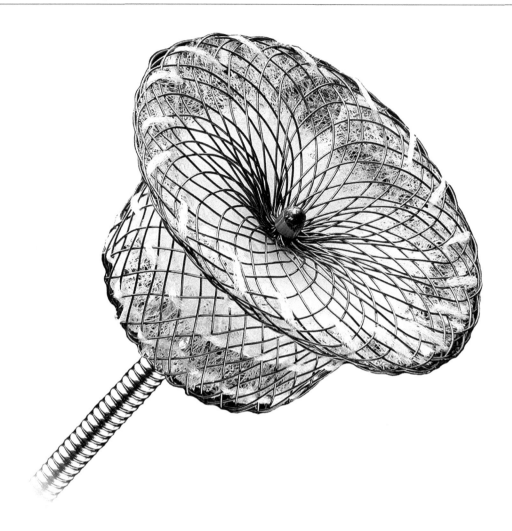

Figure 37.3 Amplatzer duct occluder. (Courtesy of St. Jude Medical.)

vein. Once the delivery sheath has been passed across the defect from the pulmonary artery to the aorta, the disc of the device is deployed in the aorta, and the whole system is pulled back until it is wedged in the ductus. Occlusion of the ductus is confirmed by aortography before the cable is detached. The procedure is a very viable and convenient alternative to surgical closure.

AORTIC COARCTATION

Another relatively common congenital anomaly (5%–7% of congenital heart disease) that can present for the first time in adulthood is coarctation of the aorta. This most commonly results in a focal stricture of the descending thoracic aorta, adjacent to the ductus arteriosus or its remnant, the ligamentum arteriosum. It can also be associated with hypoplasia of the aortic arch or descending aorta or narrowing of the abdominal aorta. Coarctation has an incidence of approximately 3 per 10,000 births and may be associated with other congenital cardiac disorders including bicuspid aortic valve and dilatation of the ascending aorta, VSD, PDA, atrioventricular cushion defects and left heart hypoplasia. It may also be associated with intracranial aneurysms. It is most commonly first recognised in young adults with hypertension but may also cause lower limb claudication. Treatment is recommended if there is a >20 mmHg peak-to-peak gradient across the coarctation.[24]

Surgical resection with interposition grafting, and patch aortoplasty have been described but carry a risk of paraparesis due to spinal cord ischaemia, recoarctation and aneurysm formation. Balloon aortic angioplasty was described in 1982,[25] and endovascular stent placement in 1991.[26] Aortic wall complications (dissection, aneurysm formation) and recoarctation remain potential complications. In the COAST trial,[27] the Numed (Hopkinton, NY) Cheatham Platinum stent was evaluated in 105 children and adults. There were no deaths or serious adverse events. All patients had an immediate reduction in blood pressure difference between upper and lower limbs. At 2-year follow-up, aneurysms were identified in 6 patients (5.7%) and stent fractures in 11 patients (10.5%). More recently, covered stents have been used in an attempt to reduce the incidence of aortic wall injury and late aneurysm formation.[28,29] To date, however, there does not appear to be a difference in acute or long-term incidence of aortic wall injury.[28] Observational data suggest that the larger access diameter required for delivery of the coated stent might also be associated with an increased risk of femoral arterial injury.[29]

REFERENCES

1. Kaplan S. Congenital heart disease in adolescents and adults: Natural and postoperative history across age groups. *Cardiol Clin.* 1993;11(4):543–556.
2. Bridges ND, Hellenbrand W, Latson L, Filiano J, Newburger JW, Lock JE. Transcatheter closure of patent foramen ovale after presumed paradoxical embolism. *Circulation.* 1992;86(6):1902–1908.
3. Ende DJ, Chopra PS, Rao PS. Transcatheter closure of atrial septal defect or patent foramen ovale with the buttoned device for prevention of recurrence of paradoxic embolism. *Am J Cardiol.* 1996;78(2):233–236.
4. Rome JJ, Keane JF, Perry SB, Spevak PJ, Lock JE. Double-umbrella closure of atrial defects. Initial clinical applications. *Circulation.* 1990;82(3):751–758.
5. Sharafuddin MJ, Gu X, Titus JL, Urness M, Cervera-Ceballos JJ, Amplatz K. Transvenous closure of secundum atrial septal defects: Preliminary results with a new self-expanding nitinol prosthesis in a swine model. *Circulation.* 1997;95(8):2162–2168.
6. Thanopoulos BD, Laskari CV, Tsaousis GS, Zarayelyan A, Vekiou A, Papadopoulos GS. Closure of atrial septal defects with the Amplatzer occlusion device: Preliminary results. *J Am Coll Cardiol.* 1998;31(5):1110–1116.
7. Windecker S, Meier B. Percutaneous patent foramen ovale (PFO) closure: It can be done but should it? *Catheter Cardiovasc Interv.* 1999;47(3):377–380.
8. Jalal Z, Hascoet S, Gronier C, Godart F, Mauri L, Dauphin C, et al. Long-term outcomes after percutaneous closure of ostium secundum atrial septal defect in the young: A nationwide cohort study. *JACC Cardiovasc Interv.* 2018;11(8):795–804.
9. Konstantinides S, Geibel A, Olschewski M, Gornandt L, Roskamm H, Spillner G, et al. A comparison of surgical and medical therapy for atrial septal defect in adults. *N Engl J Med.* 1995;333(8):469–473.
10. Hagen PT, Scholz DG, Edwards WD. Incidence and size of patent foramen ovale during the first 10 decades of life: An autopsy study of 965 normal hearts. *Mayo Clin Proc.* 1984;59(1):17–20.
11. Lynch JJ, Schuchard GH, Gross CM, Wann LS. Prevalence of right-to-left atrial shunting in a healthy population: Detection by Valsalva maneuver contrast echocardiography. *Am J Cardiol.* 1984;53(10):1478–1480.
12. Johnson BI. Paradoxical embolism. *J Clin Pathol.* 1951;4(3):316–332.
13. Nellessen U, Daniel WG, Matheis G, Oelert H, Depping K, Lichtlen PR. Impending paradoxical embolism from atrial thrombus: Correct diagnosis by transesophageal echocardiography and prevention by surgery. *J Am Coll Cardiol.* 1985;5(4):1002–1004.
14. Webster MW, Chancellor AM, Smith HJ, Swift DL, Sharpe DN, Bass NM, et al. Patent foramen ovale in young stroke patients. *Lancet.* 1988;2(8601):11–12.
15. Mugge A, Daniel WG, Angermann C, Spes C, Khandheria BK, Kronzon I, et al.

Atrial septal aneurysm in adult patients: A multicenter study using transthoracic and transesophageal echocardiography. *Circulation*. 1995;91(11):2785–2792.

16. Han YM, Gu X, Titus JL, Rickers C, Bass JL, Urness M, et al. New self-expanding patent foramen ovale occlusion device. *Catheter Cardiovasc Interv*. 1999;47(3):370–376.

17. Mas JL, Derumeaux G, Guillon B, Massardier E, Hosseini H, Mechtouff L, et al. Patent foramen ovale closure or anticoagulation vs. antiplatelets after stroke. *N Engl J Med*. 2017;377(11):1011–1021.

18. Saver JL, Carroll JD, Thaler DE, Smalling RW, MacDonald LA, Marks DS, et al. Long-term outcomes of patent foramen ovale closure or medical therapy after stroke. *N Engl J Med*. 2017;377(11):1022–1032.

19. Sondergaard L, Kasner SE, Rhodes JF, Andersen G, Iversen HK, Nielsen-Kudsk JE, et al. Patent foramen ovale closure or antiplatelet therapy for cryptogenic stroke. *N Engl J Med*. 2017;377(11):1033–1042.

20. Kitagawa T, Durham LA, 3rd, Mosca RS, Bove EL. Techniques and results in the management of multiple ventricular septal defects. *J Thorac Cardiovasc Surg*. 1998;115(4):848–856.

21. Hijazi ZM, Hakim F, Al-Fadley F, Abdelhamid J, Cao QL. Transcatheter closure of single muscular ventricular septal defects using the Amplatzer muscular VSD occluder: Initial results and technical considerations. *Catheter Cardiovasc Interv*. 2000;49(2):167–172.

22. McElhinney DB. Small and preterm infants: The shrinking frontier of transcatheter patent ductus arteriosus closure. *Catheter Cardiovasc Interv*. 2017;89(6):1066–1068.

23. Masura J, Walsh KP, Thanopoulous B, Chan C, Bass J, Goussous Y, et al. Catheter closure of moderate- to large-sized patent ductus arteriosus using the new amplatzer duct occluder: Immediate and short-term results. *J Am Coll Cardiol*. 1998;31(4):878–882.

24. Warnes CA, Williams RG, Bashore TM, Child JS, Connolly HM, Dearani JA, et al. ACC/AHA 2008 guidelines for the management of adults with congenital heart disease: A report of the American College of Cardiology/American Heart Association task force on practice guidelines (Writing Committee to develop guidelines on the management of adults with congenital heart disease). Developed in collaboration with the American Society of Echocardiography, Heart Rhythm Society, International Society for Adult Congenital Heart Disease, Society for Cardiovascular Angiography and Interventions, and Society of Thoracic Surgeons. *J Am Coll Cardiol*. 2008;52(23):e143–e263.

25. Lock JE, Bass JL, Amplatz K, Fuhrman BP, Castaneda-Zuniga W. Balloon dilation angioplasty of aortic coarctations in infants and children. *Circulation*. 1983;68(1):109–116.

26. O'Laughlin MP, Perry SB, Lock JE, Mullins CE. Use of endovascular stents in congenital heart disease. *Circulation*. 1991;83(6):1923–1939.

27. Meadows J, Minahan M, McElhinney DB, McEnaney K, Ringel R. Intermediate outcomes in the prospective, multicenter coarctation of the aorta stent trial (COAST). *Circulation*. 2015;131(19):1656–1664.

28. Sohrabi B, Jamshidi P, Yaghoubi A, Habibzadeh A, Hashemi-Aghdam Y, Moin A, et al. Comparison between covered and bare Cheatham-Platinum stents for endovascular treatment of patients with native post-ductal aortic coarctation: Immediate and intermediate-term results. *JACC Cardiovasc Interv*. 2014;7(4):416–423.

29. Taggart NW, Minahan M, Cabalka AK, Cetta F, Usmani K, Ringel RE. Immediate outcomes of covered stent placement for treatment or prevention of aortic wall injury associated with coarctation of the aorta (COAST II). *JACC Cardiovasc Interv*. 2016;9(5):484–493.

38

Mitral valvuloplasty: The Inoue balloon dilatation technique

PAUL ROY

INTRODUCTION

Percutaneous transvenous mitral valvuloplasty (PTMV) was first introduced into clinical practice by Inoue and colleagues in 1984 and is now a safe and effective therapy that replaces the need for surgery in many patients with symptomatic mitral stenosis. Worldwide, a procedural success rate greater than 95% has been achieved, with operator experience a determining factor in this outcome.

MITRAL STENOSIS

In normal adults the mitral valve orifice is $4–6\ cm^2$. When the orifice is reduced to approximately $2\ cm^2$ (which is considered mild mitral stenosis) blood flow from the left atrium to the left ventricle occurs only if propelled by an abnormal pressure gradient. When the mitral valve opening is reduced to $1\ cm^2$ (which is considered severe mitral stenosis) a left atrial pressure of approximately 25 mmHg is required to maintain a normal cardiac output. This elevated left atrial pressure in turn raises pulmonary venous and capillary pressures, reducing pulmonary compliance and causing exertional dyspnoea.

PATIENT SELECTION

Once the symptomatic patient has been assessed clinically, careful selection is required to ensure that the valve is suitable for this procedure. Commissural splitting is the dominant mechanism by which mitral valve area is increased by the balloon. Therefore, the extent of fusion, fibrosis or calcification of one or both commissures is a major determinant of the outcome of mitral valvotomy. Patients with pliable valves without severe sub-valvular lesions are ideal candidates, whereas patients with poorly-mobile mitral leaflets, severely fused commissures and significant sub-valvular lesions may obtain less than optimal results and are at higher risk of developing mitral regurgitation.

ECHOCARDIOGRAPHY

Echocardiography allows careful analysis of mitral valve morphologies. Echocardiographic scoring systems based on qualitative assessment of leaflet and sub-valvular morphology were devised to predict the outcome of mitral valvotomy. The specific importance of commissural morphology was for some time neglected but Inoue considered this an important determinant. Echocardiographic studies have confirmed the importance of commissural morphology to the extent that before undertaking mitral balloon valvuloplasty, more reliance is now placed on echocardiographic evaluation of commissural morphology than on other echo-scoring mechanisms.

The procedure is not usually performed if there is more than trivial to mild mitral regurgitation. Presence of thrombus in the left atrial appendage is a relative contraindication. Patients with atrial fibrillation are usually subjected to a transoesophageal echo-Doppler study prior to the procedure to ensure that there is no left atrial thrombus likely to become dislodged. As the atrial septum is punctured during the procedure, any thrombus in the left atrium can easily be dispersed into the circulation. This may be caused either by the transeptal needle if thrombus is on the atrial septum, or by the wire or balloon should either of these enter into the left atrial appendage. If thrombus is present, the patient should be treated with warfarin for 2–3 months, then reassessed by transoesophageal echo before the procedure is undertaken.

Generally, symptoms do not occur until the orifice of the mitral valve is less than 1.5 cm^2 but disabling symptoms do sometimes occur in patients performing heavy physical work with a mitral orifice larger than 1.5 cm^2. In patients whose valve morphology is not ideal for balloon dilatation, associated illnesses prohibiting open heart surgery may nonetheless favour the balloon method. Occasionally pulmonary oedema may result during pregnancy from severe mitral stenosis. In this situation the balloon procedure can be performed as an ideal alternative to surgery. With a pregnant patient it is preferable to wait until after 5 months, when the impact of any x-ray irradiation on the foetus is minimal.

THE PROCEDURE

Patients are admitted to hospital on the day of the procedure having had a transoesophageal echocardiogram and assessment prior to admission.

Echo-Doppler is usually performed in the catheterisation laboratory at the same time as the mitral procedure. A 6F pigtail catheter is passed to the left ventricle via a right femoral artery percutaneous puncture. The purpose of this catheter is to measure left ventricular pressure for estimation of the mitral gradient. It also permits the operator to see exactly where the aorta lies in order to avoid damage during transeptal puncture. Right heart catheterisation is then performed via a sheath from the right femoral vein, and a pigtail catheter is used to perform a right atrial angiogram before commencing.

The next part of the procedure, perforating the inter-atrial septum, is the most delicate and one where an inexperienced operator is most likely to experience serious difficulty, as it requires experience to safely perform a transeptal puncture. The two major problems inherent in this technique are cardiac perforation and puncture of an inappropriate atrial septal site. The former may lead to the serious complications of cardiac tamponade and the latter leads to difficulties in subsequently trying to manoeuvre the Inoue balloon catheter across the mitral orifice.

A simple method is used by Inoue to locate the site of trans-septal puncture, the foramen ovale: by applying a slightly complicated formula, examining flow of contrast from the right atrium through the pulmonary circulation into the left atrium indicates approximately where the foramen ovale is situated on the atrial septum. First, a Brockenbrough needle is passed via the venous sheath into the right atrium and the tip is placed against the selected puncture site. Normally at the point of needle puncture a distinct pulsation can be felt, particularly when there is a high left atrial pressure. When the operator is satisfied with the intended puncture site, the needle is advanced 1 cm across the septum and blood is withdrawn. Measurement of left atrial pressure at this point confirms that the catheter is in the appropriate site. A small amount of pure contrast is also injected, further confirming the left atrial position of the needle tip. Should it transpire that the needle tip is in the aorta or the pericardium, provided the needle only is advanced at this stage, generally no problem will result. It is therefore important at this point not to push the catheter over the needle point until the operator is certain of the position of the needle tip.

Precautionary measurement of right atrial pressure on entry into the right atrium allows the operator to observe any subsequent rise in right atrial pressure that could indicate tamponade from an inappropriate puncture.

If no blood is aspirated when the needle is first passed through the chosen site, this indicates that the needle has either dissected the high septum or is caught in a thickened septum. Staining of the septum with injection of a small amount of contrast easily distinguishes the two.

When the high septum is dissected, myocardial staining spreads in a vertical fashion. In this situation the needle needs to be withdrawn and septal puncture made at a lower site.

When the needle is caught in the thickened septum, the stain takes a more horizontal orientation. If this occurs, it requires some experience to decide whether to persist in this area or attempt puncture at another site. It is not possible to differentiate dissection of the high septum from entrapment of the needle in a thick septum by pressure monitoring alone.

Heparin is usually given at a dose of 5,000 units at the commencement of the procedure with a further 5,000 units once septal puncture is safely performed. While this may appear excessive in the small female patient, it removes the risk that can result if a lengthy delay occurs in trying to cross the mitral orifice with the Inoue catheter. If this occurs, extra heparin is required.

Once septal puncture has been safely performed, the long guiding stilette of the Inoue apparatus is passed into the left atrium. This is an ingenious needle with a long soft curved tip that sits safely in the left atrium but with a very rigid distal end of the shaft allowing passage of the Inoue balloon into the left atrium.

THE INOUE BALLOON

The Inoue balloon has a 12F polyvinyl tube shaft with a co-axial double lumen. The inner lumen of the catheter permits pressure measurement and blood sampling and insertion of metal tube, guide wire or stiletto. The outer lumen connects proximally with a two-way stopcock used to connect the catheter to an inflation/deflation syringe and a vent, distally mounted with a balloon at the end of the shaft.

The balloon is made of double layers of latex tubing and can be transformed into various shapes from its natural form to serve different functions. The balloon is stiffened and slenderised when the rubber balloon is stretched by inserting a metal tube. In this shape the balloon is passed across the atrial septum to minimise the size of the hole used to enter the left atrium. Once in the left atrium, the stretching metal tube is withdrawn and the balloon assumes a more semi-circular shape. Usually at this point a recording of the pressure gradient across the mitral valve is made using the lumen of the Inoue balloon to measure left atrial pressure and the pigtail balloon in the left ventricle to measure left ventricular pressure (Figure 38.1a and b).

Now the balloon is ready to be passed across the mitral valve. A slightly differently shaped wire is then inserted into the Inoue balloon. This wire allows various manoeuvres to be made to attempt to cross the mitral valve with the Inoue balloon. Before commencing this part of the procedure, the distal section of the Inoue balloon is inflated to prevent the balloon slipping back across the atrial septal puncture. Difficulties are sometimes encountered trying to cross the mitral valve. Occasionally a slippery black guide wire through the Inoue lumen allows easier crossing, and very occasionally, use of the Mullins sheath has been described to cross a difficult valve.

Balloon inflation

The Inoue balloon has an ingenious feature called differential compliance that allows the more distal half of the balloon to inflate first when dye is injected into the balloon. Once the distal half of the balloon is inflated, the balloon is pulled back against the mitral valve orifice and the proximal half of the balloon is then inflated. Usually an obvious constriction is seen as a waist in the middle of the balloon where the balloon sits across the mitral valve (Figure 38.1c). This serves to locate the balloon snugly across the valve. Further inflation dilates the waist. It is this third inflation that dilates the mitral opening, splitting the commissures.

Balloon size is chosen according to the patient's height. There is a set formula for this, which is obtained from the manufacturer's information in the balloon kit.

Following the first inflation, it is important to re-measure the pressure gradient across the valve. If the gradient has fallen to less than 5 mmHg this would generally be considered a satisfactory result. It is important at this stage to monitor the v wave in the left atrial trace, which gives a measure of any increasing degree of mitral regurgitation. It may be necessary to slowly increase the size of the Inoue balloon

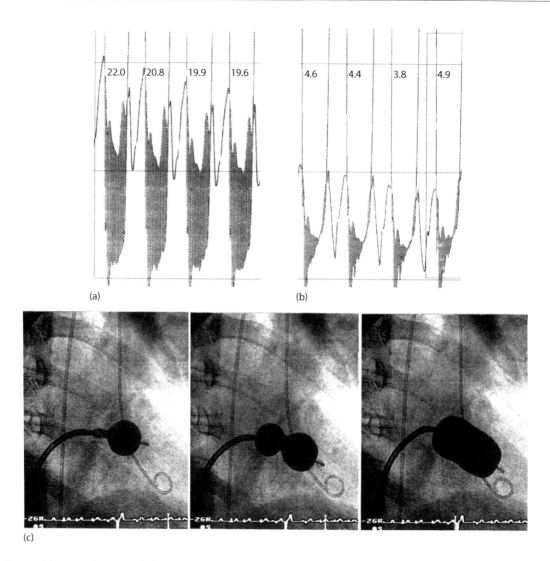

Figure 38.1 Simultaneous left ventricular and left atrial pressure tracings in a patient with severe mitral stenosis before and after mitral balloon valvuloplasty. Mean gradient across the mitral valve (shaded area) was 20.9 mmHg before the procedure (a) and 4.6 mmHg after balloon dilatation (b). (c) The three stages of Inoue balloon inflation. The first inflation dilates the distal end of the balloon, allowing positioning against the mitral orifice. The second inflation dilates the proximal end, locking the waist across the mitral valve. Commissural splitting occurs with the third inflation, which dilates the waist.

until an adequate result is obtained. At first sign of any rise in the v wave, no further dilatation should be made; otherwise, severe mitral regurgitation may occur due to oversplitting of the commissures.

Balloon removal

Once a satisfactory result is achieved, before removing the Inoue balloon catheter from the left atrium, a stretching metal tube needs to be carefully reinserted to slenderise the balloon for withdrawal across the atrial septum from the femoral vein. A 9F sheath is usually inserted over the guide wire after removal of the Inoue balloon, which allows the patient to be immediately removed from the catheter table. Compression of the femoral artery and vein is done in the recovery area.

Prospective randomised clinical trials comparing valvuloplasty and surgical closed mitral commissurotomy have shown no difference in early results or late clinical follow-up, assessed by calculation of mitral valve area during cardiac catheterisation at 7 months and at 3.5 years following the procedures; thus PTMV is now providing results that are comparable with those obtained by surgical closed valvotomy, with low morbidity and mortality. In most countries, cost of the procedure is a fraction of that of surgical treatment and hospital stay is reduced to 24 hours. Prior to the Inoue design, mitral valvuloplasty was undertaken with double balloon techniques that were quite cumbersome. It is a genuine tribute to Kanji Inoue that the methodology has been simplified to such an extent by his ingenious device.

FURTHER READING

Carroll JD, Feldman T. Percutaneous mitral balloon valvotomy and the new demographics of mitral stenosis. *JAMA*. 1993;270(14):1731–1736.

Chen G-Y, Tseng C-D, Chiang F-T, Hsu K-L, Lo H-M, Tseng Y-Z, et al. Congenital mitral stenosis: Challenge of percutaneous transvenous mitral commissurotomy. *Int J Cardiol*. 1997;60(1):99–102.

Inoue K, Owaki T, Nakamura T, Kitamura F, Miyamoto N. Clinical application of transvenous mitral commissurotomy by a new balloon catheter. *J Thorac Cardiovasc Surg*. 1984;87(3):394–402.

Lock JE, Khalilullah M, Shrivastava S, Bahl V, Keane JF. Percutaneous catheter commissurotomy in rheumatic mitral stenosis. *N Engl J Med*. 1985;313(24):1515–1518.

Lokhandwala YY, Banker D, Vora AM, Kerkar PG, Deshpande JR, Kulkarni HL, et al. Emergent balloon mitral valvotomy in patients presenting with cardiac arrest, cardiogenic shock or refractory pulmonary edema. *J Am Coll Cardiol*. 1998;32(1):154–158.

Members ATF, Vahanian A, Alfieri O, Andreotti F, Antunes MJ, Barón-Esquivias G, et al. Guidelines on the management of valvular heart disease (version 2012) The Joint Task Force on the Management of Valvular Heart Disease of the European Society of Cardiology (ESC) and the European Association for Cardio-Thoracic Surgery (EACTS). *Eur Heart J*. 2012;33(19):2451–2496.

Moore P, Adatia I, Spevak PJ, Keane JF, Perry SB, Castaneda AR, et al. Severe congenital mitral stenosis in infants. *Circulation*. 1994;89(5):2099–2106.

Nishimura RA, Otto CM, Bonow RO, Carabello BA, Erwin JP, Guyton RA, et al. 2014 AHA/ACC guideline for the management of patients with valvular heart disease: A report of the American College of Cardiology/American Heart Association Task Force on Practice Guidelines. *J Am Coll Cardiol*. 2014;63(22):e57–e185.

Sutaria N, Elder A, Shaw T. Long term outcome of percutaneous mitral balloon valvotomy in patients aged 70 and over. *Heart*. 2000;83(4):433–438.

39

Transcatheter aortic valve implantation

DAVID A. ROY

INTRODUCTION

Since the first transcatheter aortic valve implantation (TAVI) in 2002,[1] more than 300,000 of these procedures have been performed worldwide. This has resulted in a substantial number of published case series, registries, and randomised controlled trials (RCTs). Diversity in technique and TAVI devices as well as disparity in the learning curve may potentially explain some of the discrepancies in outcomes that have been reported but with time, published data clearly show that outcomes for patients undergoing

TAVI are improving. This improvement has been largely due to better devices, growing operator experience and gradual changes to the TAVI procedure itself. TAVI is also being used in an off-label fashion for patients without native aortic valve stenosis, giving rise to new indications and options for treating patients with valvular disease. This chapter outlines the background, development and current contemporary practice with TAVI as a therapeutic modality for patients with aortic valve disease.

AORTIC STENOSIS (AS)

Calcific AS is a slowly progressive disorder with a disease continuum that ranges from mild valve thickening without obstruction of blood flow, termed aortic sclerosis, to severe calcification with impaired leaflet motion, or AS. Historically, this process was thought to be 'degenerative' because of time-dependent wear-and-tear of the leaflets with passive calcium deposition. Now, there are substantial clinical data and histopathological evidence suggesting that calcific AS is an active process similar to atherosclerosis, with lipoprotein deposition, chronic inflammation, and active leaflet calcification.[2,3]

The normal aortic valve consists of four clearly defined tissue layers: the endothelium, fibrosa, spongiosa, and ventricularis. The ventricularis, on the ventricular side of the leaflet, is composed of elastin-rich fibres that are aligned in a radial direction, perpendicular to the leaflet margin. The fibrosa, on the aortic side of the leaflet, comprises primarily fibroblasts and collagen fibres arranged circumferentially, parallel to the leaflet margin. The spongiosa is a layer of loose connective tissue at the base of the leaflet, between the fibrosa and ventricularis, composed of fibroblasts, mesenchymal cells, and a mucopolysaccharide-rich matrix. At their base, the valve leaflets are attached to a dense collagenous network, called the annulus, which facilitates their attachment to the aortic root and the dissipation of mechanical force. These layers work in concert to provide tensile strength and pliability for decades of repetitive motion.[2–5]

CAUSES AND SYMPTOMS OF AS

The most common causes of AS include senile calcific degeneration of the valve, congenitally bicuspid aortic valve and rheumatic aortic valve disease. In industrialised countries rheumatic fever and rheumatic valvular disease are rare, and rheumatic AS is uncommon. A congenitally bicuspid aortic valve is the second most common congenital cardiac anomaly (second only to mitral valve prolapse) and approximately one-third of these patients will develop AS in their lifetimes. This usually occurs in the fourth to sixth decade of life. In patients older than 65, senile calcification of a tri-leaflet aortic valve is by far the commonest cause of AS.

In the past few decades, landmark studies have described the common risk factors for calcific AS as identified by large epidemiological cohort studies. These include: hyperlipidaemia, hypertension, male gender, renal failure, and diabetes. These studies suggest the traditional risk factors for cardiovascular atherosclerosis are important in the development of calcific AS.[4,6]

DIAGNOSIS AND ASSESSMENT OF AS

Standard measures of AS severity are the maximum velocity (V_{max}) across the stenotic valve, the mean transaortic valve pressure gradient (ΔP mean) calculated with the Bernoulli equation, and the functional aortic valve area (AVA) calculated with the continuity equation. Echocardiographic ΔP mean and AVA calculations have been well validated against invasive measurements and are now the clinical standard of care. AVA calculation is especially important when transaortic volume flow rate is higher than normal (as with coexisting aortic regurgitation) or lower than normal (as with left ventricular dysfunction or a small normally functioning left ventricle [LV]) because transaortic velocities and gradients vary with volume flow rate. In patients with mixed stenosis and regurgitation, the diagnosis of severe valve disease will be evident on the basis of a high transaortic gradient. However, with a low transaortic flow rate, severe AS might be missed if only velocity or pressure gradient data are considered.

MEDICAL MANAGEMENT OF AS

The natural history of untreated AS has been well documented. Classic natural history studies by Ross and Braunwald, Frank et al., and Rapapport have shown that once symptoms such as congestive cardiac failure, syncope or angina develop, the longevity of the patient is shortened significantly.[5,7,8]

There are currently no effective medical treatment options in the treatment of severe AS. Systemic arterial hypertension should be treated cautiously and any hypotension avoided. According to latest evidence-based guidelines,[9] routine endocarditis antibiotic prophylaxis is no longer recommended. Although the active valvular disease process is characterised by lipid accumulation, inflammation and calcification, statin therapy does not reduce disease progression in patients with severe AS.[10,11]

SURGICAL MANAGEMENT OF AS: AORTIC VALVE REPLACEMENT (AVR)

In the 1950s and 1960s, early surgical techniques for treatment of AS included surgical balloon valvuloplasty, valvotomy and valve-sparing surgical debridement of calcium deposits, which was sometimes performed in addition to comissurotomy, particularly in patients with rheumatic AS. The first surgical valve replacements of diseased human heart valves were performed in 1960. In the past five decades, cardiothoracic surgeons have made important advances in the operative techniques and post-operative care of patients with valvular heart disease. Biomedical engineers, in collaboration with cardiologists and cardiothoracic surgeons, have developed both mechanical and bioprosthetic/xenograft valve options for surgical aortic valve replacement.[12-16] Standard access for AVR is through a full median sternotomy, a maximally invasive approach. During AVR, the patient's circulation is maintained using cardiopulmonary bypass; thus, stable haemodynamic function can be guaranteed throughout the procedure. Most importantly, the calcified and degenerated aortic valve cusps are excised during conventional AVR, followed by implantation of a xenograft or mechanical prosthesis using standard suturing techniques.

MINIMALLY INVASIVE AVR AND SUTURELESS VALVES

Minimally invasive access techniques are aimed at reducing the length of incision in order to minimise further the effects of surgical trauma. For so-called minimally invasive AVR, most surgeons use a partial upper mini-sternotomy with a 'J' incision to the third or fourth intercostal space. Cannulation for cardiopulmonary bypass can be accomplished directly through the incision or by means of a femoral venous percutaneous puncture and direct aortic access. Overall, results of minimally invasive AVR are comparable to a complete sternotomy approach.[17,18] In a meta-analysis of 4586 patients (2054 mini-sternotomy vs. 2532 full sternotomy) mini-sternotomy was proven to be as safe as conventional sternotomy for AVR, without increased risk of death or any other major complication.[18] Sutureless valves aim for a fast and reliable implantation after resection of the degenerative calcified native aortic valve. Implantation of sutureless valves is performed by means of a conventional sternotomy or by a minimally invasive approach. Sutureless valves may allow for a more rapid AVR and eventually for a broader penetration of the minimally invasive surgical technique. There may be a specific subset of patients that could particularly benefit from sutureless valves—for example, those at higher surgical risk who require a fast procedure through a smaller incision. In addition, patients with a small aortic root—an anatomical characteristic that can be technically challenging in some patients—would be suitable candidates for sutureless devices.[19]

Patients certainly benefit from preserved stability of the lower sternum, and thus may benefit from improved mobilisation and faster recovery to hospital discharge. Mini-sternotomy remains a significantly invasive approach, however, mandating general anaesthesia and cardiopulmonary bypass. This needs to be kept in mind, particularly when considering surgical AVR for higher-risk patients.

BALLOON AORTIC VALVULOPLASTY

The first use of balloon dilatation (Figure 39.1) to treat AS was reported in 23 paediatric patients in 1984.[20] Soon after, Alain Cribier performed the first balloon aortic valvuloplasty (BAV)/percutaneous transluminal aortic valvuloplasty (PTAV) in an adult with calcific AS in Rouen in September 1985.[21] This technique was reserved for patients with so called non-operable AS, which in the 1980s meant any patient over the age of 75. BAV was associated with midterm improvement in quality of life,[22] explaining its rapid adoption and explosive growth worldwide. However, a lack of survival benefit and a recurrence rate of 80% at 1 year[23,24] led to a dramatic decline in its use.

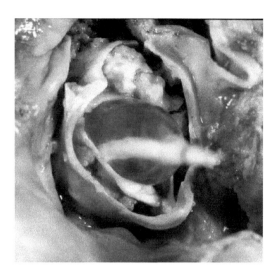

Figure 39.1 Example of balloon dilatation of a stenosed aortic valve.

DEVELOPMENT OF TAVI

By the 1970s, a number of novel projects aimed at treating aortic regurgitation, and explored the concept of a stented valve.[25-27] In 1989, a balloon-expandable catheter-mounted stented valve was implanted within the aorta of pigs by Henning-Rud Andersen. This was performed using an original model handmade mesh containing a porcine valve. The results, published in 1992, were not immediately followed by any work towards human application of this technique.[28]

Various experimental concepts emerged, but these were not developed into models for human use.[29,30] In 2000, Philip Bonhoeffer developed a stented valve made of a bovine jugular vein conduit inserted in a platinum-iridium stent, which was implanted in the pulmonary artery of lambs. Bonhoeffer then performed the first human implantation of this device in a right ventricle to pulmonary artery conduit in 2000,[31,32] which was followed by great interest in the technology not only for this indication, but for other transcatheter valve indications.

Bonhoeffer's work paved the way for the first transcatheter aortic valve implant to be performed by Alain Cribier and his team in 2002. This was performed as an antegrade approach via trans-septal puncture, and the patient survived for 4 months post procedure but succumbed due to complications related to leg ischaemia.[1] A feasibility study

in Europe and Canada soon followed. This prosthesis was balloon expandable, and by 2004 a second self-expanding transcatheter valve had been developed, with early success via a retrograde femoral approach.[33] Refined versions of the balloon expandable and self-expanding transcatheter valves were commercially available by 2007. Since then TAVI has enjoyed an exponential rise in the field of AS, with more than 10 devices now available for use across the globe.

EVIDENCE BASE FOR TAVI

The early days of TAVI

Two devices emerged and became available for compassionate use or as part of registry studies—the Edwards Sapien valve (Edwards Lifesciences, Irvine, California) and the CoreValve (Medtronic Inc, Minneapolis, Minnesota). Data from early registries included patient cohorts consisting of surgically inoperable patients or patients at very high surgical risk. Even in this very high-risk subset of patients, early procedural results were encouraging. The Source registry published outcomes from 2007–2011 on 1,038 patients treated with the Edwards Sapien valve at 32 centres. Results showed total Kaplan Meier 1-year survival of 76.1% overall, 72.1% for transapical and 81.1% for transfemoral patients, and 73.5% of surviving patients were in New York Heart Association (NYHA) class I or II at 1 year. Stroke occurred in 10.2% of patients.[34] A similar registry report using the CoreValve system is the CoreValve Multicentre, Expanded Evaluation Registry.[35] This reported 646 patients and 30-day outcomes. Procedural success was 97%; procedural mortality was 1.5%; 30-day all-cause mortality was 8%; and the combination of death, stroke and myocardial infarction was 9.3%. With this third-generation 18F device the vascular complication rate was low at 1.9%. The incidence of stroke at 30 days was 1.9%, and the requirement for a new permanent pacemaker (PPM) was 9.3%.

These early registries used first-generation TAVI devices, large delivery systems requiring large diameter vascular sheaths, and less sophisticated deployment mechanisms with fewer valve sizes to cover the ranges of aortic annulus anatomy. There was also a 'learning curve', with procedural success rates clearly improving with operator and institutional experience.

The Placement of Aortic Transcatheter Valves (PARTNER) trial was the first RCT comparing TAVI to surgery.[36] At 30 days, TAVI had a lower rate of all-cause death than surgery (3.4 vs. 6.5%; $p = 0.007$), a higher rate of vascular complications (11 vs. 3.2%; $p \leq 0.001$) and a similar risk of stroke. At 1 year all cause death was similar (24.2% vs. 26.8%; $p = 0.44$; $p = 0.001$ for non-inferiority) with an increased risk of stroke 5.1% vs. 2.4%; $p = 0.07$). There was a second cohort of patients undergoing TAVI who could not have surgery due to extreme risk, and these patients were compared to standard medical therapy (PARTNER Cohort B study).[37] This study showed that at 1 year death following TAVI was lower (30.7% vs. 50.7%; $p < 0.001$) as was the risk of death or repeat hospitalisation (42.5% vs. 71.6%; $p < 0.001$).

Intermediate and low risk evidence

In 2016, the PARTNER 2 trial published the results of 2032 randomised patients with symptomatic severe AS at intermediate perioperative risk (estimated perioperative mortality ~4% to 8%) to TAVI or surgical AVR.[38] At 2 years, TAVI was non-inferior to surgical AVR with respect to the primary endpoint, with very similar rates of all-cause mortality or disabling stroke in both groups. Furthermore, TAVI and surgical AVR resulted in similar rates of improvement in clinical heart failure as well as echocardiographic valvular function. Most importantly, there was a borderline significant ($p = 0.06$) interaction between TAVI access approach and the primary endpoint, with a 4% absolute decrease in the primary endpoint with transfemoral TAVI and a 4% absolute increase in the primary endpoint with transthoracic TAVI, suggesting that transfemoral TAVI may actually be superior to surgical AVR while transthoracic TAVI may be inferior (with the pooled combination of the two resulting in noninferiority). Complications more prevalent with open AVR included a 30% higher rate of major bleeding, a 2% higher rate of acute kidney injury, and a 16% higher rate of incident atrial fibrillation. Conversely, TAVI was associated with a 3% increase in major vascular complications.

A small, randomised study of low-risk patients undergoing TAVI has already been published, with inconclusive results due to underpowering.[39] In the Nordic Aortic Valve Intervention Trial (NOTION), no significant difference was found between TAVI and surgical AVR for the composite rate of death from any cause, stroke or MI after 1 year, although the study numbers were low (280 patients randomised). Large randomised trials are underway with both the Evolut-R valve and the Sapien3 valve, and have both finished enrollment.

CONTEMPORARY TAVI PRACTICE

Patient selection for TAVI

Patient selection for TAVI has matured from a procedure bordering on futility in extreme risk inoperable patients, to a procedure that offers mortality benefit without the invasiveness of surgical AVR to carefully selected patients. In its current status, TAVI is often the treatment of choice for patients with a relative degree of surgical risk that includes inoperable, high and intermediate-risk patients, while low-risk RCT data are still pending. With this in mind it is also necessary to ensure TAVI-eligible patients have the appropriate workup with multimodality imaging to ensure they are anatomically suitable for the procedure. Once this information is collected, a 'heart-team' or multidisciplinary team (MDT) discussion is mandatory, to ensure all the aspects of the patient's risk and anatomy are considered before recommending a TAVI procedure. Results of TAVI MDT discussions should be recorded, to allow for audit at a later date.

In general terms, patients should have symptomatic, severe AS as determined by imaging and clinical review before being considered for TAVI. Where suitable, patients should also have the opportunity to see a cardiothoracic surgeon to assess the relative risk for surgical aortic valve replacement prior to an open forum MDT discussion.

Given the cost of the procedure, attempts are being made to exclude patients with excessive frailty, where TAVI often offers no patient benefit. Validated frailty scoring systems like the essential frailty toolset (EFT), the Rockwood and the Katz index have all been used in trying to weed out patients where a TAVI procedure is futile, but thus far no consensus has been reached on exactly which measures/tools provide the most accurate frailty estimations.[40]

Echocardiography

The transthoracic echocardiogram (TTE) is vital in both the diagnosis of severe AS and determining a patient's anatomical suitability for a transcatheter heart valve. For patients to be eligible, they must have severe AS in the absence of other severe valvular lesions that are unlikely to improve following a TAVI procedure. If patients have severe mitral or tricuspid valve disease, for example, they should be reconsidered for a surgical approach to valve replacement if the surgical risk is not prohibitive.

The patient's LV function (ejection fraction) should be quantified by TTE to ensure careful consideration is given to the risk of rapid pacing, which if prolonged can be dangerous in the case of severely reduced LV function. The left ventricular outflow tract (LVOT) anatomy is important to visualise, as occasionally LVOT obstruction contributes to elevated valve gradients and is misdiagnosed as severe AS. LVOT obstruction caused by a bulky or sigmoid septum can occasionally cause upwards displacement and embolisation of the valve during deployment, and is necessary to identify pre-procedurally to avoid this complication. The anatomy of the valve itself, including degree of calcification, bicuspid anatomy and the presence and severity of aortic regurgitation, all provide vital pieces of information that must be carefully considered in planning any TAVI procedure.

Valve sizing was historically performed using echo, but due to the limitations of two-dimensional imaging, annulus diameters were used, which often undersized the patient's anatomy and therefore the choice of valve prosthesis.

Multi-Detector Computed Tomography (MDCT)

MDCT has emerged as having a key role in the pre-TAVI work-up of all patients having the procedure. MDCT images provide not only accurate information about the aortic valve complexity and valve size but also the entire delivery route from femoral artery to the ascending aorta (Figure 39.2).

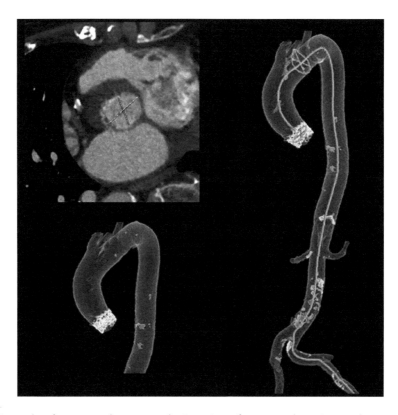

Figure 39.2 Example of computed tomography imaging of aorta and aortic annulus.

The iliac and femoral anatomy must be examined in detail in order to determine the most suitable approach for TAVI. MDCT provides information regarding minimum and maximum luminal vessel diameters, the tortuosity of the vessels, and the presence and extent, both longitudinal and circumferential, of significant calcification of the access vessels, which are major determinants for the feasibility of the TAVI procedure.

Aortic annulus dimensions can be accurately measured during the cardiac cycle by ECG-gated CT angiography, which aims to capture the images in the systolic phase at approximately 40% of the R-R interval, thus maximising the aortic valve opening. Perimeter- and area-based annulus measurements are used as reliable parameters for choosing the appropriate size of the prosthesis. Self-expanding valves tend to be sized using perimeter-based measurements, which are less affected by the cardiac cycle. Balloon expandable valves have traditionally had annulus sizing using area-based annulus measurements. These measurements are sometimes challenging, and depend on the quality of the CT scan and on the experience of the person measuring the annulus. Difficulties sometimes arise where the annulus measurement falls between two recommended valve sizes, and in these cases multiple measurements taken with an average of many can improve accuracy, but patient factors should also then be considered when deciding whether to 'size up' or 'size down'.

Accurate sizing of the annulus and visualisation of the degree, location and distribution of calcium is important in preventing paravalvular regurgitation which, if significant, can affect post-procedural outcomes.[41]

MDCT is also useful to predict and prevent some of the major complications in TAVI, namely annulus rupture and coronary occlusion. Annulus rupture occurs where heavy unilateral or focal calcification is present in a patient undergoing a balloon expandable valve. In cases where high-risk features are identified, a self-expanding TAVI system is preferred to avoid this often lethal complication. Coronary obstruction can be predicted where there are small sinuses combined with long, bulky aortic leaflets.

Last, MDCT offers an exact orthogonal visualisation of the aortic annulus, which can be used to predict the optimal angle of fluoroscopic deployment during the TAVI procedure.

TAVI PROCEDURE

Anaesthetic support

GENERAL ANAESTHESIA (GA)

It is universally accepted that anaesthetic support is necessary for TAVI procedures. Some variation exists, however, in how sedation is chosen for patients undergoing TAVI procedures. Many operators prefer the controlled element of a GA, where patients are still and all oxygenation and haemodynamic parameters are taken care of by an anaesthetist. GA also facilitates transoesophageal echocardiography (TEE), which can be useful for valve placement and the immediate diagnosis of tamponade in the case of hypotension. TEE is also useful to assess the amount of paravalvular leak (PVL) after TAVI. Excessive PVL has been shown to increase mortality.

CONSCIOUS SEDATION (CS)

Many TAVI centres now prefer local anaesthetic with CS as an alternative to GA. This technique offers a much faster recovery time, particularly for patients who may be elderly and frail to begin with, where a prolonged GA may lead to delirium or prolonged recovery. CS also helps to minimise unnecessary line placement (central and arterial lines) and reduces the need for urinary catheterisation, which causes considerable morbidity in elderly male patients. The depth of CS is highly variable, and in many cases dependent on both the individual patient needs and the anaesthetist's preference. Patient comfort can be increased by using dedicated femoral nerve blocks, which can be applied under ultrasound at the beginning of the procedure. The main benefits of CS are to reduce the need for intra-procedural inotropes, intensive care unit length of stay and hospital length of stay. The principal downside to CS is the inability to use TEE and the rare but occasional need for immediate intra-procedural conversion to GA, which may lead to increased morbidity if performed under more emergent circumstances.

To date, there are no large, randomised, controlled data to guide the anaesthetic choice between GA and CS, although large US TAVI database registry data and meta-analysis suggest CS may be the preferred approach for selected patients.[42] Despite this there are clearly patients who will require GA due to co-morbidities, or other factors including patient preference.

Vascular access

Initial TAVI devices were delivered through such large bore sheaths that they were performed via the femoral vein, using an antegrade approach. Fortunately, devices improved quickly and the maximum sheath sizes for transfemoral approach TAVI now range between 14 and 18 Fr. The transfemoral approach is by far the commonest access approach for TAVI with all institutions using this as the default approach, with alternative access approaches reserved for those with hostile iliac or femoral anatomy. Preventing vascular complications is facilitated through careful procedural planning and using the work-up imaging (in particular the CT) to decide the best access route. Vessel tortuosity, significant iliac or femoral artery stenoses, calcification and its location and the level of the femoral bifurcation are all important factors to consider when deciding where and how to obtain safe transfemoral access (Figure 39.3). The following steps could act as a guide for safe transfemoral access, although there may be many variations on this technique:

1. Examine the CT scan for calcium and significant disease. In general terms, a minimal luminal diameter of <5 to 5.5 cm will be too small for a TAVI delivery system. Significant tortuosity, particularly where the vessel is also calcified, should be avoided if possible as this increases the risk of vessel rupture/dissection or failure to advance the delivery system. A large abdominal aortic aneurysm (AAA) is a relative contraindication to transfemoral access, although the shape and anatomy of the AAA may determine whether transfemoral access may be performed through the aneurysmal segment. If there are any of the above features, consider an alternative access approach.
2. Iliac/femoral digital subtraction angiography (DSA) at the time of work-up coronary angiography is useful as an adjunct to CT-derived angiography. A wire can also be used at the time to assess how a tortuous artery may behave when a wire is placed through it.
3. Perform a contra-lateral femoral puncture first. This access is needed for the pigtail catheter, which will perform angiography throughout the procedure. Some operators use a radial approach for the second access to minimise femoral complications, but femoral access facilitates quick

access for vascular complications later, and hence is the preferred second access for most TAVI operators. While ultrasound is not essential, it is recommended for all femoral TAVI cases. Use the ultrasound to get venous access for a pacing wire (internal jugular, or transfemoral) and for the contra-lateral puncture.
4. Image the vessel to be used for the large bore access with ultrasound, up-and-over DSA from the contra-lateral access, or both. Aim to puncture the common femoral artery over the femoral head in an area free of significant calcification. Once access is achieved, pre-close the artery with two Proglide devices (or similar device, e.g. Prostar). Exchange for a stiff wire *before* inserting any large bore sheath or dilator. Use sequential dilators to minimise arterial trauma before the final sheath is inserted, then give intravenous (IV) heparin aiming for an activated clotting time (ACT) of 250–300 seconds prior to inserting a TAVI delivery system.

Aortography

An aortogram image in a projection that shows all three aortic cusps in equal portions forming the line of the aortic annulus should be sought (Figure 39.4). Often, this angle may be in a shallow left anterior oblique (LAO) projection with some cranial or caudal angulation. This view is important to determine prior to commencing valve delivery to ensure the valve will be deployed in the correct position with respect to the annulus. TAVI workup CT should be able to predict the optimal deployment angle.

Crossing the aortic valve

Crossing the aortic valve can be performed in a number of different ways, with most operators becoming proficient at their own individual techniques. The commonest technique is to use an AL-1 shaped coronary catheter, aimed toward the left coronary cusp, and sweep the catheter across the annulus while probing the valve with a straight tipped wire. Once the valve is crossed, the catheter is advanced into the LV cavity. If the valve is difficult to cross, a hydrophilic wire or different catheter angle can be used. An alternative

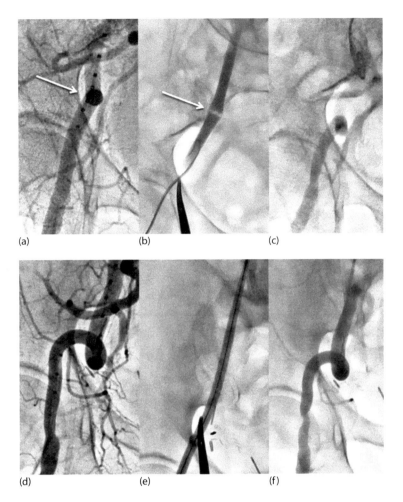

(a)   (b)   (c)

(d)   (e)   (f)

Figure 39.3 Transcatheter aortic valve implantation in patients with iliofemoral tortuosity. A patient with tortuosity of his external iliac artery (a, arrow) that straightened out after it was crossed with the wire and the sheath. However, the sheath kinked (b, arrow), but the procedure was successfully carried out after the sheath was replaced. Contralateral angiography showed minimal stenosis after closure with ProGlide system (Abbott Vascular, Abbott Park, Illinois) (c). Extensive tortuosity of the external iliac artery (d) that straightened out with an Amplatz Extra Stiff Wire (Cook Medical Inc., Bloomington, Indiana) and an 18-F Edwards sheath (Edwards Lifesciences, Irvine, California) (e). Crossover angiography confirmed a good result after closure (f). (From Toggweiler, S. et al., *JACC Cardiovasc. Interv.*, 6, 643–653, 2013.)

is to place a pigtail in the right coronary cusp and use this to determine the root anatomy and anatomic landmarks—this technique may be useful in difficult to cross bicuspid anatomy.[43] Some operators use a pigtail and straight wire technique, similar to that used in routine angiography. Whatever technique is used, it is important to be vigilant with the straight wire in the LV, as wire perforation can occur, leading to pericardial tamponade.

TAVI delivery wire

Standard stiff guidewires were not designed for TAVI, or indeed for use within the LV, and have design flaws that make them unsuitable for TAVI procedures. The major design flaw involves the transition point from 'stiff' to 'soft' wire portion. The Amplatz extra-stiff, the Lunderquist and the Amplatz stiff wires share the common feature of a stainless steel core that terminates some distance

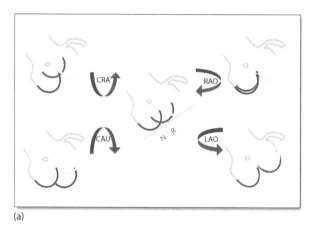

(a)

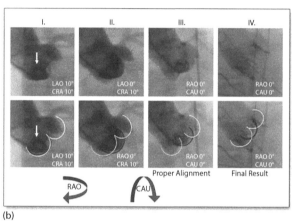

(b)

Figure 39.4 (a) Suggested scheme for determining the optimal coplanar implant view, showing the 'follow the right cusp' rule pointing to proper alignment in the case of normal aortic root anatomy. (b) Example of normal aortic root anatomy: Images are provided without (upper images) and with (lower images) a schematic overlay. The white arrow indicates the pigtail catheter. Panels I through III show fluoroscopy-guided alignment of the aortic plane; panel IV shows the final result. (*Abbreviations:* CAU, caudal; CRA, cranial; L, left cusp; LAO, left anterior oblique; N, non-coronary cusp; R, right cusp; RAO, right anterior oblique.) (From Kasel, A.M. et al., *JACC Cardiovasc. Imaging.*, 6, 274–275, 2013.)

(e.g. 1, 3 or 6 cm) from the proximal tip of the wire. The tip itself is comprised of a coiled floppy segment. There is therefore a discrete transition point at which the wire can form a sharp bend or kink and the shoulder so formed can cause traumatic injury to the ventricle. Furthermore, standard wires come out of their respective packaging as a straight wire, which the operator must then shape to form a loop in an attempt to minimise the risk of LV trauma. This shaping process can be very inconsistent, and often the same operator will not be able to replicate the exact same shape during each procedure. Figure 39.5 compares suboptimal wire shaping and position for TAVI with operator shaped curves and optimal wire shaping using a dedicated TAVI wire.[44]

Dedicated TAVI guidewires are now used by most operators now for TAVI procedures. The two commercially available options included the Confidawire (Medtronic Inc, Minneapolis, Minnesota) or the Safari (Boston Scientific, Marlborough, Massachusetts). Both of these wires share a stiff shaft to ease trackability of the delivery system and a pre-shaped coil with a smooth transition from stiff shaft to soft tip through the coiled segment.

The TAVI wire can be delivered either through a pigtail catheter or through the AL-1 catheter after crossing the valve. This should be performed in a right anterior oblique projection to ensure the wire sits in the mid to apical LV, ready for pre-TAVI balloon valvuloplasty or the TAVI delivery device.

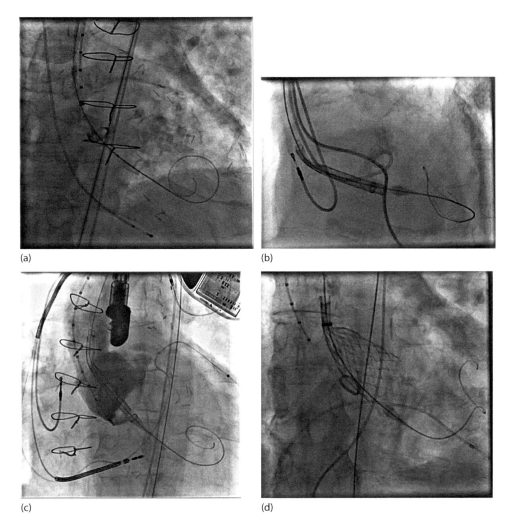

(a)

(b)

(c)

(d)

Figure 39.5 Angiographic images of various stages during deployment of the Corevalve Evolut valve. **(a)** Initial approach from aortic arch, **(b)** Positioning of valve apparatus across aortic valve, **(c)** Aortic angiogram confirming exact location of prosthetic valve just before deployment and **(d)** Sheath withdrawal showing near-complete deployment of new valve.

Pre-TAVI balloon aortic valvuloplasty

Predilatation with an aortic semi-compliant balloon is performed prior to TAVI and after deployment of the stiff TAVI wire in the LV. Generally, this step should be performed using a balloon sized to the smallest annulus diameter dimension, to avoid unnecessary trauma to the aortic valve apparatus and aortic root. Often, operators will choose an even smaller sized balloon, particularly given the predilatation is only being performed to facilitate the TAVI procedure. Rapid ventricular pacing is implemented at the time of balloon inflation, with the aim to drop the blood pressure enough (usually 40–60 mmHg systolic) to

stabilise the balloon across the valve during inflation without embolisation of the balloon itself into the aorta.

In the early years of TAVI, predilatation using balloon aortic valvuloplasty was considered a mandatory step before TAVI, since it facilitates valve crossing and prosthesis delivery, ensures optimal valve expansion and improves haemodynamic stability during valve deployment. However, as a result of procedural evolution over time, direct TAVI (without pre-implantation balloon aortic valvuloplasty) has emerged as an option to simplify the procedure and to avoid potential valvuloplasty-related complications. Several real-world retrospective studies have shown that direct TAVI (with both self-expanding and balloon-expandable prostheses) is feasible, safe and associated with outcomes similar to standard TAVI with pre-implantation balloon aortic valvuloplasty.[45,46] The DIRECTTAVI randomised study is enrolling patients to explore this concept, but many operators have already switched to performing predilatation-only on selected patients.

In certain situations, particularly where there is heavy calcification concurrent with the use of self-expanding valves, predilatation may still be preferred.

INDIVIDUAL TAVI DEVICES AND THEIR MECHANISMS/ DEPLOYMENT TIPS

The Evolut-R and Evolut-Pro valves

The Evolut family of TAVI is a third-generation self-expanding valve based on the original CoreValve concept. The Evolut-R (Medtronic Inc, Minneapolis, Minnesota) is easy to use and forgiving, with a recapture mechanism allowing for accurate valve positioning (Figure 39.6). Sizes ranging from 23 to 29 mm can be deployed through a 14 Fr in-line sheath with the 34 mm device requiring a 16 Fr sheath.

The Evolut-Pro (Medtronic Inc, Minneapolis, Minnesota) has added a skirt to the distal end of the prosthesis with an adaptive seal, with the aim to limit PVL.

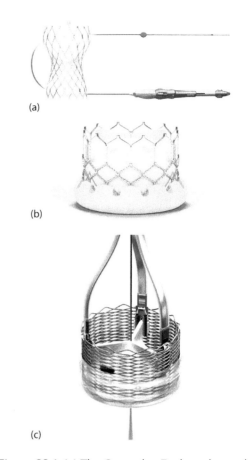

(a)

(b)

(c)

Figure 39.6 (a) The Corevalve Evolut valve and delivery sheath. (b) Sapien 3. (c) Lotus valve.

The Sapien 3 (S3) valve

The Sapien 3 valve (Edwards Lifesciences, Irvine, California) has improved a number a features from the Sapien XT, with the major factor being the addition of a skirt to prevent PVL (Figure 39.6). The frame has also changed, with a large cell design at the top to facilitate coronary flow and coronary access. The deployment mechanism has also changed from a straight balloon to a tapered or dog-boned balloon to allow early valve fixation and prevent valve dislocation/embolisation. The S3 system is delivered through an expandable 14 Fr E-sheath, which is a significant improvement on early devices.

THE LOTUS VALVE

The Lotus valve (Boston Scientific, Marlborough, Massachusetts) has a number of unique features that makes it different by design to other balloon expandable or self-expanding valve mechanisms (Figure 39.6). The Lotus valve uses a mechanical deployment mechanism that allows for full valve deployment and valve functional assessment prior to release, with the option of recapture in situations of malplacement. It was the first valve to use Adaptive Seal™ technology that was designed to minimise PVL by conforming to various types of anatomies to create a strong and secure seal. The Lotus Edge valve, the second generation of this device, has a number of improvements including a depth guard system to minimise LVOT interaction and lower post procedure pacemaker requirements.

THE ACCURATE NEO VALVE

The ACCURATE Neo Aortic Valve (Boston Scientific, Marlborough, Massachusetts) with Transfemoral and Transapical Delivery Systems is a self-expanding, supra-annular valve, offering an intuitive procedure with predictable release, stable positioning, and has demonstrated excellent clinical outcomes (Figure 39.6). The transfemoral system uses a two step top-down deployment, which is different from other self-expanding systems that deploy from the LVOT upwards. Initial results with this valve have been favourable, with lower pacemaker requirements than the other self-expanding devices, although no RCTs have been undertaken.

PORTICO VALVE

The Portico valve (Abbott, Abbott Park, Illinois) is a self-expanding nitinol valve with the ability to fully recapture the valve and reposition the valve in situ. It has a gradual deployment mechanism and a functioning valve during deployment, which allows for haemodynamic stability during the TAVI procedure. To date there have been no RCTs with this device.

Vascular closure

By far the most commonly used device is the Perclose Proglide (Abbott, Abbott Park, Illinois), and two of these devices are required for large vessel closure. Usually, the femoral artery is punctured and dilated with a standard arterial sheath. Then, the Proglide device is advanced over the guidewire, and the first suture is deployed slightly angulated at the 10 o'clock position. Guidewire access is maintained, and a second Proglide device is inserted and deployed at the 2 o'clock position. The regular J wire is then exchanged for a stiffer wire, and the large sheath is advanced under fluoroscopy. After conclusion of the procedure, the introducer sheath is slowly removed, but the guidewire is left to maintain access. The sutures are tightened. In case of sufficient haemostasis, the guidewire can be removed and the sutures are further tightened using the knot pusher to ensure approximation of the knot to the vessel wall. Should haemostasis fail, it is possible to implant a third (or fourth) Proglide over the guidewire.[47]

CURRENT TAVI LIMITATIONS

Conduction disturbances requiring a permanent pacemaker

The need for a PPM due to new atrioventricular conduction disturbances is one of the most frequent complications post TAVI. In both registry data and RCTs, PPM rates have been significantly higher than that for surgery, due to the proximity of the left ventricular outflow tract (LVOT) and aortic valve with the bundle of His and AV node. The mechanism seems to be one of trauma to this region in the case of balloon-expandable valves, while for self-expanding valves the mechanism is likely due to ongoing force exerted by the nitinol frame.

PPM implantation rates vary between studies and have improved over time with newer generation devices. A change in practice in all devices of implanting higher, with less valve protruding into the LVOT, has also led to a lower need for post procedure PPM. In the early studies, the rate of PPM was 5%–12% after implantation of an Edwards Sapien valve versus 24%–33% following CoreValve.[33,34] These numbers have improved significantly over time, with the currently available Sapien 3 valve now showing pacing rates of 12%, and the Evolut-R valve of 16.4%.[48,49] The Lotus valve, which uses mechanical deployment and is comprised of a sub-annular valve mechanism, still has one of the highest quoted PPM rates in registry studies—28.9% in the extended REPRISE II registry.[50]

It is unclear whether PPM implantation should be considered a major complication, but certainly procedural cost, length of stay and in-hospital morbidity are increased when post-procedure permanent pacing is required. The PARTNER study also showed increased rates of re-hospitalisation and increased mortality with the need for post-procedure PPM.[51]

Vascular complications

Vascular complications (VC) following TAVI are common and are one of the leading procedural causes of morbidity and mortality. Early TAVI devices involved the use of very large calibre sheaths 18–24 Fr for delivery system introduction, which led to the relatively high rates of major vascular complications in early TAVI studies. TAVI was also frequently being performed routinely via femoral artery surgical cutdown in some centres, which added to procedural morbidity and length of hospital stay. The way VC were being reported also varied in early studies, until the advent of the valve academic research consortium (VARC) and now the VARC2 criteria, which make it possible to compare VC outcomes across studies.[52–54]

VC have improved significantly in TAVI for a number of reasons. First and most importantly, the current commercially available devices frequently only require a 14 Fr sheath, which is a major improvement on the 24 Fr sheath of early Edwards Sapien devices. Second, operators and heart teams are improving their skills in patient selection, excluding patients with vascular access that is likely to be unfavourable for TAVI. This improvement has also been made possible with more experience in the interpretation of peripheral CT angiography data, in particular the extent and sites of calcification and tortuosity.

From the Partner 2 study, the vascular complication rates for transfemoral procedures are low, with 7.9% of patients having a major vascular complication at 30 days.[38]

Techniques of managing VC have also improved with improving operator experience. Crossover balloon techniques using peripheral balloons are useful and can overcome the need for surgical intervention when complete closure is not achieved with percutaneous closure devices.

Paravalvular leak

PVL was the Achilles heel of early TAVI, and is still quoted by some surgeons as a reason not to consider TAVI as a realistic therapy for low risk patients. Given that the native aortic valve is not removed during TAVI (as compared to surgical AVR) there is risk that the TAVI prosthesis will not be able to expand uniformly due to eccentric calcifications and there will therefore be PVL. Trivial or mild PVL has been quoted to be present in up to 61% patients post TAVI, which differs from surgery, where PVL is almost never present post-operatively. Whether mild PVL is benign or not is contentious, but certainly moderate or severe PVL is associated with an increased cardiovascular mortality across TAVI studies.[55,56]

PVL can result from patient factors, such as severe or very eccentric leaflet calcification, or a bicuspid valve, or from procedural factors like valve position or the prosthesis size and specific device selection. Sizing has improved with the use of CT annulus measurement, where echocardiographic sizing during early TAVI often undersized the annulus, and which led to valve undersizing and higher rates of PVL. Figure 39.7 shows different mechanisms of PVL.

PVL has been a major driver of new generation device improvements, with valve skirts now present on the Sapien 3, Evolut-Pro and Lotus Edge devices. Re-capturable valves have become standard for the self-expanding mechanically expanding technologies, allowing operators to reposition the valve in cases where valve malpositioning leads to PVL. An increased number of available valve sizes has also led to lower PVL rates by allowing for more precision when sizing TAVI devices.

Current PVL rates for the newest generation devices are favourable, with the Sapien 3 showing significant PVL rates of 2.6% and the Evolut Pro showing no significant PVL in early published data.[48,57]

PVL can be hard to quantify, particularly with variations in contrast volume for aortography, variations in pigtail catheter placement, angulation and TEE use. Simultaneous haemodynamic pressure tracing examination with a catheter in the LV and aorta is vital to confirm severe aortic regurgitation is not present post procedure. To adjust the gradient for the respective systolic blood pressure of the patient, one can calculate the dimensionless aortic regurgitation index according to the following formula: $[(DBP - LVEDP)/SBP] \times 100$.[55]

Stroke

Early TAVI studies showed a relatively high risk of stroke, which has been a major concern going forward with the treatment of patients with this therapy. The PARTNER study showed a rate of major stroke of 5.1% at 1 year in cohort A.[37] The risk of stroke was higher after TAVI than with AVR, and hence there persisted a belief that stroke was more likely after TAVI than with AVR. In addition, clinically silent brain infarctions seen on magnetic resonance imaging are associated with neurocognitive function changes and these silent infarctions are common after TAVI and surgical AVR.[58]

The risk of stroke has reduced significantly. However, both registry and RCT data show stroke risks are lower with newer generation valves and are also lower in trials examining TAVI in intermediate-risk populations.[38,39,48,49,57]

Embolic Protection Devices (EPD) offer a potential mechanism to reduce stroke by preventing the embolisation of thrombotic or calcific debris during TAVI. EPDs which have been studied thus far include deflections devices, transcatheter filters or

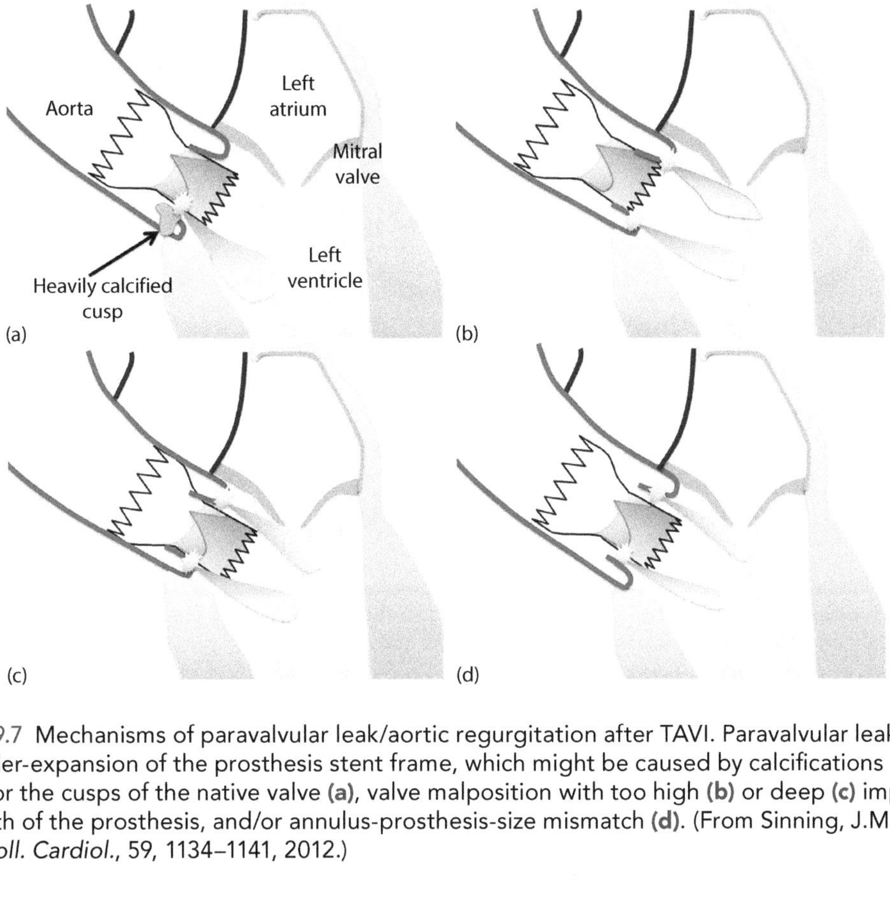

Figure 39.7 Mechanisms of paravalvular leak/aortic regurgitation after TAVI. Paravalvular leak results from under-expansion of the prosthesis stent frame, which might be caused by calcifications of the annulus or the cusps of the native valve (a), valve malposition with too high (b) or deep (c) implantation depth of the prosthesis, and/or annulus-prosthesis-size mismatch (d). (From Sinning, J.M. et al., J. Am. Coll. Cardiol., 59, 1134–1141, 2012.)

transcatheter cerebral embolic protection. To date, none of the studies comparing the use of EPDs during TAVI versus controls has shown statistical significance in preventing stroke, although some have shown a trend toward reduced cerebral ischaemic lesion volume on magnetic resonance imaging.[59–61]

OFF-LABEL TAVI TREATMENTS

Bicuspid aortic valves

A bicuspid aortic valve is the most common congenital cardiac anomaly, with an estimated incidence of 0.4%–2.25% in the general population. Bicuspid anatomy actually comprises a spectrum of deformed aortic valves, presenting on gross examination with two functional cusps forming a valve mechanism with less than three zones of parallel apposition between cusps. Bicuspid valves are most commonly classified using the Sievers method (Figure 39.8), where phenotypes were classified according to (1) numbers of raphes, (2) spatial

position of the cusps or raphes, (3) functional status of the valve. The first characteristic was found to be the most significant it terms of how the anomaly affects the valve anatomy and three major types are described: type 0 (no raphe), type 1 (one raphe) and type 2 (two raphes), as shown in Figure 39.8.[62]

Bicuspid aortic anatomy has been excluded from the landmark RCTs involving TAVI and, despite favourable results from registries and observational reports, it continues to be considered a relative contraindication in recent guidelines. However, up to 20% of clinically relevant BAV stenoses occur in octogenarians and, furthermore, in light of recent evidence demonstrating TAVI to be a valid alternative to surgery for intermediate risk patients and potentially low risk populations, younger patients with BAV are increasingly referred for consideration of TAVI.

Selection of the type and size of the TAVI device in treating bicuspid stenosis can be difficult. The bicuspid aortic valve annulus often has an elliptical shape and relatively larger size compared with

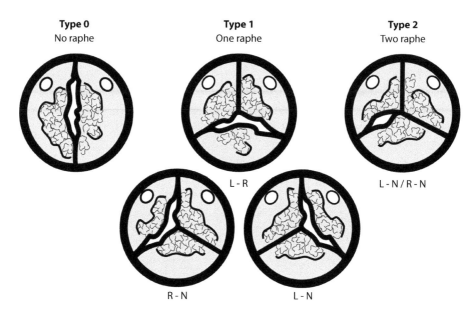

Figure 39.8 Classification of bicuspid valves according to the description of Sievers et al. (*Abbreviations:* BAV, bicuspid aortic valve; L, left coronary cusp; N, non coronary cusp; R, right coronary cusp.) (From Sievers, H.H. et al., *J. Thorac. Cardiovasc. Surg.*, 133, 1226–1233, 2007; Mylotte, D. et al., *J. Am. Coll. Cardiol.*, 64, 2330–2339, 2014. With permission.)

tricuspid valves, and is more likely to exhibit severe eccentric calcification. In addition, it is often associated with a dilated, horizontal ascending aorta, and effaced sinuses. All of this may hinder valve positioning and expansion, which could impair normal valve functioning and significantly increase PVL. In addition, the risk of coronary obstruction is not negligible in BAV, as leaflet fusion tends to result in longer leaflets.

While bicuspid aortic valve anatomy is more challenging, registry data suggest good results can be achieved with TAVI procedures, particularly with newer generation devices.[63,64]

TAVI for native aortic regurgitation

There is minimal published clinical evidence of the use of TAVI for native aortic regurgitation (NAR), and thus far there have been RCTs. There are a number of reasons why TAVI has not been used routinely for patients with NAR. First, the prevalence of NAR is lower than that of AS, and early TAVI devices were designed to treat only AS. Second, although AS is predominantly caused by calcification and degeneration of the valve, NAR is

caused by a heterogenous group of aetiologies and affects younger patients, the majority of whom are clearly surgically operable. Furthermore, a proportion of patients with NAR have pathologies involving dilatation of the ascending aorta, mandating surgical treatment. Finally, patients with NAR have more complex and diverse anatomy, making transcatheter treatment with the currently available devices extremely challenging. Figure 39.9 shows the use of the two-pigtail technique, during TAVI for NAR.

A number of isolated case reports describing use of TAVI for this indication have been reported, with successful TAVI implantation in very high-risk patients in whom surgery was not possible.[65–67] The majority of these reports describe the use of a self-expanding CoreValve TAVI prosthesis in special circumstances. Use of the balloon expandable Edwards prosthesis (Edwards Lifesciences) and the JenaValve (JenaValve Technology GmbH, Munich, Germany) have also been described for NAR in patients with a left ventricular assist device (LVAD), where even moderate aortic regurgitation can result in malfunction of the LVAD device.[68]

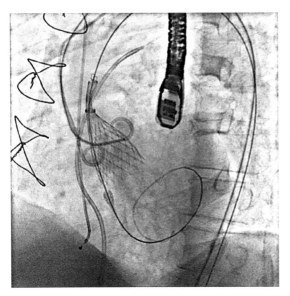

Figure 39.9 The two-pigtail technique. In cases of severe native aortic regurgitation without annulus or valve leaflet calcification, the two-pigtail technique can be used to outline the aortic annulus. One pigtail is placed in the non-coronary cusp and the other in the right coronary cusp.

THE TWO-PIGTAIL TECHNIQUE

In cases of severe native aortic regurgitation without annulus or valve leaflet calcification, the two-pigtail technique can be used to outline the aortic annulus. One pigtail is placed in the non-coronary cusp and the other in the right coronary cusp.[69]

The first series to explore the use of TAVI for NAR examined 43 patients treated with the CoreValve device for pure NAR without AS.[69] The clinical outcomes of this study were acceptable but while implantation of a TAVI was successful in 97.7% of cases, the VARC defined procedural success was only 74.4% due to the need for a second valve and ≥grade II residual aortic regurgitation post procedure. Also of interest was the finding that the need for a second valve was limited to patients without aortic valve calcification. This study demonstrated the feasibility of this technique and highlighted the potential procedural difficulties in treating NAR with TAVI. A further registry using second generation TAVI devices showed encouraging outcomes for patients with NAR, albeit with similar concerns regarding lack of calcification and valve movement during the procedure.[70]

Valve-in-valve TAVI

Surgical bioprosthetic valves (Figure 39.10a) are often preferred over metallic valves for elderly patients or those who are unsuitable for long term anticoagulation with warfarin. During the last decade, the relative use of bioprosthetic aortic valves has increased by nearly 80%. Improvements in surgical techniques and valve durability are likely to have fuelled this increase. Bioprosthetic valve failure usually occurs within 8–15 years and the actuarial freedom from reoperation for a failing bioprosthetic valve is approximately 95%, 90% and 70% at 5, 10 and 15 years respectively.[71] The operative mortality for a redo aortic valve surgery is 2%–7%, but this can increase to more than 30% for high-risk patients.

Because TAVI in a surgical bioprosthetic valve represents a minimally invasive alternative to conventional redo surgery, it may prove to be safer, and just as effective as redo surgery.[72]

One of the major advantages of valve-in-valve TAVI is the ability to accurately size the valve, due to the known bioprosthetic valve construction and dimensions. A clearly visible, precise, circular neo-annulus is also a significant advantage in valve-in-valve TAVI where a stented bioprosthetic valve has been used. This allows for TAVI deployment with minimal (and in some cases zero) contrast use. Examples of valve-in-valve cases using commonly available TAVI devices in different surgical bioprosthetic valves are shown in Figure 39.10b.

The VIVID registry has been an invaluable tool in collecting outcomes and implantation techniques in different failing surgical bioprosthetic valves.[73,74] This registry highlighted the importance of initial surgical valve size in determining haemodynamic outcomes post procedure and helping to predict patient prosthesis mismatch. In smaller bioprostehtic valve sizes, a self-expanding prosthesis like the Evolut system offers better haemodynamics and lower gradients due to its supra-annular function.

Coronary obstruction is a major concern in small aortic root anatomy, particularly in patients with a native BAV as the sino-tubular junction is often effaced. Of most concern is where patients have had a stented, externally mounted bioprosthetic valve such as the Mitroflow or Trifecta valve, where the surgical leaflets may be pushed aside to block the coronary ostia. MDCT is imperative in these cases

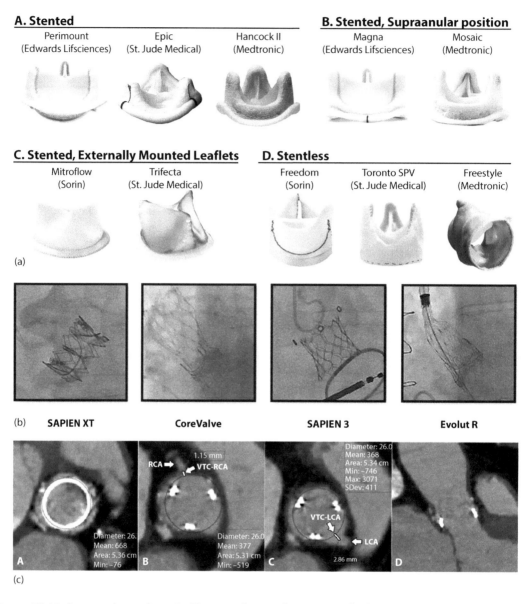

Figure 39.10 Commonly used surgical bioprosthetic valves. Stented valves **(a)** tend to be the easiest for the surgeon to implant and also the easiest to perform valve-in-valve TAVI, given the highly visible stented frame and relatively low risk of coronary obstruction. These valves have somewhat worse haemodynamic profiles, however, and are often undersized at the time of surgery. Stented supra-annular valves **(b)** behave in a very similar manner to stented bioprosthetics, albeit with the haemodynamic advantage of a supra-annular valve. Stented, externally mounted bioprosthetic leaflets **(c)** give the best post-operative haemodynamics, but in small anatomy can be the most risky cases for coronary obstruction when valve-in-valve TAVI is performed. Stentless valves **(d)** are commonly used when there is bicuspid valve anatomy or ascending aortic pathology, and are the most challenging for valve-in-valve procedures due to lack of fluoroscopic landmarks at the bioprosthetic neo-annulus.

and the risk of coronary obstruction may be determined by creating a virtual TAVI ring according to the planned valve size, and then calculating the distance from this to the coronary ostia (Virtual TAVI to Coronary Distance or VTC) as shown in Figure 39.10c. If the VTC is <4 mm, the patient is at increased risk for coronary obstruction and TAVI should either be reconsidered or performed using coronary protection or chimney stenting.[75] Coronary protection can be performed by inserting a guiding catheter in the coronary artery at risk, with a coronary wire across an undeployed stent. The stent is kept in place through the TAVI procedure and only pulled back and deployed if coronary obstruction occurs. When deploying the stent, it must be pulled back so that the proximal portion is in the aorta, and used as a scaffold or chimney to prevent the bioprosthetic leaflet sitting across the sinus and preventing coronary artery flow.

Alternative access TAVI

Between 5%–10% of patients referred for TAVI have unsuitable iliac/femoral anatomy for trans-femoral access. This means that they either have to be reconsidered for surgery, or an alternative access site needs to be considered to deliver the prosthesis.

TRANS-APICAL TAVI

The first alternative access approach described was via the trans-apical route, which has the advantage of providing a straight, direct short access to the aortic valve via the LV apex. This technique requires cardiothoracic surgical access, using a technique of access that is not an everyday approach for most cardiothoracic surgeons, and hence there is a learning curve for surgeons new to this approach. Trans-apical TAVI was developed with the Edwards Sapien family of valves but has also been used with the Symetis accurate valve and the Jena Valve TA system.[76,77]

DIRECT AORTIC/TRANS-AORTIC TAVI

Direct aortic TAVI makes sense as an alternative approach to be performed by cardiothoracic surgeons as it involves a limited sternotomy or hemisternotomy, which is a routine approach for any cardiothoracic surgeon and hence there is no significant learning curve. The ideal position to puncture the aorta can be achieved using fluoroscopy, where at least 7 cm above the aortic annulus provides enough room for most delivery systems to function appropriately. This technique provides an easily achievable perpendicular approach to the annulus, which is sometimes hard to achieve from the trans-femoral approach. This, and the one-to-one torque advantage mean that direct aortic approach TAVI is often more stable at the time of deployment, with less likelihood of valve migration/embolisation. Both the direct aortic and trans-apical approaches are maximally invasive and therefore require intensive care post operatively, with longer in-hospital stay.[78]

SUBCLAVIAN/AXILLARY APPROACH

Use of the axillary and subclavian artery is familiar to cardiac surgeons. It has been advocated for routine use in cannulation for cardiopulmonary bypass during thoracic aortic surgery and where conventional ascending aortic cannulation is contra-indicated. Its use as an alternative entry point to the vasculature is therefore appealing in endovascular procedures. The subclavian and axillary approaches to TAVI provide a less invasive access approach than trans-apical or direct aortic access, but are limited to patients without significant tortuosity or calcification, similarly to the trans-femoral approach.

Relative contraindications to this approach are the presence of an ipsilateral pacemaker or the presence of an ipsilateral internal mammary artery coronary bypass graft.[79]

TRANSCAVAL APPROACH

In recent years, a new technique has been described using access from the right femoral venous approach and then approaching the aorta via the inferior vena cava using a direct guided puncture, in patients with unsuitable iliac/femoral anatomy. This technique was refined in animals, and works by the assumption that the inferior vena cava pressure is lower than the retroperitoneal pressure, and hence bleeding occurs into the IVC as a fistula, rather than into the retroperitoneal space. The puncture is then closed using a nitinol cardiac occluder, which seals over time, sealing the fistula. This technique was published in 100 patients with promising results, and warrants further study and experience.[80]

THE FUTURE OF TAVI

TAVI is currently the standard of care for high-risk and inoperable surgical patients, but already many institutions are treating patients at intermediate risk after the results of recent trials in these patient cohorts. Whether TAVI will overtake surgical AVR as the gold standard is uncertain, and may depend on many factors, including proven long-term valve durability and favourable results in low-risk TAVI versus surgery trials.

For now, surgical AVR remains the gold standard until some of the TAVI limitations allow this therapy to penetrate fully into the low-risk patient cohorts and until then, appropriate risk stratification and MDT/heart team discussion is necessary to determine individual patients' optimal therapies based on their risk scores and co-morbidities.

REFERENCES

1. Cribier A, Eltchaninoff H, Bash A, Borenstein N, Tron C, Bauer F, et al. Percutaneous transcatheter implantation of an aortic valve prosthesis for calcific aortic stenosis: First human case description. *Circulation.* 2002;106(24):3006–3008.
2. Freeman RV, Otto CM. Spectrum of calcific aortic valve disease: Pathogenesis, disease progression, and treatment strategies. *Circulation.* 2005;111(24):3316–3326.
3. Dweck MR, Boon NA, Newby DE. Calcific aortic stenosis: A disease of the valve and the myocardium. *J Am Coll Cardiol.* 2012;60(19):1854–1863.
4. Stewart BF, Siscovick D, Lind BK, Gardin JM, Gottdiener JS, Smith VE, et al. Clinical factors associated with calcific aortic valve disease. Cardiovascular Health Study. *J Am Coll Cardiol.* 1997;29(3):630–634.
5. Ross J, Jr., Braunwald E. Aortic stenosis. *Circulation.* 1968;38(1 Suppl):61–67.
6. Otto CM, Lind BK, Kitzman DW, Gersh BJ, Siscovick DS. Association of aortic-valve sclerosis with cardiovascular mortality and morbidity in the elderly. *N Engl J Med.* 1999;341(3):142–147.
7. Rapaport E. Natural history of aortic and mitral valve disease. *Am J Cardiol.* 1975;35(2):221–227.
8. Frank S, Johnson A, Ross J, Jr. Natural history of valvular aortic stenosis. *Br Heart J.* 1973;35(1):41–46.
9. Plicht B, Lind A, Erbel R. Infective endocarditis: New ESC guidelines 2015. *Internist (Berl).* 2016;57(7):675–690.
10. Cowell SJ, Newby DE, Prescott RJ, Bloomfield P, Reid J, Northridge DB, et al. A randomized trial of intensive lipid-lowering therapy in calcific aortic stenosis. *N Engl J Med.* 2005;352(23):2389–2397.
11. Thiago L, Tsuji SR, Nyong J, Puga ME, Gois AF, Macedo CR, et al. Statins for aortic valve stenosis. *Cochrane Database Syst Rev.* 2016;9:Cd009571.
12. Harken DE, Black H, Taylor WJ, Thrower WB, Soroff HS. The surgical correction of calcific aortic stenosis in adults; results in the first 100 consecutive transaortic valvuloplasties. *J Thorac Surg.* 1958;36(6):759–773; discussion 73–76.
13. Harken DE, Taylor WJ, Lefemine AA, Lunzer S, Low HB, Cohen ML, et al. Aortic valve replacement with a caged ball valve. *Am J Cardiol.* 1962;9:292–299.
14. Henry WL, Bonow RO, Borer JS, Kent KM, Ware JH, Redwood DR, et al. Evaluation of aortic valve replacement in patients with valvular aortic stenosis. *Circulation.* 1980;61(4):814–825.
15. Schwarz F, Baumann P, Manthey J, Hoffmann M, Schuler G, Mehmel HC, et al. The effect of aortic valve replacement on survival. *Circulation.* 1982;66(5):1105–1110.
16. Brose S, Autschbach R, Rauch T, Engel M, Mohr FW. Patient-adapted valve selection: Biological vs. mechanical heart valve replacement in aortic valve diseases. *Z Kardiol.* 2001;90 Suppl 6:48–57.

17. ElBardissi AW, Shekar P, Couper GS, Cohn LH. Minimally invasive aortic valve replacement in octogenarian, high-risk, transcatheter aortic valve implantation candidates. *J Thorac Cardiovasc Surg.* 2011;141(2):328–335.

18. Brown ML, McKellar SH, Sundt TM, Schaff HV. Ministernotomy versus conventional sternotomy for aortic valve replacement: A systematic review and meta-analysis. *J Thorac Cardiovasc Surg.* 2009;137(3):670–679.e5.

19. Martens S, Sadowski J, Eckstein FS, Bartus K, Kapelak B, Sievers HH, et al. Clinical experience with the ATS 3f Enable(R) Sutureless Bioprosthesis. *Eur J Cardiothorac Surg.* 2011;40(3):749–755.

20. Lababidi Z, Wu JR, Walls JT. Percutaneous balloon aortic valvuloplasty: Results in 23 patients. *Am J Cardiol.* 1984;53(1):194–197.

21. Cribier A, Savin T, Saoudi N, Rocha P, Berland J, Letac B. Percutaneous transluminal valvuloplasty of acquired aortic stenosis in elderly patients: An alternative to valve replacement? *Lancet.* 1986;1(8472):63–67.

22. Letac B, Cribier A, Koning R, Bellefleur J-P. Results of percutaneous transluminal valvuloplasty in 218 adults with valvular aortic stenosis. *Am J Cardiol.* 1988;62(9):598–605.

23. Percutaneous balloon aortic valvuloplasty. Acute and 30-day follow-up results in 674 patients from the NHLBI Balloon Valvuloplasty Registry. *Circulation.* 1991;84(6):2383–2397.

24. Lieberman EB, Bashore TM, Hermiller JB, Wilson JS, Pieper KS, Keeler GP, et al. Balloon aortic valvuloplasty in adults: Failure of procedure to improve long-term survival. *J Am Coll Cardiol.* 1995;26(6):1522–1528.

25. Moulopoulos SD, Anthopoulos L, Stamatelopoulos M, Stefadouros, M. Catheter-Mounted Aortic Valves. *Ann Thorac Surg.* 1971;(11):423–430.

26. Davies H, Anthony G, Missen K, Blandford G, Roberts CI, Lessof HL, et al. Homograft replacement of the aortic valve. *Am J Cardiol.*1968;(22):195-217.

27. Phillips SJ, Ciborski M, Freed, PS, Cascade PM, Jaron D. A Temporary Catheter-Tip Aortic Valve: Hemodynamic Effects on Experimental Acute Aortic Insufficiency. *Ann Thorac Surg.* 1976;21(2):134–137.

28. Andersen HR, Knudsen LL, Hasenkam JM. Transluminal implantation of artificial heart valves. Description of a new expandable aortic valve and initial results with implantation by catheter technique in closed chest pigs. *Eur Heart J.* 1992;13(5):704–708.

29. Pavcnik D, Wright KC, Wallace S. Development and initial experimental evaluation of a prosthetic aortic valve for transcatheter placement. Work in progress. *Radiology.* 1992;183(1):151–154.

30. Sochman J, Peregrin JH, Rocek M, Timmermans HA, Pavcnik D, Rosch J. Percutaneous transcatheter one-step mechanical aortic disc valve prosthesis implantation: A preliminary feasibility study in swine. *Cardiovasc Intervent Radiol.* 2006;29(1):114–119.

31. Bonhoeffer P, Boudjemline Y, Saliba Z, Hausse AO, Aggoun Y, Bonnet D, et al. Transcatheter implantation of a bovine valve in pulmonary position: A lamb study. *Circulation.* 2000;102(7):813–816.

32. Bonhoeffer P, Boudjemline Y, Saliba Z, Merckx J, Aggoun Y, Bonnet D, et al. Percutaneous replacement of pulmonary valve in a right-ventricle to pulmonary-artery prosthetic conduit with valve dysfunction. *Lancet.* 2000;356(9239):1403–1405.

33. Grube E, Laborde JC, Zickmann B, Gerckens U, Felderhoff T, Sauren B, et al. First report on a human percutaneous transluminal implantation of a self-expanding valve prosthesis for interventional treatment of aortic valve stenosis. *Catheter Cardiovasc Interv.* 2005;66(4):465–469.

34. Thomas M, Schymik G, Walther T, Himbert D, Lefevre T, Treede H, et al. One-year outcomes of cohort 1 in the Edwards SAPIEN Aortic Bioprosthesis European Outcome (SOURCE) registry: The European registry of transcatheter aortic valve implantation using the Edwards SAPIEN valve. *Circulation.* 2011;124(4):425–433.

35. Piazza N, Grube E, Gerckens U, den Heijer P, Linke A, Luha O, et al. Procedural and 30-day outcomes following transcatheter aortic valve implantation using the third generation (18 Fr) corevalve revalving system: Results from the multicentre, expanded evaluation registry 1-year following CE mark approval. *Euro Interven.* 2008;4(2):242–249.

36. Smith CR, Leon MB, Mack MJ, Miller DC, Moses JW, Svensson LG, et al. Transcatheter versus surgical aortic-valve replacement in high-risk patients. *N Engl J Med.* 2011;364(23):2187–2198.

37. Leon MB, Smith CR, Mack M, Miller DC, Moses JW, Svensson LG, et al. Transcatheter aortic-valve implantation for aortic stenosis in patients who cannot undergo surgery. *N Engl J Med.* 2010;363(17):1597–1607.

38. Leon MB, Smith CR, Mack MJ, Makkar RR, Svensson LG, Kodali SK, et al. Transcatheter or surgical aortic-valve replacement in intermediate-risk patients. *N Engl J Med.* 2016;374(17):1609–1620.

39. Thyregod HG, Steinbruchel DA, Ihlemann N, Nissen H, Kjeldsen BJ, Petursson P, et al. Transcatheter versus surgical aortic valve replacement in patients with severe aortic valve stenosis: 1-year results from the all-comers NOTION randomized clinical trial. *J Am Coll Cardiol.* 2015;65(20):2184–2194.

40. Afilalo J, Lauck S, Kim DH, Lefevre T, Piazza N, Lachapelle K, et al. Frailty in older adults undergoing aortic valve replacement: The Frailty-AVR study. *J Am Coll Cardiol.* 2017;70(6):689–700.

41. Jabbour A, Ismail TF, Moat N, Gulati A, Roussin I, Alpendurada F, et al. Multimodality imaging in transcatheter aortic valve implantation and post-procedural aortic regurgitation: Comparison among cardiovascular magnetic resonance, cardiac computed tomography, and echocardiography. *J Am Coll Cardiol.* 2011;58(21):2165–2173.

42. Hyman MC, Vemulapalli S, Szeto WY, Stebbins A, Patel PA, Matsouaka RA, et al. Conscious sedation versus general anesthesia for transcatheter aortic valve replacement: Insights from the National Cardiovascular Data Registry Society of Thoracic Surgeons/American College of Cardiology Transcatheter Valve Therapy Registry. *Circulation.* 2017;136(22):2132–2140.

43. Kasel AM, Shivaraju A, von Scheidt W, Kastrati A, Thilo C. Anatomic guided crossing of a stenotic aortic valve under fluoroscopy: "Right cusp rule, part III". *JACC Cardiovasc Interv.* 2015;8(1 Pt A):119–120.

44. Roy DA, Laborde JC, Sharma R, Jahangiri M, Brecker SJ. First-in-man assessment of a dedicated guidewire for transcatheter aortic valve implantation. *Euro Interven.* 2013;8(9):1019–1025.

45. Grube E, Naber C, Abizaid A, Sousa E, Mendiz O, Lemos P, et al. Feasibility of transcatheter aortic valve implantation without balloon pre-dilation: A pilot study. *JACC Cardiovasc Interv.* 2011;4(7):751–757.

46. Auffret V, Regueiro A, Campelo-Parada F, Del Trigo M, Chiche O, Chamandi C, et al. Feasibility, safety, and efficacy of transcatheter aortic valve replacement without balloon predilation: A systematic review and meta-analysis. *Catheter Cardiovasc Interv.* 2017;90(5):839–850.

47. Toggweiler S, Leipsic J, Binder RK, Freeman M, Barbanti M, Heijmen RH, et al. Management of vascular access in transcatheter aortic valve replacement: Part 1: Basic anatomy, imaging, sheaths, wires, and access routes. *JACC Cardiovasc Interv.* 2013;6(7):643–653.

48. Wendler O, Schymik G, Treede H, Baumgartner H, Dumonteil N, Ihlberg L, et al. Source 3 registry: Design and 30-day results of the European postapproval registry of the latest generation of the Sapien 3 transcatheter heart valve. *Circulation.* 2017;135(12):1123–1132.

49. Kalra SS, Firoozi S, Yeh J, Blackman DJ, Rashid S, Davies S, et al. Initial experience of a second-generation self-expanding transcatheter aortic valve: The UK & Ireland Evolut R Implanters' registry. *JACC Cardiovasc Interv.* 2017;10(3):276–282.

50. Meredith Am IT, Walters DL, Dumonteil N, Worthley SG, Tchetche D, Manoharan G, et al. Transcatheter aortic valve replacement for severe symptomatic aortic

stenosis using a repositionable valve system: 30-day primary endpoint results from the REPRISE II study. *J Am Coll Cardiol.* 2014;64(13):1339–1348.

51. Nazif TM, Dizon JM, Hahn RT, Xu K, Babaliaros V, Douglas PS, et al. Predictors and clinical outcomes of permanent pacemaker implantation after transcatheter aortic valve replacement: The PARTNER (Placement of AoRtic TraNscathetER Valves) trial and registry. *JACC Cardiovasc Interv.* 2015;8(1 Pt A):60–69.

52. Stahli BE, Bunzli R, Grunenfelder J, Buhler I, Felix C, Bettex D, et al. Transcatheter aortic valve implantation (TAVI) outcome according to standardized endpoint definitions by the Valve Academic Research Consortium (VARC). *J Invasive Cardiol.* 2011;23(8):307–312.

53. Kappetein AP, Head SJ, Genereux P, Piazza N, van Mieghem NM, Blackstone EH, et al. Updated standardized endpoint definitions for transcatheter aortic valve implantation: The Valve Academic Research Consortium-2 consensus document (VARC-2). *Eur J Cardiothorac Surg.* 2012;42(5):S45–S60.

54. Zhang S, Kolominsky-Rabas PL. How TAVI registries report clinical outcomes: A systematic review of endpoints based on VARC-2 definitions. *PLOS ONE.* 2017;12(9):e0180815.

55. Sinning JM, Hammerstingl C, Vasa-Nicotera M, Adenauer V, Lema Cachiguango SJ, Scheer AC, et al. Aortic regurgitation index defines severity of peri-prosthetic regurgitation and predicts outcome in patients after transcatheter aortic valve implantation. *J Am Coll Cardiol.* 2012;59(13):1134–1141.

56. Hayashida K, Lefevre T, Chevalier B, Hovasse T, Romano M, Garot P, et al. Impact of post-procedural aortic regurgitation on mortality after transcatheter aortic valve implantation. *JACC Cardiovasc Interv.* 2012;5(12):1247–1256.

57. Forrest JK, Mangi AA, Popma JJ, Khabbaz K, Reardon MJ, Kleiman NS, et al. Early outcomes with the evolut PRO repositionable self-expanding transcatheter aortic valve with pericardial wrap. *JACC Cardiovasc Interv.* 2018;11(2):160–168.

58. Alassar A, Soppa G, Edsell M, Rich P, Roy D, Chis Ster I, et al. Incidence and mechanisms of cerebral ischemia after transcatheter aortic valve implantation compared with surgical aortic valve replacement. *Ann Thorac Surg.* 2015;99(3):802–808.

59. Heuser RR. SENTINEL: The tip of the iceberg in transcatheter cerebral embolic protection. *J Am Coll Cardiol.* 2017;69(21):2679.

60. Van Mieghem NM, van Gils L, Ahmad H, van Kesteren F, van der Werf HW, Brueren G, et al. Filter-based cerebral embolic protection with transcatheter aortic valve implantation: The randomised MISTRAL-C trial. *Euro Interven.* 2016;12(4):499–507.

61. Haussig S, Mangner N, Dwyer MG, Lehmkuhl L, Lucke C, Woitek F, et al. Effect of a Cerebral protection device on brain lesions following transcatheter aortic valve implantation in patients with severe aortic stenosis: The CLEAN-TAVI randomized clinical trial. *JAMA.* 2016;316(6):592–601.

62. Sievers HH, Schmidtke C. A classification system for the bicuspid aortic valve from 304 surgical specimens. *J Thorac Cardiovasc Surg.* 2007;133(5):1226–1233.

63. Mylotte D, Lefevre T, Sondergaard L, Watanabe Y, Modine T, Dvir D, et al. Transcatheter aortic valve replacement in bicuspid aortic valve disease. *J Am Coll Cardiol.* 2014;64(22):2330–2339.

64. Yoon SH, Lefevre T, Ahn JM, Perlman GY, Dvir D, Latib A, et al. Transcatheter aortic valve replacement with early- and new-generation devices in bicuspid aortic valve stenosis. *J Am Coll Cardiol.* 2016;68(11):1195–1205.

65. Dhillon PS, Kakouros N, Brecker SJ. Transcatheter aortic valve replacement for symptomatic severe aortic valve regurgitation. *Heart.* 2010;96(10):810.

66. Dumonteil N, Marcheix B, Lairez O, Laborde JC. Transcatheter aortic valve implantation for severe, non-calcified aortic regurgitation and narrow aortic root: Description from a case report of a new approach to potentially avoid coronary artery obstruction. *Catheter Cardiovasc Interv.* 2013;82(2):E124–E127.

67. Yeow WL, Roberts-Thomson P, Shetty S, Yong G. Expanding role for transcatheter aortic valve replacement: Successful

transfemoral implantation of a medtronic core valve for severe aortic regurgitation. *Heart Lung Circ.* 2012;21(11):754–758.

68. Ribichini F, Faggian G, Pesarini G, Milano A, Gottin L, Vassanelli C. Bail-out transcatheter aortic valve implantation to reduce severe acute aortic regurgitation in a failing homograft secondary to HeartMate II ventricular assistance device. *Cardiovasc Revasc Med.* 2014;15(5):295–297.

69. Roy DA, Schaefer U, Guetta V, Hildick-Smith D, Mollmann H, Dumonteil N, et al. Transcatheter aortic valve implantation for pure severe native aortic valve regurgitation. *J Am Coll Cardiol.* 2013;61(15):1577–1584.

70. Sawaya FJ, Deutsch MA, Seiffert M, Yoon SH, Codner P, Wickramarachchi U, et al. Safety and efficacy of transcatheter aortic valve replacement in the treatment of pure aortic regurgitation in native valves and failing surgical bioprostheses: Results from an International Registry Study. *JACC Cardiovasc Interv.* 2017;10(10):1048–1056.

71. Piazza N, Bleiziffer S, Brockmann G, Hendrick R, Deutsch MA, Opitz A, et al. Transcatheter aortic valve implantation for failing surgical aortic bioprosthetic valve: From concept to clinical application and evaluation (part 1). *JACC Cardiovasc Interv.* 2011;4(7):721–732.

72. Piazza N, Bleiziffer S, Brockmann G, Hendrick R, Deutsch MA, Opitz A, et al. Transcatheter aortic valve implantation for failing surgical aortic bioprosthetic valve: From concept to clinical application and evaluation (part 2). *JACC Cardiovasc Interv.* 2011;4(7):733–742.

73. Dvir D, Webb JG, Bleiziffer S, Pasic M, Waksman R, Kodali S, et al. Transcatheter aortic valve implantation in failed bioprosthetic surgical valves. *JAMA.* 2014;312(2):162–170.

74. Dvir D, Webb J, Brecker S, Bleiziffer S, Hildick-Smith D, Colombo A, et al. Transcatheter aortic valve replacement for degenerative bioprosthetic surgical valves: Results from the global valve-in-valve registry. *Circulation.* 2012;126(19):2335–2344.

75. Ribeiro HB, Rodes-Cabau J, Blanke P, Leipsic J, Kwan Park J, Bapat V, et al. Incidence, predictors, and clinical outcomes of coronary obstruction following transcatheter aortic valve replacement for degenerative bioprosthetic surgical valves: Insights from the VIVID registry. *Eur Heart J.* 2018;39(8):687–695.

76. Wendler O, Walther T, Schroefel H, Lange R, Treede H, Fusari M, et al. The SOURCE Registry: What is the learning curve in trans-apical aortic valve implantation? *Eur J Cardiothorac Surg.* 2011;39(6):853–859; discussion 9–60.

77. Wendler O, Walther T, Schroefel H, Lange R, Treede H, Fusari M, et al. Transapical aortic valve implantation: Mid-term outcome from the SOURCE registry. *Eur J Cardiothorac Surg.* 2013;43(3):505–511; discussion 11–12.

78. Soppa G, Roy D, Brecker S, Jahangiri M. Early experience with the transaortic approach for transcatheter aortic valve implantation. *J Thorac Cardiovasc Surg.* 2012;143(5):1225–1227.

79. Petronio AS, De Carlo M, Giannini C, De Caro F, Bortolotti U. Subclavian TAVI: More than an alternative access route. *Euro Interven.* 2013;9 Suppl:S33–S37.

80. Greenbaum AB, Babaliaros VC, Chen MY, Stine AM, Rogers T, O'Neill WW, et al. Transcaval access and closure for transcatheter aortic valve replacement: A prospective investigation. *J Am Coll Cardiol.* 2017;69(5):511–521.

81. Kasel AM, Cassese S, Leber AW, von Scheidt W, Kastrati A. Fluoroscopy-guided aortic root imaging for TAVR: "Follow the right cusp" rule. *JACC Cardiovasc Imaging.* 2013;6(2):274–275.

40

Transcatheter interventions for mitral and tricuspid regurgitation

DAVID W. M. MULLER

INTRODUCTION

The prevalence of atherosclerotic coronary disease has fallen progressively since the 1960s.[1] Conversely, the prevalence of valvular heart disease is increasing, in spite of a decline in rheumatic valve disease in industrialised countries.[2] In particular, severe, symptomatic mitral regurgitation (MR) is an increasingly frequent cause of hospitalisation for congestive cardiac failure, and is associated with a high mortality.[3-5] While medical therapies, such as beta-blockers and inhibitors of the renin-angiotensin-aldosterone pathways, have improved the outlook for patients with MR and cardiac failure,[6,7] surgical correction of severe MR remains the mainstay of treatment for eligible patients.[8,9] Recent surveys have suggested, however, that up to 50% of patients with an indication

for mitral valve surgery are not referred because of advanced age, co-morbidities or the perception of a low likelihood of benefit.[10,11] For these patients, transcatheter therapies offer a potential alternative to surgery.

PATHOGENESIS OF MITRAL VALVE DISEASE

Mitral valve competence is dependent on multiple factors including the size of the mitral annulus, the architecture of the valve leaflets, the integrity of the chordae and papillary muscles, and the size and shape of the left ventricle (LV). Dysfunction at any level can lead to severe mitral regurgitation (MR) (Table 40.1). Rheumatic mitral valve disease typically causes thickening and calcification of the leaflets, with commissural fusion and

Table 40.1 Pathogenesis of mitral valve regurgitation

A. Primary mitral regurgitation
  Fibro-elastic deficiency
  Myxomatous degeneration (Barlow's syndrome)
  Rheumatic heart disease
  Endocarditis – infective, non-infective
  Connective tissue disorders
  Mitral annular/leaflet calcification
  Congenital (e.g. cleft leaflet)
  Radiation injury
B. Secondary mitral regurgitation
  Leaflet tethering
  • Ischemic fibrous scarring and shortening
  • Regional LV dilatation
  • Papillary muscle displacement or rupture
  Annular dilatation
  • Global LV dysfunction (ischemic, non-ischemic)
  • Atrial fibrillation

Abbreviation: LV, left ventricular.

valve stenosis. This is often associated with thickening and calcification of the subvalvar apparatus. Retraction of the leaflets can lead to valve incompetence and MR. Infective endocarditis causes valve dysfunction by destruction of the leaflets or support structures. Rheumatic and infective mitral regurgitation have typically been excluded from the novel transcatheter valve therapies because of the potential for embolisation from the valve, or infection of the prosthesis.

Non-rheumatic, non-infective mitral regurgitation can be broadly classified into primary (or degenerative) MR and secondary (or functional) MR. Primary MR results from degenerative changes in the mitral leaflets or support structures (Table 40.1). Fibro-elastic deficiency refers to a spectrum of abnormalities ranging from elongation of the chordae with mild leaflet prolapse, to chordal rupture with a flail leaflet, to multiple ruptured chords involving several segments (scallops) of both leaflets. The leaflets themselves may be thickened and expanded (myxomatous). At the extreme, both leaflets may be enlarged, thickened, billowing and very redundant (Barlow's syndrome). Secondary MR arises when changes in left ventricular (LV) architecture cause a failure of leaflet coaptation. The valve leaflets in this

condition are typically normal. Previous inferior wall infarction, for example, may cause expansion of the postero-basal segment of the myocardium. This results in shortening of the posterior chords and tethering of the posterior leaflet, with a lack of coaptation due to over-riding of the anterior leaflet. The result is an eccentric, posteriorly-directed jet of MR. If both leaflets are tethered, as occurs in more extensive LV infarction or non-ischaemic cardiomyopathies, leaflet mal-coaptation is often symmetrical and the resulting MR is central. As the failing LV dilates, the mitral annular dimension increases, causing further failure of leaflet coaptation. Annular dilatation and severe MR can also occur in the presence of a normal LV in the context of longstanding atrial fibrillation (AF) (Table 40.1).

SURGERY FOR MITRAL VALVE REGURGITATION

Indications for mitral valve surgery have been well defined.[8,9] In primary MR, surgery is recommended (class 1, level of evidence B) for patients with severe, symptomatic MR and LV ejection fraction (LVEF) >30%.[9] It is also recommended for asymptomatic patients with left ventricular impairment (LVEF 30%–60% or LV end-systolic diameter >40 mm). It is recommended that surgery be considered in asymptomatic patients with preserved LV function when there is a high likelihood of valve repair, and in patients with new onset AF or a resting pulmonary artery systolic pressure >50 mm Hg (class IIa, level of evidence B).[9] Contemporary techniques allow the majority of patients with primary MR to undergo valve repair rather than valve replacement, with the expectation of excellent long-term results.[12] These techniques include partial leaflet resection, chordal replacement using polytetrafluoroethylene (ePTFE) neochords, and ring annuloplasty.[13] In high volume centres, valve repair is commonly performed using minimally invasive endoscopic or robot-assisted techniques.[14,15]

Indications for surgery in secondary MR are less certain. It is understood that the additional volume overload of severe MR complicates management and worsens the prognosis of patients with a failing left ventricle, but it is less clear that correcting the MR provides long-term symptomatic benefit or an increase in survival. Recent surgical data have also cast doubt on the efficacy of surgical valve repair in this context. In a randomised, controlled trial conducted by the Cardiothoracic Surgical Trial Network (CSTN), patients with ischaemic MR were randomly assigned to undergo valve replacement or valve repair. While there was a trend for higher mortality rates in the replacement group at 30 days (4.0% vs. 1.6%, $p = $ NS) and at 12 months (17.6% vs. 14.3%, $p = $ NS), the incidence of recurrent moderate or severe MR at 2 years was 58.8% in the repair group, compared with 3.8% in the replacement group ($p < 0.001$).[16] This was associated with an increased need for heart failure (HF) hospitalisation in the repair group. While there was no difference in LV remodelling between the two groups, post-hoc analysis suggested that the best LV outcome occurred in patients with a durable effective mitral repair. Mitral valve surgery for severe secondary MR is recommended for patients undergoing concomitant coronary or aortic valve surgery (class IIa, level of evidence C), and for patients with

symptoms refractory to optimal medical therapy (class IIb, level of evidence B). When surgery is performed, it is recommended consideration be given to chordal-sparing MV replacement rather than annuloplasty repair (class IIa, level of evidence B-R).[9] Current surgical techniques used to treat secondary MR include a downsized complete ring annuloplasty with or without chordal elongation or patch augmentation of the posterior leaflet.[17]

TRANSCATHETER MITRAL VALVE REPAIR

Transcatheter techniques for treating mitral valve regurgitation can be divided into interventions to repair the valve, and transcatheter valve replacement. Transcatheter repair techniques aim to increase leaflet apposition by (i) direct approximation of prolapsing or tethered leaflets (edge-to-edge repair), (ii) indirect annuloplasty, (iii) direct annuloplasty, or (iv) chordal repair (Figure 40.1).

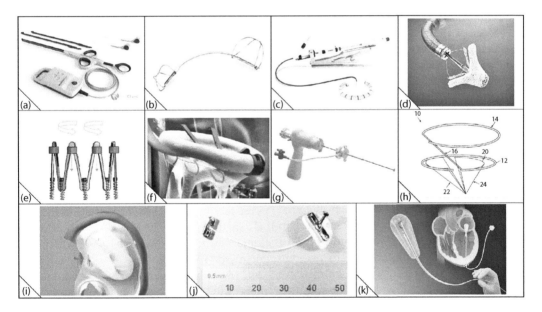

Figure 40.1 Transcatheter mitral valve repair devices. (a) Neochord DS1000. (b) CARILLON Mitral Contour System. (c) Cardioband. (d) MitraClip. (e) IRIS. (f) Amend. (g) TSD-5. (h) MISTRAL. (i) ARTO. (j) TASRA. (k) MitraSpacer. [a] Courtesy of NeoChord Inc., St. Louis Park, MN; [b] Cardiac Dimensions Inc., Kirkland, WA; [c] Edwards Lifesciences, Irvine, CA; [d] Abbott Vascular, Santa Clara, CA; [e] Millipede Medical, Santa Rosa, CA; [f] ValCare Medical, Herzliya Pituach, Israel; [g] Harpoon Medical, Baltimore, MD; [h] Mitralix Ltd., Rehovot, Israel; [i] MVRx Inc., Belmont, AC; [j] MitraSpan Inc., Belmont, MA; [k] Cardiosolutions Inc., West Bridgewater, MA; Reprinted from *Euro Interven.*, 13, AA51–AA59, 2017. With permission from Europa Digital and Publishing.

Edge-to-edge repair

Transcatheter edge-to-edge mitral repair is based on a surgical technique described by Otavio Alfieri.[18-20] The technique has been used to surgically treat complex primary MR, including severe myxomatous disease,[20] with good long-term results, particularly when edge-to-edge suturing is combined with a ring annuloplasty.[19] In 2003, St Goar and colleagues reported successful transcatheter edge-to-edge mitral repair in a porcine model via a femoral venous approach.[21] Further development led to the MitraClip Endovascular Cardiovascular Valve Repair System (Abbott Laboratories, Abbott Park, IL), which has now been used to treat more than 65,000 patients. The device consists of a polyester-covered, cobalt chromium, v-shaped clip attached to a delivery catheter that is introduced through a 24F steerable guiding catheter (Figure 40.1). The guiding catheter is introduced via the femoral vein, across the atrial septum, into the left atrium using standard trans-septal techniques. Using transoesophageal (TEE) guidance, the clip is opened in the left atrium, aligned so that the arms are perpendicular to the line of coaptation, and advanced across the valve into the left ventricle. The open clip is then retracted, grasping the anterior and posterior leaflets at the site of maximum regurgitation, and closed to create a double mitral orifice. If necessary, the clip can be reopened, repositioned and closed again. In approximately 50% of cases, a second clip is required to maximise the reduction in MR. Accurate positioning of the clip has been greatly facilitated in recent years by use of 3-D TEE.[22]

After an initial feasibility phase, MitraClip was evaluated in a randomised comparison of transcatheter mitral repair and mitral valve surgery in the EVEREST II trial.[23] The pivotal study included 279 patients in a 2:1 randomisation. Patients were excluded from the study if they had a mitral valve area <4.0 cm², a leaflet flail width >15 mm or flail gap >10 mm, or severe leaflet tethering with a coaptation depth >11 mm or length <2 mm. The majority of the patients (73%) had primary MR. At 30 days, the primary safety endpoint, a composite of multiple endpoints including the need for transfusion >2 units, occurred in 9.6% of the Mitraclip group compared with 57% in the surgical arm. The difference was largely due to the difference in need for transfusion. The primary efficacy endpoint of

MitraClip was considered to be non-inferior to surgery (72.4% vs. 87.8%). At 5 years, freedom from death, mitral valve surgery and 3+ or 4+ MR in the as-treated population was 44.2% in the percutaneous group compared with 64.3% in the surgical group ($p = 0.01$), largely due to the more frequent need for surgery for residual or recurrent MR in the MitraClip group during the first 6 months post-procedure.[24] Based on the results of the trial, MitraClip was approved in the US by the Food and Drug Administration for treatment of primary, but not secondary, MR. Large registries suggest that Mitraclip is effective in secondary MR,[25] and can be used successfully by experienced operators in many of the subgroups excluded in the EVEREST trial. In Europe, no distinction is drawn between primary and secondary MR. The European guidelines recommend consideration be given to transcatheter edge-to-edge repair for inoperable or high surgical risk patients with either primary or secondary MR (class IIa, level of evidence C).[8] The value of MitraClip therapy for secondary MR has been formally evaluated in a number of randomised clinical trials (Table 40.2). The COAPT trial (Cardiovascular Outcomes Assessment of the MitraClip Percutaneous Therapy for Heart Failure Patients with Functional Mitral Regurgitation; NCT01626079) randomised 614 patients with moderate to severe or severe MR to MitraClip or optimal medical therapy (Table 40.2). In a roll-in phase, 51 patients with severe secondary MR were treated with MitraClip in a single-arm registry. At two years, 80.8% had MR<2+, the two-year mortality was 23.9%, and 37.0% required heart failure hospitalisation.[26] Outcome data from the COAPT trial[27] and a similar French trial (MITRA-FR)[28] were recently published. The results of the two trials are discrepant. The MitraFR trial included 304 patients with severe secondary MR who were randomised to Mitraclip or to medical therapy. Severe MR was defined as an effective regurgitant orifice area (EROA) >0.20 cm² or a regurgitant volume >30 mL per beat. The LVEF was between 15% and 40% (mean 33.1%), and the mean LV end-diastolic volume index was 135.4 mL/m². The trial showed no difference in the primary endpoint of death or hospitalisation for heart failure at 12 months (54.6% in the intervention group vs. 51.3% in the control group, $p = 0.53$).[28] In contrast, the COAPT trial showed a striking benefit for Mitraclip intervention in severe secondary MR. In this study,

Table 40.2 Randomised, controlled trials of transcatheter mitral (MitraClip) valve intervention

Trial	COAPT	Reshape-HF2	Mitra-FR	Matterhorn
Patient number/ site number	614/100	420/50	304/22	210/15
Control arm	GDMT + CRT	GDMT + CRT	GDMT + CRT	MV surgery
LVEF (%)	20–50	15–40	15–40	20–45
Primary efficacy	HF hospitalisation	Death or HF hospitalisation	Death or HF hospitalisation	Death, HF hospitalisation, CVA, LVAD
Follow-up (years)	5	1	2	1
Enrolment	Completed	Ingoing	Completed	Ongoing

Abbreviations: COAPT, Cardiovascular Outcomes Assessment of mitraclip Therapy; CVA, cerebrovascular acci-
dent; CRT, cardiac resynchronisation therapy; GDMT, guideline directed medical therapy; HF, heart failure;
LVAD, left ventricular assist device; LVEF, left ventricular assist device; MV, mitral valve.

patients were included after a period of intensive guideline-directed medical therapy. The mean LVEF was similar to that in the MitraFR trial (31.3%), but the LV volumes were lower, and the EROA was greater (0.41 vs. 0.31 cm^2). The MR grade post-Mitraclip was <1+ in 82.3% and <2+ in 95.0% in COAPT compared with 75.6% and 91.9%, respectively in the MitraFR trial. In COAPT, the primary endpoint (hospitalisation for heart failure within two years) occurred at a rate of 35.8% per patient-year in the device group compared with 67.9% in the medically treated group (hazard ratio, 0.53; 95% confidence interval 0.40–0.70, $p < 0.001$) (Figure 40.2).[27] Multiple other secondary endpoints were also strongly in favour of the interventional arm. The differences in outcome between these trials will be debated for some time. Two additional trials of MitraClip for secondary MR are ongoing (Table 40.2).

The MitraClip System has changed little since its introduction. Conformite Europeenne (CE) mark approval for the original device was obtained in 2008. Small changes were made to the system in 2016 (MitraClip NT). In 2017, the delivery system was redesigned and the MitraClip NTR and XTR were introduced to improve the delivery system performance. Whereas the total clip length of the NT and NTR systems is 15 mm, the XTR has a clip length of 18 mm, increasing the coaptation length from 9 mm to 12 mm. The larger size potentially improves the depth of leaflet capture, and increases the number of patients considered eligible for treatment.

A recently introduced alternative to the MitraClip is the PASCAL Mitral Repair System (Edwards Lifesciences, Irvine CA).[25] The system has broader clips (paddles) than MitraClip, a central spacer, and independent action of the two arms. The device is designed to increase the applicability of transcatheter mitral repair to complex anatomy including wide coaptation gaps and severe leaflet tethering. The first-in-man experience with this device was reported by Praz and colleagues.[25] Successful device implantation occurred in 23 of 23 patients, with residual MR<2+ in 96%.

Indirect annuloplasty

Downsizing mitral annuloplasty has been a central component of surgical techniques for the management of MR for a long period. Controlling annular size has also been considered important in transcatheter therapies, particularly for secondary MR. The CARILLON Mitral Contour System (Cardiac Dimensions, Kirkland, WA) consists of a double-anchor nitinol device that is placed in the coronary sinus from the internal jugular vein through a 9F delivery catheter (Figure 40.1).[29] The distal anchor is advanced to the level of the anterior commissure and deployed by retraction of the delivery catheter. Traction is then applied to the system, plicating the periannular tissues and shortening the septo-lateral dimension of the annulus. Three-dimensional (3D)-TEE is used to monitor changes in the annular dimensions and the severity of MR. Once optimal reduction in annular size is achieved, the proximal anchor is deployed and locked into position. If the result is not optimal, the system can be recaptured and redeployed, or removed. This is important because of the potential for flow-limitation in the adjacent circumflex coronary artery, and because the system

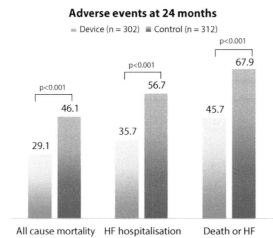

Adverse events at 24 months

Device (n = 302) Control (n = 312)

All cause mortality: 29.1, 46.1 (p<0.001)
HF hospitalisation: 35.7, 56.7 (p<0.001)
Death or HF hospitalisation: 45.7, 67.9 (p<0.001)

Figure 40.2 Cumulative incidence of all cause mortality, heart failure (HF) hospitalisation, and death or HF hospitalisation at 24 months in the COAPT trial. For each endpoint, outcomes were statistically better for patients undergoing trans-catheter mitral repair with guideline-directed medical therapy (MitraClip-device group) than for the group treated with medical therapy alone (control group). (Adapted from Stone, G.W. et al., N. Engl. J. Med., 2018.)

may be ineffective if the coronary sinus lies above the plane of the annulus. In the AMADEUS trial, the CARILLON device was successfully implanted in 30 of 48 patients. In 18 patients, the device could not be deployed (n = 5) or was removed because of inadequate reduction in MR of coronary artery compromise.[29] In those patients in whom the device was successfully implanted, there was a sustained reduction in annular dimensions and improvement in MR severity at 6 months. This was associated with an improved NYHA class, 6-minute walk test and quality of life score.[29] Similar outcomes were obtained in subsequent non-randomised trials.[30,31] The device is currently being evaluated in a double-blind, randomised trial of 120 patients with secondary MR, the REDUCE-FMR trial (ClinicalTrials.gov NCT02325830).[32] All patients will undergo invasive evaluation including coronary sinus venography. Those with appropriate anatomy will be randomly assigned in a 3:1 allocation to undergo device implantation, or to have no device implanted.

Other indirect annuloplasty systems include the ARTO device (MVRx Inc., Belmont, CA, USA) (Figure 40.1). The system connects a T-bar anchor

in the coronary sinus with a suture attached to an atrial septal anchor using magnet-tipped catheters. Tensioning of the suture results in shortening of the antero-posterior diameter of the annulus. Preliminary data from the feasibility study (MAVERIC trial, ClinicalTrials.gov NCT02302872) showed a high procedural success rate with an improvement in MR severity (90% grade 3–4+ at baseline vs. 80% grade 1–2+ at 6 months).[33]

Direct mitral annuloplasty

A major limitation of the indirect annuloplasty approach is the lack of direct relationship between the plane of the annuloplasty and the plane of the annulus. This issue is best addressed by the direct annuloplasty techniques, which aim to address the annulus itself, rather than surrounding tissues. The most advanced of these systems is the Cardioband Mitral Repair System, which received CE Mark approval in 2015 and was recently acquired by Edwards Lifesciences (Irvine, CA). The system includes a polyester sleeve that is deployed via trans-femoral, trans-septal access through a 25F delivery catheter (Figure 40.2). The sleeve is anchored to the annulus using a series of 6 mm-long metal anchors, which are screwed into the annulus sequentially from the anterior commissure, posteriorly towards the posterior commissure. When the final anchor is implanted adjacent to the posterior commissure, the length of the sleeve is adjusted using a size adjustment tool that cinches the annulus by drawing the anchors closer together. The system was evaluated in a feasibility study of 31 patients with severe secondary MR.[34] Procedural success was achieved in 100% with a >30% reduction in septo-lateral dimension of the annulus. This was associated with a reduction in MR>3+ from 77.4% to 10.7% (p < 0.001) at 30 days and a reduction in NYHA class, increase in 6-minute walk time and improved quality of life score.[34] The system is currently being evaluated in the ACTIVE trial (ClinicalTrials.gov NCT03016975), a randomised pivotal trial of 375 patients with severe secondary MR and heart failure in a 2:1 allocation against guideline-directed medical therapy. The estimated primary completion date is 2020.

Other direct annuloplasty systems that are undergoing clinical evaluation include the Millipede IRIS system (Boston Scientific, Marlborough, MA, USA), a system that can be deployed surgically or via the trans-femoral, trans-septal route. It is a complete, semi-rigid ring with a 'zig-zag' design that is held in place by 8 stainless steel anchors screwed directly into the annulus (Figure 40.1). Actuation of the device shortens the septo-lateral dimension of the annulus.[35] The Mitralign Direct Annuloplasty System (Mitralign, Tewksbury, MA) places anchors in the posterior annulus via retrograde left ventricular access. Radiofrequency energy is used to facilitate crossing of the annulus with a 0.019 in wire, followed by a pledget delivery catheter. Pairs of pledgeted sutures are placed at the P1/P2 and P2/P3 scallops. A locking device is delivered over the two sutures and tensioned, plicating the posterior annulus and reducing the annular size.[36] In a feasibility study of 71 patients with secondary MR, the device success rate was 70.4%. Cardiac tamponade occurred in 4 patients (8.9%). Both antero-posterior and septo-lateral dimensions were reduced. At 6 months, severity of MR improved in treated patients by a mean of 1.3 grades.[36]

Transcatheter chordal repair

While annuloplasty techniques are particularly valuable for patients with secondary MR, transcatheter therapies directed at repairing elongated or ruptured mitral chords are more appropriate in primary MR. To date, these interventions have been performed in the beating heart via transapical access.[37,38] The Transapical Artificial Chordae Tendinae (TACT) trial[38] enrolled 30 patients with posterior leaflet prolapse in a trial evaluating the NeoChord system (NeoChord, Inc., Minneapolis, MN). The system enables PTFE neo-chordae to be attached to the free edge of the posterior leaflet and fixed to the left ventricular apex. The chordal length can be adjusted under physiological conditions thereby optimising control of the MR. In the TACT trial,[38] acute procedural success was achieved in 86.7%. MR<2+ was achieved in 5 of the first 15 patients (33.3%) and 12 of the last 14 patients (85.7%). The Harpoon Mitral Valve Repair System (Harpoon Medical Inc., Baltimore, MD) is a similar system and has also recently completed a feasibility study. The Mitral TransApical NeoChordal Echo-Guided Repair (TRACER) trial enrolled 30 patients with posterior leaflet prolapse and severe MR.[37] Technical success was achieved in 93% with an average of 3.9 pairs of implanted

ePTFE chords. At 6 months, 85% of the patients had MR grade <1+.

TRANSCATHETER MITRAL VALVE REPLACEMENT (TMVR)

The mitral valve repair techniques described above all reduce the severity of MR, and improve symptoms and measures of quality of life. Recent evidence has suggested, however, that reducing the severity of MR from severe to moderately severe may not be adequate, as there does seem to be a survival disadvantage to having moderately severe residual MR, even in the elderly. In an analysis of data from 1,867 patients in the Transcatheter Valve Therapies Registry of the Society of Thoracic Surgery and American College of Cardiology (STS/ACC TVT Registry),[39] the cumulative incidences of death at 1 year for patients with residual MR grade <1, grade 2, and grade >3 were 21.7%, 29.2% and 48.9%, respectively ($p < 0.0001$). The combined endpoint of death or heart failure at 1 year occurred in 35.7%, 39.2%, and 54.4% respectively ($p < 0.0001$). Importantly, multivariate analysis of predictors of 1-year mortality showed that the hazard ratio for grade 0 or grade 1 residual MR was substantially lower than for grade 2 residual MR ($p = 0.0004$).[39] These findings raise the question of whether transcatheter mitral valve replacement (TMVR), rather than repair, might have an important role to play, particularly in patients with complex anatomy in whom the likelihood of achieving residual grade 0 or 1 MR is low. Numerous TMVR systems are in clinical or pre-clinical development with several now having published the results of initial feasibility studies (Figure 40.3). It is clear, however, that the engineering requirements for transcatheter mitral valve replacement are considerably more challenging than for aortic valve implantation. Implanting a valve in the mitral position requires consideration of the potential for valve instability and embolisation, para-valvular regurgitation and hemolysis, left ventricular outflow obstruction (due to a combination of the bulk of the device and to systolic anterior motion (SAM) of the anterior mitral leaflet), distortion or disruption of myocardial contractility, coronary flow limitation, erosion of surrounding structures, and conduction disturbance. The large mitral annular size also limits options for the access route. Initial efforts to deliver transcatheter mitral valve prostheses have been restricted to trans-apical and trans-atrial approaches, but recent

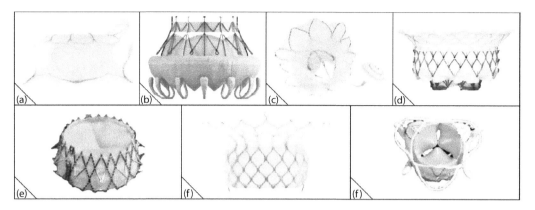

Figure 40.3 Transcatheter mitral valve replacement devices. (a) Tiara. (b) CardiAQ. (c) Tendyne. (d) Intrepid. (e) Navi. (f) HighLife. (g) Caisson TMVR. [a] Courtesy of Neovasc Inc., Richmond, BC; [b] Edwards Lifesciences, Irvine, CA; [c] Abbott Vascular, Santa Clara, CA; [d] Medtronic, Minneapolis, MN; [e] NaviGateCardiac Structures Inc., Lake Forest, CA; [f] HighLife SAS, Paris, France; [g] Caisson Interventional LLC [now LivaNova], Maple Grove, MN; Reprinted from *Euro Interven.*, 13, AA51–AA59, 2017. With permission from Europa Digital and Publishing.

and future design changes will allow trans-femoral venous, trans-septal delivery, albeit using very large delivery catheters.

The Tendyne valve system

The Tendyne prosthesis consists of two self-expanding nitinol frames and a trileaflet porcine pericardial valve (Figure 40.3).[40] The outer frame has a D-shape that is aligned with the aorto-mitral curtain, which forms the anterior margin of the mitral annulus. The valve is deployed through a 34 or 36F delivery sheath that is advanced through the valve to the left atrium from the left ventricular apex. As the delivery catheter is retracted, the partially open valve is oriented using 3D TEE guidance, withdrawn into the annulus, and then fully deployed without the need for rapid ventricular pacing. The valve is held in position by a braided high-molecular weight polyethylene tether that is attached to an epicardial pad at the ventricular access site. Tension on the tether can be adjusted to ensure the valve is seated securely on the floor of the left atrium with no para-valvular regurgitation. The epicardial pad also acts as a closure device to minimise bleeding from the ventriculotomy site. A major advantage of the system is that even after it has been fully deployed and secured in position, it can be recaptured, and redeployed or retrieved without the need for open cardiac surgery.

The valve has been implanted in more than 150 patients. Thirty-day outcome data for 30 patients enrolled in the Global Feasibility Study have been reported.[40] The age of the cohort was 75.6 ± 5.7 years and 83.3% were men. The majority (76.7%) had secondary MR. Successful device implantation was achieved in 28 of the 30 patients (93.3%). In one patient, the device was removed after implantation due to left ventricular outflow obstruction. In the other, the device could not be seated in a stable position because of a non-coaxial access site. There were no procedural deaths, strokes or myocardial infarctions. At 30 days, one patient had mild residual MR but the remainder had no MR. There was an associated reduction in left ventricular volumes, improved NYHA class, and an improved quality of life score.[40] At one year, all-cause mortality in this cohort was 16.7% and heart failure hospitalisation was required in 23.3%. In the Tendyne Expanded Feasibility Study, similar findings were apparent in 100 patients with a high procedural success rate (96%), low 30-day mortality (6.0%), and grade 0 residual MR in 98.0%.[41] These changes were again associated with positive LV remodelling, improved symptoms and an improved quality of life. A pivotal, randomised controlled comparison of the Tendyne TMVR device and mitral valve surgery (SUMMIT) will commence in late 2018.

The Medtronic Intrepid™ valve

The Intrepid valve (Medtronic Cardiovascular, Santa Rosa, CA) is a self-expanding, double-frame nitinol device with a central bovine pericardial trileaflet valve (Figure 40.3).[42] Both frames are circular. The valve is deployed via trans-apical access using a 35F delivery sheath. Fixation of the valve is achieved through a combination of oversizing, engagement of the stiffer ventricular portion with the subannular space, and a series of small cleats on the outer frame that engage the mitral leaflets.[42] Successful valve implantation was achieved in 48 of 50 patients but required circulatory support using an intra-aortic balloon pump or extracorporeal membrane oxygenation in 7 patients. There were 3 procedural deaths due to access site bleeding, and 1 due to refractory heart failure. Subsequent echocardiography showed grade 0 or 1 residual MR in all patients with implants. There was, however, a small increase in LV end-systolic dimension (51 ± 9 vs. 48 ± 10 mm at baseline, $p < 0.0001$), and a decline in LV ejection fraction ($36.2 \pm 10.2\%$ vs. $43.6 \pm 2.1\%$ at baseline, $p < 0.0001$). The Intrepid valve is now undergoing evaluation in a randomised pivotal trial (APOLLO) comparing TMVR with surgical valve repair or replacement. After an initial roll-in phase, 650 patients with primary or secondary MR will be assigned in a 1:1 randomisation to TMVR or surgery. Patients who are not considered surgically eligible will be included in a single-arm registry ($n = 550$).

The Neovasc Tiara™ valve

The Tiara valve (Neovasc Inc., Richmond, British Columbia, Canada) is also deployed trans-apically (Figure 40.3). It is a single-frame, self-expanding, asymmetric, D-shaped nitinol prosthesis that is delivered through a 32F delivery catheter. It is fixed in position by ventricular anchors or tabs, which engage the fibrous trigones of the annulus. It has an atrial skirt to minimise paravalvular leakage. To date, 58 patients have been enrolled under compassionate use protocols ($n = 22$), in the TIARA-1 Early Feasibility Study ($n = 20$), or in the CE Mark TIARA-II study ($n = 16$) (Banai S, Structural Heart Disease Summit, Chicago 2018). The majority of patients have had secondary or mixed pathology MR. There were no peri-procedural deaths or strokes but 3 patients required conversion to open surgery due to valve malposition. There has been no long-term valve dysfunction.

Other TMVR devices

Several other TMVR devices are undergoing early clinical feasibility or pre-clinical studies (Figure 40.3).[43] The CardiaQ system (Edwards Lifesciences, Irvine, CA, USA) can be deployed trans-apically or trans-septally through a 33F delivery catheter. The first human implantation was performed in 2012. A second-generation device is currently being evaluated.[44] The Caisson valve (LivaNova Caisson Interventional, LLC, Austin, TX, USA) is a docking system that is deployed in two stages trans-septally. The anchoring component is a PTFE covered, self-expanding nitinol frame that is held in place by 4 sub-annular feet and 3 atrial holding loops. The valve is D-shaped and houses a porcine pericardial valve. The anchoring component and the valve can both be retrieved before final deployment. Enrollment in a clinical feasibility study is ongoing. Like the Caisson valve, the HighLife TMVR system (HighLife SAS, Paris, France) is a two-component system. A sub-annular ring is initially deployed via an 18F femoral artery sheath, followed by placement of the self-expanding valve via trans-apical or trans-atrial access. The nitinol frame houses a bovine pericardial valve.[45] Other systems undergoing initial clinical studies include the M3 valve (Edwards Lifesciences, Irvine, CA, USA), the Navi valve (NaviGate Cardiac Structures Inc., Lake Forest, CA, USA), the Cardiovalve (Edwards Lifesciences, Irvine, CA, USA) and the Cephea valve (Cephea Valve Technologies, San Jose, CA, USA).

TRICUSPID VALVE INTERVENTIONS

Severe tricuspid valve regurgitation (TR), like severe MR, is a cause of considerable morbidity and mortality due to increasing volume overload, progressive RV dilatation, eventual right heart failure, and a low cardiac output state. Although it is commonly associated with left sided valve pathology, primary or isolated TR does occur (Table 40.3). The importance of persisting TR after correction of left sided valve disease has been highlighted recently. A report from the STS/ACC TVT Registry[46] confirmed previous observations suggesting an important influence of moderately

Table 40.3 Pathogenesis of tricuspid valve regurgitation

A. Primary tricuspid regurgitation
- Iatrogenic (endomyocardial biopsy, pacemaker/defibrillator leads)
- Congenital heart disease (Ebstein's anomaly, TV hypoplasia, DOTV)
- Infective endocarditis
- Rheumatic heart disease
- Myxomatous degeneration
- Carcinoid
- Radiation injury
- Trauma

B. Secondary tricuspid valve regurgitation (annular dilatation, RV dysfunction)
- Aortic or mitral valve disease
- Severe LV dysfunction
- Pulmonary hypertension (PE, chronic lung disease, primary PHT)
- Atrial fibrillation
- Global RV dysfunction/cardiomyopathy
- Left to right cardiac shunt (ASD, VSD, APVD)
- Endomyocardial fibrosis

Abbreviations: APVD, anomalous pulmonary venous drainage; ASD, atrial septal defect; DOTV, double outlet tricuspid valve, LV, left ventricular; PE, pulmonary embolism; PHT, pulmonary hypertension; RV, right ventricular; TV, tricuspid valve.

severe or severe residual TR on outcome after transcatheter aortic valve implantation (TAVI). In the study of 34,576 patients, adjusted 1-year mortality was worse for patients with severe TR (hazard ratio (HR) 1.29, 95% confidence interval (CI: 1.11–1.50), as was heart failure readmission (HR: 1.27, 95% CI: 1.04–1.54).[46] Similarly, in 1,867 patients in the STS/ACC TVT Registry, severe residual TR after transcatheter MV repair was an independent predictor of 1-year mortality (HR: 1.91, 95% CI: 1.42–2.55; $p < 0.001$), and the combined endpoint of 1-year death and heart failure rehospitalisation (HR: 1.89; 95% CI: 1.49–2.39; $p < 0.001$).[39]

Transcatheter therapies for TR are still very much in their infancy.[47] Treatment of the tricuspid valve, like the mitral valve, poses several anatomical challenges including the very large size of the annulus, the low flow velocity and low valve opening pressure, conformational changes during the cardiac cycle, the absence of annular and leaflet calcification, and the proximity of the conduction pathways

(atrio-ventricular (AV) node and Bundle of His) in the Koch triangle, and of the right coronary artery in the AV groove adjacent to the annulus.[48] Moreover, because of the very large annular size (normal area >9 cm^2) and the anterior location of the valve, conventional intra-procedural imaging including TEE can be challenging. Nonetheless, several repair systems and a small number of tricuspid valve replacements have been evaluated clinically.[49]

TRANSCATHETER TRICUSPID VALVE REPAIR

TriClip

Adaptation of the MitraClip System (Abbott Vascular, Santa Clara, CA, USA) to the tricuspid valve has become the dominant treatment approach for severe TR (Figure 40.4).[47] This has been facilitated by miskeying the delivery system (i.e. inserting the clip 90° counterclockwise from the recommended locking position), and by the use of the MitraClip XTR, the larger arms of which enable capture of leaflets in the setting of a large coaptation gap. Outcome data from a multicentre European registry showed a procedural success rate of 97% in 64 patients, 22 of whom also underwent transcatheter mitral valve repair.[50] Further data will be available following completion of the TRILUMINATE CE Mark trial (ClinicalTrials.gov, NCT03227757). A dedicated Triclip system is under development.

The Forma Repair System

The Forma Repair System (Edwards Lifesciences, Irvine, CA, USA) is designed to occupy the coaptation gap in severe TR using a foam-filled balloon spacer anchored to the right ventricular (RV) apex (Figure 40.4). The system is advanced from the left subclavian vein through a 20–24F introducer sheath. Adverse outcomes reported in the US Early Feasibility Study included RV perforation and device migration.[51] Further data will be available from the ongoing European SPACER trial (ClinicalTrials.gov, NCT02787408).

The TriCinch system

The TriCinch system (4Tech Cardio Ltd, Galway, Ireland) consists of a nitinol coil fixation device (i.e. attached to the TV annulus adjacent to the

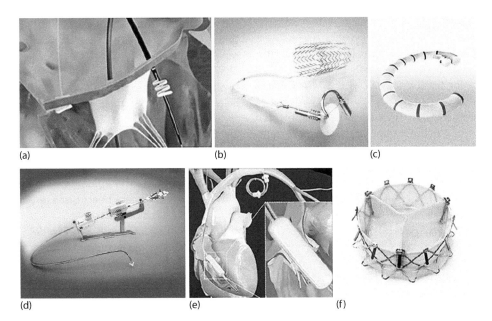

Figure 40.4 Emerging transcatheter technologies for tricuspid valve regurgitation. (a) Trialign device (Mitralign Inc). (b) TriCinch system (4Tech Cardio). (c) Cardioband (Edwards Lifesciences). (d) MitraClip system (AbbottVascular). (e) FORMA tricuspid repair system (Edwards Lifesciences). (f) Gate tricuspid atrioventricular valved stent (NaviGate Cardiac Structures Inc.). (Reprinted from Kalra, A. et al., *Methodist Debakey Cardiovasc J.*, 13, 120–125, 2017. With permission.)

antero-posterior commissure), and a band connected to a self-expanding stent. After fixation of the coil to the annulus, the band is pulled caudally, bringing the anterior leaflet closer to the septum. Tension is maintained on the band by deployment of the stent in the hepatic region of the inferior vena cava (Figure 40.4). The system is delivered through a 26F catheter advanced from the femoral vein. A first-generation of the device was evaluated in the PREVENT study (ClinicalTrials. gov NCT2098200). The device was successfully implanted in 18 of 24 patients with at least one grade reduction in TR severity in the majority. A second-generation device with a modified fixation device that is deployed from the endocardium through the RV wall to the pericardial space is being evaluated in an ongoing clinical trial.

The Trialign system

The Trialign system (Mitralign Inc., Tewksbury, MA) aims to plicate the posterior TV annulus using pledgeted sutures implanted from the ventricular side of the annulus through a catheter

advanced from the right internal jugular vein. Pledgets are placed at the antero-posterior and postero-septal commissures (Figure 40.4). Tensioning of the attached sutures plicates the posterior annulus, creating a bicuspid valve.[51] The system is currently undergoing evaluation in US (SCOUT) and European (SCOUT II) trials.

Cardioband

Like the Cardioband Mitral Repair System, the Cardioband Tricuspid Repair Sytem (Edwards Lifesciences, Irvine, CA) involves placement of a series of anchors extending from the antero-septal commissure, around the free wall of the RV to the septal annulus (Figure 40.4). Tensioning of the device plicates the annulus, reducing leaflet malcoaptation and the severity of TR. The system is delivered through a 24F catheter in the femoral vein. Thirty-day outcomes of the initial feasibility study (REPAIR study; NCT02981953) showed a 100% procedural success with two peri-procedural deaths and one stroke. There was an average reduction of septo-lateral diameter of 17%.[49]

Millipede IRIS

The Millipede IRIS system (Boston Scientific, Marlborough, MA, USA) has been evaluated as a treatment for the TV as well as the MV. Devices have been implanted surgically and will be available for transcatheter use. The system has the potential advantage of providing a docking platform for subsequent valve implantation if adequate control of the TR cannot be achieved with annuloplasty alone.

TRICUSPID VALVE REPLACEMENT

The NaviGate prosthesis

The NaviGate Tricuspid prosthesis (NaviGate Cardiac Structures, Lake Forest, CA, USA) is a dedicated valve consisting of a low-profile, tapered, cone-shaped frame with a trileaflet pericardial valve (Figure 40.4) that is available in sizes from 36 to 52 mm. It is delivered through a 42F sheath via a trans-atrial or internal jugular venous approach. In a series of 11 patients, successful device implantation was achieved in 10 (91%) with few device-related complications.[49]

Bicaval valve implantation

Valve implantation in the inferior vena cava or both vena cavae has been proposed as a means of symptom control in severe TR. The Sapien 3 balloon-expandable valve has been used for this purpose but is limited by the relatively small size of the largest available valve compared to the size of the vena cavae, which are commonly >30 mm in diameter. A dedicated self-expanding valve (TricValve, P&F, Vienna, Austria) has also been used for bicaval interventions.[52] In the small experience to date, concerns about the impact of right-atrial ventricularisation and persisting RV dilatation on outcome have not materialised.[53,54]

CONCLUSIONS

The last decade has seen explosive growth in the number of interventions evaluated for mitral and tricuspid valve disease. Although these lag well behind the number of aortic valve interventions over the same period, the need for transcatheter mitral and tricuspid therapies is no less critical. Important questions remain unanswered. These

include the optimal timing of treatment, anatomical criteria for patient selection, repair versus replacement, and appropriate post-intervention pharmacotherapy. Ongoing trials will contribute to the understanding of the problem, and should help answer many of the remaining questions.

REFERENCES

1. Dalen JE, Alpert JS, Goldberg RJ, Weinstein RS. The epidemic of the 20th century: Coronary heart disease. *Am J Med.* 2014;127(9):807–812.
2. Soler-Soler J, Galve E. Worldwide perspective of valve disease. *Heart.* 2000;83(6):721–725.
3. Grigioni F, Enriquez-Sarano M, Zehr KJ, Bailey KR, Tajik AJ. Ischemic mitral regurgitation: Long-term outcome and prognostic implications with quantitative doppler assessment. *Circulation.* 2001;103(13):1759–1764.
4. Nasser R, Van Assche L, Vorlat A, Vermeulen T, Van Craenenbroeck E, Conraads V, et al. Evolution of functional mitral regurgitation and prognosis in medically managed heart failure patients with reduced ejection fraction. *JACC Heart Fail.* 2017;5(9):652–659.
5. Tribouilloy C, Rusinaru D, Grigioni F, Michelena HI, Vanoverschelde JL, Avierinos JF, et al. Long-term mortality associated with left ventricular dysfunction in mitral regurgitation due to flail leaflets: A multi-center analysis. *Circ Cardiovasc Imaging.* 2014;7(2):363–370.
6. Cioffi G, Tarantini L, De Feo S, Pulignano G, Del Sindaco D, Stefenelli C, et al. Pharmacological left ventricular reverse remodeling in elderly patients receiving optimal therapy for chronic heart failure. *Eur J Heart Fail.* 2005;7(6):1040–1048.
7. Seneviratne B, Moore GA, West PD. Effect of captopril on functional mitral regurgitation in dilated heart failure: A randomised double blind placebo controlled trial. *Br Heart J.* 1994;72(1):63–68.
8. Baumgartner H, Falk V, Bax JJ, De Bonis M, Hamm C, Holm PJ, et al. 2017 ESC/EACTS guidelines for the management of valvular heart disease. *Eur Heart J.* 2017;38(36):2739–2791.

9. Nishimura RA, Otto CM, Bonow RO, Carabello BA, Erwin JP, 3rd, Fleisher LA, et al. 2017 AHA/ACC focused update of the 2014 AHA/ACC guideline for the management of patients with valvular heart disease: A report of the American College of cardiology/American heart association task force on clinical practice guidelines. *J Am Coll Cardiol.* 2017;70(2):252–289.

10. Mirabel M, Iung B, Baron G, Messika-Zeitoun D, Detaint D, Vanoverschelde JL, et al. What are the characteristics of patients with severe, symptomatic, mitral regurgitation who are denied surgery? *Eur Heart J.* 2007;28(11):1358–1365.

11. Goel SS, Bajaj N, Aggarwal B, Gupta S, Poddar KL, Ige M, et al. Prevalence and outcomes of unoperated patients with severe symptomatic mitral regurgitation and heart failure: Comprehensive analysis to determine the potential role of MitraClip for this unmet need. *J Am Coll Cardiol.* 2014;63(2):185–186.

12. David TE, Armstrong S, McCrindle BW, Manlhiot C. Late outcomes of mitral valve repair for mitral regurgitation due to degenerative disease. *Circulation.* 2013;127(14):1485–1492.

13. Holubec T, Sundermann SH, Jacobs S, Falk V. Chordae replacement versus leaflet resection in minimally invasive mitral valve repair. *Ann Cardiothorac Surg.* 2013;2(6):809–813.

14. Adams DH, Anyanwu AC. Seeking a higher standard for degenerative mitral valve repair: Begin with etiology. *J Thorac Cardiovasc Surg.* 2008;136:551–556.

15. Bush B, Nifong LW, Alwair H, Chitwood WR. Robotic mitral valve surgery: Current status and future directions. *Ann Cardiothorac Surg.* 2013;2(6):814–817.

16. Goldstein D, Moskowitz AJ, Gelijns AC, Ailawadi G, Parides MK, Perrault LP, et al. Two-year outcomes of surgical treatment of severe ischemic mitral regurgitation. *N Engl J Med.* 2016;374(4):344–353.

17. Glower DD. Surgical approaches to mitral regurgitation. *J Am Coll Cardiol.* 2012;60(15):1315–1322.

18. Alfieri O, Maisano F, De Bonis M, Stefano PL, Torracca L, Oppizzi M, et al. The double-orifice technique in mitral valve repair: A simple solution for complex problems. *J Thorac Cardiovasc Surg.* 2001;122(4):674–681.

19. De Bonis M, Lapenna E, Lorusso R, Buzzatti N, Gelsomino S, Taramasso M, et al. Very long-term results (up to 17 years) with the double-orifice mitral valve repair combined with ring annuloplasty for degenerative mitral regurgitation. *J Thorac Cardiovasc Surg.* 2012;144(5):1019–1024.

20. Maisano F, Schreuder JJ, Oppizzi M, Fiorani B, Fino C, Alfieri O. The double-orifice technique as a standardized approach to treat mitral regurgitation due to severe myxomatous disease: Surgical technique. *Eur J Cardiothorac Surg.* 2000;17(3):201–205.

21. St Goar FG, Fann JI, Komtebedde J, Foster E, Oz MC, Fogarty TJ, et al. Endovascular edge-to-edge mitral valve repair: Short-term results in a porcine model. *Circulation.* 2003;108(16):1990–1993.

22. Wunderlich NC, Beigel R, Ho SY, Nietlispach F, Cheng R, Agricola E, et al. Imaging for mitral interventions: Methods and efficacy. *JACC Cardiovasc Imaging.* 2018;11(6):872–901.

23. Feldman T, Foster E, Glower DD, Kar S, Rinaldi MJ, Fail PS, et al. Percutaneous repair or surgery for mitral regurgitation. *N Engl J Med.* 2011;364(15):1395–1406.

24. Feldman T, Kar S, Elmariah S, Smart SC, Trento A, Siegel RJ, et al. Randomized comparison of percutaneous repair and surgery for mitral regurgitation: 5-year results of EVEREST II. *J Am Coll Cardiol.* 2015;66(25):2844–2854.

25. Praz F, Spargias K, Chrissoheris M, Bullesfeld L, Nickenig G, Deuschl F, et al. Compassionate use of the PASCAL transcatheter mitral valve repair system for patients with severe mitral regurgitation: A multicentre, prospective, observational, first-in-man study. *Lancet.* 2017;390(10096):773–780.

26. Mack M, Abraham W, Lindfield J, Weissman N, Marx S, Ellis J, et al. Cardiovascular outcomes assessment of MitraClip therapy in heart failure patients with functional mitral regurgitation (the COAPT trial): Baseline characteristics and preliminary 2-year outcomes of the roll-in cohort. *J Am Coll Cardiol.* 2017;70(18 suppl B):B60.

27. Stone GW, Lindenfeld J, Abraham WT, Kar S, Lim DS, Mishell JM, et al. Transcatheter mitral-valve repair in patients with heart failure. *N Engl J Med.* 2018;379;2307–2318.

28. Obadia JF, Messika-Zeitoun D, Leurent G, Iung B, Bonnet G, Piriou N, et al. Percutaneous repair or medical treatment for secondary mitral regurgitation. *N Engl J Med.* 2018;379:2297-2306.

29. Schofer J, Siminiak T, Haude M, Herrman JP, Vainer J, Wu JC, et al. Percutaneous mitral annuloplasty for functional mitral regurgitation: Results of the CARILLON mitral annuloplasty device European Union Study. *Circulation.* 2009;120(4):326–333.

30. Lipiecki J, Siminiak T, Sievert H, Muller-Ehmsen J, Degen H, Wu JC, et al. Coronary sinus-based percutaneous annuloplasty as treatment for functional mitral regurgitation: The TITAN II trial. *Open Heart.* 2016;3(2):e000411.

31. Siminiak T, Wu JC, Haude M, Hoppe UC, Sadowski J, Lipiecki J, et al. Treatment of functional mitral regurgitation by percutaneous annuloplasty: Results of the TITAN trial. *Eur J Heart Fail.* 2012;14(8):931–938.

32. Goldberg SL, Meredith I, Marwick T, Haluska BA, Lipiecki J, Siminiak T, et al. A randomized double-blind trial of an interventional device treatment of functional mitral regurgitation in patients with symptomatic congestive heart failure-trial design of the REDUCE-FMR study. *Am Heart J.* 2017;188:167–174.

33. Rogers JH, Thomas M, Morice MC, Narbute I, Zabunova M, Hovasse T, et al. Treatment of heart failure with associated functional mitral regurgitation using the ARTO system: Initial results of the first-in-human MAVERIC trial (mitral valve repair clinical trial). *JACC Cardiovasc Interv.* 2015;8(8):1095–1104.

34. Nickenig G, Hammerstingl C, Schueler R, Topilsky Y, Grayburn PA, Vahanian A, et al. Transcatheter mitral annuloplasty in chronic functional mitral regurgitation: 6-month results with the CardioBand percutaneous mitral repair system. *JACC Cardiovasc Interv.* 2016;9(19):2039–2047.

35. Rogers JH, Boyd WD, Smith TW, Bolling SF. Early experience with Millipede IRIS transcatheter mitral annuloplasty. *Ann Cardiothorac Surg.* 2018;7:780-786.

36. Nickenig G, Schueler R, Dager A, Martinez Clark P, Abizaid A, Siminiak T, et al. Treatment of chronic functional mitral valve regurgitation with a percutaneous annuloplasty system. *J Am Coll Cardiol.* 2016;67(25):2927–2936.

37. Gammie JS, Bartus K, Gackowski A, D'Ambra MN, Szymanski P, Bilewska A, et al. Beating-heart mitral valve repair using a novel ePTFE cordal implantation device: A prospective trial. *J Am Coll Cardiol.* 2018;71(1):25–36.

38. Seeburger J, Rinaldi M, Nielsen SL, Salizzoni S, Lange R, Schoenburg M, et al. Off-pump transapical implantation of artificial neo-chordae to correct mitral regurgitation: The TACT trial (Transapical Artificial Chordae Tendinae) proof of concept. *J Am Coll Cardiol.* 2014;63(9):914–919.

39. Sorajja P, Vemulapalli S, Feldman T, Mack M, Holmes DR, Jr., Stebbins A, et al. Outcomes with transcatheter mitral valve repair in the United States: An STS/ACC TVT Registry report. *J Am Coll Cardiol.* 2017;70(19):2315–2327.

40. Muller DW, Farivar RS, Jansz P, Bae R, Walters D, Clarke A, et al. Transcatheter mitral valve replacement for patients with symptomatic mitral regurgitation: A feasibility trial. *J Am Coll Cardiol.* 2017;69(4):381–391.

41. Sorajja P, Moat N, Badhwar V, Walters D, Paone G, Muller D. First 100 patients treated with the tendyne transcatheter mitral prosthesis: Results from the global feasibility study. *J Am Coll Cardiol.* 2018;In press.

42. Bapat V, Rajagopal V, Meduri C, Farivar RS, Walton A, Duffy SJ, et al. Early experience with new transcatheter mitral valve replacement. *J Am Coll Cardiol.* 2018;71:12-21.

43. Natarajan D, Joseph J, Denti P, Redwood S, Prendergast B. The big parade: Emerging percutaneous mitral and tricuspid valve devices. *Euro Interven.* 2017;13(Aa):Aa51–Aa9.

44. Barbanti M, Tamburino C. Transcatheter mitral valve implantation: Cardiaq. *Euro Interven.* 2016;12(Y):Y73–Y74.

45. Barbanti M, Piazza N, Mangiafico S, Buithieu J, Bleiziffer S, Ronsivalle G, et al. Transcatheter mitral valve implantation using the HighLife system. *JACC Cardiovasc Interv.* 2017;10(16):1662–1670.

46. McCarthy FH, Vemulapalli S, Li Z, Thourani V, Matsouaka RA, Desai ND, et al. Association of tricuspid regurgitation with transcatheter aortic valve replacement outcomes: A report from the the Society of Thoracic Surgeons/American College of Cardiology Transcatheter Valve Registry. *Ann Thorac Surg.* 2018;105(4):1121–1128.

47. Taramasso M, Hahn RT, Alessandrini H, Latib A, Attinger-Toller A, Braun D, et al. The The International Multicenter Trivalve Registry: Which patients are undergoing transcatheter tricuspid repair? *JACC Cardiovasc Interv.* 2017;10(19):1982–1990.

48. Pozzoli A, Zuber M, Reisman M, Maisano F, Taramasso M. Comparative anatomy of mitral and tricuspid valve: What can the interventionlist learn from the surgeon. *Front Cardiovasc Med.* 2018;5:80.

49. Asmarats L, Puri R, Latib A, Navia JL, Rodes-Cabau J. Transcatheter tricuspid valve interventions: Landscape, challenges, and future directions. *J Am Coll Cardiol.* 2018;71(25):2935–2956.

50. Nickenig G, Kowalski M, Hausleiter J, Braun D, Schofer J, Yzeiraj E, et al. Transcatheter treatment of severe tricuspid regurgitation with the edge-to-edge mitraclip technique. *Circulation.* 2017;135(19):1802–1814.

51. Taramasso M, Calen C, Guidotti A, Kuwata S, Biefer HRC, Nietlispach F, et al. Management of tricuspid regurgitation: The role of transcatheter therapies. *Interv Cardiol.* 2017;12(1):51–55.

52. Lauten A, Ferrari M, Hekmat K, Pfeifer R, Dannberg G, Ragoschke-Schumm A, et al. Heterotopic transcatheter tricuspid valve implantation: First-in-man application of a novel approach to tricuspid regurgitation. *Eur Heart J.* 2011;32(10):1207–1213.

53. Lauten A, Figulla HR, Unbehaun A, Fam N, Schofer J, Doenst T, et al. Interventional treatment of severe tricuspid regurgitation: Early clinical experience in a multicenter, observational, first-in-man study. *Circ Cardiovasc Interv.* 2018;11(2):e006061.

54. Lauten A, Dreger H, Schofer J, Grube E, Beckhoff F, Jakob P, et al. Caval valve implantation for treatment of severe tricuspid regurgitation. *J Am Coll Cardiol.* 2018;71(10):1183–1184.

55. Kalra A, Uberoi AS, Latib A, Khera S, Bhatt DL, Reardon MJ et al. Emerging transcatheter options for tricuspid regurgitation. *Methodist Debakey Cardiovasc J.* 2017;13:120–125.

41

Transcatheter left atrial appendage occlusion

ROBERTO SPINA, DAVID W. M. MULLER AND BRENDAN GUNALINGAM

INTRODUCTION

Atrial fibrillation (AF) is the most common cardiac arrhythmia globally.[1] The estimated number of individuals with AF globally in 2010 was 33.5 million (20.9 million men and 12.6 million women), with both incidence and prevalence increasing because of an aging population (in high-income countries) and due to the epidemiological transition from communicable to non-communicable diseases (in middle- and low-income countries). In the United States alone, AF prevalence is projected to increase from 5.2 million in 2010 to 12.1 million cases in 2030.[2] The health burden associated with AF, measured as disability-adjusted life-years, increased by 18.8% in men and 18.9% in women from 1990 to 2010.[1] AF also imposes a significant

economic burden, both through its direct health costs, and through the opportunity costs represented by loss of productivity.

AF significantly increases the risk of stroke.[3] Oral anticoagulation with warfarin substantially reduces the risk of stroke in patients with AF,[4,5] but it is associated with a significant risk for haemorrhagic complications, inconvenience and interactions with other medications.[6,7] The novel anticoagulants—factor Xa thrombin or thrombin inhibitors—have obviated some of the shortcomings of warfarin therapy, but are themselves associated with a non-negligible risk of bleeding and concern remains regarding the lack of universally available reversal agents.[8–11]

Surgical, pathological, and transoesophageal studies have determined that in non-valvular AF, around 90% of cardiac thrombi arise from the left atrial appendage.[12,13] Occlusion of left atrial appendage closure has therefore emerged as a therapeutic modality to reduce the risk of systemic thromboembolism in atrial fibrillation. Historically, left atrial appendage occlusion (LAAO) was performed surgically, often during concomitant coronary artery bypass grafting or valvular or other open-heart interventions. In the last decade, percutaneous transcatheter techniques have become available to exclude the atrial appendage. Several devices have been tested and used in humans, but the two devices most commonly used worldwide currently are the Watchman device (Boston Scientific, Natick, MA, USA) and the Amplatzer Plug (St Jude Medical, St Paul, MN, USA).

LEFT ATRIAL APPENDAGE: STRUCTURE, FUNCTION, AND ROLE IN THROMBOEMBOLISM

Anatomy

The left atrial appendage is the remnant of the embryonic left atrium that develops in the third week of gestation. The left atrial cavity proper develops later and is formed from the outgrowth of the pulmonary veins.[14] The LAA is a long, tubular, structure with a narrow neck and a crenelated lumen (Figure 41.1). In contrast, the right appendage is broad and triangular with a wide neck.[14] Both the right and left appendages are trabeculated. The LAA lies within the pericardium, and abuts the pulmonary artery superiorly and the free wall of the left ventricle inferomedially. The LAA is separated from the orifices of the left pulmonary veins by an infolding of the lateral atrial wall called the left lateral ridge, or warfarin (or coumadin) ridge.[15] Substantial variation exists in the morphology of the LAA. In a study of 45 Chinese patients with a history of atrial fibrillation,[16] invasive angiographic imaging of the left atrial appendage demonstrated a considerable morphological variability in terms of its size, shape and number of lobes (Figure 41.1).

Physiology

The contractile function of the left atrial appendage in sinus rhythm includes a phase of forward flow (out of the appendage) occurring soon after the start of transmitral flow in early diastole, followed by a short phase of backward flow (into the appendage). Coincident with atrial systole is a further phase of forward flow owing to contraction of the appendage, followed by another phase of backward flow possibly caused by elasticity of the appendage.[14] In atrial fibrillation, blood flow velocities are generally lower compared to sinus rhythm, less predictable, and more highly variable.[18] Low LAA blood flow velocities are significant predictors of thrombus formation, independent of various haemostatic variables indicating platelet or coagulation activation.[19] Almost uniformly, the presence of LAA thrombus is accompanied by extreme LAA dysfunction, manifested as a low-to-absent LAA flow velocity profile.[20]

The atria and the atrial appendages are the site of production of atrial natriuretic peptide (ANP), brain natriuretic peptide (BNP) and C-type natriuretic peptide (CNP). The natriuretic hormones have potent natriuretic, and diuretic, vasodilator activity, and play a major role in salt-water homeostasis.[21] The highest concentration of ANP-containing atrial granules is found in the atrial appendages.[22] Animal and human studies have demonstrated that the surgical removal of the atrial appendages blunts ANP secretion, natriuresis, and diuresis in response to plasma volume expansion.[23,24]

Role in thrombogenesis

Surgical, pathological, and transoesophageal studies have determined that in non-valvular AF, 90% of cardiac thrombi arise from the left atrial appendage in non-rheumatic atrial fibrillation.[12,13,25] In atrial fibrillation associated with rheumatic heart disease, around 60% of the thrombi are located in the LAA.[12,26] Poor contractile function of the appendage, the presence of spontaneous echocardiographic contrast, and specific Doppler flow signals have been associated with increased risk of left atrial appendage thrombus formation.

LAA OCCLUSION

Surgical LAA occlusion

Surgical exclusion of the LAA has traditionally been performed in patients with atrial fibrillation at moderate or high risk of thromboembolism undergoing coronary artery or valvular heart

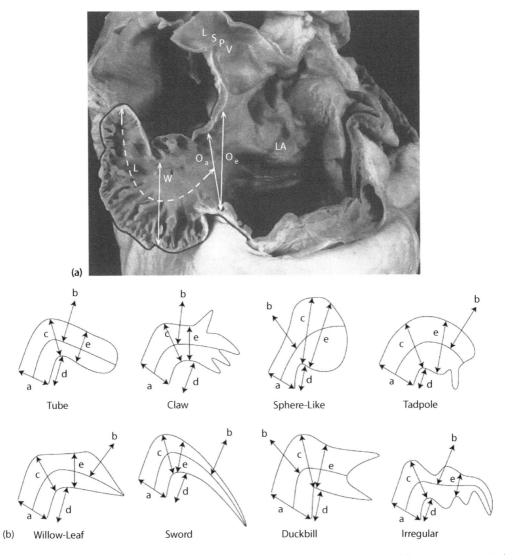

Figure 41.1 **(a)** Left atrial appendage (LAA) anatomy in a cadaveric specimen. (*Abbreviations:* LA, Left atrium; LSPV, Left superior pulmonary vein; L, Length; W, Width.) **(b)** Schematic representation of the morphological variability of the left atrial appendage. ([a] Reprinted from Veinot, J.P. et al., *Circulation.*, 96, 3112–3115, 1997. With permission; Courtesy of Wolters Kluwer; [b] Reprinted from Shi, A.W. et al., *J. Int. Med. Res.* 40, 1560–1567, 2012. With permission; Courtesy of Sage Publishing, UK.)

surgery. The LAA Occlusion Study (LAAOS) is the first randomised study of surgical LAA occlusion in patients undergoing concurrent coronary artery bypass surgery with staples or sutures versus control.[27] Seventy-seven patients were randomised to undergo either occlusion ($n = 52$) or control (no occlusion; $n = 25$). By TEE, occlusion was successful in 29 (66%) patients. Two ischemic strokes occurred in the immediate perioperative period. Both patients had undergone LAA occlusion. After a follow-up period of 13 ± 7 months, no additional stroke events were reported in either occlusion or control groups. A small follow-up trial, the LAAOS II study, randomised 26 patients to LAA occlusion, and 25 to oral anticoagulation.[28] At 12 months, the composite outcome of death, myocardial infarction, stroke, non-CNS embolism, and major bleeding was largely similar between groups. Three strokes occurred in the oral anticoagulation group, one in the LAA occlusion group.

Several studies have called into question the effectiveness of surgical ligation of the left atrial appendage in occluding the LAA in the medium-to-long term. A study by Kanderian et al. examined a total of 137 of 2,546 patients who underwent surgical LAA closure from 1993 to 2004.[29] Of the 137 patients, 52 (38%) underwent excision and 85 (62%) underwent exclusion. Only 55 of 137 (40%) of closures were successful by TEE examination. LAA thrombus was present in 28 of 68 patients (41%) with unsuccessful LAA exclusion versus none with excision.

Transcatheter LAA occlusion

Trans-catheter LAAO has emerged as an alternative to systemic anticoagulant therapy in the last decade. Although several closure devices have been developed, the systems most widely adopted worldwide are the Watchman (Boston Scientific, Natick, MA, USA) and the Amplatzer cardiac plug (St Jude Medical, Minneapolis, MN).

The first percutaneous LAA occlusion device: PLAATO

The PLAATO LAA transcatheter occlusion (PLAATO System, ev3 Inc., Plymouth, MN) was the first to be studied in clinical trials (Figure 41.2). The device consisted of a self-expanding nitinol cage (range of diameter 15–32 mm) covered with expanded polytetrafluoroethylene in order to close off blood flow into the remaining part of the LAA. The device was deployed via a transeptal approach under TEE guidance. In the first multicentre study, LAA occlusion was achieved successfully in 97.5% of patients, with a 5.5% major adverse event rate.[30] In a 5-year non-randomised follow-up study of patients undergoing LAA occlusion with the PLAATO device, the annualised stroke/transient ischemic attack (TIA) rate was 3.8%. The anticipated stroke/TIA rate (with the CHADS2 scoring method) for the study cohort was 6.6%/year.[31] The device was withdrawn from the market for commercial reasons.

The Watchman device

The second percutaneous LAA occlusion device to appear on the market was the Watchman device, which consists of a self-expanding nitinol frame designed to conform to the appendage anatomy and reduce embolisation risk. The frame is covered with a permeable (160 mm) polyethylene terephthalate (PET) membrane designed to block emboli and promote healing. There are 10 active fixation anchors at the nitinol frame perimeter, designed to engage LAA tissue for device stability (Figure 41.3).

The Watchman device has been used in more than 20,000 patients worldwide and is the only closure device to have been tested in randomised

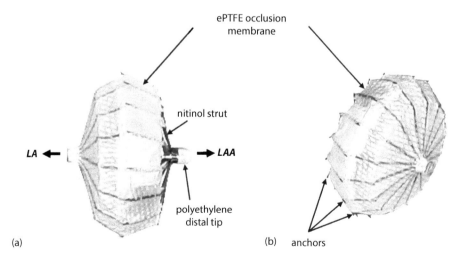

Figure 41.2 PLAATO device consisting of a nitinol cage structure covered with ePTFE. (a) Lateral view. (b) Front surface (LA-facing side). (Reprinted from Nakai, T. et al., *Circulation*., 105, 2217–2222, 2002. With permission; Courtesy of Wolters Kluwer.)

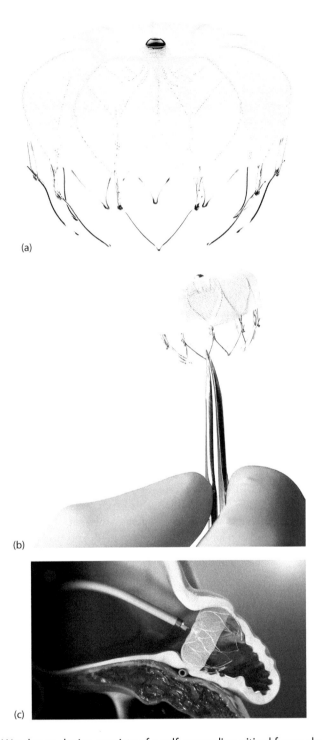

(a)

(b)

(c)

Figure 41.3 (a–c) The Watchman device consists of a self-expanding nitinol frame designed to conform to the appendage anatomy and reduce embolisation risk. The frame is covered with a permeable (160 mm) polyethylene terephthalate (PET) membrane designed to block emboli and promote healing. There are 10 active fixation anchors at the nitinol frame perimeter, designed to engage LAA tissue for device stability. (Courtesy of Boston Scientific. ©2018 Boston Scientific Corporation or its affiliates. All rights reserved.)

clinical trials. The PROTECT AF pivotal clinical trial randomised 463 patients with non-valvular AF and a CHADS$_2$ (congestive heart failure, hypertension, age ≥75 years, diabetes mellitus, and prior stroke or transient ischemic attack) score ≥1 to LAA occlusion with the Watchman device, and 244 to oral anticoagulation with dose-adjusted warfarin. LAAO with the Watchman proved to be non-inferior to warfarin in preventing stroke in non-valvular AF patients at 12 months.[33] In addition, long-term follow-up up to 3.8 years of the PROTECT AF trial patients confirmed the non-inferiority of device therapy.[34] However, concerns were raised regarding patient selection criteria and relatively high rate of procedural events, prompting a second randomised trial, the PREVAIL trial.[35] In the latter study, 269 patients were assigned to the intervention group, and 138 to long-term warfarin therapy. Although the procedural safety improved significantly and LAA occlusion was proven to be non-inferior to warfarin for non-procedural ischaemic stroke prevention, non-inferiority was not achieved for the overall efficacy endpoint. Both PROTECT AF and PREVAIL trials were followed by investigational devices exemption registries (CAP 1 (2008–2010, n = 566) and CAP 2 (2012–2014, n = 579), respectively), to allow continued access to the Watchman device and to gain further safety and efficacy data on the device.[36] Five-year outcomes data from the PROTECT AF and PREVAIL trials and meta-analyses of trial and registry data demonstrated improved rates of haemorrhagic stroke, cardiovascular/unexplained death and non-procedural bleeding compared to warfarin.[37,38]

Amplatzer cardiac plug and amulet devices

The AMPLATZER™ Cardiac Plug (ACP; St Jude Medical, St Paul, MN, USA) is a self-expandable device, based on the well-established Amplatzer occluder technology and specifically designed for LAAO, which has demonstrated favourable feasibility and safety results in observational studies. The ACP consists of self-expanding nitinol mesh forming a lobe and disk, connected by a central articulating waist (Figure 41.4). The second-generation ACP, Amulet (St Jude Medical), has a wider lobe, longer waist, recessed proximal end screw, and more stabilising wires. These features improve the stability of Amulet and theoretically may reduce

thrombus formation on the atrial side of the device. Amulet also comes in 8 sizes and accommodates larger LAAs (up to 32 mm).

Since the launch of the ACP in 2008, over 7,000 devices have been implanted worldwide. The ACP was initially evaluated in several small retrospective registries, mostly involving single-centre experiences in Europe, Canada, Asia, and Latin America.[39] In aggregate, >1,100 patients were included in these registries, showing good safety profile (serious pericardial effusion 1.7%, device embolisation 1.1%, ischemic stroke 0.4%), and procedural success (96.4%). More recently, Tsikas et al presented the results of the pooled experience of a total of 1,047 consecutive patients undergoing LAA occlusion at 22 centres.[40] This large multicentre study confirmed the results of previous analyses (procedural success 97.3%, periprocedural major adverse events 4.5%). One-year all-cause mortality was 4.2% (none device-related). The annual rate of systemic thromboembolism was 2.3% (31/1,349 patient-years), whereas the annual rate of major bleeding was 2.1% (28/1,349 patient-years).

The U.S. pivotal ACP randomised-controlled trial commenced enrolment in early 2013, randomising AF patients with CHADS2 ≥2 to ACP versus anticoagulation (warfarin or dabigatran) in a 2:1 ratio. However, due to slow enrolment and imminent FDA approval of WATCHMAN, this study was discontinued in December 2013 after enrolment of 80 patients. The study is being redesigned, and it is anticipated that the new randomised study will involve a noninferiority comparison to the Watchman device.

OTHER DEVICES

Hybrid endovascular and epicardial LAA closure: The LARIAT system

The LARIAT (SentreHeart, Redwood City, CA, USA) system accomplishes percutaneous delivery of a suture that snares the LAA epicardially, at its os, via trans-septal and pericardial access.

Price et al.[41] published the multicentre retrospective U.S. experience of 154 patients who underwent the Lariat procedure. Technical success was 94%, but a significant number of procedures (14%) were complicated by major adverse events including pericardial effusion requiring

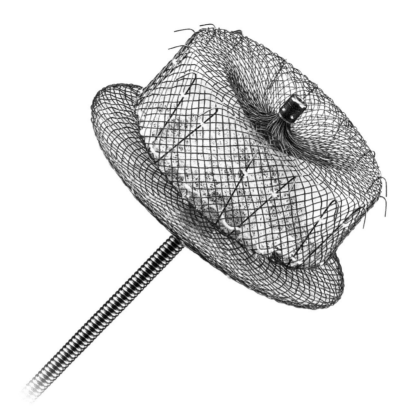

Figure 41.4 The Amplatzer Cardiac Plug is made of a flexible braided Nitinol mesh. The lobe conforms to the inner wall of the LAA and requires only a minimum depth of 10 mm for deployment, providing secure placement in a shallow landing zone. The device can be fully recaptured and repositioned for precise placement. (Courtesy of Abbott Cardiovascular.)

intervention (10.4%); bleeding requiring transfusion (4.5%); and emergent cardiac surgery (2.0%). At a median follow-up of 112 days, death, myocardial infarction or stroke occurred in 2.9%. TEE follow-up was performed in 63 patients revealing residual leak in 20%, and presence of thrombus in 4.8%. Even though its technical success is acceptable, the Lariat procedure is still in its infancy and is associated with significant adverse effects.

LAA closure in clinical guidelines

The relevant European Society of Cardiology and the American Heart Association/American College of Cardiology guidelines suggest that left atrial appendage occlusion may be considered to reduce stroke in patients for whom oral anticoagulation is contra-indicated (Grade IIB),[42] and that

surgical excision of the LAA may be considered in patients undergoing cardiac surgery or thoracoscopic atrial fibrillation surgery (Grade IIB).[43]

AREAS OF UNCERTAINTY AND FUTURE DIRECTIONS

LAA occlusion and prevention of ischemic stroke

The raison d'être of LAA closure devices is to prevent thrombus forming in the left atrial appendage and subsequent systemic and cerebral embolism. Therefore, one would expect LAA closure to be associated with a lower risk of ischemic, cardioembolic stroke. Puzzlingly, however, a meta-analysis of the results of the two device trials and their associated registries concluded that although all-cause stroke and systemic embolism was similar between both strategies (1.7% vs. 1.8%/100 PY; HR: 0.96; 95% CI: 0.60–1.54; p = 0.87), there were more ischemic strokes in the device group (1.6% vs. 0.95% /100 PY; HR: 1.71; p = 0.08).[37] One explanation for this finding is that a number of ischemic strokes occurred in the peri-procedural period, and included procedure-related air embolism. When the analysis is confined to the longer term, on the other hand, device and oral anticoagulation have similar rates of (ischemic) stroke.[37]

In contrast, analysis of the pooled data revealed that haemorrhagic stroke occurred significantly less frequently in the LAAO group at a rate of 0.15 per 100 PY for device versus 0.96 for warfarin.[44] By demonstrating that the rates of haemorrhagic stroke are reduced compared to the warfarin arm, these device trials have also highlighted another desirable feature of left atrial appendage occlusion: By removing the need for long-term anticoagulation, LAAO offers patients a clear benefit in terms of reduction of bleeding risk. Indeed, in the PREVAIL trial, the rates of warfarin discontinuation were 92%, 98%, and 99% at 45 days, 6 and 12 months, respectively.

Post-procedure anticoagulation following Watchman device deployment

Following Watchman device deployment, OAC is recommended for 45 days post-procedure, in addition to antiplatelet therapy, to allow for device endothelialisation and prevent device thrombosis and associated stroke. Patients randomised to the LAA closure arm in the PROTECT AF and PREVAIL trials received concomitant warfarin after Watchman implantation for 6 weeks. However, patients with absolute contra-indications to oral anticoagulation because of life-threatening haemorrhagic events, who would stand to benefit most from LAAO, were excluded from these trials. The safety and efficacy of Watchman device deployment without warfarin transition has not been evaluated extensively. The non-randomised ASAP study examined the safety and efficacy of LAA closure in 150 non-valvular AF patients with a contraindication for warfarin therapy.[45] Patients only received antiplatelet agents after Watchman implantation. The ASAP study demonstrated that warfarin-eligible and warfarin-ineligible patients experienced similar efficacy and

safety event rates. Based on the result of the ASAP study, it appears reasonable to treat warfarin-ineligible patients with the Watchman device without oral anticoagulation cover post-procedure. The ASAP-TOO study is multinational, multicentre prospective randomised trial currently recruiting patients.[46] The trial is designed to establish the safety and effectiveness of the Watchman left atrial appendage closure device in patients with non-valvular AF who are deemed ineligible for OAC. This trial will answer the question whether Watchman device implantation is safe and effective without warfarin transition.

Alternative trans-catheter LAA closure systems do not require anticoagulation with warfarin post-procedure. The PLAATO and Amplatzer cardiac plug devices both required antiplatelet therapy only post-procedure.

Device related thrombosis

The prevalence of TEE-proven device-related thrombus (DRT) in the PROTECT-AF was 27/485 (5.7%) of patients. DRT was present at 45 days in 1.4% of patients, with higher prevalence at 6 and 12 months (3.9% and 2.5% of patients, respectively). The primary efficacy event of stroke, systemic embolism, and death occurred at a rate of 3.4 per 100 patient-years in the DRT subgroup and is between the event rate of the two arms of the entire trial cohort (2.2% for device vs. 3.7% for warfarin per 100 patient-years) after 5 years of follow-up.[47] Three device thrombosis events were associated with ischemic stroke. Of the 150 patients enrolled in the ASAP registry, there were 6 cases (4%) of device-related thrombus on the device face, but only 1 resulted in clinical sequela (an ischemic stroke.)[45]

In the multicentre registry involving Amplatzer device,[40] a thrombus related to the device was observed in 28/632 patients (4.4%). DRT was not associated with any adverse event at follow-up. A recent small series of LAA closure with a new device requiring only antiplatelet therapy post-procedure, the Amplatzer Amulet device, has reported high adherent thrombus rates (16.7%) without associated adverse sequelae.[48] Device-related thrombus and its associated potential adverse effects are important issues that require further investigation in a field that is moving towards less intense anticoagulation regimens post LAAO.

Comparison with novel anticoagulants

Novel oral anticoagulants (NOACs), including the direct thrombin inhibitor dabigatran and the factor Xa inhibitors apixaban, edoxaban, and rivaroxaban, have emerged in recent years as suitable alternatives to vitamin K antagonists for stroke prevention in AF, and their use in clinical practice is increasing rapidly. A meta-analysis based of the pivotal studies of warfarin vs. NOACs found that NOACs significantly reduced stroke or systemic embolic events compared with warfarin, mainly driven by a reduction in haemorrhagic stroke.[49] Mortality was 10% lower in patients randomised to NOAC therapy and intracranial haemorrhage was halved, while gastrointestinal bleeding events were more frequent.[49] Transcatheter LAAO has only been tested against warfarin, and therefore an interest has arisen as to how it would perform against the NOACs. The multicentre randomised Prague-17 clinical trial is currently recruiting and will address that issue.[50]

CONCLUSION

Transcatheter left atrial appendage occlusion has emerged in the last decade as a safe and effective alternative to oral anticoagulation with warfarin to prevent ischemic stroke in patients with non-valvular atrial fibrillation. Most of the clinical benefit appears to derive from a reduction in haemorrhagic stroke. The Watchman device is the only system that has been studied in randomised clinical trials, and is the most widely adopted device worldwide, but other transcatheter devices have emerged in recent years. Unresolved issues include the optimal antithrombotic and anticoagulation regimen post left atrial appendage occlusion, the clinical significance of device-related thrombosis, the selection of patients, and the untested performance of LAA occlusion devices compared to the novel anticoagulants.

REFERENCES

1. Chugh SS, Havmoeller R, Narayanan K, Singh D, Rienstra M, Benjamin EJ, et al. Worldwide epidemiology of atrial fibrillation A Global Burden of Disease 2010 Study. *Circulation.* 2014;129:837–847.
2. Colilla S, Crow A, Petkun W, Singer DE, Simon T, Liu X. Estimates of current and future incidence and prevalence of atrial fibrillation in the U.S. Adult Population. *Am J Cardiol.* 2013;112:1142e1147.
3. Wolf PA, Abbott RD, Kannel WB. Atrial fibrillation as an independent risk factor for stroke: The Framingham Study. *Stroke.* 1991;22: 983–988.
4. Hylek EM, Go AS, Chang Y, et al. Effect of intensity of oral anticoagulation on stroke severity and mortality in atrial fibrillation. *N Engl J Med.* 2003;349:1019–1026.
5. Mant J, Hobbs FR, Fletcher K, Roalfe A, Fitzmaurice D, Lip GY, et al. Warfarin versus aspirin for stroke prevention in an elderly community population with atrial fibrillation (the Birmingham Atrial Fibrillation Treatment of the Aged Study, BAFTA): A randomised controlled trial. *Lancet.* 2007;370:493–503.
6. Hylek EM, Evans-Molina C, Shea C, Henault LE, Regan S. Major hemorrhage and tolerability of warfarin in the first year of therapy among elderly patients with atrial fibrillation. *Circulation.* 2007;115: 2689–2696.
7. Flaherty M, Kissela B, Woo D, Kleindorfer D, Alwell K, Sekar P, et al. The increasing incidence of anticoagulant-associated intracerebral hemorrhage. *Neurology.* 2007;68: 116–121.
8. Connolly SJ, Ezekowitz MD, Yusuf S, Eikelboom J, Oldgren J, Parekh A, et al. Dabigatran versus warfarin in patients with atrial fibrillation. *N Engl J Med.* 2009;361(12):1139–1151.
9. Patel MR, Mahaffey KW, Garg J, Pan G, Singer DE, Hacke W, et al. Rivaroxaban versus warfarin in nonvalvular atrial fibrillation. *N Engl J Med.* 2011;365(10):883–891.
10. Granger CB, Alexander JH, McMurray JJ, Lopes RD, Hylek EM, Hanna M, et al. Apixaban versus warfarin in patients with atrial fibrillation. *N Engl J Med.* 2011;365(11):981–992.
11. Giugliano RP, Ruff CT, Braunwald E, Murphy SA, Wiviott SD, Halperin JL, et al. Edoxaban versus warfarin in patients with atrial fibrillation. *N Engl J Med.* 2013;369(22):2093–2104.

12. Manning WJ, Weintraub RM, Waksmonski CA, Haering JM, Rooney PS, Maslow AD et al. Accuracy of transoesophageal echocardiography for identifying left atrial thrombi. *Ann Intern Med.* 1995;123:817–822.

13. Blackshear JL, Odell JA. Appendage obliteration to reduce stroke in cardiac surgical patients with atrial fibrillation. *Ann Thorac Surg.* 1996;61:755–759.

14. Al-Saady NM, Obel OA, Camm AJ. Left atrial appendage: Structure, function, and role in thromboembolism. *Heart.* 1999;82:547–555.

15. Cabrera JA, Saremi F, Sanchez-Quintana D. Left atrial appendage: Anatomy and imaging landmarks pertinent to percutaneous transcatheter occlusion. *Heart* 2014;100:1636–1650.

16. Shi AW, Chen ML, Yang B, Cao KJ, Kong XQ. A morphological study of the left atrial appendage in Chinese patients with atrial fibrillation. *J Int Med Res.* 2012;40(4):1560–1567.

17. Veinot JP, Harrity PJ, Gentile F, Khandheria BK, Bailey KR, Eickholt JT, et al. Anatomy of the normal left atrial appendage: A quantitative study of age-related changes in 500 autopsy hearts: Implications for echocardiographic examination. *Circulation.* 1997;96:3112–3115.

18. Agmon Y, Khandheira BK, Gentile F, Seward JB. Echocardiographic assessment of the left atrial appendage. *J Am Coll Cardiol.* 1999;34(7):1867–1877.

19. Heppell RM, Berkin KE, McLenachan JM, Davies JA. Haemostatic and haemodynamic abnormalities associated with left atrial thrombosis in non-rheumatic atrial fibrillation. *Heart.* 1997;77:407–411.

20. García-Fernández MA, Torrecilla EG, San Román D, Azevedo J, Bueno H, Moreno MM, et al. Left atrial appendage Doppler flow patterns: Implications on thrombus formation. *Am Heart J.* 1992;124:955–961.

21. Levin ER, Gardner DG, Samson WK. Natriuretic peptides. *N Engl J Med.* 1998; 339(5):321–328.

22. Hamid Q, Wharton J, Terenghi G, Hassall CJ, Aimi J, Taylor KM, et al. Localization of atrial natriuretic peptide mRNA and immunoreactivity in the rat heart and human atrial appendage. *Proc Natl Acad Sci USA.* 1987;84:6760–6764.

23. Stewart JM, Dean R, Brown M, Diasparra D, Zeballos GA, Schustek M, et al. Bilateral atrial appendectomy abolishes increased plasma atrial natriuretic peptide release and blunts sodium and water excretion during volume loading in conscious dogs. *Circ Res.* 1992;70:724–732.

24. Omari BO, Nelson RJ, Robertson JM. Effect of right atrial appendectomy on the release of atrial natriuretic hormone. *J Thorac Cardiovasc Surg.* 1991;102:272–279.

25. Thambidorai SK, Murray RD, Parakh K, Shah TK, Black IW, Jasper SE, et al. Utility of transesophageal echocardiography in identification of thrombogenic milieu in patients with atrial fibrillation (an ACUTE ancillary study). *Am J Cardiol.* 2005; 96:935–941.

26. Mahajan R, Brooks AG, Sullivan T, Lim HS, Alasady M, Abed HS, et al. Importance of the underlying substrate in determining thrombus location in atrial fibrillation: Implications for left atrial appendage closure. *Heart.* 2012;98(15):1120–1126.

27. Healey JS, Crystal E, Lamy A, Teoh K, Semelhago L, Hohnloser SH, et al. Left Atrial Appendage Occlusion Study (LAAOS): Results of a randomized controlled pilot study of left atrial appendage occlusion during coronary bypass surgery in patients at risk for stroke. *Am Heart J.* 2005;150(2):288–293.

28. Whitlock RP, Vincent J, Blackall MH, Hirsh J, Fremes S, Novick R, et al. Left Atrial Appendage Occlusion Study II (LAAOS II). *Can J Cardiol.* 2013;29(11):1443–1447.

29. Kanderian AS, Gillinov AM, Pettersson GB, Blackstone E, Klein AL. Success of surgical left atrial appendage closure: Assessment by transesophageal echocardiography. *J Am Coll Cardiol.* 2008;52(11):924–929.

30. Ostermayer SH, Reisman M, Kramer PH, Matthews RV, Gray WA, Block PC, et al. Percutaneous left atrial appendage transcatheter occlusion (PLAATO system) to prevent stroke in high-risk patients with non-rheumatic atrial fibrillation: Results from the international multi-center feasibility trials. *J Am Coll Cardiol.* 2005;46(1):9–14.

31. Block PC, Burstein S, Casale PN, Kramer PH, Teirstein P, Williams DO, Reisman M. Percutaneous left atrial appendage occlusion for patients in atrial fibrillation suboptimal for warfarin therapy: 5-year results of the PLAATO (Percutaneous Left Atrial AppendageTranscatheter Occlusion) Study. *JACC Cardiovasc Interv.* 2009;2(7):594–600.

32. Nakai T, Lesh MD, Gerstenfeld EP, Virmani R, Jones R, Lee RJ. Percutaneous left atrial appendage occlusion (PLAATO) for preventing cardioembolism: First experience in canine model. *Circulation.* 2002;105(18):2217–2222. Accessed 13 February 2018.

33. Holmes DR, Reddy VY, Turi ZG, Doshi SK, Sievert H, Buchbinder M, et al. Percutaneous closure of the left atrial appendage versus warfarin therapy for prevention of stroke in patients with atrial fibrillation: A randomised non-inferiority trial. *Lancet.* 2009;374:534–542.

34. Reddy VY, Sievert H, Halperin J, Doshi SK, Buchbinder P, Nuzil K, et al. Protect AF steering ommitee Investigators. Percutaneous left atrial appendage closure vs warfarin for atrial fibrillation: A randomized clinical trial. *JAMA.* 2014; 312(19):1988–1998.

35. Holmes DR, Kar S, Price MJ, Whisenant B, Sievert H, Doshi SK, Huber K, Reddy VY. Prospective randomized evaluation of the Watchman left atrial appendage closure device in patients with atrial fibrillation versus long-term warfarin therapy: The PREVAIL trial. *J Am Coll Cardiol.* 2014;64:1–12.

36. Reddy VY, Holmes D, Doshi SK, Neuzil P, Kar S. Safety of percutaneous left atrial appendage closure: Results from the WATCHMAN Left Atrial Appendage System for Embolic Protection in Patients with AF (PROTECT AF) clinical trial and the Continued Access Registry. *Circulation.* 2011;123(4):417–424.

37. Reddy VY, Doshi SK, Kar S, Gibson DN, Price MJ, Huber K, et al. PREVAIL and PROTECT AF investigators. 5-year outcomes after left atrial appendage closure: From the PREVAIL and PROTECT AF trials. *J Am Coll Cardiol.* 2017;70(24):2964–2975.

38. Sahay S, Nombela-Franco L, Rodes-Cabau J, Jimenez-Quevedo P, Salinas P, Biagioni C, et al. Efficacy and safety of left atrial appendage closure versus medical treatment in atrial fibrillation: A network meta-analysis from randomised trials. *Heart.* 2017;103(2):139–147.

39. Urena M, Rodés-Cabau J, Freixa X, Saw J, Webb JG, Freeman M, et al. Percutaneous left atrial appendage closure with the AMPLATZER cardiac plug device in patients with nonvalvular atrial fibrillation and contraindications to anticoagulation therapy. *J Am Coll Cardiol.* 2013;62:96–102.

40. Tzikas A, Shakir S, Gafoor S, Omran H, Berti S, Santoro G, et al. Left atrial appendage occlusion for stroke prevention in atrial fibrillation: Multicentre experience with the AMPLATZER Cardiac Plug. *Euro Intervent.* 2016;11:1170–1179.

41. Price MJ, Gibson DN, Yakubov SJ, Schultz JC, Di Biase L, Natale A, et al. Early safety and efficacy of percutaneous left atrial appendage suture ligation: Results from the U.S. transcatheter LAA ligation consortium. *J Am Coll Cardiol.* 2014;64(6):565–572.

42. Kirchhof P, Benussi S, Kotecha D, Ahlsson A, Atar D, Casadei B, Castella M. 2016 ESC Guidelines for the management of atrial fibrillation developed in collaboration with EACTS. *Eur Heart J.* 2016; 37:2893–2962.

43. January CT, Wann LS, Alpert JS, Calkins H, Cigarroa JE, Conti JB, et al. 2014 AHA/ACC/HRS guideline for the management of patients with atrial fibrillation: Executive summary: A report of the American College of Cardiology/American Heart Association Task Force on practice guidelines and the Heart Rhythm Society. *Circulation.* 2014;130:2071–2104.

44. Price MJ, Reddy VY, Valderrábano M, Halperin JL, Gibson DN, Gordon N, et al. Bleeding outcomes after left atrial appendage closure compared with long-termwarfarin: A pooled, patient-level analysis of the WATCHMAN randomized trial experience. *JACC Cardiovasc Interv.* 2015;8(15):1925–1932.

45. Reddy VY, Möbius-Winkler S, Miller MA, Neuzil P, Schuler G, Wiebe J, et al. Left atrial appendage closure with the

Watchman device in patients with a contraindication for oral anticoagulation: The ASAP study (ASA Plavix feasibility study with watchman left atrial appendage closure technology). *J Am Coll Cardiol.* 2013;61(25):2551–2556.

46. Holmes DR, Reddy VY, Buchbinder M, Stein K, Elletson M, Bergmann MW, et al. The Assessment of the Watchman Device in Patients Unsuitable for Oral Anticoagulation (ASAP-TOO) trial. *Am Heart J.* 2017;189:68–74.

47. Main ML, Fan D, Reddy VY, Holmes DR, Gordon NT, Coggins TR, et al. Assessment of device-related thrombus and associated clinical outcomes with the WATCHMAN left atrial appendage closure device for embolic protection in patients with atrial fibrillation (from the PROTECT-AF Trial). *Am J Cardiol.* 2016;117(7):1127–1134.

48. Sedaghat A, Schrickel J, Andrié R, Schueler R, Nickenig G, Hammerstingl C. Thrombus formation after left atrial appendage occlusion with the Amplatzer amulet device. *Catheter Cardiovasc Interv.* 2017;90(5):E111–21.

49. Ruff CT, Giugliano RP, Braunwald E, Hoffman EB, Deenadayalu N, Ezekowitz MD, Et al. Comparison of the efficacy and safety of new oral anticoagulants with warfarin in patients with atrial fibrillation: A meta-analysis of randomised trials. *Lancet.* 2014;383:955–962.

50. Osmancik P, Tousek P, Herman D, Neuzil P, Hala P, Stasek J, et al.; PRAGUE-17 Investigators. Interventional left atrial appendage closure vs novel anticoagulation agents in patients with atrial fibrillation indicated for long-term anticoagulation (PRAGUE-17 study). *Am Heart J.* 2017;183:108–114.

42

Cardiac surgery and percutaneous cardiac interventions

ARJUN IYER AND PAUL JANSZ

INTRODUCTION

Cardiac surgery has been the cornerstone for treatment of valvular pathology until recently, with the advent of new percutaneous cardiac interventions, which have now progressed to include percutaneous therapy for valve disease. This evolution has been instrumental in allowing alternative treatment options for patients deemed high-risk for surgical intervention, and is now at a stage where percutaneous valve therapy has its own role in the armamentarium against heart disease. With ongoing trials underway, the evidence base continues to be consolidated. In this chapter, an overview of the current place of percutaneous therapy for aortic and mitral valve pathology, and the hybrid approach to coronary disease, is presented.

AORTIC STENOSIS

Aortic stenosis is the most common valvular heart pathology in the developed world, with approximately 7% of the general population over the age of 65 afflicted with this degenerative process.[1] Beginning as aortic sclerosis, gradual narrowing of the aortic valve orifice causes a pressure gradient between the left ventricle (LV) and aorta. To cope with this gradient, the heart compensates with progressive myocardial hypertrophy, thereby preventing the onset of symptoms. A point is reached in this process, however, where there is loss of compliance due to severe hypertrophy, with subsequent myocardial dysfunction. The onset of this, combined with progressive narrowing of the aortic valve, results in worsening symptoms and subsequent risk to life. Once symptomatic, prognosis deteriorates quickly. Following onset of symptoms, ranging from angina and syncopal episodes to heart failure, survival is limited to between 2 and 5 years.[2]

Bearing a class IA indication in the 2014 American College of Cardiology/American Heart Association (ACC/AHA) guidelines,[3] and with a clearly defined mortality benefit and a low mortality and morbidity to low-risk patients, surgical aortic valve replacement has been the mainstay treatment for severe symptomatic aortic stenosis. Following the first successful surgical replacement in 1960, today 75,000 patients undergo surgical aortic valve replacement each year in the United States.[4]

The limitation of surgical aortic valve replacement is evident in the nearly 30% of referred patients that are deemed too high-risk for surgical intervention.[5] With numerous comorbidities, advanced age, left ventricular dysfunction and general frailty, these patients carry a significantly elevated mortality and morbidity risk for surgical aortic valve replacement (SAVR).

This subset of patients rejected for surgical intervention has formed the basis for development of alternative approaches to the correction of aortic valve stenosis. Use of balloon aortic valvuloplasty was trialed, and it demonstrated lowered gradients and clinical and functional improvement.[6] However, high rates of restenosis within months to years, and the recurrence of aortic regurgitation limited any mortality benefit and its widespread use. The next stage in the evolution of non-surgical percutaneous therapies was the development of transcatheter aortic valve implantation or replacement (TAVI/TAVR).

TAVI

In 1987, large vascular stents that allowed access to the aortic valve were created, paving the way for the first series of percutaneously inserted bioprosthetic aortic valve replacements in animal models.[7,8] The 'first-in-man' TAVI was performed in 2002 by Alain Cribier and colleagues.

In a 57-year-old male with a bicuspid aortic valve stenosis, a percutaneous valve was inserted via a transvenous, antegrade approach that presented several challenges.[9] Subsequently, Webb and associates successfully demonstrated the safety and feasibility of the transfemoral approach for TAVI.[10]

Indications for aortic valve replacement

With progression of surgical and percutaneous aortic valve replacements and improving outcomes, guidelines have adapted with changes to the indications for replacement. The 2014 ACC/AHA guidelines for AVR have evolved, with TAVI now considered the choice of intervention in the following scenarios[3]:

1. Patients considered to be at prohibitive risk of surgery, but with a post-TAVI survival of >12 months (class I indication).
2. As an alternative to SAVR in patients considered to be at high risk for surgery (Class II indication).

The above class I and II indications for TAVI represent a real paradigm shift, with the emergence of TAVI as a legitimate alternative to surgical valve replacement.

It is increasingly evident that the most important development in decision making about SAVR vs. TAVI is the establishment of the 'heart valve team', a combination of several medical and other health care professionals, and improvements in TAVI outcomes have been heavily influenced by this multidisciplinary approach.[11]

Vascular access for TAVI

TAVI is technically possible in the majority of aortic stenosis patients; however, the limiting factor remains safe and adequate vascular access. The use of larger sheaths and catheters increases the risk of vascular complications, which have a significant impact on mortality, both early and late. Major vascular complications in the pioneering study of TAVI, the PARTNER trial, occurred in 15.3% of patients.[12] More contemporary data, with better vascular assessment and patient selection and smaller calibre devices, has lowered this rate to 7.9%.[13]

The imaging modality of choice in assessment of vascular access, specifically the iliofemoral system and abdominal aorta, is best achieved with multidetector computed tomography (MDCT) using three-dimensional (3D) volume-rendering imaging and multiplanar reformats.[14] Computed tomography (CT) imaging is used to assess luminal size, calcification, plaque burden, vessel tortuosity and high-risk features of complex atheroma and dissection. It is suggested that a sheath to femoral artery size ratio of 1.12 or greater is associated with a higher rate of vascular complications and 30-day mortality.[15] Use of this information for screening, along with smaller sheaths and percutaneous repair techniques, has lowered rates of vascular TAVI access site complications.

While contrast CT imaging is the imaging modality of choice, other options include magnetic resonance imaging (MRI) and angiography. These alternatives are used in the setting of absolute contraindications to MDCT, specifically the use of 80–120 mL of low-osmolar iodinated contrast. Some protocols have been established to minimise the risk of contrast nephropathy by using direct power injection of diluted contrast.[14–18]

In the case of non-viable femoral access, alternative vascular access sites can be considered. In this setting, a multidisciplinary procedural approach is used, with surgical input for vascular access as required. Each option is addressed below.

TRANSFEMORAL ACCESS

The femoral artery is the preferred and most widely-used access site for TAVI. Under local anaesthesia, percutaneous approaches to the femoral artery and suture pre-closure techniques are the preferred options for entry and closure.

Figures of up to 20% of cases needing elective surgical exposure or conversion to surgical exposure are quoted, especially with increasing complexity of the patient population.[19,20] The main concern with femoral access is damage to the iliofemoral vessels. Current TAVI catheters range in size between 14 and 20 French and require a minimal vessel diameter of 5.5–6.5 mm, with limited calcification and tortuosity. Surgical cut-down is indicated in obese patients, and in the presence of femoral grafts/stents or situations where a high femoral puncture is desired.[21]

The older age of the TAVI population is also associated with a greater prevalence of peripheral vascular disease. While use of smaller catheters and complete percutaneous approaches have lowered rates of vascular complications, significant calcification, tortuosity and atherosclerosis should be approached with great caution, and alternative access sites should be considered.

TRANSAPICAL ACCESS

This approach is recommended in the setting of severe peripheral vascular disease or severely calcified porcelain thoracic aorta.[22,23] Initially described by Ye in 2006,[24] the transapical left ventricular approach requires general anaesthesia and is best performed in a hybrid theatre. A left anterolateral thoracotomy is performed via the 5th or 6th intercostal space, the pericardium is opened and the LV apex exposed. Subsequent puncture and sheath insertion is followed by a guidewire across the aortic valve prior to the usual technique for retrograde valve deployment (see Figure 42.1).

TRANSAXILLARY/SUBCLAVIAN ACCESS

This technique is used in the setting of contraindications to transfemoral and transapical approaches. Gaining approval in 2010, it is usually approached with a cutdown surgical technique. Dissection past the pectoralis major muscle with careful avoidance of the brachial plexus allows relatively easy access to the subclavian artery at the deltopectoral groove. Contraindications for its use include luminal diameter less than 6 mm, severe calcification and tortuosity, and any narrowing along its course. Either side can be used; however, the right subclavian access creates more difficulty when the plane of the valve to the horizontal is greater than 30°. Challenges with left subclavian artery access include compromise of the left internal mammary artery (LIMA) graft, if this exists.[25]

TRANS-AORTIC ACCESS

The proximal aorta is accessed through either a right anterior thoracotomy or a hemisternotomy, depending on the location of the aorta in relation to the sternum. Placement of a pursestring suture and a sheath through the ascending aorta allows easy deployment of the valve. For most TAVI devices, the aortic access site needs to be approximately 6 cm above the annular plane to allow device deployment. Advantages of this approach include familiarity for the cardiac surgeon, avoiding smaller femoral or subclavian arteries, and a more direct approach to

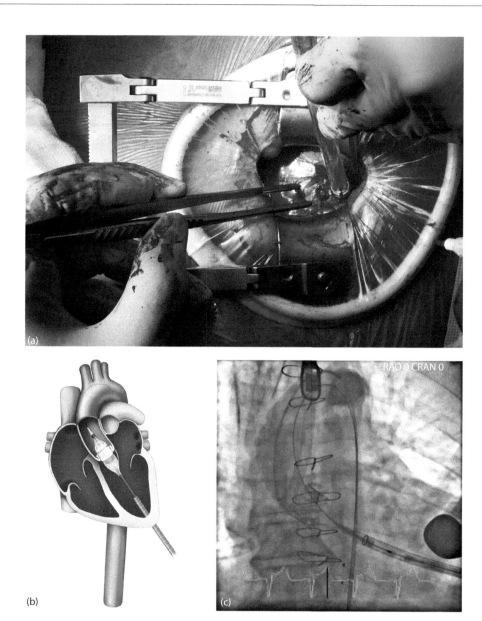

Figure 42.1 (a) Apical approach showing delivery sheath insertion through the left ventricular apex using the Octopus clamp. (b) Schematic showing balloon inflation and deployment of Edwards Sapien valve via the trans-apical approach. (c) Angiogram showing position of apical delivery sheath post-deployment of Edwards Sapien valve. ([b] Courtesy of Edwards Lifesciences LLC, Irvine, CA.)

the aortic root, allowing more precise placement in the horizontal root.[26] It has also been associated with more favourable outcomes when compared to the transapical approach, with less bleeding, myocardial injury and intensive care stay.[27]

OTHER ACCESS SITES

Some authors have suggested the transcarotid approach, but this is reliant on the patient tolerating temporary unilateral carotid artery occlusion and an adequate anterior communicating artery at the Circle of Willis.[28] This approach is not widely used, with only a few case series reported.

TRANSCAVAL ACCESS

When comparing access sites, the transfemoral route is associated with lower 30 days and 1 year mortalities. Comparing transfemoral with transapical approaches, there is lower 30 days mortality with transfemoral access. A recent paper comparing transfemoral with transaortic and transapical approaches suggested a trend towards higher 30 days and 1 year mortalities with the latter, suggesting that the transaortic approach should be the second-line choice after transfemoral access.[29]

Types of TAVI valves

Several percutaneous valves have attained European approval; however, the majority of the published data and Food and Drug Administration (FDA) approval has been achieved for two main percutaneous devices—the Medtronic CoreValve Revalving system and the Edwards Sapien system. Both these valves have proven effective in the Pivotal and Partner trials

EDWARDS SAPIEN VALVE

The Sapien valve is a balloon-expandable, trileaflet check bovine pericardial valve on a stainless-steel framework. It is available in two forms, namely the Sapien XT and the Sapien 3. Sizes range from 20 to 29 mm and both can be deployed via all the main access sites—transfemoral, transapical, trans-subclavian and transaortic. Both valves can be used for valve-in-valve procedures, while the Sapien 3 valve has a lower profile, improved delivery catheter and a polyethylene terephthalate outer skirt, all contributing to lower vascular complications and a reduction in paravalvular leak.[30]

PARTNER TRIAL

The Placement of AoRTic traNscathetER Valve (PARTNER) trial was a randomised, prospective trial assessing the Sapien valve. It was divided into two substudies, PARTNER A and PARTNER B. Partner A compared TAVI (transapical or transfemoral) with SAVR in high-risk patients who were deemed to have an operative risk >15%. Assessing 699 patients between the two arms of Partner A, there was no difference in mortality at 30 days, 1 or 5 years. Higher rates of stroke and transient ischemic attack were noted with TAVI at 30 days, but this difference no longer existed at 5 years. More frequent vascular complications were noted with TAVI, while there was more bleeding and atrial fibrillation with the surgical arm. Higher rates of moderate/severe

paravalvular leak existed with the TAVI groups, and this extended out to 5 years and was associated with higher mortality.[31]

The Partner B trial assessed TAVI against medical therapy for patients deemed inoperable. Assessing 358 patients, there was a significantly lower mortality in the TAVI group at 1 year (30.7% for TAVI vs. 50.7% with medical therapy including balloon valvotomy; $p < 0.001$). This mortality benefit extended out to 5 years (71.8% vs. 93.6%; $p < 0.0001$).[32]

The next stage was assessment of intermediate-risk patients, determined as a Society of Thoracic Surgery (STS) mortality score of approximately 6%. PARTNER 2 compared the Sapien XT valve with SAVR in this population.[13] There was no difference in mortality or stroke between the groups, but the TAVI cohort had less severe bleeding, atrial fibrillation, and acute renal injury. The SAVR cohort had fewer vascular complications and less paravalvular regurgitation, which when moderate or greater was associated with higher mortality at 2 years. The next generation Sapien valve 3 addresses this, with smaller sheath size contributing to lower vascular complications, and a skirt mechanism that reduces the rate of paravalvular leak.[33] These improvements and the favourable mortality rates of Partner 2 have paved the way for the Sapien 3 valve to be approved for use in intermediate-risk patients in the US.

COREVALVE REVALVING SYSTEM

The CoreValve system, containing a self-expanding nitinol frame, consists of a trileaflet porcine pericardial tissue valve. It is available in sizes ranging from 23 to 34 mm and is approved for valve-in-valve replacement. The latest generation CoreValve, the Evolut R, has a low profile and is the only repositionable and recapturable device available in the US.[30] From the Australian perspective, Sapien 3 and Evolut-R have been approved for reimbursement, and the Portico, Accurate, and Lotus valves are all commercially available.

COREVALVE PIVOTAL TRIAL

A non-inferiority trial performed at 45 different sites across the US, the Pivotal trial, compared TAVI using the CoreValve with SAVR in patients with severe aortic stenosis and increased risk of death from surgery. Seven hundred and ninety five patients were assessed and there was a significant trend towards lower mortality in the TAVI group at 1 and 2 years when evaluating all cause-mortality.[34]

CHOICE TRIAL

This trial compared the self-expanding CoreValve with the balloon-inflatable Sapien XT valve in high-risk patients with severe aortic stenosis. There was no difference in mortality or stroke at 1 year, but there was a higher need for pacemakers, more aortic regurgitation and valve embolisation, and a need for more than one valve with the self-expanding CoreValve.[35]

Future of TAVI

The current-generation Sapien 3 valve addresses some of the complications demonstrated in the PARTNER 2 trial—use of smaller sheath size works towards minimising vascular complications and its skirt mechanism allows lower rates of paravalvular leaks. This improvement, and the improved mortality rates of PARTNER 2, support TAVI being first-line therapy for intermediate-risk patients. Furthermore, the FDA has recently approved clinical trials to assess TAVI in low-risk surgical patients, evaluating the newer-generation devices of the repositionable CoreValve Evolut R and the lower profile Edwards Sapien 3 systems (PARTNER 3 trial). Another device being evaluated is the LOTUS valve system in the REPRISE III trial, and this offers another repositionable device. The improving TAVI technology will no doubt result in improved outcomes, and the future of this percutaneous modality looks bright and set to change the landscape of aortic valve treatment.

PERCUTANEOUS MITRAL VALVE THERAPY

Balloon valvuloplasty for selected mitral stenosis (MS) patients has long been established as an important arm in the treatment for this pathology (see Chapter 38), whereas percutaneous treatment of mitral regurgitation (MR) is novel and not well-established yet. The mitral annulus is variable and asymmetrical, and usually lacks annular calcification for device fixation (an important aspect of fixation for aortic transcatheter valves), and these

factors all contribute to the challenge of developing a reliable percutaneous option for MR.

Mitral valve anatomy

The mitral valve is a complex structure that consists of two leaflets, each subdivided into segments commonly referred to as scallops. The larger anterior leaflet lies close to the aorta, while the smaller posterior leaflet is positioned posterolaterally. The leaflets are anchored to the LV by chords running from the edge of the leaflets to two papillary muscles. The mitral leaflets are attached to the saddle-shaped mitral annulus, which plays an important role in myocardial contraction and left ventricular function.

MR is the primary pathology targeted by novel percutaneous therapies now discussed in this chapter. Pathology can originate from changes in the mitral leaflets or changes in the mitral annulus, causing failure of leaflet apposition and resulting in valvular regurgitation.

MR

MR is broadly divided into two categories—primary (or degenerative) and secondary (or functional) MR. Primary mitral valve disease is a result of abnormal thickening, redundancy, perforations or abnormalities in the subvalvular supporting structures, namely the papillary muscles and chords. Broadly referred to as fibro-elastic deficiency or myxomatous change, there exists a spectrum of disorders ranging from single-segment prolapse from chordal elongation, to severe bileaflet prolapse referred to as Barlow's disease.

Secondary MR is a consequence of either ischaemic or non-ischaemic left ventricular dysfunction. Regurgitation results from failure of leaflet coaptation from ventricular dilatation and remodelling as a result of dilated cardiomyopathy or myocardial infarction, or from atrial dilatation caused by long-standing atrial fibrillation. Ischaemic MR is broadly categorised under secondary MR, and is a result of leaflet tethering and papillary muscle displacement.

The approach to the surgical repair of these pathologies varies. Degenerative MR is addressed through leaflet plication, resection or chordal reconstruction combined with annuloplasty rings. Functional MR with central MR usually requires an annuloplasty ring, while ischaemic MR is addressed with a combination of coronary revascularisation and annuloplasty interventions. The aim has been to reproduce such reliable repair techniques via percutaneous approaches. A few of the currently available percutaneous options are discussed in the following.

MitraClip

The MitraClip is the most successful and widely-used percutaneous delivery device for mitral regurgitation, and is the only currently available device for MR with FDA approval. Its mechanism is based around a surgical technique, referred to as the Alfieri 'edge-to-edge' stitch, where the middle scallops of the anterior and posterior leaflets are sutured together to allow a double-barrel opening with enough orifice area to avoid mitral stenosis.[36] While the benefits of this techniques have

been debated due to variable results with certain pathologies and the risk of mitral stenosis, its use combined with an annuloplasty ring has been demonstrated to have good survival and freedom from re-operations.[37]

Performed under general anaesthesia with fluoroscopic and transoesophageal guidance, the MitraClip device consists of a steerable guide catheter, a clip delivery system and an implantable clip. The clip itself is made up of two polypropylene fabric-covered cobalt chromium arms with grippers at their ends for leaflet fixation.[38] Femoral venous puncture is followed by trans-septal puncture. After being aligned above the mitral valve perpendicular to the line of coaptation, it is advanced across the mitral valve and deployed (Figure 42.2). The degree of MR is then assessed,

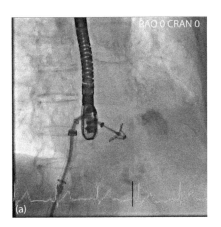
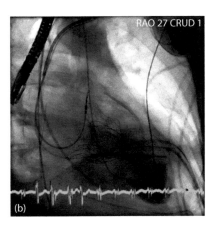
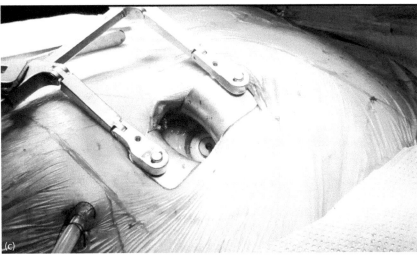

Figure 42.2 **(a)** Angiogram showing deployment of Mitraclip device via trans-septal approach. **(b)** Angiogram showing Tendyne device in situ. **(c)** External view of Tendyne apical tether attached to apex of left ventricle.

and if unacceptable, the device can be re-opened, re-positioned and redeployed, or alternatively additional clips can be deployed.

Indications

The MitraClip device (Figure 42.2a) is used worldwide for both degenerative and functional MR; however, FDA approval is at present only for primary degenerative MR. The 2014 AHA/ACC and 2012 European Society of Cardiology guidelines[3,39] recommend their use in:

- Severely symptomatic (New York Heart Association Class III or IV) heart failure despite medical therapy
- Chronic severe (3 to 4+) primary (degenerative) mitral regurgitation (MR)
- Favourable anatomy for the repair procedure
- Reasonable life expectancy
- Prohibitive surgical risk due to comorbidities

The anatomical considerations for use of MitraClip in MR are important to establish the effectiveness of this therapy.[40] These include:

- Planimetered mitral valve area (in parasternal short axis view at tips of the mitral valve, see Chapter 38) $\geq$4.0 cm^2.
- Minimal leaflet calcification in the grasping area.
- If leaflet flail is present, width of the flail segment <15 mm and flail gap of <10 mm. Flail gap was defined as the greatest distance between the ventricular side of the flail segment and the atrial side of the opposing leaflet (measured in the four-chamber long axis and left ventricular outflow tract views).
- Jet of MR may be central and large (>6 cm^2 or >30% of left atrial area) or smaller if eccentric and encircling the left atrium.

Currently, it is advised that all patients considered for MitraClip should be discussed at a multidisciplinary meeting involving the heart team. In general, it has been suggested that prohibitive surgical risk is a Society of Thoracic Surgeons (STS) risk score of >6% mortality. Additional factors that must be considered in calculating patient risk beyond what is captured by the STS score include patient frailty, severe pulmonary hypertension, porcelain aorta and severe liver disease.[3,39]

Trials

EVEREST 1 trial: This was a prospective multicentre single-arm feasibility trial consisting of 107 patients treated with Mitraclip therapy.[41] Demonstrating no procedural mortality and in-hospital mortality of <1%, procedural success was 74%. However, 17% of these patients needed mitral valve surgery during the 1 year follow up period. Despite this, this trial demonstrated the feasibility of this therapy for primary MR.

EVEREST II trial: This large randomised, prospective, multicentre trial compared Mitraclip to mitral valve surgery in 279 patients with moderate/severe MR.[42] Primary efficacy endpoint was freedom from death, from surgery for mitral valve dysfunction and from grade 3+ or 4+ MR at 12 months. Safety endpoint was defined as major adverse events at 30 days. While overall mortality was similar at 12 months, the primary endpoint was more frequent in the surgical arm (73% vs. 55%) due to higher rates of subsequent surgery for mitral valve dysfunction in the MitraClip arm (20% vs. 2%). At 4 years, surgery for mitral valve dysfunction was needed in 25% of patients treated with MitraClip (5.5% in the surgical arm). However, the majority of these occurred in the first 6 months and therefore it appeared that if a good outcome was achieved procedurally, the likelihood of needing surgery for recurrent MR was very low. Safety endpoint favoured the Mitraclip group (48% vs. 15%), mainly due to the need for blood transfusion with surgery. Subgroup analysis of data from the EVEREST II trial suggested that patients over the age of 70 and those with functional MR or poor LV dysfunction had comparable long-term results to surgical repair.[41,42]

Secondary/functional MR

Secondary MR represents a high-risk cohort where the presence of LV dysfunction and ischaemia contribute to significantly increased risk and poorer survival. No therapy, surgical or otherwise, has demonstrated a survival benefit in this group. Observational data suggests that selected patients with secondary MR benefit from MitraClip therapy, with an improvement in heart failure symptoms but no evidence of improved survival.

A subgroup analysis of 327 high-risk patients (STS score >12%) in the EVEREST II trial was performed[43]—70% of these patients had secondary MR. MitraClip therapy was associated with an acute reduction in MR to 2+ or less in 86%, >80% of patients were in NYHA class I/II at 12 months post-procedure, and annual hospitalisation fell significantly.

While the above and similar studies[44] demonstrate high rates of technical success in secondary MR, and improvement in symptoms in this group, there is no clear consensus about its use in this setting. Ongoing randomised trials are underway to further define the role of Mitraclip in heart failure and secondary MR.

Complications

The overall complication rate in EVEREST II was 15%–19% at 30 days,[41,43] mainly due to the need for blood transfusion. As stated earlier, rates of transfusion, however, are significantly lower than with surgical intervention. Other issues, occurring rarely, include partial clip detachment, device embolisation and development of mitral stenosis.

Thus, MitraClip has become established as a useful therapy in treating severe MR and there now exists a reasonable clinical experience worldwide across numerous registries. While surgical repair remains the treatment of choice in MR due to lower rates of subsequent intervention, studies to date do not demonstrate any mortality difference between surgery and percutaneous therapy. The role of this therapy at present is limited to patients deemed too high-risk and unsuitable for surgical intervention.

Transcatheter mitral valve replacement (TMVR)

The heavy burden of MR is widely accepted, affecting 6% of patients over the age of 75 in the developed world.[45] A large proportion of these patients who require intervention are not suitable for surgical therapy. While use of MitraClip has progressed extensively in the last decade, it is limited to anatomically and clinically suitable patients. With significant experience and progress with transcatheter aortic valve replacement, there has been a substantial investment in similar interventions for the mitral valve. While there are numerous transcatheter mitral valve replacement (TMVR) devices in development, the device at the forefront of this therapy is the Tendyne TMVR.

Numerous challenges exist in the development of a TMVR, especially when compared with similar devices in the aortic position. The absence of calcium to allow anchorage, asymmetry of the valves, varied aetiologies and risk of excess radial force in the mitral position are a few of the issues making TMVR a more challenging prospect.[46]

Tendyne mitral valve systems

The Tendyne valve is deployed via a trans-apical approach using a 32 Fr sheath. The valve consists of two nitinol self-expanding stents, one for attachment of the pericardial leaflets, and the other to conform to the mitral annulus. A polyethylene terephthalate fabric cuff covers the outer stent, and the stent is anchored in place using a pad and braided fibre tethered to the left ventricular apex (Figure 42.2b and c). It is a retrievable and repositionable valve.[47] Care must be taken in the setting of large anterior leaflets and a narrow left ventricular outflow tract as there is a risk of obstruction with these larger prostheses.

St Vincent's Hospital, Sydney, has been one of the leading investigator centres for this device.[48] The Tendyne Global Feasibility Study involved 30 patients with high surgical risk stratification, with the majority having secondary MR.[48] Successful valve implantation was achieved in 93% of patients. Primary performance endpoints of successful valve implantation and freedom from cardiovascular mortality and device dysfunction were achieved in 86.7% of patients. These excellent outcomes, albeit in an early feasibility study, demonstrate much promise for this device in mitral valve pathology. Several questions are yet to be addressed, including the possible impact of the apical tethering mechanism on mild worsening of left ventricular function and the optimal anticoagulation regimen for this bulky device. The next decade, with plans for a pivotal trial, will determine its role in percutaneous mitral valve therapy.

HYBRID CORONARY ARTERY REVASCULARISATION

The approach to multivessel coronary artery disease is evolving. While coronary artery bypass grafting (CABG) has been the mainstay treatment of multivessel disease, it has several disadvantages. A big achievement of surgery has been grafting of the LIMA graft to the left anterior descending (LAD) coronary artery, achieving a patency of greater than 90% at 10 years.[49–51] This graft is undoubtedly the reason for the mortality benefit associated with surgery. Surgery, however, is maximally invasive, requiring a median sternotomy in order to access all coronary territories. In addition, multiple grafts are usually performed using cardiopulmonary bypass and cessation of cardiac activity requiring ascending aorta cross-clamping. All of these contribute to the increased risk of complications, namely stroke,[52–54] prolonged recuperation following sternotomy, and saphenous vein conduit harvest site complications. While traditionally the issue with regards to percutaneous coronary intervention (PCI) has been the higher rates of re-intervention with PCI, progress with newer generation drug eluting stents (DES) has arrived at a stage now where they achieve significantly improved longer term patency rates similar to or even better than those of saphenous vein grafts.

With the aim of reducing the risks of surgical intervention but to continue to maximise the unrivaled benefit of the LIMA-LAD graft, a hydrid approach was investigated in the 1990s. The concept was first described by Angelini and colleagues in 1996.[55] Using a sternum-sparing minimally invasive approach, the LIMA conduit is harvested and anastomosed to the LAD artery. This is frequently performed via a small left mini-thoracotomies in the 5th intercostal space, using a surgical robot. Single-lung ventilation, CO_2 insufflation and the robot console are used to harvest the mammary artery and perform a beating-heart anastomosis. The operation can be performed with or without cardiopulmonary bypass via peripheral cannulation.

The remaining coronary territories, namely the circumflex and the right coronary arteries, can then be addressed with DES. Outcomes with DES are much improved, as seen in a large meta-analysis comparing DES with CABG in 2011.[56] This study demonstrated lower cardiac, cerebrovascular events and mortality at 30 days with DES, while there were lower rates of revascularisation and the same cardiac and cerebrovascular events at 12 months with bypass grafting. Hybrid approaches may well combine the respective benefits of PCI with DES and surgical grafting.

Patient selection is important in this population. The Syntax and Syntax II score are both useful adjuncts in identifying patients at high risk of PCI, specifically left main disease, diabetes, impaired LV function, complex anatomy for PCI and renal dysfunction.[57] Once there is a medical indication for intervention (mortality benefit/symptoms), and there is perceived benefit from a LIMA-LAD graft, patients can be considered for hybrid revascularisation. The important considerations are whether the patient has suitable anatomy for a minimally invasive LIMA-LAD graft and appropriate coronary technical anatomy for PCI therapy to other areas. In addition, the need for single-lung ventilation precludes patients with severe pulmonary disease, and the effects of post-operative dual antiplatelet therapy must be considered.

There have not been any large randomised trials to compare hybrid revascularisation, but smaller studies have demonstrated it to be a safe and effective alternative to complete surgical coronary revascularisation.[58] Lower rates of blood transfusion and earlier return to work have been demonstrated in the hybrid group, but at the expense of higher procedural and hospital costs.[59]

The combined surgical and percutaneous approach appears a promising option in the therapy against coronary disease. By employing the benefits of both arms, a mortality benefit can be achieved while limiting the morbidity of surgery. Further well-designed trials to assess outcomes are needed to best determine the suitable target population for this novel approach to revascularisation.

CONCLUSION

Percutaneous therapy has evolved to form an important arm in the treatment against cardiac pathology. Surgery does remain the gold standard treatment for these pathologies; however, avoidance of maximally invasive sternotomy, especially in patients at high risk of complications, is an important consideration. It is thus paramount that all higher-risk cases be discussed as part of a multidisciplinary approach with a heart team—this is vital in the decision making of surgical versus percutaneous approaches, and in determining the ideal vascular approach for percutaneous therapy. While TAVI is firmly established as treatment for aortic stenosis, MitraClip and the transcatheter mitral valves are gaining momentum and establishing their evidence base in primary and in secondary mitral valve pathology. Hybrid coronary revascularisation sums up the beautiful interplay and benefits of surgical and percutaneous therapy in the same setting—by using the strengths of each approach, combination therapy that allows maximal benefit and least risk is potentially offered. The changing landscape provides an exciting time in percutaneous cardiac interventions, and the combined approach of surgeons and interventional cardiologists in achieving clinical excellence with this novel therapy is paramount for its continued success.

REFERENCES

1. Eveborn GW, Schirmer H, Heggelund G. The evolving epidemiology of valvular aortic stenosis. The Tromso Study. *Heart*. 2013;99(6):396–400.
2. Ross J, Braunwald E. Aortic stenosis. *Circulation*. 1968;38:V-61–V-67.
3. Nishimura RA, Otto CM, Bonow RO, Carabello BA, Erwin JP, Guyton RA, et al. 2014 AHA/ACC guideline for the management of patients with valvular heart disease: A report of the American College of Cardiology/American Heart Association Task Force on Practice Guidelines. *J Am Coll Cardiol*. 2014;63(22):e57–185.
4. Harken DE, Taylor WJ, Lefemine AA, Lunzer S, Low HB, Cohen ML, et al. Aortic valve replacement with a gaged ball valve. *Am J Cardiol*. 1962;9(2):292–299.
5. Lung B, Cachier A, Baron G, Messika-Zeitoun D, Delahaye F, Tornos P, et al. Decision-making in elderly patients with severe aortic stenosis: Why are so many denied surgery? *Eur Heart J*. 2005;26(24):2714–2720.
6. Cribier A, Saoudi N, Berland J, Savin T, Rocha P, Letac B. Percutaneous transluminal valvuloplasty of acquired aortic stenosis in elderly patients: An alternative to valve replacement? *Lancet*. 1986;327(8472):63–67.
7. Sigwart U, Puel J, Mirkovitch V, Joffre F, Kappenberger L. Intravascular stents to prevent occlusion and restenosis after transluminal angioplasty. *N Engl J Med*. 1987;316(12):701–706.
8. Andersen HR, Knudsen LL, Hasenkam JM. Transluminal implantation of artificial heart valves description of a new expandable aortic valve and initial results with implantation by catheter technique in closed chest pigs. *Eur Heart J*. 1992;13(5):704–708.
9. Cribier A, Eltchaninoff H, Bash A, Borenstein N, Tron C, Bauer F, et al. Percutaneous transcatheter implantation of an aortic valve prosthesis for calcific aortic stenosis - first human case description. *Circulation*. 2002;106:3006–3008.
10. Webb JG, Chandavimol M, Thompson CR, Ricci DR, Carere RG, Munt BI, et al. Percutaneous aortic valve implantation retrograde from the femoral artery. *Circulation*. 2006;113(6):842–850.
11. Agarwal S, Tuzcu EM, Krishnaswamy A, Schoenhagen P, Stewart WJ, Svensson LG, et al. Transcatheter aortic valve replacement: Current perspectives and future implications. *Heart*. 2015;101(3):169–177.
12. Généreux P, Webb JG, Svensson LG, Kodali SK, Satler LF, Fearon WF, et al. Vascular complications after transcatheter aortic valve replacement: Insights from the Partner (Placement of Aortic Transcatheter Valve) Trial. *J Am Coll Cardiol*. 2012;60(12):1043–1052.
13. Leon MB, Smith CR, Mack MJ, Makkar RR, Svensson LG, Kodali SK, et al. Transcatheter or surgical aortic-valve replacement in intermediate-risk patients. *N Engl J Med*. 2016;374(17):1609–1620.
14. Toggweiler S, Gurvitch R, Leipsic J, Wood DA, Willson AB, Binder RK, et al. Percutaneous aortic valve replacement: Vascular outcomes with a fully percutaneous procedure. *J Am Coll Cardiol*. 2012;59(2):113–118.
15. Okuyama K, Jilaihawi H, Kashif M, Takahashi N, Chakravarty T, Pokhrel H, et al. Transfemoral access assessment for transcatheter aortic valve replacement: Evidence-based application of computed tomography over invasive angiography. *Circ Cardiovasc Imaging*. 2014;8(1):e001995.

16. Kurra V, Schoenhagen P, Roselli EE, Kapadia SR, Tuzcu EM, Greenberg R, et al. Prevalence of significant peripheral artery disease in patients evaluated for percutaneous aortic valve insertion: Preprocedural assessment with multidetector computed tomography. *J Thorac Cardiovasc Surg.* 2009;137(5):1258–1264.

17. Masson J-B, Kovac J, Schuler G, Ye J, Cheung A, Kapadia S, et al. Transcatheter aortic valve implantation: Review of the nature, management, and avoidance of procedural complications. *JACC: Cardiovasc Interv.* 2009;2(9):811–820.

18. Hayashida K, Lefèvre T, Chevalier B, Hovasse T, Romano M, Garot P, et al. Transfemoral aortic valve implantation new criteria to predict vascular complications. *JACC Cardiovasc Interv.* 2011;4(8):851–858.

19. Ludman PF, Moat N, de Belder MA, Blackman DJ, Duncan A, Banya W, et al. Transcatheter aortic valve implantation in the united kingdom: Temporal trends, predictors of outcome, and 6-year follow-up: A report from the UK. Transcatheter Aortic Valve Implantation (Tavi) Registry, 2007 To 2012. *Circulation.* 2015;131(13):1181–1190.

20. Gilard M, Eltchaninoff H, Iung B, Donzeau-Gouge P, Chevreul K, Fajadet J, et al. Registry of transcatheter aortic-valve implantation in high-risk patients. *N Engl J Med.* 2012;366(18):1705–1715.

21. Toggweiler S, Webb JG. Challenges in transcatheter aortic valve implantation. *Swiss Med Wkly.* 2012;142:W13735.

22. Lichtenstein SV, Cheung A, Ye J, Thompson CR, Carere RG, Pasupati S, et al. transapical transcatheter aortic valve implantation in humans: Initial clinical experience. *Circulation.* 2006;114(6):591–596.

23. Walther T, Möllmann H, van Linden A, Kempfert J. Transcatheter aortic valve implantation transapical: Step by step. *Semin Thorac Cardiovasc Surg.* 2011;23(1):55–61.

24. Ye J, Cheung A, Lichtenstein SV, Carere RG, Thompson CR, Pasupati S, et al. Transapical aortic valve implantation in humans. *J Thorac Cardiovasc Surg.* 2006;131(5):1194–1196.

25. Fraccaro C, Napodano M, Tarantini G, Gasparetto V, Gerosa G, Bianco R, et al. Expanding the eligibility for transcatheter aortic valve implantation the trans-subclavian retrograde approach using: The iii generation corevalve revalving system. *JACC Cardiovasc Interv.* 2009;2(9):828–833.

26. Pascual I, Carro A, Avanzas P, Hernández-Vaquero D, Díaz R, Rozado J, et al. Vascular approaches for transcatheter aortic valve implantation. *J Thorac Dis.* 2017;9(Suppl 6):S478–S487.

27. Lardizabal JA, O'Neill BP, Desai HV, Macon CJ, Rodriguez AP, Martinez CA, et al. The transaortic approach for transcatheter aortic valve replacement: Initial clinical experience in the United States. *J Am Coll Cardiol.* 2013;61(23):2341–2345.

28. Guyton RA, Block PC, Thourani VH, Lerakis S, Babaliaros V. Carotid artery access for transcatheter aortic valve replacement. *Catheter Cardiovasc Interv.* 2013;82(4):E583–E586.

29. Arai T, Romano M, Lefèvre T, Hovasse T, Farge A, Le Houerou D, et al. Direct comparison of feasibility and safety of transfemoral versus transaortic versus transapical transcatheter aortic valve replacement. *JACC Cardiovasc Interv.* 2016;9(22):2320–2232.

30. Arora S, Misenheimer JA, Ramaraj R. Transcatheter aortic valve replacement: Comprehensive review and present status. *Tex Heart Inst J.* 2017;44(1):29–38.

31. Mack MJ, Leon MB, Smith CR, Miller DC, Moses JW, Tuzcu EM, et al. 5-year outcomes of transcatheter aortic valve replacement or surgical aortic valve replacement for high surgical risk patients with aortic stenosis (partner 1): A randomised controlled trial. *Lancet.* 2015;385(9986):2477–2484.

32. Kapadia SR, Leon MB, Makkar RR, Tuzcu EM, Svensson LG, Kodali S, et al. 5-year outcomes of transcatheter aortic valve replacement compared with standard treatment for patients with inoperable aortic stenosis (Partner 1): A randomised controlled trial. *Lancet.* 2015;385(9986):2485–2491.

33. Amat-Santos IJ, Dahou A, Webb J, Dvir D, Dumesnil JG, Allende R, et al. Comparison of hemodynamic performance of the

balloon-expandable Sapien 3 versus Sapien xt transcatheter valve. *Am J Cardiol.* 2014;114(7):1075–1082.

34. Adams DH, Popma JJ, Reardon MJ, Yakubov SJ, Coselli JS, Deeb GM, et al. Transcatheter aortic-valve replacement with a self-expanding prosthesis. *N Engl J Med.* 2014;370(19):1790–1798.

35. Abdel-Wahab M, Neumann F-J, Mehilli J, Frerker C, Richardt D, Landt M, et al. 1-year outcomes after transcatheter aortic valve replacement with balloon-expandable versus self-expandable valves: Results from the choice randomized clinical trial. *J Am Coll Cardiol.* 2015;66(7):791–800.

36. Maisano F, Schreuder JJ, Oppizzi M, Fiorani B, Fino C, Alfieri O. The double-orifice technique as a standardized approach to treat mitral regurgitation due to severe myxomatous disease: Surgical technique. *Eur J Cardiothorac Surg.* 2000;17(3):201–205.

37. Maisano F, Torracca L, Oppizzi M, Stefano P, d'Addario G, La Canna G, et al. The edge-to-edge technique: A simplified method to correct mitral insufficiency. *Eur J Cardiothorac Surg.* 1998;13(3):240–245; Discussion 245–246.

38. Bhamra-Ariza P, Muller DW. The MitraClip experience and future percutaneous mitral valve therapies. *Heart Lung Circ.* 2014;23(11):1009–1019.

39. Vahanian A, Alfieri O, Andreotti F, Antunes MJ, Barón-Esquivias G, et al. Guidelines on the management of valvular heart disease (version 2012): The Joint Task Force on the Management of Valvular Heart Disease of the European Society of Cardiology (ESC) and the European Association for Cardio-Thoracic Surgery (EACTS). *Eur Heart J.* 2012;33(19);2451–2496.

40. Feldman T, Kar S, Rinaldi M, Fail P, Hermiller J, Smalling R, et al. Percutaneous mitral repair with the mitraclip system: Safety and midterm durability in the initial Everest (Endovascular Valve Edge-To-Edge Repair Study) cohort. *J Am Coll Cardiol.* 2009;54:686–694.

41. Feldman T, Foster E, Glower DD, et al. Percutaneous repair or surgery for mitral regurgitation. *N Engl J Med.* 2011;364(15):1395–1406.

42. Mauri L, Foster E, Glower DD, et al. 4-year results of a randomized controlled trial of percutaneous repair versus surgery for mitral regurgitation. *J Am Coll Cardiol.* 2013;62(4):317–328.

43. Glower DD, Kar S, Trento A, et al. Percutaneous mitral valve repair for mitral regurgitation in high-risk patients: Results of The Everest Ii Study. *J Am Coll Cardiol.* 2014;64(2):172–181.

44. Auricchio A, Schillinger W, Meyer S, et al. Correction of mitral regurgitation in nonresponders to cardiac resynchronization therapy by mitra-clip improves symptoms and promotes reverse remodeling. *J Am Coll Cardiol.* 2011;58(21):2183–2189.

45. Enriquez-Sarano M, Avierinos Jf, Messika-Zeitoun D, et al. Quantitative determinants of the outcome of asymptomatic mitral regurgitation. *N Engl J Med.* 2005;352(9):875–883.

46. Alkhouli M, Alqahtani F, Aljohani S. Transcatheter mitral valve replacement: An evolution of a revolution. *J Thorac Dis.* 2017;9(Suppl 7):S668–S672.

47. Moat NE, Duncan A, Quarto C. Transcatheter mitral valve implantation: Tendyne. *Eurointervention.* 2016;12(Y):Y75–Y77.

48. Muller DWM, Farivar RS, Jansz P, et al. Transcatheter mitral valve replacement for patients with symptomatic mitral regurgitation: A global feasibility trial. *J Am Coll Cardiol.* 2017;69(4):381–391.

49. Bypass Angioplasty Revascularization Investigation (BARI) Investigators. The final 10-year follow-up results from the BARI randomized trial. *J Am Coll Cardiol.* 2007;49(15):1600–1606.

50. Serruys PW, Morice MC, Kappetein AP. Percutaneous coronary intervention versus coronary-artery bypass grafting for severe coronary artery disease. *N Engl J Med.* 2009;360(10):961–972.

51. Bypass Angioplasty Revascularization Investigation (BARI) Investigators. comparison of coronary bypass surgery with angioplasty in patients with multivessel disease. *N Engl J Med.* 1996;335(4):217–225.

52. Sabik JF 3rd, Lytle BW, Blackstone EH, et al. Comparison of saphenous vein and internal thoracic artery graft patency by coronary system. *Ann Thorac Surg.* 2005;79(2):544–551; Discussion 544–551.

53. Palmerini T, Biondi-Zoccai G, Riva DD, et al. Risk of stroke with percutaneous coronary intervention compared with on-pump and off-pump coronary artery bypass graft surgery: Evidence from a comprehensive network meta-analysis. *Am Heart J.* 2013;165(6):910–917.E14.

54. Farkouh ME, Domanski M, Sleeper LA. Strategies for multivessel revascularization in patients with diabetes. *N Engl J Med.* 2012;367(25):2375–2384.

55. Angelini GD, Wilde P, Salerno TA, et al. Integrated left small thoracotomy and angioplasty for multivessel coronary artery revascularisation. *Lancet.* 1996;347(9003):757–758.

56. Yan TD, Padang R, Poh C, et al. Drug-eluting stents versus coronary artery bypass grafting for the treatment of coronary artery disease: A meta-analysis of randomized and nonrandomized studies. *J Thorac Cardiovasc Surg.* 2011;141(5):1134–1144.

57. Lee MS, Faxon DP. Revascularization of left main coronary artery disease. *Cardiol Rev.* 2011;19(4):177–183.

58. Halkos ME, Vassiliades TA, Douglas JS, et al. Hybrid coronary revascularization versus off-pump coronary artery bypass grafting for the treatment of multivessel coronary artery disease. *Ann Thorac Surg.* 2011;92(5):1695–16701; Discussion 1701–1702.

59. Bachinsky WB, Abdelsalam M, Boga G, et al. Comparative study of same sitting hybrid coronary artery revascularization versus off-pump coronary artery bypass in multivessel coronary artery disease. *J Interv Cardiol.* 2012;25(5):460–468.

PART 7

Interventions for arrhythmias

43

The electrophysiology laboratory

DENNIS L. KUCHAR

INTRODUCTION

Electrophysiology (EP) is the science of recording, analysis, and interpretation of the electrocardiogram (ECG) via surface and intracardiac electrodes. Patients with heart rhythm disturbances are studied and treated in the EP laboratory. Invasive EP involves recording spontaneous and pacing-induced intracardiac electrical activation patterns and their study in a controlled environment. If an arrhythmia is suspected, diagnostic tests including measurement of conduction intervals in response to pacing, and programmed electrical stimulation of the heart may be performed to determine the source of the arrhythmia. Therapeutic procedures performed in the EP laboratory include transcatheter radiofrequency ablations, implantations of permanent pacemakers and defibrillators, overdrive pacing and electrical cardioversions.

This chapter outlines the basic functions of the EP laboratory and describes equipment used, types of procedures performed, and the reasons for doing so. For the beginner, this is a concise and simple introduction into a complex and fast-growing branch of cardiology.

DIAGNOSIS OF ARRHYTHMIA

Patients with heart rhythm disturbances are studied and treated in the electrophysiology (EP) laboratory. The usual symptoms caused by cardiac arrhythmias include palpitations, chest pain, exertional dyspnoea, dizziness and syncope. Cardiac arrest may relate to a rapid arrhythmia usually ventricular in origin, or to a profound bradycardia. If an arrhythmia is suspected, diagnostic tests including measurement of conduction intervals in response to pacing and programmed electrical stimulation of the heart may be performed to determine the source of symptoms. Therapeutic procedures performed in the electrophysiology laboratory include transcatheter radiofrequency ablations, implantations of permanent pacemakers and defibrillators, overdrive pacing and electrical cardioversions.

Invasive electrophysiology studies (EPS) involve the recording of spontaneous and pacing-induced intracardiac electrical activation patterns and their study in a controlled environment. The aim is to investigate the electrical aspects of abnormal electrical heart activity for diagnostic, therapeutic and/or prognostic purposes. EPS may be performed:

1. To establish the site of origin and the mechanism of a tachycardia or bradycardia (e.g. the cause of a cardiac arrest or to assess a documented arrhythmia in which the diagnosis may not be apparent from the surface ECG
2. To guide in the treatment of arrhythmias (e.g. drug therapy or other interventions such as implantation of defibrillators, radiofrequency ablation, surgery)
3. To assess the likelihood of future arrhythmic events

ELECTROPHYSIOLOGIC EVALUATION OF CARDIAC CONDUCTION AND RHYTHM IN THE EP LABORATORY

The electrophysiology study

The EP study is conducted to:

1. Provoke and examine an arrhythmia under controlled conditions
2. Acquire more accurate, detailed information than with any other diagnostic test
3. Choose the most effective treatment
4. In many cases, provide treatment (i.e. catheter ablation) during the same session

During the study, special electrode catheters (long, flexible wires) are inserted into veins and are guided into the heart. These catheters sense electrical impulses and may also be used to stimulate different areas of the heart. Sites that are causing serious arrhythmias can be localised and, if appropriate, ablated.

Implantable loop recorders

If EP testing does not reveal a definite cause for presumed arrhythmic symptoms (e.g. palpitations, syncope), an event monitor can be used to identify the culprit cardiac rhythm. A symptom-rhythm correlate can be confidently obtained using an implantable ECG monitor that can be surgically placed or 'injected' subcutaneously. The device is capable of automatic detection of arrhythmias according to set programmed criteria and can also be activated when the patient experiences symptoms. The device can then be interrogated by the physician or a recording can be downloaded to a home monitor that can then transmit the recording over the internet to an arrhythmia interpretation service.

The tilt table test

Vasovagal syncope (neurocardiogenic syndrome or vasodepressor syncope) is a relatively common syndrome seen in young people, more commonly in women. The clinical setting is usually related to standing for a prolonged period of time in a crowded environment e.g. inside a bus, train or underground railway system or following situations such as fright, a dentist's chair or the sight of blood. The patient may feel dizzy or short of breath. A 'black screen' may occur in front of the eyes followed by a fall to the ground with a brief period of loss of consciousness. It may be preceded by an awareness of a faster heart beat and nausea and sweatiness. This is usually a benign situation and the patient wakes in seconds to minutes. If examined during that time, the patient will usually have hypotension and bradycardia. A vasovagal episode is the most common cause of syncope in otherwise healthy young persons. Investigation is mainly to exclude other causes of syncope (e.g. arrhythmias, drugs, epilepsy).

A cardiovascular cause of syncope can be identified in a significant number of patients by use of electrophysiologic studies or the head-up tilt test. Tilt testing with or without isoprenaline or nitroglycerine can provoke hypotension and bradycardia in patients with neurocardiogenic mechanisms of syncope. It must be emphasised, however, that syncope can be a sign of more sinister heart disease, particularly in patients with structural heart disease. These patients should be considered for investigation with electrophysiological testing.

THERAPEUTIC INTERVENTIONS

Catheter ablation

This technique is designed to cure certain types of tachycardia. From ECG tracings, it may be possible to identify patients suitable for this technique. There are two broad types of tachycardia that may be suitable for treatment. These are supraventricular tachycardia (SVT) and ventricular tachycardia (VT). These are discussed in Chapters 19 and 20 in more detail.

SVT comprises abnormal heart rhythms that either originate in the atria, causing the heart to beat rapidly (may be regular or irregular beating), or may arise because of an abnormal extra connection between the atrium and ventricle, leading to a short circuit in the heart. SVT may be due to a bypass tract or to a double circuit in the central electrical junction in the heart, the AV node. Other types of SVT amenable to ablation include atrial fibrillation, atrial tachycardia and flutter. Sites of ablation may be the abnormal pathway or the normal electrical system itself. If the normal electrical system is the target, a permanent pacemaker may also be required.

VT is an abnormal rapid beating of the ventricles and may result from scarring in the heart from a heart attack, or it may be seen in young people with structurally normal hearts. A small area in the ventricle is the usual target for ablation in these cases. The ablation procedure is very similar to the EP study. Special insulated wires (catheters) make it possible to study heart rhythm disturbances under controlled conditions, and the doctor can identify the heart rhythm disturbance and determine whether to go ahead with the ablation procedure.

Atrial fibrillation (AF)

This can be approached by electrically isolating the pulmonary veins using either radiofrequency energy or by applying cryogenic energy via a balloon-tipped catheter to freeze the atrial tissue. This is effective as a large proportion of patients with paroxysmal AF have a trigger in one or other of the pulmonary veins. Electrical isolation impairs the ability for the fibrillatory impulses to reach the bulk of atrial tissue, causing AF. More extensive ablation of atrial tissue is often used if isolation alone is ineffective.

His bundle ablation

His bundle ablation (HBA) is a procedure used to stop A-V conduction in atrial fibrillation, flutter (when flutter ablation is not indicated) or tachycardia. A permanent pacemaker (PPM) must be inserted. A ventricular pacing catheter and an ablation catheter are inserted via the femoral vein. The ablation catheter is positioned on or proximal to the area of recording of the His bundle electrogram and the conductive tissue is destroyed by application of radiofrequency energy so the abnormal atrial rhythm is not conducted through to the ventricles.

Permanent pacemaker implantation

Presence of symptoms remains the most common indication for pacemaker treatment. Symptomatic bradycardia is the term used to identify clinical manifestations associated with a heart rate that does not allow cardiac output to meet physiologic demands. The aim of the procedure is to ensure optimal heart rate in a heart with a conduction deficit. Duration of the implant procedure is 1–2 hours depending on the number of leads and difficulty of access. Local anaesthetic (usually Marcain 0.4%) is administered at the site. It is an aseptic procedure, in which the medical practitioner scrubs, gowns and gloves. Cutdown cannulation of the cephalic vein and/or percutaneous cannulation of the sub-clavian vein provides access to the right atrium and ventricle. Pacing leads are then inserted into the heart via this access and the lead parameters measured via alligator leads and the pacing system analyser (PSA). The pacing device is then connected to the lead(s), inserted into a pre-pectoral pocket, and the wound closed. A drain may be required, particularly if the patient has been anticoagulated. Antibiotic prophylaxis, usually a cephalosporin, is given routinely, and occasionally with gentamicin cover. If penicillin allergy is suspected a skin test for drug reaction is performed with the cephalosporin. Cardioversion may (rarely) be required to continue the procedure (e.g. in the event of VF or VT). Recent developments to reduce infection and bleeding risk include an antibiotic sleeve (Tyrx, Medtronic) that encapsulates the generator, and a fibrinogenic implant (Tachosil, Medtronic), respectively.

Internal cardioverter defibrillator (ICD) implantation

The ICD may be used in patients with prior cardiac arrest or ventricular tachycardia (secondary prevention) or in patients deemed to be at high risk of these events (primary prevention). The anti-tachycardia pacemaker is an important adjunct to ICD therapy for patients with frequent episodes of well-tolerated VT. Some devices have the facility to perform anti-tachycardia pacing as well as delivering shocks, while others may be shock-only devices (uncommonly used in recent times).

Cardiac resynchronisation for heart failure

Patients with dilated cardiomyopathy and end-stage heart failure may benefit from synchronised biventricular pacing (ASBP). Suitable patients usually have a significant intra-ventricular conduction delay often manifested as a wide LBBB. With marked conduction delay, left ventricular contraction may be dyssynchronous and left ventricular stroke volume may improve by simultaneously activating both the left ventricular septum and lateral wall, thereby improving the ejection fraction. This type of pacing can be used in a defibrillator system (CRT-D) or as a pacing only device (CRT-P).

EQUIPMENT

The equipment used in the EP laboratory comprises cardiac electrodes that are placed in various heart chambers, recording equipment, a programmed stimulator and fluoroscopic equipment to facilitate positioning of the catheters. An electrical defibrillator is essential to rapidly treat any life-threatening arrhythmias that may result during cardiac stimulation. The room should be treated as a sterile operating facility particularly if used for pacemaker and defibrillator implants. This includes air filtration and following routine infection control procedures between cases. Operating theatre apparel is worn by all staff.

Catheter electrodes: These consist of between 2 and 20 electrodes in various configurations. These allow stimulation usually from the distal electrode pair and simultaneous recording from the other electrodes facilitating rapid mapping of arrhythmia circuitry.

Recording equipment: This is generally able to record and process electrical signals. Multiple intracardiac and external surface ECG leads can be recorded simultaneously and saved to a hard drive or external memory source for later analysis. An electric junction box interfaces the signals from the electrodes into the recording system. Sophisticated mapping systems have been developed to facilitate real-time recording and mapping of arrhythmia substrates.

Electroanatomic mapping: Systems are designed to enhance the ability to define arrhythmia substrates and demonstrate realtime heart structures in three dimensions (3D). The mapping electrode (Biosense Webster) has a magnetic sensor within the shaft near the catheter tip and together with an external, ultralow magnetic field emitter provide a precise 3-D map of the position of the catheter. Electrograms can be recorded simultaneously with the position in space generating an anatomic map. The catheter can be placed back to any desirable position, a particularly important feature in mapping. In addition, the catheter may be moved in the absence of fluoroscopy, thereby saving unnecessary radiation exposure. The catheter, because of its ability to map the virtual anatomy, can display the cardiac dimensions and with a prior template derived from a CT or MRI scan, accurately reflect catheter position relative to specific cardiac structures such as pulmonary veins, the left atrial appendage and ventricular aneurysms.

Noncontact endocardial mapping, using an intracavitary multielectrode probe is also available (Ensite, St Jude Medical). It can generate endocardial electrograms reconstructed using inverse solution methods. Endocardial potentials and activation sequences can be reconstructed from intracavitary probe signals; beat-to-beat activation sequences of the entire chamber are then generated, facilitating mapping of arrhythmia circuits.

Programmed stimulator: This is an electrical device that is able to deliver timed electrical stimulation to the heart to facilitate pacing of individual chambers and delivery of additional extrastimuli in order to induce arrhythmias. These may be mechanically or digitally operated.

X ray equipment: Fluoroscopy facilitates entry and placement of the catheters to the cardiac chambers from the entry vein or artery. Multiplane capability is an advantage for optimal catheter placement. Pulsed fluoroscopy allows a reduced dose of radiation without compromising image quality. Cinefluoroscopy is useful for recording sites of catheter placement and for imaging of vessels such as the coronary sinus branches used for cannulation of the veins for left ventricular stimulation and recording.

Defibrillator: This should be readily accessible and preferably attached to shocking electrodes affixed to the patient.

LABORATORY PERSONNEL

A minimum of two nurses (trained in catheterisation/EP skills) should accompany the trained electrophysiologist. A cardiac fellow training in the discipline of EP is usually at hand. An EP technician and/or additional electrophysiologist is often available for more complex EP studies and catheter ablation. A cardiac technician (often from a pacemaker manufacturing company) is often on hand for pacemaker and defibrillator implants to facilitate lead evaluation at the time of implant.

Ready access to an anaesthetist, cardiac surgeon and biomedical engineer is important for urgent backup should they be required for patient care or equipment malfunction.

The nurses are generally responsible for patient welfare, administration of antibiotics, sedation and analgesia and for constant observation and recording of patient vital signs.

CARDIAC CATHETERISATION

Femoral venous and arterial access are generally used to introduce the catheters, but upper extremity (basilar, subclavian) and cervical vessels (internal jugular) may be accessed. The catheters are generally inserted using the Seldinger technique after local anaesthetic infiltration. Vascular ultrasound may be used to reduce risk of inadvertent puncture of the incorrect vessel. A subxiphoid introducer can be placed to allow for epicardial cardiac mapping if required.

Catheters are generally introduced into the high right atrium, His bundle region, right ventricle and coronary sinus.

POTENTIAL COMPLICATIONS

Complications may arise from the catheterisation procedure itself or from the consequences of electrical stimulation. Complication rates tend to be higher in elderly patients and those undergoing catheter ablation.

Vascular complications

This includes local haemorrhage from the vessel puncture site if the artery is deliberately or inadvertently punctured, particularly when the patient is on anticoagulants. Haemostasis is usually achieved by local pressure at the puncture site. Use of vascular ultrasound to cannulate the vessel may reduce risk of accidental puncture.

Thromboembolism

In situ deep venous thrombosis at catheter entry sites is rarely seen and may be minimised by the use of systemic heparinisation, particularly in cases where a catheter is used in left-heart studies and in right-heart studies of very long duration, and especially in a patient with a history of or high risk of thromboembolism.

Arrhythmias

Induced arrhythmias are commonly seen and can often be terminated by stimulation. Electrical cardioversion can be immediately applied should a haemodynamically significant arrhythmia, unresponsive to pacing manoeuvres, occur.

Atrial fibrillation is particularly common and is usually transient, lasting a few seconds to several minutes. If the fibrillation is well tolerated haemodynamically, no active therapy need be undertaken, but DC cardioversion or chemical reversion (usually with intravenous flecainide) can be applied.

Complications of left sided studies

Introduction of catheters in the left atrium and ventricle may be associated with additional complications, including strokes, systemic emboli, and protamine reactions during reversal of heparinisation. Inadvertent puncture of adjacent femoral vein and artery may result in an arterio-venous fistula. Specific complications related to ablation of left atrium and pulmonary veins include atrio-oesophageal fistula and gastric dysmotility.

Pericardial tamponade

Perforation of the ventricle or atrium resulting in tamponade is a possibility and will often require pericardiocentesis or intraoperative repair. This is more likely to result as a complication of ablation procedures.

FURTHER READING

Andrade JG, Bennett MT, Deyell MW, Hawkins N, Krahn AD, Macle L, et al. *The Clinical Cardiac Electrophysiology Handbook*: Minneapolis: Cardiotext Publishing; 2016. 384p.

Electrophysiology Lab virtual tour. https://www.youtube.com/watch?v=cE9Y-yWoqB0.

Fogoros RN, Mandrola JM. *Fogoros' Electrophysiologic Testing* 6th ed. Hoboken, NY:Wiley-Blackwell; 2017. 416p.

Glover BM, Brugada P. *Clinical Handbook of Cardiac Electrophysiology*. Cham, Switzerland: Springer International; 2016. 271p.

Ho RT. *Electrophysiology of Arrhythmias: Practical Images for Diagnosis and Ablation.* Philadelphia, PA: Lippincott Williams & Wilkins; 2009. 384p.

Josephson ME. *Clinical Cardiac Electrophysiology: Techniques and Interpretations.* 4th ed. Philadelphia, PA: Lippincott Williams & Wilkins; 2008. 912 p.

Klein GJ, Gula LJ, Leong-Sit P, Manlucu J, Skanes AC, Yee R. *Electrophysiological Maneuvers for Arrhythmia Analysis*. Minneapolis: Cardiotext Publishing; 2014. 208p.

Sra JS, Akhtar M, Natale A, Wilber DJ. *Practical Electrophysiology*. Minneapolis: Cardiotext Publishing; 2014. 624p.

Tung R, Frankel D. *Essential Concepts of Electrophysiology through Case Studies.* Minneapolis: CardioText Publishing; 2015. 336p.

44

Catheter ablation therapy

WILLIAM LEE AND BRUCE WALKER

INTRODUCTION

Treatment of cardiac arrhythmias by catheter-directed ablation therapy (CAT) is a rapidly developing field in cardiology. Originally, in the early 1980s this involved delivery of high-energy direct current shocks to cardiac tissue,[1] whereas now discrete therapy is delivered using radiofrequency (RF) energy or refrigerant to heat or cool the cardiac tissue. Regardless of the method, the principle of CAT remains the same, which is to create electrically-inert lesions within cardiac tissue, either to destroy or electrically isolate arrhythmogenic substrates within the myocardium, while avoiding damage to surrounding healthy tissue. The advent of modern technology has allowed for more discrete lesions to be created, as well as higher imaging and electrical mapping resolution, greatly improving the safety and efficacy of this therapy.

INDICATIONS FOR ABLATION

Arrhythmias that can be treated by CAT are wide-ranging and as a result, so too are the methods and techniques employed to perform this procedure. It should be noted, however, that there are inherent risks in performing any procedure and it is recommended that other non-invasive, low-risk therapies be considered before undergoing CAT. Critical to reducing complications is the choice in approach to performing any CAT procedure and the correct identification of the arrhythmia requiring treatment.

In general terms, arrhythmias requiring CAT are fast arrhythmias (tachyarrhythmias). These tachyarrhythmias are caused by two different mechanisms: (1) Automaticity, where a focal collection of cells is able to depolarise independently of, and faster than, the heart's normal pacemaker system; (2) re-entry, where anatomical

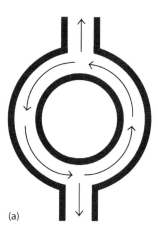 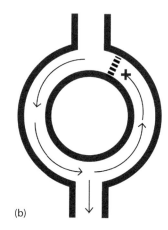

(a)   (b)

Figure 44.1 Conceptual example of re-entry tachycardia. (a) The electrical wave of depolarisation continuously activates in a circus movement. As the depolarising wavefront travels around the circuit, the myocardium behind the wavefront has time to repolarise and recover, ready to depolarise again when the wavefront reaches it. As a result, the re-entry circuit continuously activates without end. (b) Ablation of one limb of the re-entry circuit (dashed line) results in block of conduction through that area, thereby preventing breaking the circuit and preventing continuous activation.

or functional circuits exist in the heart that allow continual activation of the heart as the wave of depolarisation travels around the circuit (Figure 44.1a). In practice, tachycardias are separated anatomically into supraventricular and ventricular tachycardias.

Supraventricular tachycardias

Tachyarrhythmias that originate in cardiac structures above the ventricles (atria and atrio-ventricular junctions) are grouped as supraventricular tachycardias. From most common to least common, the supraventricular tachycardias amenable to CAT include:

Atrioventricular (AV) nodal re-entry tachycardia: A re-entry tachycardia where two limbs of conduction exist around the AV node.

AV re-entry tachycardia: A re-entry tachycardia where an accessory pathway connecting the atria and ventricles exists, separate to the normal cardiac conduction system.

Atrial flutter: A re-entry tachycardia where anatomical structures (either congenital or acquired) create re-entry circuits within the atria. The most common of these is typical right atrial flutter (Figure 44.2), described in more detail below.

Atrial fibrillation: Disorganised rapid electrical activation of the atria, leading to non-coordinated ineffective contraction of the atria. Most commonly, focal autonomic triggers of this tachycardia are found in the insertion sites of the pulmonary veins; however, other focal trigger sites do exist.

Atrial tachycardia: Autonomic rapidly firing foci or localised re-entry within the atria, resulting in a tachycardia.

Ventricular tachycardias

As the name suggests these are arrhythmias that originate in the ventricles of the heart. Most commonly, ventricular tachycardias amenable to ablation are re-entrant circuits caused by scar tissue from previous myocardial infarction, or from dilated cardiomyopathies, or from infiltrative diseases such as sarcoidosis. Autonomic foci that cause ventricular ectopic beats have been shown to trigger episodes of ventricular tachycardia. Therefore, these foci can often be targeted to prevent initiation of the arrhythmia.

Other ablation targets

In some instances, there is no obvious ablation target to treat an arrhythmia, so non-diseased

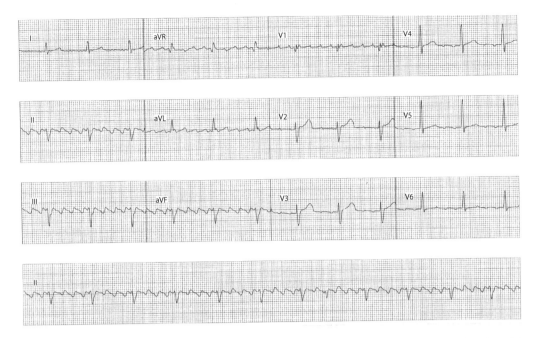

Figure 44.2 Typical atrial flutter with characteristic 'saw-tooth baseline' pattern seen in lead II of the electrocardiogram.

cardiac tissue can be targeted to try to prevent arrhythmias. An example of this is His bundle ablation, where the normal connection between the atria and ventricles is abolished to prevent transmission of abnormally fast atrial arrhythmias (such as atrial fibrillation) to the ventricles. In this particular example, insertion of a permanent pacemaker is mandatory to maintain ventricular contraction.

CATHETERS

As CAT is an invasive procedure, it involves insertion of one or more catheters inside the heart. Catheters are insulated electrical wires attached to an exposed platinum electrode that contacts the intracardiac surface of the heart at the distal end. On the proximal end they are connected to a recording device that can both sense electrical activity and deliver electrical impulses. There are two basic categories of catheters: (1) mapping catheters that detect electrical activity from different points within the heart, and (2) ablation catheters that create ablation

lesions either via RF energy to heat, or via refrigerant to cool the myocardium.

Mapping catheters

As previously mentioned, critical to the safety and success of an ablation procedure is the correct identification and localisation of the offending arrhythmia. Choice of mapping catheter is often at the discretion of the operating specialist and what is appropriate for the procedure. As such, there is a wide range in choice of mapping catheters, from simple fixed-curve quadripolar catheters that provide four points of information, to more complex steerable decapolar (10 points) and duodecapolar (20 points) (Figure 44.3a) catheters. As technology continues to progress and miniaturise, these options can only increase. There also exist specially shaped, purpose-built catheters for specific procedures such as lasso-shaped (20 points), penta-ray (five-fingered, 20 points,) and basket-shaped (64 points) (Figure 44.3b) catheters.

As this technology increases, one limitation is the human brain's ability to rapidly process the

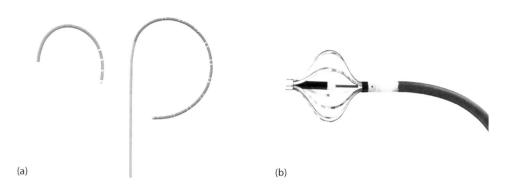

(a)   (b)

Figure 44.3 Examples of different multipolar mapping catheters. **(a)** Linear mapping catheters: quadripolar (left) and duodecapolar (right). **(b)** Multi-point 'Orion-Hero' catheter. (Courtesy of Boston Scientific. ©2018 Boston Scientific Corporation or its affiliates. All rights reserved Boston, MA.)

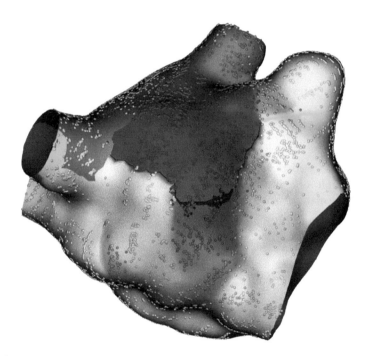

Figure 44.4 Rhythmia™ mapping system, electro-anatomical map of the left atrium. This electro-anatomical map was constructed using an Orion-hero™ mapping catheter. Dots represent data points collected and used to create the map. Colour mapping: red-yellow-green-blue-violet represents early to late timing of electrical activation.

masses of data that are acquired; therefore, more sophisticated computer processing is required to accurately process these data and present information in a comprehensive and comprehensible format. Several integrated magnetic navigational mapping systems exist, such as CARTO (Biosense Webster, CA, USA), Ensite (St Jude Medical, MN, USA) and Rhythmia (Boston Scientific, MA, USA). These complex systems can track the precise location of mapping catheter data points and ablation catheters within the heart. This allows operators to gather large amounts of intracardiac electrophysiological data and generate precise electro-anatomical maps of the heart (Figure 44.4). These maps can then be used to help operators navigate within the heart to find precise critical areas for ablation.

Ablation catheters

Similar to mapping catheters, there exists a wide variety of ablation catheters designed for different tasks. The simplest form of these catheters is a unipolar catheter designed to deliver RF energy at the tip of the catheter, earthed to a large grounding patch (typically placed on the patient's thigh), which allows for highly accurate single-point lesion formation. Often, however, adequate lesion formation is limited by excessive heating of the superficial cardiac tissue, leading to damage to the superficial endocardium without adequate deep-lesion formation. The solution to this is the use of irrigated-tip catheters that use saline to cool the tip of the ablation catheter to reduce superficial tissue heating while allowing greater energy delivery to the deeper layers of cardiac tissue. The consequence of deeper, larger lesion formation is the risk of damage to surrounding structures such as the normal cardiac conduction system (Figure 44.5a and b). The solution is to use bipolar catheters that deliver RF energy between two electrodes at the tip of the catheter, allowing for significantly smaller, more accurate lesions.

In the same way, rather than using RF energy to heat, refrigerant can be used to cool the catheter tip and freeze the cardiac tissue. The advantage of this technology is that the cardiac tissue can be cooled to −28°C to create a temporary lesion prior to cooling to <40°C to create a permanent lesion, allowing the operator to test a lesion and, if needed, to avoid damage to surrounding cardiac structures. With both RF and cryoablation catheters, adequate tip-to-tissue contact is required for optimal lesion formation. This is limited by risk of physical trauma to cardiac tissue if too much force is applied, and therefore many catheters also provide the ability to measure contact force between the catheter tip and cardiac tissue. Purpose-built catheters also exist for specific uses, such as balloon catheters designed to inflate and fit within the antrum of the pulmonary veins, and deliver cooling refrigerant to create a ring-like lesion within the muscular sleeve of the pulmonary veins (Figure 44.5c).

PROCEDURAL APPROACH

Patient preparation

Preparation for a CAT procedure often begins well in advance of the procedure itself. As much confirmatory information about the arrhythmia requiring ablation, in the form of an electrocardiogram (ECG), Holter monitor or other cardiac monitor data, should be gathered before the procedure to confirm the type of arrhythmia requiring ablation, to confirm that it is amenable to ablation and to understand the location from which the arrhythmia originates so as to determine the ablation site. Despite this exhaustive preparatory work, often further invasive intra-cardiac electrophysiology studies with provocative testing to try to induce

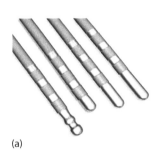
(a)

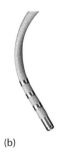
(b)

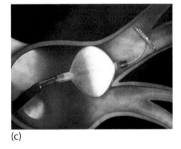
(c)

Figure 44.5 Examples of ablation catheters. (a) Standard solid-tip ablation catheters of different shapes and sizes. (b) Open-tip irrigation catheter. Note holes at the tip of the catheter that facilitate irrigation cooling of local tissue during RF ablation. (c) Arctic Front Advance™ cryo-ablation balloon with integrated lasso mapping catheter placed in the pulmonary vein antrum. ([a] Courtesy of Boston Scientific. ©2018 Boston Scientific Corporation or its affiliates. All rights reserved; [b] Courtesy of Medtronic Australasia, Sydney, NSW, Australia.)

the arrhythmia in question are required to gather sufficient information prior to the ablation.

In addition to this, the medical history of the patient is often paramount to the safety of the procedure, including cardiac and respiratory function, myocardial ischaemia, electrolyte imbalance, ongoing pharmacotherapy and previous adverse reactions to medications. Prior to the procedure the patient is required to fast for at least 6 hours to prevent airway complications such as aspiration pneumonia or pneumonitis that might result from the anaesthesia. Temporary cessation of anti-arrhythmic drugs that may interfere with electrophysiological studies and provocative testing of the heart should also be considered prior to the procedure. Patients who take oral anticoagulation should have their anticoagulation status reviewed beforehand. In some cases (particularly atrial fibrillation and atrial flutter), patients continue their anticoagulation therapy owing to the risk of embolic events post-ablation, whereas in other arrhythmias it may be appropriate to cease anticoagulation temporarily to reduce the risk of bleeding. Patients taking novel oral anticoagulants (non-warfarin anticoagulants, see Chapter 23) and who require ongoing anticoagulation should have their medication ceased and anticoagulation bridged with heparin or a heparin analogue, or in some cases transitioned to warfarin several months beforehand. A transoesophageal echocardiogram (TEE) may be required to exclude the presence of preformed thrombus within the heart. During the procedure, the patient is often lightly sedated; however, in more prolonged or complex procedures, a general anaesthetic may be required. Defibrillator pads are often applied as a safety precaution, in the event that inducing an arrhythmia may require direct current shock to terminate.

Intracardiac access

The approach to the heart is often via the right or left femoral vessels, located in the right/left groin. In most procedures the femoral vein is accessed by the Seldinger technique (see Chapter 25). This involves using a large-bore needle that is then exchanged for a guidewire that is used to guide a sheath into the femoral vein to maintain access to the femoral vein lumen. Several access sheaths may be inserted, depending on how many catheters are required to be inserted into the heart. The number and location of these sheaths is determined by the type of procedure being performed. In simpler procedures where access to the right side of the heart is required, access sheaths are placed in the femoral vein. However, access to the left ventricle may be required, in which case an access sheath may be placed in the femoral artery. On some occasions the target of ablation is not accessible from within the heart and external access is required to ablate the epicardium. In this case, a needle is used to access the pericardial space within the pericardial sac, and then a sheath is placed within the pericardial space to allow catheter access.

Access to the left atrium or left ventricle can also be achieved by trans-septal catheterisation. Commonly for ablation of atrial fibrillation, access is gained by crossing the interatrial septum. In this case a similar technique is used, where a long needle is inserted into the heart via the femoral vein and used to puncture the interatrial septum, which is then exchanged for a guidewire to guide a long sheath across the interatrial septum. Such techniques are associated with a small but significant risk of serious complication and require a considerable degree of operator expertise and training.

Catheter placement

As with all aspects of CAT, the specific arrhythmia in question will determine the catheter placement. One or more mapping catheters are placed proximal and distal to the site of ablation. These are used both in sensing the electrical depolarisation wavefront within the myocardium, as well as stimulating the myocardium to initiate a wave of depolarisation. Integral to this is the ability to sense the before-and-after area of ablation, in order to accurately measure the time taken for the depolarising electrical wave to travel from the point proximal to the ablation site to the point distal to the ablation site. This is required to be able to objectively determine the success of an ablation, and is discussed in the subsequent section.

X-ray fluoroscopy, as well as careful observation of intracardiac ECGs, is used to guide the careful and accurate placement of catheters inside the heart. Occasionally, for more complex procedures such as trans-septal catheterisation, TEE or intracardiac echocardiogram guidance is required for better three-dimensional (3D) resolution of the catheter position. Three-dimensional precision guidance of ablation catheters without use of fluoroscopy can also be achieved using the previously mentioned

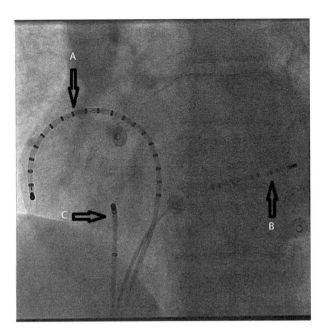

Figure 44.6 Fluoroscopic example of catheter placement for a typical atrial flutter ablation. **(a)** A duo-decapolar catheter placed in the right atrium from the lateral wall (left side) around to the septal wall (right side). **(b)** A decapolar catheter placed in the coronary sinus. **(c)** An ablation catheter positioned at the ablation target: The cavo-tricuspid isthmus.

integrated magnetic navigational mapping systems and thus limit the patient's exposure to X-ray radiation.

In Figure 44.6, a typical example of fluoroscopic X-ray of an atrial flutter ablation is shown. A duo-decapolar catheter is placed on the lateral wall of the right atrium and a second decapolar catheter is placed in the ostium of the coronary sinus. This gives multiple points of reference proximal and distal to the ablation target, which is the cavo-tricuspid isthmus, a narrow band of muscular tissue between the inferior vena cava and the tricuspid annulus.

ABLATION TARGETS AND MARKERS OF ABLATION SUCCESS

As previously mentioned, the goal of CAT is to create electrically-inert lesions within the myocardium. Focal point ablation can be used to target specific areas within the heart, such as autonomously activating tissue, causing ventricular ectopy. In contrast, linear ablation can be used to create lines of lesions in order to electrically isolate certain parts of the myocardium, such as isolating triggers of atrial fibrillation by encircling the pulmonary veins.

Macro-reentrant circuits such as atrial flutter, AV nodal re-entry tachycardia (AVNRT) and atrioventricular re-entry tachycardia (AVRT) do not require complete isolation of the circuit, but rather blockade of one limb of the reentrant circuit in order to break the circus movement of the depolarisation wave front (Figure 44.1b). In this case, often ablation lines are created to connect electrically inert anatomical structures such as heart valves or the fibrous skeleton of the heart. Therefore, the ablation target very much depends on the type of arrhythmia and the location of its origin.

The objective indicators of ablation success are: (1) electrical quiescence in the area of ablation, demonstrated by reduction in electrical signal amplitude; (2) electrical isolation of the area in question, demonstrated by the inability to detect remote native or paced depolarisation signals from within the isolated area; (3) electrical block across a line of ablation, demonstrated by delayed or widely split detection of native or paced depolarisation signals from one side of the line of block to the other side; (4) inability to induce the targeted arrhythmia when previously it was easily induced. Consequently, precise measurements or conduction times and provocative pacing intervals, as well as use of chronotropic medications,

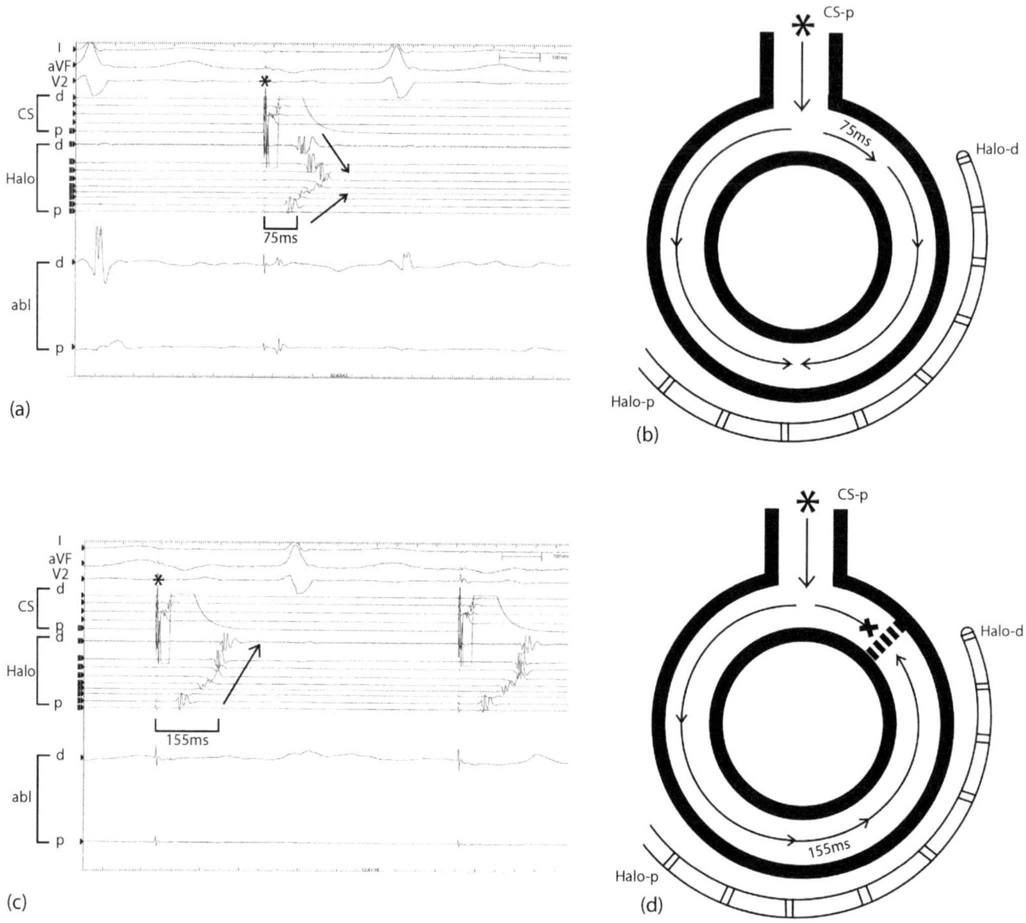

Figure 44.7 Intracardiac electrograms demonstrating objective measures of ablation success. **(a)** Pre-ablation pacing beat is initiated in the proximal coronary sinus (CS-p) marked by the asterisk (*). The subsequent depolarisation wave is detected in the right atrial catheter (Halo) moving in 2 opposing directions as indicated by the arrows. The conduction time from CS-p to the lateral wall of the right atrium (Halo-d) is 75 ms. **(b)** Conceptual view of the right atrium. Pacing (*) from CS-p initiates the wave of depolarisation that travels down both limbs of the circuit. Conduction time from CS-p to Halo-d is short at 75 ms due to the short distance of travel. **(c)** Post-ablation, the same pacing beat at CS-p now takes 155 ms to be detected in Halo-d. The wave of depolarisation travels in one direction as indicated by the arrows. **(d)** Conceptual view of the right atrium post-ablation. The pacing beat (*) can only travel down one limb of the circuit due to ablation block in the opposite limb. This results in a longer distance of travel and therefore a longer conduction time of 155 ms between CS-p and Halo-d. (Surface ECG: Lead I (I), lead aVF (aVF), lead V2 (V2). Intracardiac electrograms: Coronary sinus catheter (CS), distal portion of catheter (d), proximal portion of catheter (p). Right atrial catheter (Halo), distal portion of catheter (d), proximal portion of catheter (p). Ablation catheter: (abl), distal portion of catheter (d), proximal portion of catheter (p).

are required both before and after ablation in order to demonstrate one or more of the above objective outcomes to unequivocally measure ablation success.

In our above example of typical atrial flutter, the ablation target is the cavo-tricuspid isthmus, a narrow band of tissue between the inferior vena cava and the tricuspid annulus. Mapping catheters are placed on either side of the ablation target and conduction. A >50% increase in conduction time between the two electrodes on either side of the ablation line, a change in the activation pattern in the mapping electrodes (Figure 44.7), and a failure to induce atrial flutter with provocative pacing are all indicators of ablation success, giving a <5% chance of recurrence of atrial flutter.[1,2]

POTENTIAL COMPLICATIONS OF CATHETER ABLATION THERAPY

As with any invasive procedure, there is an inherent risk of complications, ranging from minor bruising or bleeding at the access site to major complications resulting in emergency rescue surgery, permanent disability, or death. As one would expect, major complication is more likely in high-risk complex cases, such as ablation of ventricular tachycardia, where patients are often frail with poor cardiac function and multiple comorbidities, and the ablation targets are difficult to reach or locate. Often, but not without exception, certain complications are more common depending on the specific area of the heart being ablated, due to ablation damage to nearby heart structures. For example, heart block is more common when ablating near the AV node (e.g. for AVNRT or for septal accessory pathways), and pulmonary vein stenosis is more likely to result from ablation within the pulmonary venous ostium during pulmonary vein isolation as treatment for atrial fibrillation. Transient ischaemic attack (TIA) or stroke is more likely to occur when operating in the left-sided chambers of the heart.

The rate of major complication on average ranges between 0.6% and 6%[3,4] including: death, stroke, complete heart block, cardiac tamponade, valve damage, myocardial infarction, pneumothorax, embolic events and damage to vascular structures.[5] Again, more complex procedures are more likely to have complications that are specific to that procedure. For example, left atrial ablation to isolate pulmonary veins has inherent risks which are less common in other procedures such as: Pericarditis (3.1%), permanent phrenic nerve palsy (0.4%), pulmonary vein stenosis (0.3%), TIA/stroke (0.1%) and atrio-oesophageal fistula (<0.1%).[6] It should be noted, however, that the risk of complication can often be modulated by the experience of the operator performing the procedure, as well as the expertise and volume of cases of the centre in which the procedure is done.[7] For our own centre, St Vincent's Hospital Sydney Australia, a recent internal review demonstrated a complication rate of 0.5% over 15 months.

While not a complication per se, often the most disappointing result of CAT is no result at all, as in failure to ablate, or recurrence of the ablated arrhythmia. While careful measurement of the objective endpoints discussed above can significantly reduce the incidence of arrhythmia recurrence, transient block with tissue recovery or muscle regrowth into the ablated area can occur and is unpredictable in nature. Successful ablation without recurrence varies depending on the complexity of the procedure as well as the complexity of the patient. Less complex procedures such as AV node ablation or atrial flutter ablation have reported success rates of 90%–95%,[1,8] with a recurrence of atrial flutter in 4% of patients. In comparison, more complex procedures such as pulmonary vein isolation, in pooled data, have shown an average absence of recurrence rate of 57% after the first procedure, and 77% after multiple procedures.[9]

One important distinction to make is the identification of recurrence of a previous arrhythmia compared with the iatrogenic creation of a new arrhythmia. Incomplete ablation or modification of an ablated tissue, as well as gaps in ablation lines, can lead to a new arrhythmia rather than a simple recurrence of the previous arrhythmia. Careful study of surface ECGs as well as intracardiac electrophysiological studies should be performed and compared with pre-ablation ECGs to distinguish between these two often subtly different arrhythmias. The importance of this distinction is that redo ablation of the same area may not fix an iatrogenically created arrhythmia, and occasionally new lines of ablation in sites distal to the original ablation must be created to treat the arrhythmia.

CONCLUSION

Catheter ablation therapy is a growing field within the physician's armament for treating cardiac arrhythmias. From humble and narrowly prescribed beginnings, this therapy has grown and rapidly expanded to include treatment for a variety of cardiac arrhythmias, with a wide range of varying techniques and equipment. The safety and efficacy of this therapy can only improve as technology continues to expand and develop.

REFERENCES

1. Morady F. Catheter ablation of supra-ventricular arrhythmias: State of the art. *J Cardiovasc Electrophysiol.* 2004;15 (1):124–139.
2. Oral H, Sticherling C, Tada H, Chough SP, Baker RL, Wasmer K, et al. Role of trans-isthmus conduction intervals in predicting bidirectional block after ablation of typical atrial flutter. *J Cardiovasc Electrophysiol.* 200;12 (2):169–174.
3. Hindricks, G. The Multicentre European Radiofrequency Survey (MERFS): Complications of radiofrequency catheter abla-tion of arrhythmias. The Multicentre European Radiofrequency Survey (MERFS) investigators of the Working Group on Arrhythmias of the European Society of Cardiology. *Eur Heart J.* 1993;14 (12):1644–1653.
4. Bohnen M, Stevenson WG., Tedrow UB., Michaud GF, John RM, Epstein LM, et al. Incidence and predictors of major complications from contemporary catheter ablation to treat cardiac arrhythmias. *Heart Rhythm.* 2011;8 (11):1661–1666.
5. Calkins H, Yong P, Miller JM, Olshansky B, Carlson M, Saul JP, et al. Catheter ablation of accessory pathways, atrioventricular nodal reentrant tachycardia, and the atrioven-tricular junction: Final results of a prospec-tive, multicenter clinical trial. The Atakr Multicenter Investigators Group. *Circulation.* 1999;99 (2):262–270.
6. De Greef Y, Ströker E, Schwagten B, Kupics K, De Cocker J, Chierchia G-Ba, et al. Complications of pulmonary vein isolation in atrial fibrillation: Predictors and comparison between four different ablation techniques: Results from the Middelheim PVI-registry. *EP Europace.* 2018;20(8):1279–1286.
7. De Greef Y, Tavernier R, Duytschaever M. Sequelae after AF ablation: Efficacy and Safety go Hand in Hand. *Indian Pacing Electrophysiol J.* 2012;12 (4):171–179.
8. Scheinman MM. NASPE survey on catheter ablation. *Pacing Clin Electrophysiol.* 1995;18 (8):1474–1478.
9. January, CT, Wann LS, Alpert J S, Calkins H, Cigarroa J E, Cleveland JC, Jr, et al. ACC/AHA Task Force Members. 2014 AHA/ACC/HRS guideline for the management of patients with atrial fibrillation: Executive summary: A report of the American College of Cardiology/American Heart Association Task Force on practice guidelines and the Heart Rhythm Society. *Circulation.* 2014;130 (23):2071–2104.

Index

Note: Page numbers in italic and bold refer to figures and tables, respectively.